Breast Reconstruction with Autologous Tissue

Springer Science+Business Media, LLC

Breast Reconstruction with Autologous Tissue

Art and Artistry

Stephen S. Kroll, M.D.

**M.D. Anderson Cancer Center
Department of Plastic Surgery
The University of Texas
Houston, Texas
USA**

With 634 Illustrations, 63 in Full Color

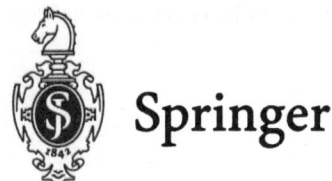 Springer

Stephen S. Kroll, M.D.
M.D. Anderson Cancer Center
Department of Plastic Surgery
The University of Texas
1515 Holcombe Boulevard
Houston, TX 77030
USA

Cover photo: Marble Amazon, 430 BC/© The Granger Collection, Ltd.

Library of Congress Cataloging-in-Publication Data
Kroll, Stephen S.
   Breast reconstruction with autologous tissue : art and artistry /
Stephen S. Kroll.
   p. cm.
Includes bibliographical references and index.
   ISBN 978-1-4757-8150-2   ISBN 978-0-387-21767-3 (eBook)
   DOI 10.1007/978-0-387-21767-3

   1. Mammaplasty.   2. Flaps (Surgery)   I. Title.
   [DNLM: 1. Mammaplasty—methods.   2. Tissue Transplantation—
methods.   3. Surgical Flaps.   WP 910 K93a 2000]
   RD539.8.K76   2000
   618.1'90592—dc21
                                                            98-51594

Printed on acid-free paper.

© 2000 Springer Science+Business Media New York
Originally published by Springer-Verlag New York, Inc. in 2000
Softcover reprint of the hardcover 1st edition 2000

Production coordinated by WordCrafters Editorial Services, Inc., and managed by Lesley Poliner; manufacturing supervised by Rhea Talbert.
Typeset by Matrix Publishing Services, Inc., York, PA.

9 8 7 6 5 4 3 2 1

ISBN 978-1-4757-8150-2   SPIN 10699039

Preface

Plastic surgery is a unique specialty that is composed of two parts: engineering and art. The engineering part is concerned with transferring tissues, keeping those tissues alive while they are healing, and minimizing donor site morbidity. This part of plastic surgery is interesting and challenging but is, in many ways, not so different from other surgical specialties. What is unique about plastic surgery is its artistic aspect: turning a flap that used to be a forehead into something that truly looks like a nose, or turning a transverse rectus abdominis myocutaneous (TRAM) flap into a breast. It is this artistry that makes successful plastic surgeons stand out from their peers. It is this artistic aspect of breast reconstruction that this book addresses.

Many books already exist about flaps, breast surgery, and breast reconstruction. This book is not meant to replace them. What is unique about this book is its focus on artistry. Before now, very little has been written on the artistic aspects of breast reconstruction. What this book provides—possibly for the first time—is some basic principles for transferring, shaping, and revising a TRAM (or other autologous tissue flap) so that it really looks like a breast that matches its opposite counterpart. As such, this book is intended to help improve the aesthetic quality of the reader's results, whatever the current level of those results might be.

Although this book includes chapters on the fundamentals of breast reconstruction and is therefore suitable for the beginning surgeon, the intended target audience is the more experienced surgeon who seeks superior aesthetic outcomes. The chapters on the free TRAM flap, breast shaping, breast revision, surgery of the opposite breast, and nipple reconstruction will be of special interest to such individuals. Although certain opinions presented here may change in years to come (or be disagreed with by some even today), I believe that everyone who performs breast reconstruction will find something useful here.

Who then should read this book? This book is for surgeons who believe in the importance of breast reconstruction and care about aesthetic outcomes. It is for surgeons who believe that they can improve and learn more about their art. It is for surgeons who want to do as much as they can to help their patients. If you are such a surgeon, this book was written for you.

Stephen S. Kroll, M.D.
M.D. Anderson Cancer Center
The University of Texas

Preface

Contents

1 Goals of Breast Reconstruction

Why Do We Reconstruct Breasts?

For most women, mastectomy is a mutilating and deforming operation that has the capacity to severely damage a woman's self-image and lead her to question her desirability as a sexual partner.[1-3] This can be true even when a loving husband (or "significant other") is providing support and when abandonment by a mate is, in reality, unlikely. Breasts are a potent symbol of femininity, and the loss of a breast can have important psychological consequences. Some women may be inhibited from entering into relationships in which their deformity might be revealed, or may withdraw from relationships with men and even other women. This isolation can be harmful not only to the patient herself but to her family, coworkers, and anyone else who depends on her. For some women, fear of possible deformity is significant enough to cause them to refuse cancer treatment, even though the absence of a breast can be easily concealed by clothing.

In theory, the loss of a breast can be corrected without difficulty using a prosthesis. Unfortunately, for many women a prosthesis is inadequate treatment. In the privacy of her bedroom, a woman who has undergone mastectomy without reconstruction is confronted by her deformity each time she undresses and is reminded that she is not only deformed but at risk for a cancer recurrence. She is limited in her selection of clothing and must be careful about choosing activities (like swimming or dancing) that might cause the prosthesis to become dislodged. Moreover, if the prosthesis is large, it may be uncomfortable, particularly in hot climates. For these and other reasons, use of an external prosthesis to replace a missing breast is not always a satisfactory option.

Breast reconstruction does not solve all the problems caused by mastectomy, but it solves many of them. A woman who has had a successful reconstruction (Fig 1-1) can usually wear almost all types of normal clothing (including many bathing suits) and participate fully in recreational activities without showing any external sign of her surgery. She is not handicapped by her cancer treatment in her daily living and is not reminded of her breast cancer except when visiting her doctors for routine checkups. She can return to an active and productive life, working and providing support to her family and friends as well as receiving it from them. This is important not only to breast cancer pa-

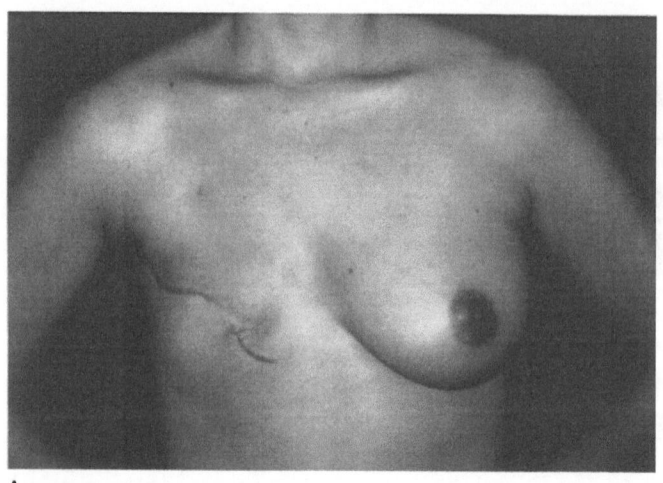

A

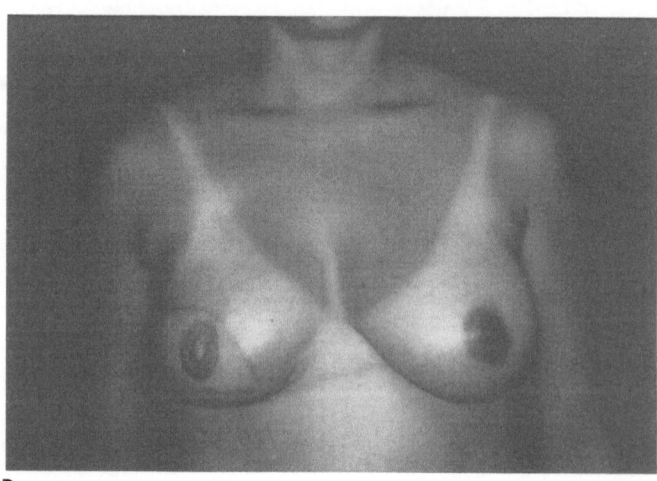

B

Fig. 1-1   (A) A 22-year-old woman following right modified radical mastectomy for breast cancer. (B) After breast reconstruction with a latissimus dorsi flap and a silicone implant. The patient sunbathes and has resumed an active life. (From Kroll SS: *Clin Plast Surg.* 1998;25:135–143. Used with permission.) See color insert, p. I-1.

tients but to society at large because breast cancer patients are often in their prime of life, and are highly productive individuals upon whom the fabric of our society depends.

Contraindications to Breast Reconstruction

The overwhelming majority of women who have had (or will need) a mastectomy can undergo successful breast reconstruction, if they choose to. Who should not be reconstructed? Women who have unrealistic expectations, and who refuse to accept the required scars, should be rejected as candidates until their expectations become realistic. This is rarely a problem in patients requesting delayed breast reconstruction, who already have scars and are likely to be pleased by any improvement in their appearance that the surgeon can provide. Unrealistic expectations can occasionally be a problem, however, for women who are requesting immediate reconstruction. Fortunately, the overwhelming majority of women who request immediate reconstruction understand that the reconstructed breast will not be flawless and that, if a flap is used, the surgeon will be required to create scars in the donor site.

Another group of women who should not have breast reconstruction are those in very poor health, who are not really candidates for any type of elective surgery. Fortunately for reconstructive surgeons, most such patients are aware of their status and do not request inappropriate reconstruction, so that rejection of such patients is rarely necessary. If a patient who is not an appropriate candidate for elective surgery does request breast reconstruction, she need not be rejected out of hand. Such a patient can be managed by gently informing her that her current medical condition does not permit breast reconstruction, but that her health may well improve, and that when it does the surgeon will be happy to revisit the issue.

The third group of patients who should not undergo breast reconstruction are those whose prognosis for survival is so abysmal that undergoing additional surgery for reconstruction is unreasonable. Patients with inflammatory breast cancer, for example, would fall into this category. Unless the reconstruction is mandatory for psychological reasons, the patient is far better served by being offered a mastectomy without reconstruction so that she can leave the hospital quickly and spend as much of her remaining time as possible with her family. If the prognosis improves at a later time, she can always undergo a delayed reconstruction, a possibility that can be suggested by the surgeon to maintain some hope.

Patient Expectations

The goal of breast reconstruction is to return the patient to a state that approximates the normal as closely as possible so that she is not handicapped in her daily living. The surgeon tries to create a breast that is shaped naturally, is soft, has sensation, moves like a real breast, and in short looks and feels like a normal breast. Ideally, the reconstructed breast should also mature with time and change with the patient's body weight, as a normal breast would.

The reconstructed breast should match the contralateral breast as closely as possible. Ideally, the reconstruction should be symmetric and attractive in the unclothed state (Fig 1-2), but in practice this goal is not always achieved even in the most experienced hands. It is therefore best for the surgeon to promise only that the patient will have good symmetry in clothing, when wearing a brassiere (Fig 1-3). This goal is usu-

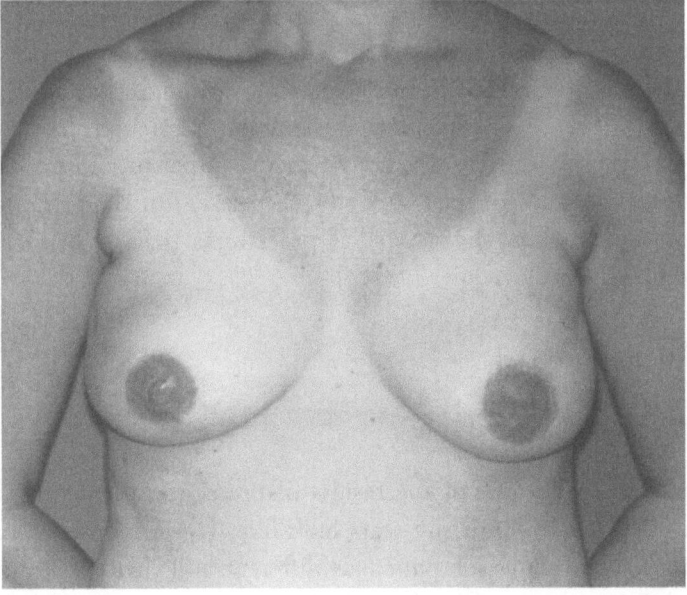

FIG. 1-2 The result of bilateral immediate breast reconstruction with free transverse rectus abdominis myocutaneous (TRAM) flaps. See color insert, p. I-2.

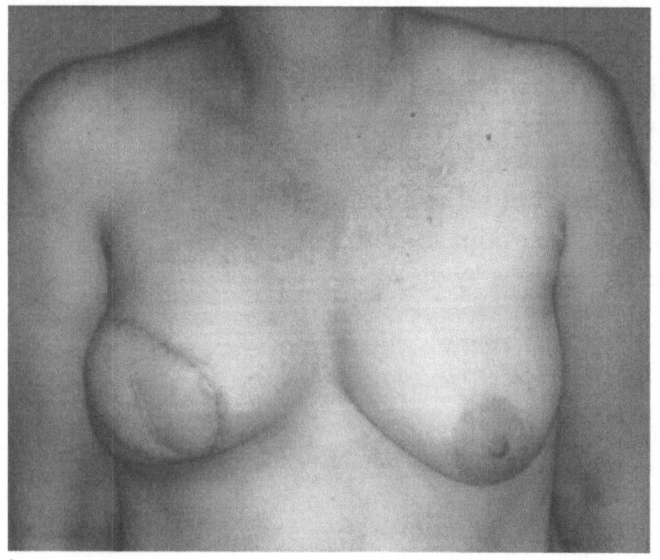
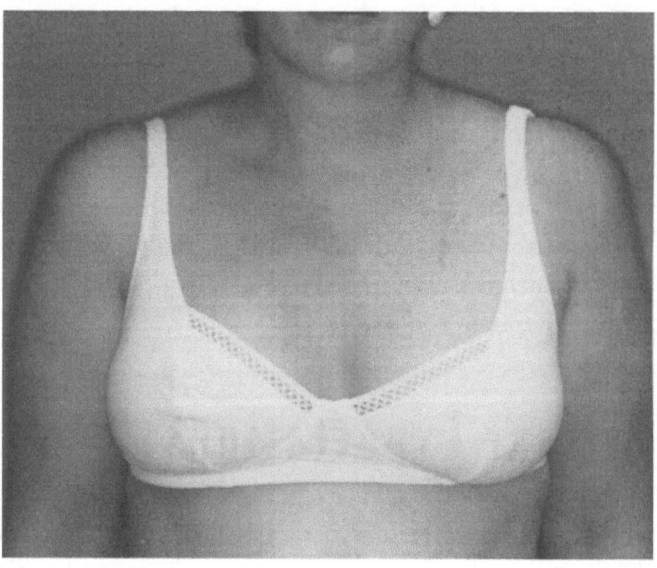

A

B

FIG. 1-3   (A) Reconstructed breast lacks symmetry. (B) Despite the imperfection, the patient has symmetry when wearing a brassiere. In her clothing she looks normal, is satisfied, and at the time of this photo had declined further revision.

ally easily met and will satisfy most patients. The surgeon naturally tries to surpass that stated goal, and often will do so. It is more practical, however, to promise less than can be delivered. In our clinic, patients are told that they will look normal in clothing but not when nude. Patients who are surprised by a result that exceeds their expectations, in our experience, are usually happy about their success and not disappointed that the surgeon did not make a more accurate forecast.

For similar reasons, it is also best to tell patients from the beginning that the breast mound will need one or more revisions to achieve a satisfactory shape. Although the surgeon always tries in the initial operation to create a mound that duplicates the contralateral breast as closely as possible, a perfect match is rarely achieved. If, owing to luck and skill, excellent symmetry is achieved in the initial procedure, no one will be disappointed because additional surgery is not necessary. On the other hand, patients and insurance companies may both rebel if procedures that were not expected and planned for are subsequently required.

Showing Photographs and Examples of Results

Patients often ask to see photos of the results of breast reconstruction, and may ask specifically to see what the donor site scars look like. Upon request, I do show them photos but caution them that each patient is different and that their own results may be significantly better or worse than those depicted in the photographs. In most cases, the scars look worse in the photographs than they do on real patients. Because of this, and for other reasons to be discussed below, I encourage patients who wish to know what our results look like to meet with other patients who have had previous transverse rectus abdominis myocutaneous (TRAM) flap reconstructions. In many cases, these successfully reconstructed patients are in the clinic for follow-up visits, and are immediately available. In most cases, they are enthusiastic supporters of breast reconstruction and are happy to be interviewed and to answer questions. In this way, prospective patients get to see both the donor scars and the reconstructed breasts, and get a more accurate and three-dimensional concept of what breast reconstruction can accomplish.

In addition to answering questions and demonstrating the location of the scars, previously reconstructed patients can help tremendously by supplying emotional support. Especially for women with newly diagnosed breast cancer, meeting with another patient who has passed successfully through all the trials posed by mastectomy and adjuvant treatment, and who has emerged happy and relatively unscathed with a soft, lifelike reconstructed breast, can be very reassuring. This reassurance comes at a time of great anxiety, when it is desperately needed. It also comes from a source that patients feel they can trust—a patient like themselves who has no incentive to mislead them. Patients often tell me how much they appreciated this support when they first came to our clinic, and frequently volunteer to help other women in the same way if ever they should be needed.

Nipple Reconstruction

Although the stated goal of breast reconstruction is to achieve a normal appearance in clothing, nipple and areolar reconstruction should be considered part of the reconstructive process and should be presented as such from the beginning. Nipple and areolar reconstruction adds significantly to the desirable illusion of normalcy, even when the reconstruction itself is imperfect (Fig 1-4). Although the nipple is concealed in pub-

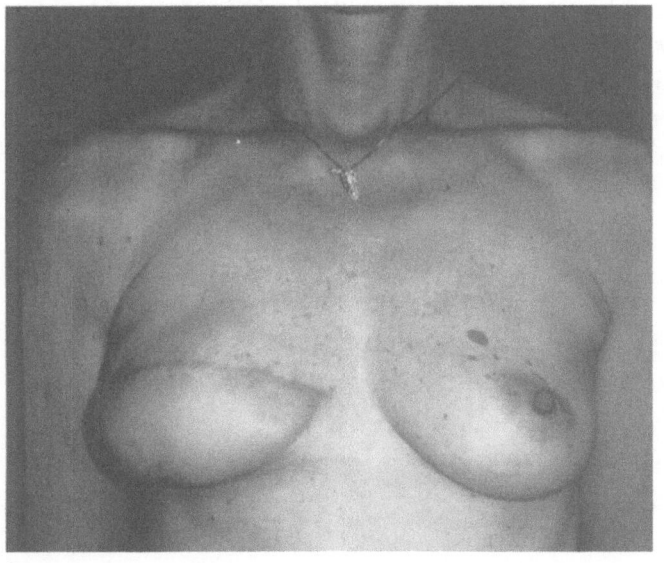
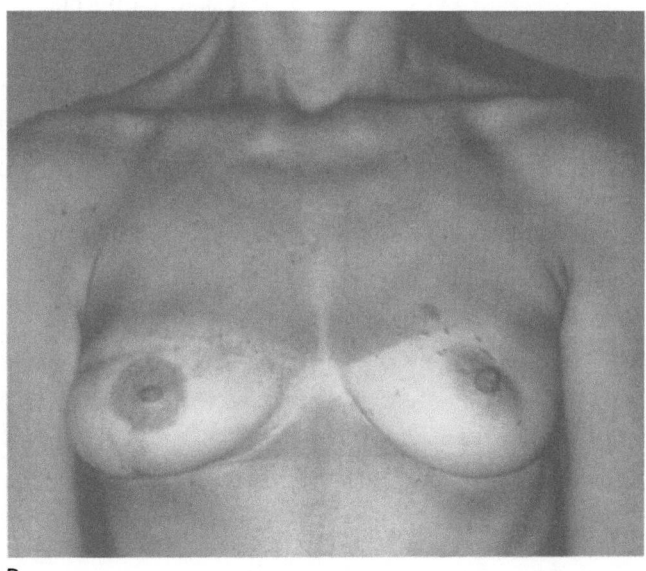

A

B

FIG. 1-4 (A) A patient after breast mound reconstruction with a free TRAM flap. (B) The same patient after revision of the breast mound and reconstruction of the nipple, showing significant improvement in her appearance. (From Kroll SS. Nipple and areolar reconstruction. In: Kroll SS, ed. *Reconstructive Plastic Surgery for Cancer.* St Louis, MO: Mosby; 1996. Used with permission.) See color insert, p. I-3.

lic, it is reassuring to the patient to know that the breast would look relatively normal in the unclothed state. Because nipple and areolar reconstruction is relatively painless, simple, and inexpensive, patients should be encouraged to undergo it whenever possible once the breast mound reconstruction has been completed.

Summary

Breast reconstruction is not cosmetic surgery. It is reconstructive surgery, performed to restore a normal form to women who have undergone mastectomy so that they will not be handicapped in their everyday living. The goal of breast reconstruction is to make women look normal in their clothing so that they can wear ordinary clothes (and most bathing suits) and do not need to wear an external prosthesis. The surgeon may try to surpass this goal and achieve the illusion of normalcy in the unclothed state (and may well succeed), but to avoid disappointment patients should not be led to expect that preoperatively. To achieve optimal results, patients usually will need to undergo at least one revision of the breast mound, followed by subsequent nipple and areolar reconstruction. To avoid conflict with patients and insurance companies, the surgeon should thoroughly explain these details before the reconstructive process begins.

References

1.   Gilboa D, Borenstein A, Floro S, Shafir R, Falach H, Tsur H. Emotional and psychological adjustment of women to breast reconstruction and detection of subgroups at risk for psychological morbidity. *Ann Plast Surg.* 1990;25:397–401.
2.   Schover LR. The impact of breast cancer on sexuality, body image, and intimate relationships. *CA Cancer J Clin.* 1991;41:112.
3.   Lasry JM, Margolese RG, Poisson R, et al. Depression and body image following mastectomy and lumpectomy. *J Chron Dis.* 1987;40:529–534.

2 Why Autologous Tissue?

Autologous tissue from the abdomen or buttocks behaves very much like normal breast tissue and is an ideal material for breast reconstruction. Reconstruction with autologous tissue is more difficult than reconstruction based on implants, however, and requires more lengthy, complex surgery. Because of that complexity, autologous tissue is used less often than implants by most plastic surgeons in community hospitals. Among surgeons who are trained to perform it, however, autologous tissue reconstruction is rapidly becoming the method of choice.[1] This chapter will explain the reasons for this preference and show why autologous tissue reconstruction is superior, in most situations, to reconstruction based on alloplastic implants.

Advantages of Implant-Based Reconstruction

Implant-based breast reconstruction, usually by tissue expansion followed by placement of an implant filled with silicone gel or saline,[2-6] is currently the most widely used method of breast reconstruction in the United States (Fig 2-1). This technique does have advantages, and for some patients—especially those for whom autologous tissue reconstruction is contraindicated because of poor health—the use of an implant can be the best choice.

The main advantage of implant-based reconstruction is simplicity. The placement of an implant or tissue expander is technically easy, requires no special equipment, and can be performed without special training by almost any plastic surgeon in virtually any hospital. The procedure itself is short, and hospitalization and recovery time is minimal. In the short term, the cost of implant-based reconstruction is lower than that of reconstruction with autologous tissue, so implant-based reconstruction is often favored by insurance companies and health maintenance organizations, who are concerned more with the short-term costs to their organization than with any long-term costs to society.

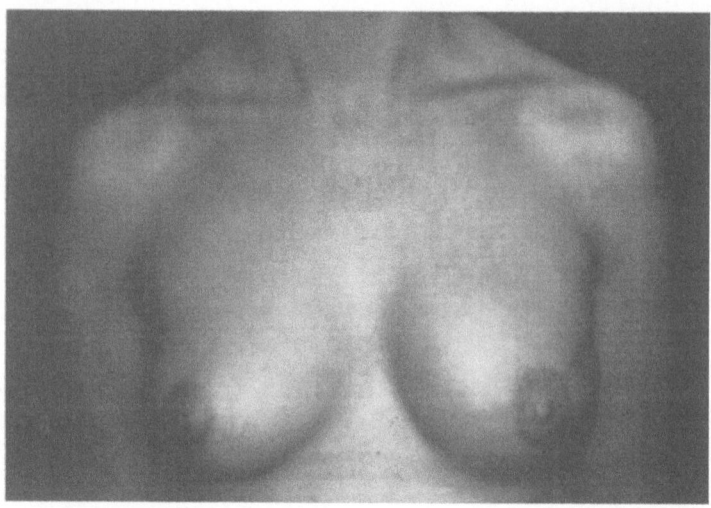

FIG. 2-1   A patient 1 year after left breast reconstruction with tissue expansion and insertion of a silicone gel-filled breast implant.

Implants also have the advantage that they can be changed if it is necessary to make the reconstructed breast moderately larger or smaller. With certain types of implants (permanent expanders), some change in volume can be accomplished without surgery by injecting saline into a subcutaneous port, provided that the port has not yet been removed. Large increases in volume, however, are usually limited by the size of the overlying skin envelope and cannot be accomplished by merely exchanging the implant for a larger one.

Implants can also be used under a latissimus dorsi (or other) flap to replace the volume of missing breast tissue while the overlying flap replaces absent breast skin (Fig 2-2).[7,8] When an implant is used for this purpose, the surgeon does not need to remove as much tissue from the back as would be required for reconstruction with autologous tissue alone. Consequently, donor site morbidity (in the back) is minimized, and the size of the reconstructed breast is not limited by the amount of available tissue.

Disadvantages of Implant-Based Reconstruction

Capsular Contracture

Unfortunately, implants also have significant disadvantages. The patient's body recognizes the prosthesis as foreign material and forms a capsule of scar tissue around it to wall off the implant and try to extrude it. Like all scar tissue, this capsule contracts; as it does the reconstructed breast becomes firmer.[8] In milder forms of capsular contracture, the appearance of the breast is altered so that it no longer feels or appears natural

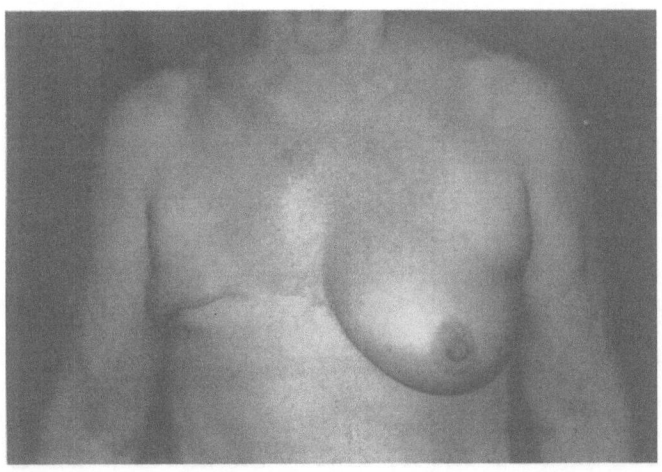
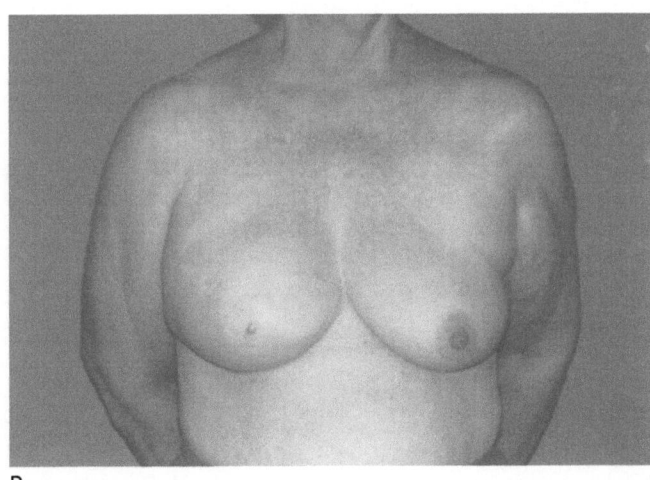

A   B

FIG. 2-2   (A) A 60-year-old woman after right modified radical mastectomy for treatment of breast cancer. (B) Seven years after reconstruction with a latissimus dorsi flap overlying a silicone gel-filled implant. (From *Plast Reconstr Surg* 1992;90:455–462. Used with permission.)

(Fig 2-3). If the capsular contracture progresses far enough, the breast can become rock-hard and painful (Fig 2-4).

Capsular contracture occurs around all breast implants, including those used for breast augmentation. In the case of breast augmentation, moderate amounts of capsular contracture are camouflaged by the overlying softness of a natural breast. In a reconstructed breast, however, there is only a thin layer of skin (and sometimes thinned, stretched-out muscle) to hide contracture-induced changes, so even a small amount of deformity becomes very apparent. For this reason, capsular contracture is a much more

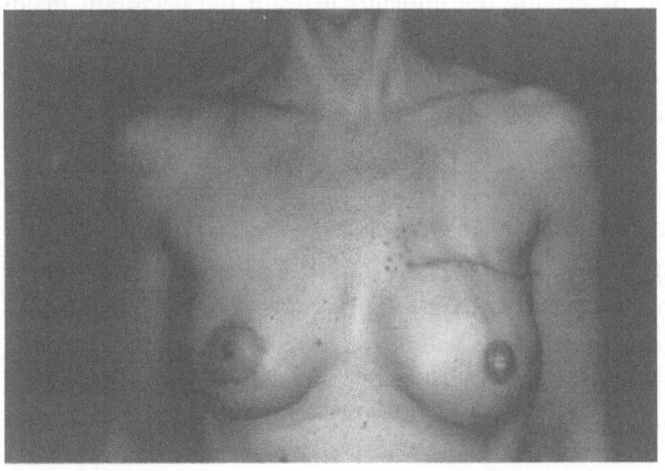
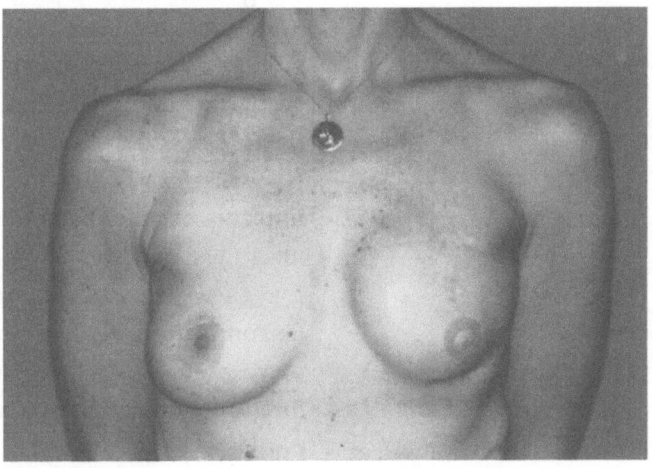

A   B

FIG. 2-3   (A) A patient 1 year after left breast reconstruction with a silicone gel-filled implant. (B) Seven years later, following radiation therapy and showing the effects of capsular contracture.

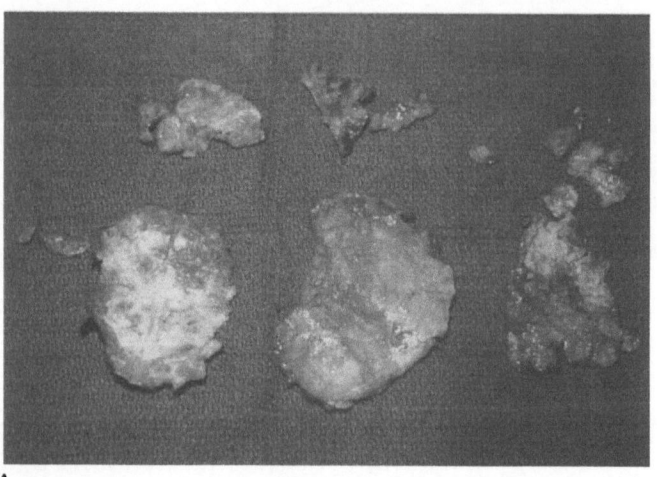
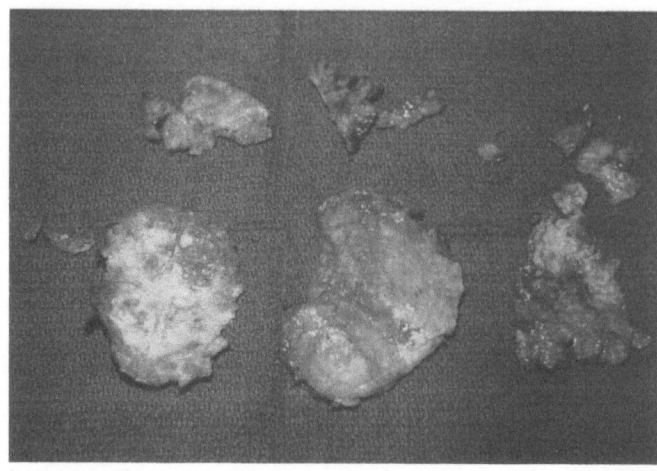

A   B

FIG. 2-4 (A) A previously irradiated patient with severe capsular contracture around a silicone gel-filled implant. The breast was hard and painful. (B) The capsule was diffusely calcified.

serious problem for breast reconstruction patients than it is for those undergoing breast augmentation.

Because the symptoms of capsular contracture increase with time, it is difficult to state its true incidence. In a series of 87 of my own patients followed for more than 1 year (with a mean follow-up of 5 years), the incidence of symptomatic capsular contracture around silicone gel-filled implants was 47.6%. When polyurethane foam-covered implants (which have a lower incidence of capsular contracture but are no longer available) are excluded, the incidence rose to 53.7%.

The incidence of symptomatic capsular contracture can be reduced somewhat by using saline-filled implants and by placing the implants beneath the pectoralis major muscle.[9] It has been claimed that this approach can reduce the rate of capsular contracture by one half. Even so, some degree of capsular contracture will occur in almost every case. When radiation therapy must be used, the incidence of symptomatic contracture rises dramatically.

Capsular contracture remains a significant obstacle to breast reconstruction using implants, even with modern prosthetic devices. I am well aware that many implant manufacturers, and even some surgeons, believe that new implants will solve the problem. Every few years, a new implant is advertised as having overcome the obstacle of capsular contracture. Perhaps some day these claims will prove correct, but as of this writing they have not, and I remain extremely skeptical that they ever will. Capsular contracture is the human body's natural response to a foreign object, and overcoming this will not be easy.

One of the difficulties in evaluating claims of a low incidence of capsular contracture is that each surgeon's definition of a capsular contracture problem is different. What one surgeon may consider a symptomatic capsular contracture that requires treatment, others might judge to be an acceptable result. Compared to a soft transverse rectus abdominus myocutaneous (TRAM) flap reconstruction, almost all implant-based reconstructions are imperfect and to some degree unlike the opposite breast. On the other hand, they can create a normal appearance in clothing, and patients are often satisfied with them even when they know that better alternatives exist. Unfortunately, no standards exist that would allow a fair comparison of results from different institutions. It is partly for this reason that the debate over the use of breast implants for reconstruction remains so far from resolution.

Other Problems

Other problems associated with breast implants include breast pain that can be present even when capsular contracture is very mild,[10] periprosthetic infection (approximately 1%), and implant leakage (approximately 1% per year). Because implant failures (leaks) tend to increase with time[11,12] and are fairly common, it is best to assume that the average implant will need to be replaced every 10 years. Thus, the costs of implant-based reconstruction, and requirements for additional surgery, will continue to accumulate indefinitely. Furthermore, if the patient gains a significant amount of weight, the opposite breast will get larger while the implant-based breast will not (Fig 2-5), causing an asymmetry that cannot always be solved simply by replacing the implant.

Finally, the relationship between the implant and the host is far more fragile than that between the patient and autologous tissue. If an implant becomes exposed because of necrosis of overlying skin, it will usually be lost (Fig 2-6). With autologous tissue, exposure of an underlying flap caused by mastectomy flap edge necrosis usually is of little consequence and does not interfere with an ultimately successful result (Fig 2-7).

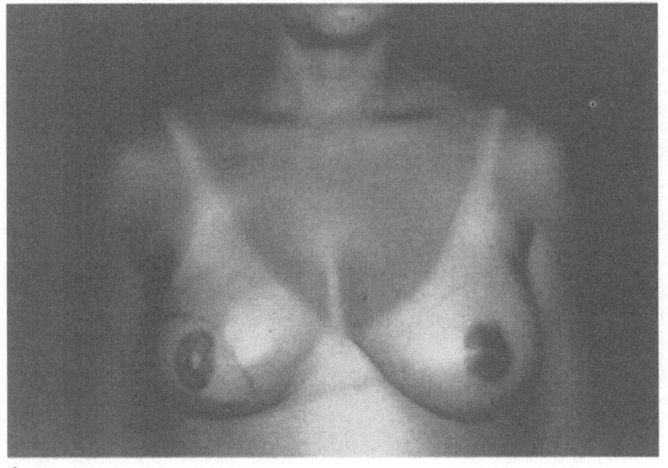
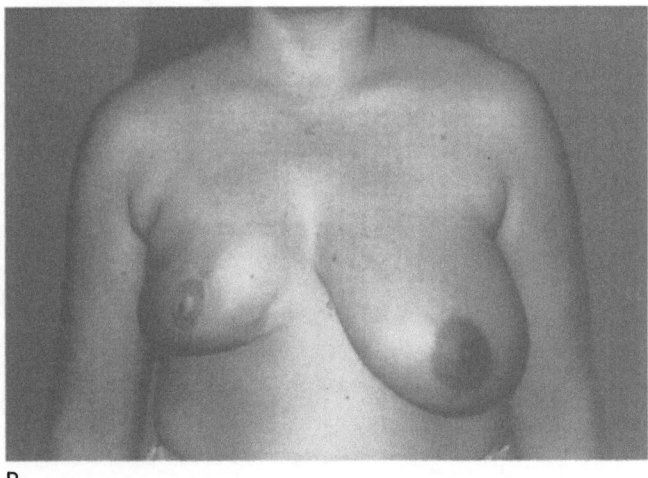

A   B

FIG. 2-5   (A) A woman 1 year after right breast reconstruction with a latissimus dorsi myocutaneous flap covering a silicone gel-filled implant. (B) The same patient 5 years later, after gaining 50 pounds. The left breast has become larger, while the right breast is unchanged. (From Kroll SS. *Clin Plast Surg.* 2998;25:135–143. Used with permission.)

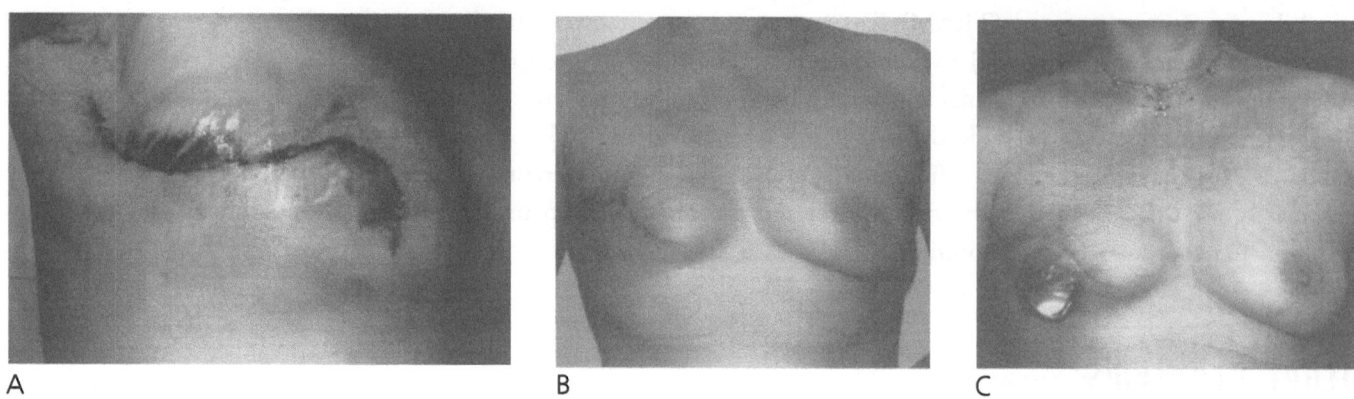

A   B   C

FIG. 2-6 (A) A patient with mastectomy flap edge necrosis following immediate reconstruction with a tissue expander. (B) One month later, after debridement of the edge necrosis and apparent healing of the wound. (C) The same patient 2 additional months later, showing implant exposure. The implant was removed, and the reconstruction ultimately failed.

Advantages of Autologous Tissue Reconstruction

Autologous fatty tissue is similar in consistency to mature breast tissue and makes an ideal substitute. Because autologous tissue is part of the patient's body, nerves can grow into it, and sensation in autologously reconstructed breasts is usually better than when implants have been used.[13] When the patient lies down, autologously reconstructed breasts

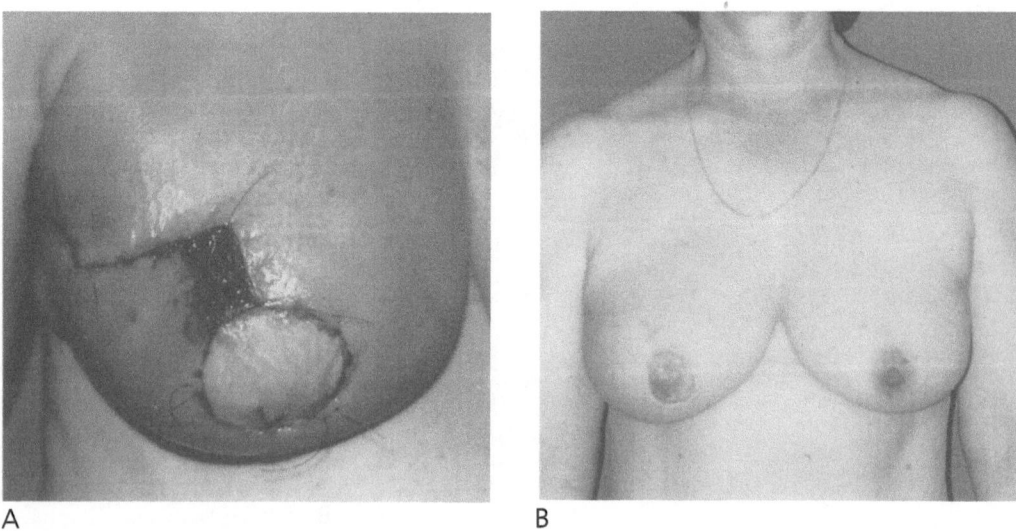

A   B

FIG. 2-7 (A) A patient with mastectomy flap edge necrosis after immediate breast reconstruction with a free TRAM flap. (B) The same patient after secondary healing, revision, and nipple reconstruction. The final result was not significantly impacted by the exposure of the underlying TRAM flap. See color insert, p. I-4.

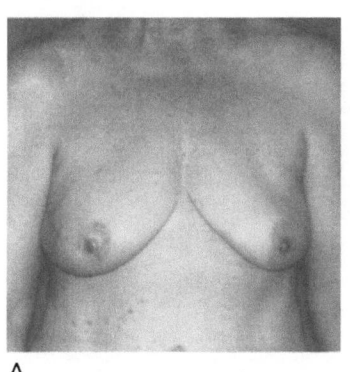
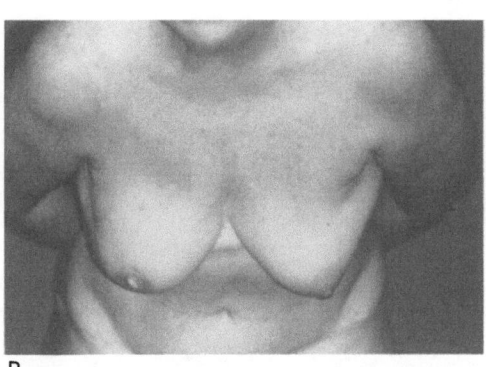
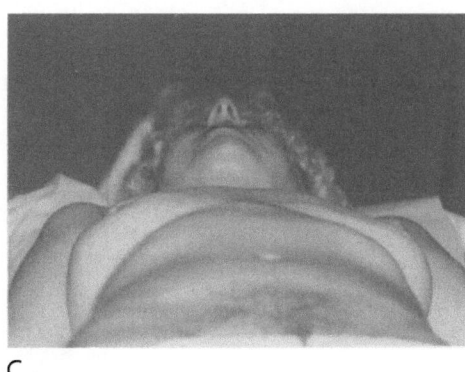

A   B   C

FIG. 2-8   (A) A 61-year-old woman after mastectomy and immediate right breast reconstruction with a free TRAM flap. (B) Same patient, bending forward. (C) When the patient is supine, the reconstructed breast falls naturally off to the side just like a real breast.

fall to the side (Fig 2-8), and they become more ptotic with time, like natural breasts. Breasts reconstructed with autologous tissue move like real breasts when the patient runs or walks and appear more natural in a bathing suit. If the patient gains or loses weight, the reconstructed breast will change along with the natural breast (although not always at the same rate). When performed properly, autologous tissue breast reconstruction almost always leads to a better-quality result than can be achieved using implants.

With autologous tissue reconstruction, in contrast to implant-based reconstruction, time can be the patient's ally; with increased follow-up scars soften and fade (Fig 2-9), sensation improves, and tissue firmness resolves. After the first year following completion of the reconstruction, additional surgery is rarely required unless the patient gains or loses a significant amount of weight or develops a new malignancy. In the long term, therefore, autologous tissue reconstruction can require less surgery than reconstruction with implants.[14]

Disadvantages of Autologous Tissue Reconstruction

Autologous tissue reconstruction is more complex, demands a longer initial hospitalization, and requires a longer recovery period than does reconstruction based on implants. The surgical procedures themselves are more difficult, and not every plastic surgeon is familiar with them. There is a "learning curve," and experience as well as training is required for the surgeon to achieve consistently good results. In the hands of poorly trained surgeons, autologous tissue reconstruction can be dangerous. Because autologous tissue can be obtained only from the patient herself, there are always some potentially deleterious changes in the donor site even when the operation is completely successful. If the donor site is not repaired properly or if too much tissue is harvested, significant morbidity can occur. Should flap loss occur, salvage is more difficult than is the case after loss of an implant, which, at least in theory, can be replaced by a new one.

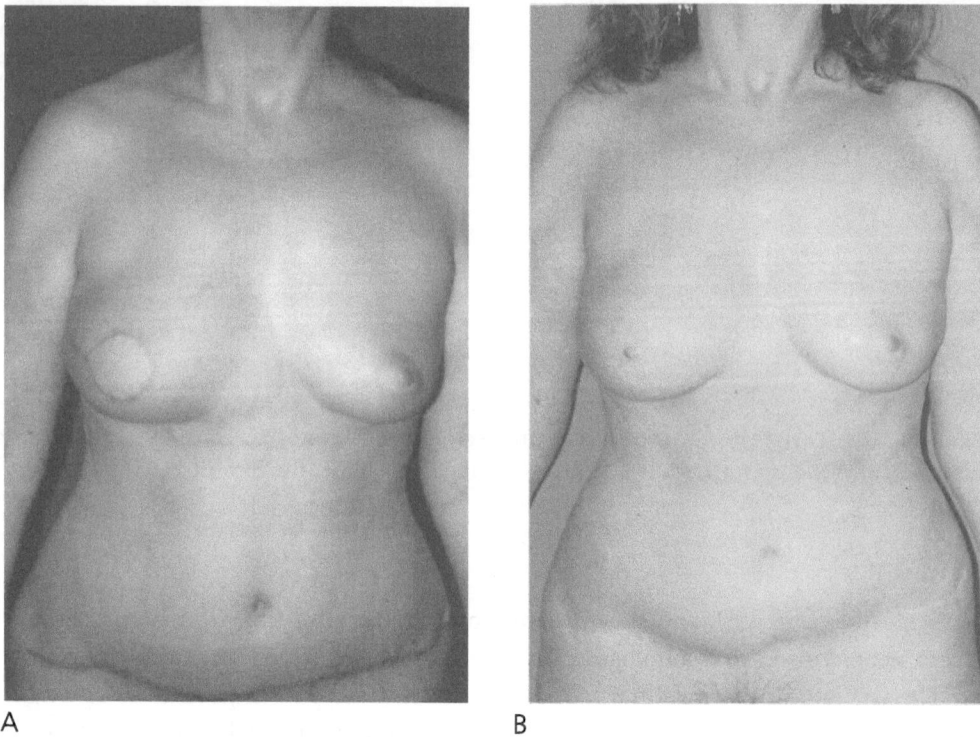

A   B

FIG. 2-9   (A) Early result of a pedicled TRAM flap breast reconstruction. (B) After 4 years, the scars have faded and the patient looks better than she did immediately after the reconstruction. See color insert, p. I-5.

Long-Term Costs of Breast Reconstruction

Implant-based reconstruction has low initial costs, but as noted above many patients will continue to need additional surgery to maintain their reconstructed breasts. Because of problems such as capsular contracture, leakage, infection, and pain, the costs of implant-based reconstruction continue to accumulate indefinitely.

At The University of Texas M. D. Anderson Cancer Center, we have analyzed the costs of breast reconstruction with tissue expansion and implants and with autologous tissue (TRAM flaps) to determine which method is more expensive in the long run. We found, as expected, that the initial hospitalization costs of implant-based reconstruction are much lower than those of reconstruction with TRAM flaps. During subsequent years, however, the costs of implant-based reconstruction accumulate at a much higher rate than do the costs of TRAM flap reconstruction, which are relatively stable. After 4 years of follow-up, the costs of implant-based reconstruction are higher than the costs of reconstruction with autologous tissue (Figs 2-10 and 2-11).[14] Although we have not yet observed significant numbers of patients for periods longer than 4 years, it seems reasonable to suppose that with additional time the cost disadvantage of implants will increase fur-

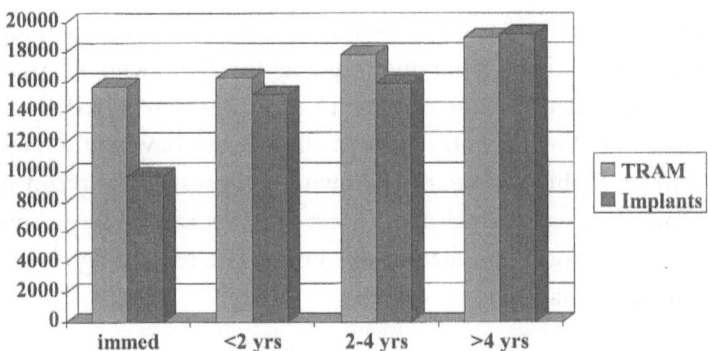

FIG. 2-10 A graphic depiction of the total corrected resource costs of unilateral mastectomy and immediate breast reconstruction in 1993 dollars, showing how the differences between implant-based and TRAM flap breast reconstruction change over time. Although the short-term costs of implant-based reconstruction are lower, after 4 years the cumulative costs are similar to or higher than the costs of TRAM flap reconstruction.

ther. If that is true, then the long-term cost of autologous tissue reconstruction will be significantly lower than that of reconstruction based on tissue expansion and implants.

Summary

Breast reconstruction can be successfully accomplished with the use of tissue expansion and implants, with flaps overlying implants, or with autologous tissue alone. We have found that autologous tissue reconstruction is more successful in creating a breast that looks and moves like a normal one, and that its use is associated with lower long-term

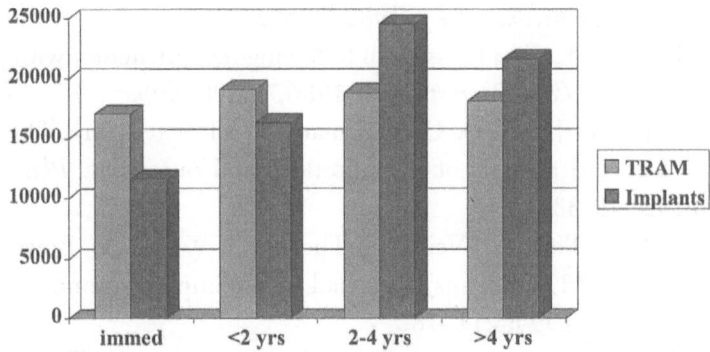

FIG. 2-11 A graphic depiction of the total corrected resource costs of bilateral mastectomy and immediate bilateral breast reconstruction in 1993 dollars, showing how the differences between implant-based and TRAM flap breast reconstruction change over time. Although the short-term costs of implant-based reconstruction are lower, after 4 years the cumulative costs are similar to or higher than the costs of TRAM flap reconstruction.

costs and fewer complications as well. For these reasons, we prefer autologous tissue reconstruction for most patients, reserving implants for those who are not good surgical candidates and those who will not consent to the surgery required for reconstruction with autologous tissue. For patients who will allow it, we have found autologous tissue reconstruction to be highly satisfactory, allowing the creation of reconstructed breasts that are often mistaken for normal ones. Most patients can undergo successful reconstruction using the methods described in this book. The remaining chapters will be devoted to showing how that is done.

References

1. Hartrampf, CR. *Hartrampf's Breast Reconstruction with Living Tissue.* New York, NY: Raven Press; 1991.
2. Radovan C. Breast reconstruction after mastectomy using the temporary expander. *Plast Reconstr Surg.* 1982;69:195.
3. Gibney J. Use of a permanent tissue expander for breast reconstruction. *Plast Reconstr Surg.* 1989;84:607–617.
4. Becker H. Breast reconstruction using an inflatable breast implant with detachable reservoir. *Plast Reconstr Surg.* 1984;73:678.
5. Slavin SA, Colen SR. Sixty consecutive breast reconstructions with inflatable expanders: a critical appraisal. *Plast Reconstr Surg.* 1990;86:910.
6. Maxwell GP, Falcone PA. Eighty-four consecutive breast reconstructions using a textured silicone expander. *Plast Reconstr Surg.* 1992;89:1022.
7. Biggs TM, Cronin ED. Technical aspects of the latissimus dorsi myocutaneous flap in breast reconstruction. *Ann Plast Surg.* 1981;6:381.
8. McCraw JB, Maxwell GP. Early and late capsular "deformation" as a cause of unsatisfactory results in the latissimus dorsi breast reconstruction. *Clin Plast Surg.* 1988;15:717–726.
9. Little JW, Golembe EV, Fisher JB. The "living bra" in immediate and delayed reconstruction of the breast following mastectomy for malignant and nonmalignant disease. *Plast Reconstr Surg.* 1981;68:392.
10. Jabalay ME, Das SK. Late breast pain following reconstruction with polyurethane-covered implants. *Plast Reconstr Surg.* 1986;78:390–395.
11. Handel N, Jenson JA, Black Q, Waisman JR, Silverstein MJ. The fate of breast implants: a critical analysis of complications and outcomes. *Plast Reconstr Surg.* 1995;96:1521–1533.
12. Netscher DT, Walker LE, Weizer G, Thornby J, Wigoda P, Bowen D. A review of 198 patients (389 implants) who had breast implants removed. *J Long-Term Eff Med Implants.* 1995;5:11–18.
13. Shaw WW, Orringer JS, Ko CY, Ratto LL, Mersmann CA. The spontaneous return of sensibility in breasts reconstructed with autologous tissues. *Plast Reconstr Surg.* 1997;99:394–399.
14. Kroll SS, Evans GRD, Reece GP, et al. Comparison of resource costs between implant-based and TRAM flap breast reconstruction. *Plast Reconstr Surg.* 1996; 97:364–372.

3 Why Use Free Flaps?

Advantages of Using Free Flaps

A t The University of Texas M. D. Anderson Cancer Center we believe that free flaps are the best choice for autologous tissue breast reconstruction in most patients.[1] There are four principal reasons for this belief. First, free flaps cause less donor site morbidity than pedicled flaps. Second, blood supply to the flap is usually more robust. Third, the use of free flaps facilitates subsequent revision of the breast mound, as I will discuss in chapter 20. Fourth, free flaps provide increased flexibility when transverse rectus abdominis myocutaneous (TRAM) flaps are not possible and other donor sites must be used. Other minor advantages include a smoother, less distorted inframammary fold. In this chapter, I will discuss these advantages of free flaps, and suggest ways to make the use of free flaps more practical, less stressful, and more successful.

Reduced Donor Site Morbidity

The most important advantage of using free flaps for breast reconstruction is reduced morbidity in the flap donor site. When a free flap is used, only that part of a muscle required to link the blood vessels of the pedicle to the vascular system of the flap must be harvested.[2] In contrast, rotational flaps usually require functional sacrifice of an entire muscle. The free TRAM flap (Fig 3-1), for example, requires sacrifice of only a fraction of the amount of rectus abdominis muscle that would be required for transfer of a pedicled TRAM flap (Figs 3-2 and 3-3). This reduced muscle loss in patients who undergo reconstruction with free TRAM flaps reduces postoperative abdominal wall weakness. Consequently, 93% of patients who have undergone breast reconstruction with free TRAM flaps are able to perform situps, while only 50% of patients who have undergone reconstruction with pedicled TRAM flaps are able to do so.[3] The difference in abdominal wall strength is particularly noticeable when the TRAM flap reconstruction has been bilateral. When bilateral pedicled TRAM flaps have been harvested, only

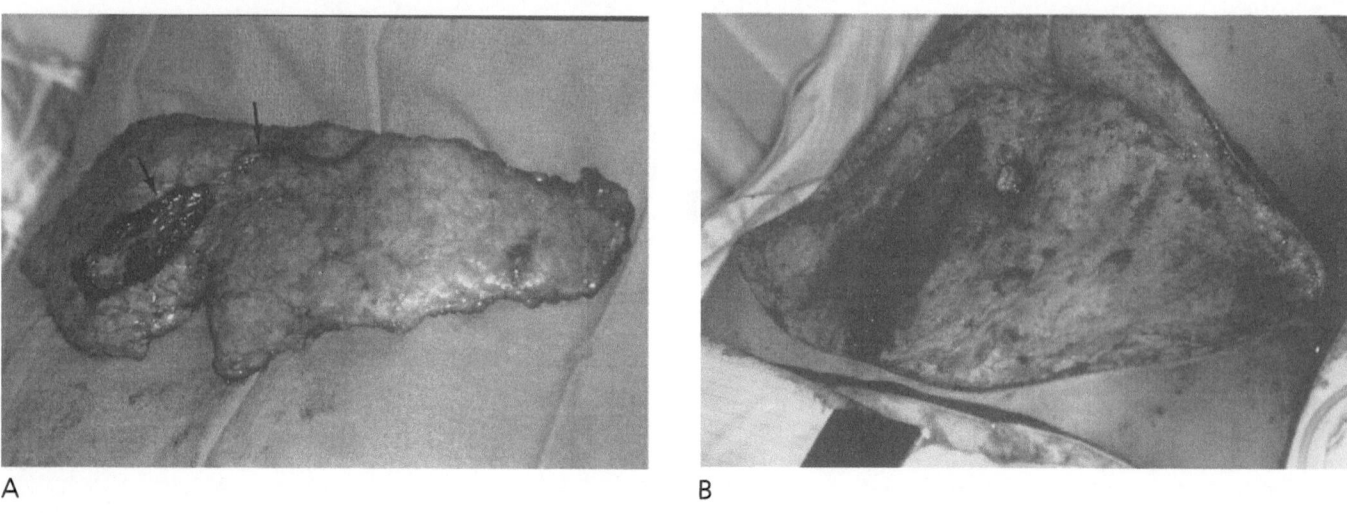

A   B

FIG. 3-1   (A) The pedicle (arrows) of a free TRAM flap: only minimal muscle tissue has been sacrificed. (B) The donor site.

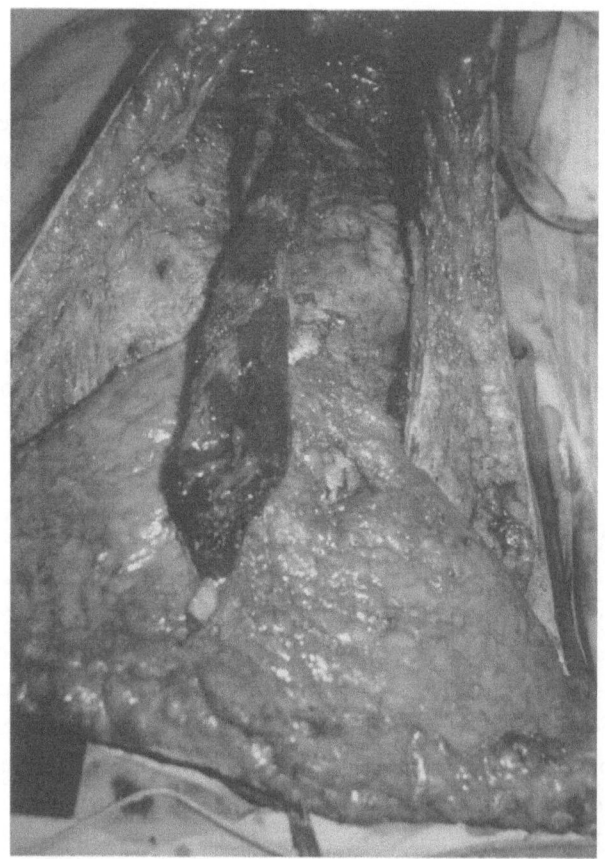

FIG. 3-2   The muscle pedicle of a conventional (pedicled) TRAM flap. A large part of the muscle has been included with the flap, inevitably causing some loss of function.

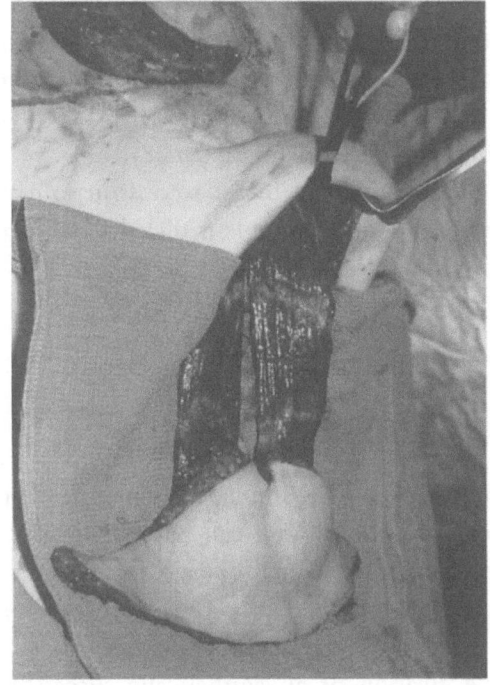 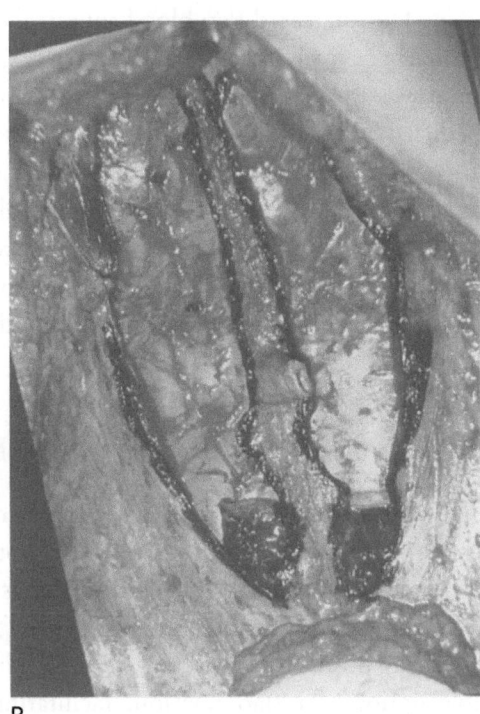

A   B

FIG. 3-3 (A) A double-pedicled conventional TRAM flap. (B) The donor site defect. Even more muscle is sacrificed in this procedure. (From Kroll SS. Breast reconstruction with the TRAM flap. In: Kroll SS, ed. *Reconstructive Plastic Surgery for Cancer.* St. Louis: Mosby; 1996. Used with permission.)

27% of our patients are able to do situps, compared to the 75% who have been able to do them after bilateral free TRAM flaps. After unilateral TRAM flap harvest, the difference in situp ability between those with free and pedicled flaps is less noticeable, presumably due to the presence of an intact rectus abdominis muscle on the opposite side.

The reduced muscle sacrifice also diminishes postoperative pain. Recovery from the surgery is more rapid and less disabling. This may not be important to every surgeon, but patients consider it compelling. For this reason alone, most patients prefer the free TRAM flap when that option is available.

Increased Flap Perfusion

The second advantage of the free TRAM flap is a more robust and efficient blood supply. The deep inferior epigastric vessels that supply blood to the free TRAM flap are larger in caliber than the superior epigastric vessels that supply the pedicled TRAM flap. Moreover, in the free TRAM flap, the flap lies in the primary territory of the deep inferior epigastric vessels, so blood does not have to pass through "choke vessels" before reaching the flap.[4] Consequently, circulation is more efficient and, compared to that of the pedicled TRAM flap, increased.

This increased flap blood supply allows the TRAM flap to be folded and sculpted more aggressively to achieve the desired shape. This increases the surgeon's options and improves the appearance of the reconstructed breast. Although some outcomes from pedicled TRAM flaps are every bit as excellent as those achieved with free flaps, the *average* outcome of free TRAM flap breast reconstruction tends to be better.

The improved flap blood supply also allows successful breast reconstruction in patients who smoke, without having to resort to the use of double-pedicled flaps (Fig 3-3). When double-pedicled flaps[5] are avoided, muscle sacrifice and donor site morbidity are significantly reduced, albeit indirectly.

Facilitation of Breast Mound Revision

The use of free tissue transfer for breast reconstruction results in a breast mound that has a superiorly based blood supply. Consequently, the mound can be revised using techniques similar to those used for breast reconstruction or mastopexy without interfering at all with the blood supply to the flap, or being impeded by the presence of an inferiorly positioned muscular pedicle. This significantly increases the number of available options for flap revision, facilitating the creation of an aesthetically successful reconstruction.

Use of Alternative Donor Sites

The routine use of free TRAM flaps, which requires a working familiarity with microsurgery, facilitates the use of other free flaps such as the inferior gluteal,[6,7] the superior gluteal,[8] and the Rubens fat pad flap.[9] This is true not only for the surgeon but also for the operating room nurses and other members of the treatment team. Although there is no rule against the use of alternative free flaps by surgeons who do not perform free TRAM flaps, surgeons who are not comfortable with free TRAM flaps are unlikely to feel comfortable attempting these other, more difficult surgical procedures. The everyday use of microsurgery removes some of the mystery from free-tissue transfer and widens the surgeon's options for breast reconstruction when a TRAM flap is not possible. The routine use of free TRAM flaps also improves the surgeon's microvascular experience and potential for success with free flap reconstruction in the head and neck, extremities, and other areas.

Less Distortion of the Inframammary Fold

Although distortion of the inframammary fold is not inevitably associated with the use of pedicled TRAM flaps, it is often seen after such reconstruction because of the need to release the medial portion of the fold and create a tunnel through it. Consequently, and because of the presence of the muscle pedicle in this tunnel, bulging of the medial portion of the inframammary fold is common. In most cases this bulging can be corrected secondarily, but sometimes the distortion will persist even after surgical removal of excess tis-

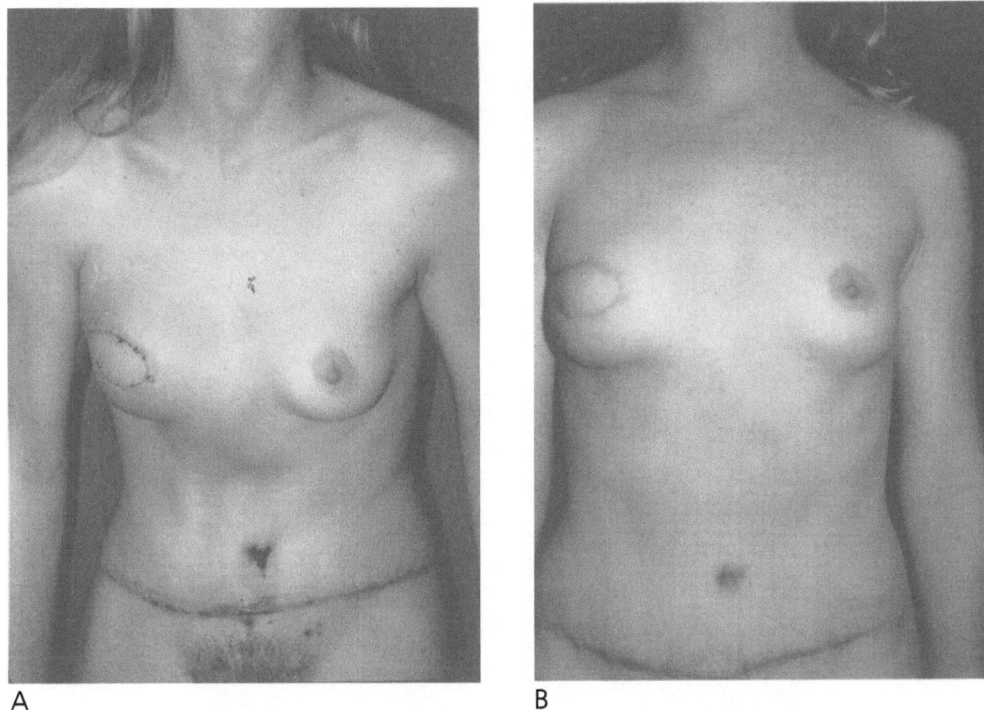

A   B

FIG. 3-4   (A) An early result of breast reconstruction with a conventional TRAM flap showing some distortion of the inframammary fold caused by the presence of the muscle pedicle. (B)
With time, much of this distortion will subside spontaneously.

sue (Fig 3-4). This type of distortion is rarely seen after a free TRAM flap, since there is
no tunnel and no need to release any part of the inframammary fold (Fig 3-5).

Making a Smaller Breast

Paradoxically, it can be more difficult to make a small breast with a TRAM flap than
to make a large one. The larger the muscle pedicle, the more difficult it is to reduce
the size of the flap without endangering blood supply. Although using a free flap does
not solve all the problems associated with making a small breast, the robust blood supply does allow more aggressive shaping and makes obtaining a symmetrical result more
likely (Fig 3-6).

Making Free Flaps More Practical

Some surgeons avoid free flaps because they see them as complex affairs that are usually not finished until late at night, are associated with high anxiety levels, and have a
high incidence of emergent returns to the operating room and failures. Usually, these

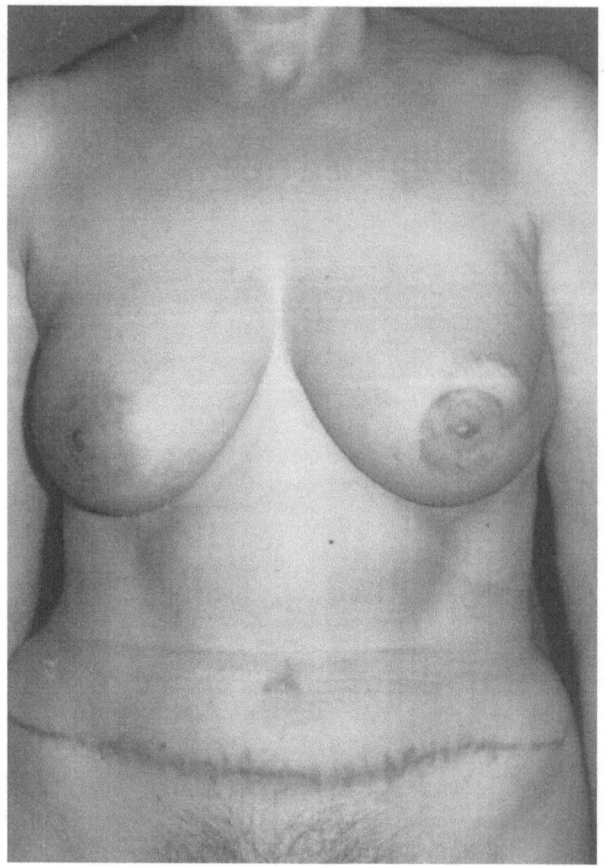

FIG. 3-5   A free TRAM flap breast reconstruction, showing a completely smooth inframammary fold. See color insert, p. I-2.

opinions have been formulated during residency training after watching relatively inexperienced surgeons struggle to overcome obstacles they were not properly trained to deal with. Free flaps do not have to be complicated and frustrating. At M. D. Anderson Cancer Center, we view free flaps as routine everyday procedures and often as the easiest way to solve a reconstructive problem. Although failures do occur, our incidence of flap loss in free flap breast reconstruction has been less than 1%,[10] a figure not substantially different from the failure rate of pedicled flaps. Free flaps can be simplified, and made more practical, by following several simple rules.

Starting Early and Finishing Early

The first rule of free flap surgery is to avoid finishing the procedure late at night. The surgeon's goal is to finish the free flap by 6 PM so that the surgical and operating room teams are not stressed by excessive overtime and can perform their functions in a routine manner. Even more important, an early finish allows detection of postoperative thrombosis or other pedicle obstruction (which usually appears in the first few hours after wound closure) before the anesthesiologists and other operating room personnel

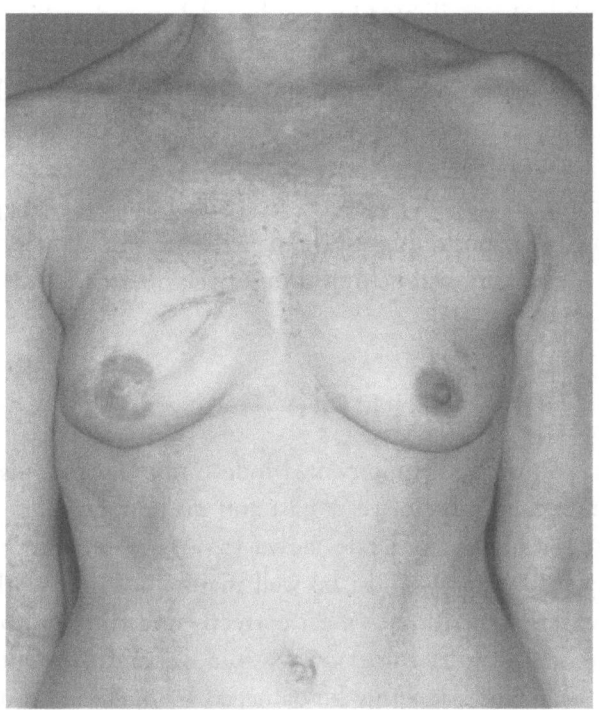

FIG. 3-6 A small breast reconstructed with a free TRAM flap. Paradoxically, this is much more difficult than reconstruction of a larger breast.

have gone home for the day. Consequently, if a return to the operating room is required it can be accomplished relatively quickly, increasing the chance of successful salvage of the flap. Moreover, a rapid and early return to the operating room avoids the need for surgery in the middle of the night, an additional source of schedule disruption and fatigue that interferes with proper function of the operating suite.

To avoid finishing free flaps late at night, every operation involving a possible free flap should be started as early as possible, as the first case of the day. This not only gives the microvascular surgeon a better chance for an early finish, but allows the most complex portion of the free flap to be completed while the daytime nurses, who are usually the most experienced and knowledgeable (and know where to find spare instruments or microscope bulbs should that be necessary) are on duty. In my experience, anastomoses that must be performed at night are often delayed by nonspecialized nurses who do not know where to locate microvascular sutures or other critical materials. That situation can usually be avoided by insisting on an early start for all complex procedures, especially those that will involve free flaps.

In our institution, no exceptions are allowed to this rule. Having a firm regulation like this discourages well-meaning colleagues from asking the microsurgeon to allow exceptions for short cases to be performed prior to the free flap as a personal favor. Invariably, the "short case" takes longer than expected and, combined with the operating room turnaround time, delays the free flap so that it finishes late. Unfortunately, most colleagues do not realize how detrimental these delays are to the success of the free flap. For that reason, it is best to have a firm rule so that exceptions cannot be made.

An early finish is also facilitated by avoiding delays and making constant progress throughout the procedure. In teaching hospitals, the surgeon may have to share parts of the operation with relatively inexperienced residents and fellows. This is permissible provided that the trainees are properly supervised and that the case is not unduly prolonged. It is the attending surgeon's responsibility, however, to ensure that adequate progress is being made. If the trainees are not capable of making adequate progress, the attending surgeon has responsibilities to the patient and to the operating room that require taking over the surgery and getting things back on schedule.

Having the Right Equipment

High success rates require good equipment. Modern microscopes, instruments, and sutures are much better than those of years past and make microsurgery easier and more successful. To ensure a high success rate, however, it is essential to have equipment of the highest quality. Moreover, it must be well maintained and work properly. Using jeweler's forceps with tips that do not meet correctly and will not hold sutures, for example, is frustrating and can lead to poor anastomoses and flap failure. Microsurgical instruments are delicate and can easily be damaged by operating room personnel during cleaning or storage. If the operating room staff is not used to working with microsurgical instruments, the surgeon needs to take a personal interest in the instruments and ensure that they are properly cared for.

Instruments used for breast reconstruction should be long enough to reach easily into the axilla (Fig 3-7). Short instruments make the surgeon struggle to reach the anastomosis, and can lead to tremor and poor technique. Longer instruments are more expensive, but are essential to achieving high success rates.

Many surgeons have successfully performed free flaps with loupes.[11] I have done this myself and agree that it is fully possible. Some would argue that an operating microscope is unnecessary, but I would not agree. A good operating microscope (Fig 3-8) provides more light, better resolution, a greater depth of focus, and a wider field of view than loupes can. A microscope also facilitates working with finer sutures, such as 10-0

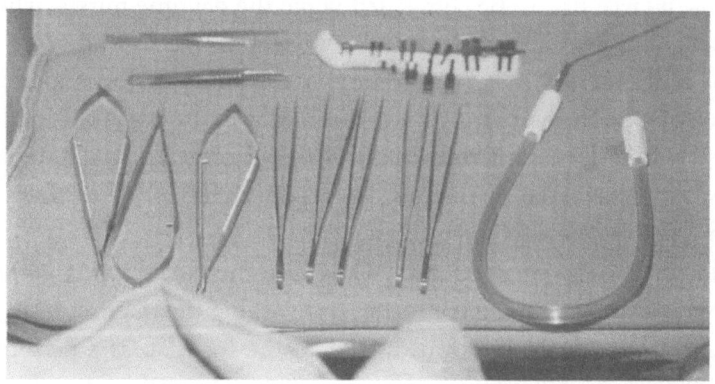

FIG. 3-7 Long (15 cm) microsurgical instruments suitable for performing anastomoses in the axilla. Instruments shorter than this greatly increase the difficulty of the anastomoses.

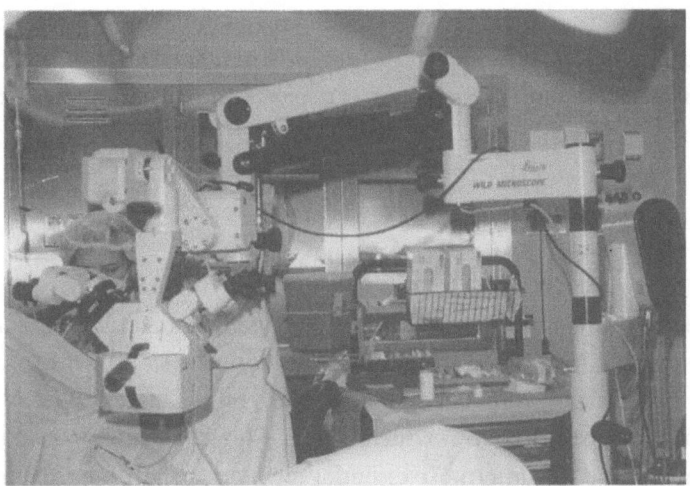

FIG. 3-8   Leica-Wild M-80 microscope. This microscope has excellent resolution and lighting, and is suitable for microvascular free tissue transfer.

nylon. Loupes are adequate when the vessels are large and the surgery is uneventful. Many excellent surgeons are getting good results with them. When an unforeseen problem arises, however, especially if it involves anastomosis of very small vessels, the microscope may allow a successful resolution when a pair of loupes might not. A good microscope reduces surgical stress and increases success rates, and in my opinion should be available in any center that plans to perform more than a few free flap procedures each year.

Using Simple and Reliable Techniques

Microsurgery is much easier and more reliable when flaps with long pedicles and large-caliber vessels are used.[10] Fortunately, the most widely used free flap for breast reconstruction is the free TRAM flap, which has a pedicle that is relatively long and easy to work with. The surgeon should take the time to dissect the pedicle (the deep inferior epigastric vessels) all the way to its origin, so that it is as long as possible. Making the pedicle long makes positioning of the flap on the chest easier and increases the caliber of the vessels. Moreover, a long pedicle facilitates positioning of the flap during the anastomoses so that the flap is not in the surgeon's way. For this reason, I prefer a long pedicle even when using the internal mammary vessels (which otherwise do not require a long pedicle) as recipients.

Having Adequate Assistance

Although it is possible to perform a free flap procedure without assistance, free flaps are much easier to do with adequate help. A well-trained assistant can make the anastomoses much easier, and can perform parts of the operation independently, greatly speeding up the procedure and increasing the chances of success. One capable assistant is all that is required for most breast reconstructions, but for bilateral reconstruction or in obese patients it is better to have two or more assistants, if possible. In that way fatigue will be less of a factor and the surgeon can pay more attention to obtaining an aesthetically good result.

Monitoring the Flap Postoperatively

Although every effort should be made to prevent pedicle obstruction, careful postoperative flap monitoring is required so that if thrombosis does occur it can be treated early enough that flap salvage is possible. There are several effective methods of monitoring flaps and some disagreement about which is best. Almost all experienced microsurgeons, however, would agree that the most essential element in flap monitoring is an experienced and intelligent nurse. Flap monitoring must be performed by someone with sufficient expertise to recognize the signs of an obstructed pedicle early enough to do something about it.

Because most episodes of thrombosis occur early in the postoperative course, we have found that hourly flap monitoring for the first 3 postoperative days is usually sufficient.[12] This monitoring is performed in a "flap unit," which is simply an ordinary group of hospital rooms where all patients who undergo free flap procedures are sent (unless they are required for other reasons to be in the intensive care unit). In that way, a small group of nurses become experts at recognizing flaps that require attention. This expertise is invaluable and has increased our success in flap salvage regardless of what monitoring technique is being used.

Summary

Provided that adequate equipment and personnel are available, free flaps can be a very practical and effective method of autologous tissue breast reconstruction. The advantages of free tissue transfer include reduced donor site morbidity, increased flap blood flow, a superiorly based blood supply that facilitates breast mound revision, and an increased choice of donor sites. At M. D. Anderson Cancer Center, the free TRAM flap is the most commonly used breast reconstruction technique, and one that has achieved excellent results with a low failure rate.

Free flaps do not necessarily have to be complex and time-consuming. With good equipment, adequate training, sufficient planning, and early start times, a procedure that includes free flaps can be completed without excessively stressing the surgeon, the patient, or the operating room team.

References

1. Schusterman MA, Kroll SS, Weldon ME. Immediate breast reconstruction: why the free TRAM over the conventional TRAM flap? *Plast Reconstr Surg.* 1992; 90:255–262.

2. Grotting JC, Urist MM, Maddox WA, Vasconez LO. Conventional TRAM flap versus free microsurgical TRAM flap for immediate breast reconstruction. *Plast Reconstr Surg.* 1989;83:842–844.

3. Kroll SS, Schusterman MA, Reece GP, Miller MJ, Robb GL, Evans GRD. Abdominal wall strength, bulging, and hernia after TRAM flap breast reconstruction. *Plast Reconstr Surg.* 1995;96:616–619.

4. Boyd JB, Taylor GI, Corlett R. The vascular territories of the superior epigastric and the deep inferior epigastric systems. *Plast Reconstr Surg.* 1984;73:1–14.

5. Ishii CH, Bostwick J, Raine TJ, Coleman JJ, Hester TR. Double-pedicle transverse rectus abdominis myocutaneous flap for unilateral breast and chest-wall reconstruction. *Plast Reconstr Surg.* 1985;76:901–907.

6. Nahai F. Inferior gluteus maximum musculocutaneous flap for breast reconstruction. *Perspect Plast Surg.* 1992;6:65.

7. Codner MA, Nahai F. The gluteal free flap breast reconstruction: making it work. *Clin Plast Surg.* 1994;21:289–296.

8. Shaw WW. Breast reconstruction by superior gluteal microvascular free flaps without silicone implants. *Plast Reconstr Surg.* 1983;72:490.

9. Hartrampf CR Jr, Noel RT, Drazan L, Elliott LF, Bennett GK, Beegle PH. Rubens fat pad for breast reconstruction: a peri-iliac soft-tissue free flap. *Plast Reconstr Surg.* 1994;93:402–407.

10. Kroll SS, Schusterman MA, Reece GP, et al. Choice of flap and incidence of free flap success. *Plast Reconstr Surg.* 1996;98:459–463.

11. Serletti JM, Deuber MA, Guidera PM, et al. Comparison of the operating microscope and loupes for free microvascular tissue transfer. *Plast Reconstr Surg.* 1995;95:270–276.

12. Kroll SS, Schusterman MA, Reece GP, et al. Timing of pedicle thrombosis and flap loss after free tissue transfer. *Plast Reconstr Surg.* 1996;98:1230–1233.

4 Immediate Breast Reconstruction

Advantages of Immediate Reconstruction

Breast reconstruction can be immediate (right after the mastectomy) or delayed (months or years later). Many years ago, virtually all breast reconstructions were delayed for fear that immediate reconstruction would compromise adjuvant treatment or make cancer follow-up more difficult. Today, those arguments are largely considered invalid, and immediate reconstruction is becoming more and more popular.[1-3] This change has occurred because immediate reconstruction has many advantages, both for the patient and for the surgeon who performs the reconstruction.

Convenience

The first advantage is patient convenience. For the patient, the prospect of waking up from the anesthetic after her mastectomy with the breast mound already reconstructed is far more attractive than that of having to return to the hospital for another major operation months or years later. A major operation, with its attendant preoperative visits, blood tests, hospital stay, and convalescence, is very inconvenient for patients, many of whom are in the prime of their lives and have significant responsibilities at work or at home. For such patients, the ability to recuperate from both the mastectomy and the breast mound reconstruction at the same time and in one hospital stay saves valuable time and is very appealing. From the patient's point of view, immediate reconstruction is always a more attractive option than reconstruction that is delayed.

Cost

The second advantage is reduced cost.[4] Because recovery from the mastectomy and the reconstruction is simultaneous, the patient requires fewer total days in the hospital than would be needed if the two procedures were done separately. Moreover, the costs of an additional anesthetic induction and required preoperative testing and office visits for the extra operation are eliminated. Finally, because immediate reconstruction is technically easier than delayed reconstruction (see below), multiple revisions are less likely to be required to achieve a satisfactory breast shape.

Safety

The third advantage is safety. Modern general anesthesia is relatively safe; however, adverse incidents, though uncommon, do occur. In eliminating one induction of general anesthesia, the risk of the reconstructive process is lowered.

Psychological Factors

The fourth advantage is the psychological one of avoiding the mental anguish of having to live with the deformity of mastectomy[5–7] for several months (or more) until a delayed reconstruction can be performed. Following mastectomy and immediate reconstruction, the patient is able to see the reconstructed breast mound as soon as she awakens from the general anesthetic, and never has to confront the deformity of an absent breast. This reduces her fear of the mastectomy, and encourages the acceptance of mastectomy when it is required.

Aesthetic Outcome

The fifth advantage is better aesthetic outcome.[8] Immediate reconstruction allows use of a skin-sparing mastectomy, which preserves the uninvolved breast skin for use in the reconstruction. If this is done correctly, preservation of the breast skin envelope and the inframammary fold makes shaping of the breast mound much easier and more accurate. Furthermore, scarring is reduced. Consequently, the aesthetic results tend to be better (Fig 4-1). Even when a skin-sparing mastectomy is not used, preservation of the inframammary fold helps the reconstructive surgeon to position the breast properly. Also, by looking at the mastectomy specimen, the reconstructive surgeon has a better idea of how much tissue will be required to replace it and achieve symmetry with the opposite breast. Immediate reconstruction also avoids the problem of established scar tissue, which in delayed reconstruction hampers expansion of the breast skin to its original dimensions and can be difficult to release adequately.

Facilitation of Free Flap Reconstruction

Finally, if a free transverse rectus abdominis myocutaneous (TRAM) flap[9–11] is to be used in the reconstruction, dissection of the thoracodorsal artery and vein for use as recipient vessels is considerably easier in immediate reconstruction. In many cases, they will already have been exposed by the oncologic surgeons during the course of an axillary dissection and will be immediately available. Even when an axillary dissection has

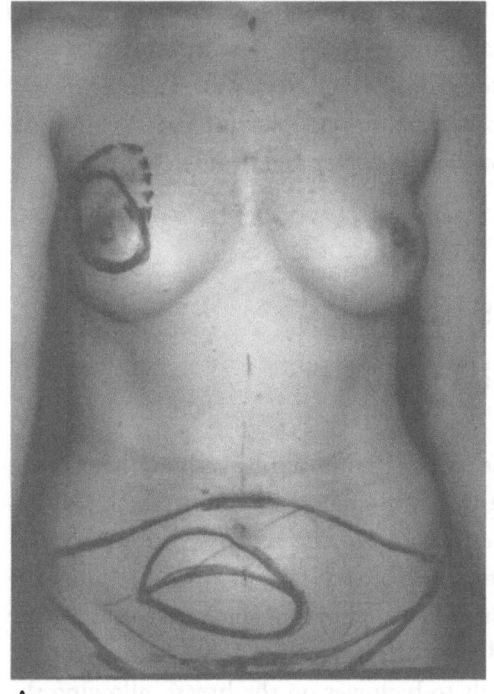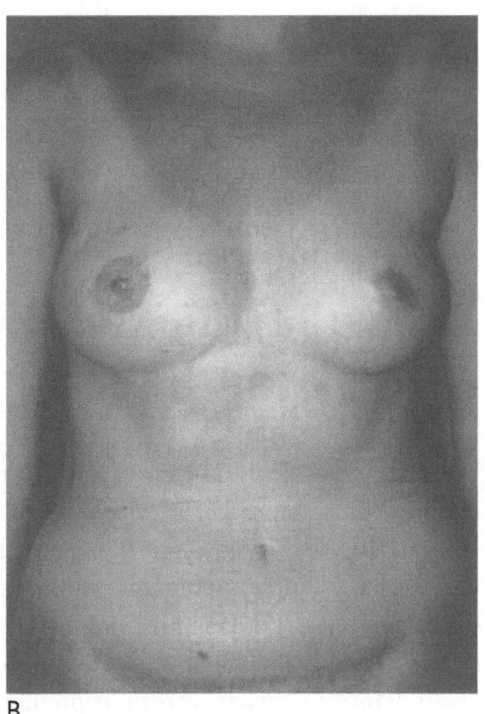

A   B

FIG. 4-1   (A) Preoperative plan for a skin-sparing mastectomy. (B) Result of immediate reconstruction with a TRAM flap. (From Kroll SS, Baldwin B. *Plast Reconstr Surg.* 1992;90: 455–462. Used with permission.) See color insert, p. I-6.

not been performed, however, they will at least not be surrounded by scar tissue from previous surgery, and their exposure will be facilitated by the dissection performed during the mastectomy.

Disadvantages of Immediate Reconstruction

A disadvantage of immediate reconstruction is that it is inconvenient for the general surgeon, who must arrange a preoperative consultation with the plastic surgeon and must schedule the mastectomy at a time when both surgeons are available. Also, if autologous tissue reconstruction is planned, the operating room will be tied up by the plastic surgeon for several hours if not for the entire day, making it impossible for the general surgeon to perform additional procedures in that room.

Immediate reconstruction ideally would not interfere with adjuvant treatment, but in practice sometimes it does. If there is partial flap necrosis or prolonged wound drainage, chemotherapy or radiotherapy may be delayed. Fortunately, these delays are usually not longer than a week or two, but there is always some risk of a more significant delay. We have found that such delays can be minimized by using flaps that have the best possible blood supply, such as free TRAM flaps.[9]

Finally, if postoperative radiotherapy will be required, the reconstructed breast will be exposed to radiation that could potentially injure it. We have found that well-vascularized autologous tissue usually tolerates radiotherapy very well, at least for the first several years;[12] however, late deleterious effects are possible, and at this time the full extent of such changes over the long term has not been determined.

Skin-Sparing Mastectomy and Role of the General Surgeon

Breast cancer is not skin cancer, and for most patients removal of overlying breast skin is unnecessary. Skin that is within 1 cm of the tumor should be removed, but otherwise the breast skin envelope can be preserved for use in the reconstruction.[13,14] Removal of the nipple, the areola, the breast, and the biopsy scar (if present) is usually sufficient (Fig 4-1). This preservation of uninvolved breast skin makes shaping of the reconstructed breast much easier and also reduces the amount of visible scarring in the breast. Moreover, what scarring is present tends to be lower on the breast, allowing the patient to wear low-cut dresses and bathing suits without showing her scars.

Immediate reconstruction with skin-sparing mastectomy is a team effort, and the general surgeon is a critical member of the team. If the general surgeon is committed to the concept of skin-sparing mastectomy and cares about the aesthetic outcome of reconstruction, the results will invariably be improved by that commitment.

The first part of the general surgeon's role is in patient selection. Not all patients are good candidates for breast reconstruction, even though most patients would prefer to have it. Ideal patients are young, healthy, and nonobese. Older patients also can be candidates, depending on their state of health and motivation. It is difficult to define universal criteria in patient selection for breast reconstruction, because patients, surgeons, and situations vary widely. In general, however, extreme obesity is a relative contraindication,[15,16] as are other major health problems. The general surgeon needs to use his or her judgment and encourage patients who would benefit the most from immediate breast reconstruction to consult the plastic surgeon and consider it.

The second part of the general surgeon's role is in choosing a plastic surgeon to work with. Not all plastic surgeons are equally committed to breast reconstruction, and not all are equally talented. The general surgeon should attempt to work with someone who is interested in breast reconstruction, willing to commit the necessary time and effort, properly trained in autologous tissue reconstruction, and artistically talented enough to achieve aesthetically successful results.

The third aspect of the general surgeon's role is in the operating room. Skin-sparing mastectomy is technically more difficult than a conventional wide-field mastectomy because of the limited incisions and longer mastectomy flaps. Additional effort and help will be needed for retraction of the skin, and it can be more difficult to visualize the depths of the wound. The general surgeon must pay attention to the inframammary fold and try not to violate it. Dissecting past the inframammary fold does not significantly increase the amount of breast tissue removed, but it does destroy an important landmark that helps the plastic surgeon to correctly position and shape the breast.

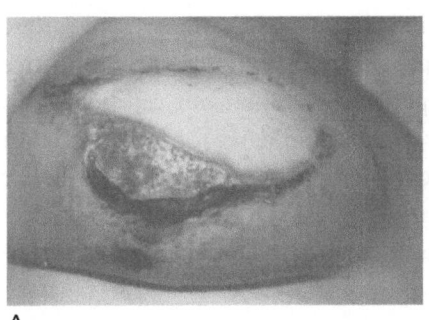 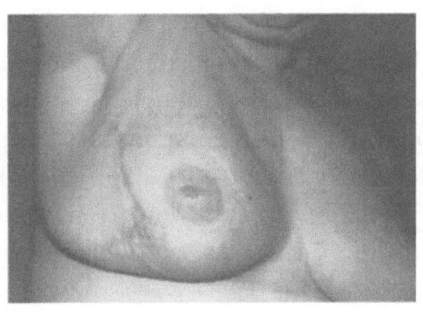 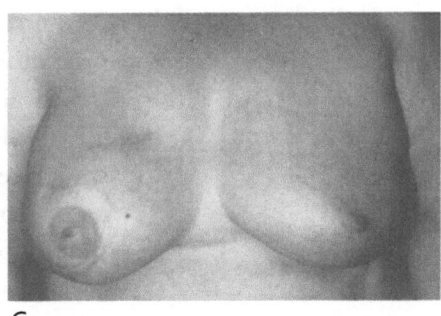

A   B   C

FIG. 4-2 (A) Mastectomy flap edge necrosis after immediate free TRAM flap breast reconstruction. (B,C) The same patient after debridement, healing, revision, and nipple reconstruction (see color insert, p. I-7). Because autologous tissue was used, the mastectomy flap necrosis did not significantly compromise the final result. (From Kroll SS. *Plast Reconstr Surg.* 1994;94:637. Used with permission.)

Similarly, the general surgeon should attempt not to dissect medially past the edge of the breast. Excessive medial dissection reduces the blood supply of the mastectomy flaps, making necrosis of them more likely. It also forces the plastic surgeon to create a new medical breast border with sutures, introducing the possibility of error and distortion.

In preserving the breast skin envelope, the general surgeon also has the responsibility for keeping it alive by maintaining its blood circulation (Fig 4-2). This is done by maintaining an adequate and uniform thickness to the flaps throughout the dissection. The thickness required varies from patient to patient. Usually a plane can be identified between the breast tissue and the subcutaneous fat. The surgeon must try to remove all the true breast tissue, while preserving as much of the subcutaneous fat as possible so that the blood supply to the mastectomy flaps is maintained.

If an axillary dissection is performed and if a free TRAM flap[9,11,17] is planned, the general surgeon should take great care to preserve the thoracodorsal vessels so that they can be used as recipients for the free flap. Injuries to these vessels, or cutting off a small branch without clipping or ligating it, can cause severe spasm that can make subsequent execution of the free flap difficult. Also, the surgeon should try to avoid tying together arterial and venous branches of the thoracodorsal vessels with one ligature very close to the main vessels because that can make separation of the thoracodorsal artery and vein (required prior to the anastomoses) technically very difficult.

Finally, the general surgeon should try to avoid tapering the breast excision so much that the plastic surgeon cannot tell exactly where the borders of the mastectomy defect are. If the edges of the mastectomy defect are obvious to the plastic surgeon, he or she can suture the autologous tissue flap to them, allowing the reconstructed breast to replace exactly what has been removed and to blend into the chest wall in a natural way.

Role of the Plastic Surgeon

The plastic surgeon also has a role in patient selection and, like the general surgeon, should select appropriate candidates and discourage those who are physiologically (but not necessarily chronologically) too old, too obese, or too unhealthy to undergo successful reconstruction. He or she also has a role in selection of the most appropriate procedure. For marginal candidates, the choice of procedure may significantly influence the chances for success. For example, very obese patients are often not candidates for TRAM flap breast reconstruction but may be appropriate candidates for reconstruction with an extended latissimus dorsi flap[18] (usually combined with a contralateral breast reduction). Similarly, patients who are in their late 60s may be better served with a simpler procedure such as an extended latissimus dorsi flap or reconstruction using an implant.

The plastic surgeon also has the responsibility to inform patients of the risks of the procedure and of the fact that revisions are usually necessary. These revisions are usually relatively minor, and many of them can be performed in the clinic or office, but patients need to be told about them in advance. Patients should be aware of what to expect in the way of donor site scars. It is often helpful if they can talk to other patients who have previously undergone the procedures.

Obviously, the plastic surgeon's role also includes actually reconstructing the breast mound, making any necessary revisions, and reconstructing the nipple/areolar complex. These procedures will be covered in subsequent chapters.

Oncologic Aspects of Immediate Reconstruction

Before immediate reconstruction became so widely available, and even today in some quarters, concerns were often raised about the oncologic risk of immediate breast reconstruction. Some oncologists worried that immediate reconstruction might increase the risk of local recurrence, particularly if a skin-sparing mastectomy were used. Recent evaluation of data at The University of Texas M. D. Anderson Cancer Center, however, has shown that for patients with early (T1 and T2) breast cancer, there are no differences in the rates of local tremor recurrence or systemic metastasis between patients who underwent skin-sparing mastectomy and those who had conventional wide-field mastectomy.[19] Moreover, the 5-year local recurrence rates (6.7% for skin-sparing mastectomy; 7% for wide-field mastectomy) are similar to those published for patients who had similar tumors treated elsewhere with mastectomy but without reconstruction.

Another possibly valid concern is that the reconstruction might make early detection of local recurrence more difficult. However, this would not be true for the great majority of local recurrences, which are superficial and are easily palpated just under the patient's skin. Superficial recurrences of that type are not hidden by the reconstructed breast and in fact are sometimes more easily detected, since the tumor is separated from the chest wall by the soft breast mound and not easily confused with scar tissue. Deep tumor recurrence on the chest wall, however, can be camouflaged by an overlying breast mound. One could argue, however, that such chest wall recurrences are manifestations of systemic disease and are not likely to be affected by early diagnosis and treatment, making early diagnosis somewhat moot. Fortunately,

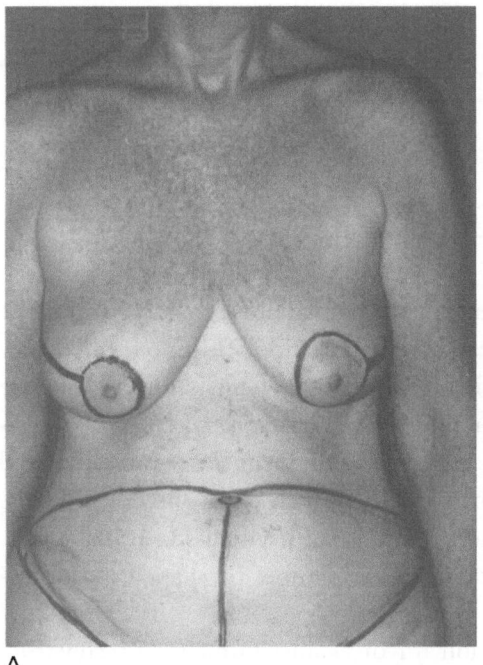 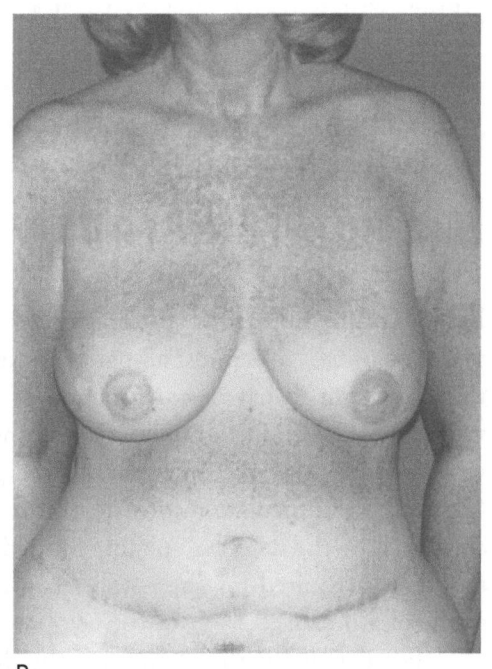

A   B

FIG. 4-3   (A) Operative plan for bilateral immediate free TRAM flap breast reconstruction in a patient with unilateral breast disease. (B) The result 1 year later. The patient has also had a hysterectomy. (From Kroll SS. *Clin Plast Surg.* 1998;25:251–259. Used with permission.)

such recurrences are rare, so their early detection is not of great importance to the majority of patients.

Bilateral Immediate Breast Reconstruction

Bilateral breast reconstruction is becoming increasingly common, both for patients with bilateral breast cancer and for some patients with unilateral tumors who are at unusually high risk for a second primary tumor in the opposite breast, such as those with familial breast cancer (Fig 4-3). Immediate breast reconstruction after bilateral skin-sparing mastectomy allows both breasts to be reconstructed simultaneously using the same reconstruction technique.[20] Usually the technique chosen in our institution is the bilateral TRAM flap, with half of the TRAM flap used for each breast. A bilateral skin-sparing mastectomy preserves some of the original breast volume in the form of the skin envelope and subcutaneous fat, reducing the amount of tissue needed for reconstruction of each breast mound. This reduction of required flap volume is not important in unilateral reconstruction, nor in bilateral reconstruction of patients who are moderately obese or even of average build. For thin patients, however, it can be very important in achieving adequate breast size when bilateral reconstruction is required.

When to Choose Immediate Reconstruction

Because of the numerous advantages described above, immediate reconstruction is the preferred option for almost all patients with early-stage (T1 and T2) tumors who know that they want to have reconstruction of their breast. If the patient is unsure that she wants reconstruction, however, the reconstruction should be deferred since it can always be done at a later time as a delayed procedure. If the patient has a very advanced (T4) tumor, immediate reconstruction may be required just to cover the defect of the chest wall. If the defect is suitably located and if there is sufficient tissue available, the flap that is required for chest wall reconstruction can sometimes be shaped into a facsimile of a breast.

For patients with T3 tumors, the decision for or against immediate reconstruction is more difficult. Patients with these more advanced malignancies are at much higher risk of developing both systemic and local recurrence, and so have a lower probability of benefiting over a long term from their breast reconstructions than do patients with early-stage tumors. Postoperative radiotherapy will probably be required, and performing immediate reconstruction mandates irradiation of the reconstructed breast. After reconstruction, the irradiation will be more difficult to administer (because the chest wall is no longer flat), and the reconstructed breast mound will be subjected to, and can be damaged by, the effects of the radiation. Delaying the reconstruction avoids these problems. On the other hand, delayed reconstruction is always technically more difficult than immediate reconstruction, and is especially so after the patient has received radiotherapy. With good technique, successful and safe irradiation of the chest wall is possible despite the presence of a reconstructed breast mound. Provided that excessive doses are not used, we have found that TRAM flaps, and especially free TRAM flaps, tolerate radiation therapy quite well. From the plastic surgeon's point of view, therefore, there is no clear argument for or against immediate reconstruction of patients with T3 breast cancers.

Our philosophy at The University of Texas M. D. Anderson Cancer Center has changed over the years, and we have become more willing to offer immediate reconstruction to some patients, especially younger ones, with T3 tumors. If the patients are strongly in favor of having immediate reconstruction, and if their prognosis is not unusually poor so there is some potential for long-term survival, we are generally willing to perform reconstruction immediately. In doing this, we must accept the likelihood of an increased incidence of tumor recurrence in our patient population, and the disappointments that will be occasionally encountered as a result. Fortunately, improved systemic adjuvant treatment has allowed many of these patients with more advanced tumors to survive in a relatively normal state for many years, despite the presence of recurrent disease. Many such patients have been very grateful for their reconstructions, and have told us that their restored breasts have made their lives better. For those patients who feel that the reconstruction is important enough to them that they are willing to accept the necessary risks, therefore, we are usually willing to perform immediate reconstruction if the patient is physically a good candidate.

When Not to Choose Immediate Reconstruction

Ambivalence

Immediate reconstruction should not be performed when the patient is ambivalent about undergoing the procedure. If the patient is unsure about having reconstruction, it is better to defer the reconstruction until the patient has lived for some time with the deformity of mastectomy and has developed the necessary motivation to become a good patient. Ambivalence about the reconstruction is a red flag for psychological instability, and such patients should be avoided until the ambivalence is clearly resolved.

Marked Obesity

Immediate reconstruction should not be performed when the patient is markedly obese (the definition of which will be given in later chapters), but has some potential for losing weight and becoming an acceptable candidate for reconstruction with a TRAM flap. If she is not likely to or unwilling to lose the excess weight, she can be evaluated for immediate reconstruction with an extended latissimus doris flap, as described in chapter 12. If she is not a good candidate for that procedure, however, the reconstruction should be deferred until the patient does lose enough weight to become an acceptable surgical candidate, even if that means deferring the reconstruction indefinitely.

Poor Tumor Prognosis

Immediate reconstruction ordinarily should not be offered to patients with such a poor prognosis for survival that they are unlikely to benefit enough from the reconstruction to justify the investment of time and effort required. A patient who becomes terminally ill just after the reconstruction has been completed has usually not received a fair return on her investment. Unless the patient refuses to undergo the necessary mastectomy unless reconstruction is also performed, she will be better served by undergoing only the mastectomy and deferring the reconstruction. If she overcomes the odds and survives longer than expected, a delayed reconstruction can always be undertaken at a later time.

Summary

Immediate breast reconstruction is more convenient for patients, less expensive, less risky, less distressing, and achieves better aesthetic results than delayed reconstruction. Immediate reconstruction can be combined with a skin-sparing mastectomy to achieve the best possible aesthetic outcome without any significantly increased risk of tumor recurrence. For the general surgeon, performing a skin-sparing mastectomy is more difficult than performing a conventional wide-field mastectomy. The way the mastectomy is performed affects the quality of the breast reconstruction result, and the general surgeon who performs a skin-sparing mastectomy is therefore an important member of the reconstructive team. Skin-sparing mastectomy also facilitates the performance of bilateral TRAM flap reconstruction, especially in thin patients.

References

1. Noone RB, Murphy JB, Spear SL, Little JW. A 6-year experience with immediate reconstruction after mastectomy for cancer. *Plast Reconstr Surg.* 1985;76:258–269.
2. Noone RB, Frazier TG, Hayward CZ. Patient acceptance of immediate reconstruction following mastectomy. *Plast Reconstr Surg.* 1982;69:632–640.
3. Grotting JC. Immediate breast reconstruction using the free TRAM flap. *Clin Plast Surg.* 1994;21:207–221.
4. Elkowitz A, Colen S, Slavin S, Seibert J, Weinstein M, Shaw W. Various methods of breast reconstruction after mastectomy: an economic comparison. *Plast Reconstr Surg.* 1993;92:77–83.
5. Gilboa D, Borenstein A, Floro S, Shafir R, Falach H, Tsur H. Emotional and psychological adjustment of women to breast reconstruction and detection of subgroups at risk for psychological morbidity. *Ann Plast Surg.* 1990;25:397–401.
6. Schover LR. The impact of breast cancer on sexuality, body image, and intimate relationships. *CA Cancer J Clin.* 1991;41:112.
7. Lasry JM, Margolese RG, Poisson R, et al. Depression and body image following mastectomy and lumpectomy. *J Chron Dis.* 1987;40:529–534.
8. Kroll SS, Coffey JA Jr, Winn RJ, Schusterman MA. A comparison of factors affecting aesthetic outcomes of TRAM flap breast reconstruction. *Plast Reconstr Surg.* 1995;96:860–864.
9. Schusterman MA, Kroll SS, Weldon ME. Immediate breast reconstruction: why the free TRAM over the conventional TRAM flap? *Plast Reconstr Surg.* 1992;90:255–262.
10. Schusterman MA, Kroll SS, Miller MJ, et al. The free TRAM flap for breast reconstruction: a single center's experience with 211 consecutive cases. *Ann Plast Surg.* 1994;32:234–242.
11. Grotting JC, Urist MM, Maddox WA, Vasconez LO. Conventional TRAM flap versus free microsurgical TRAM flap for immediate breast reconstruction. *Plast Reconstr Surg.* 1989;83:842–844.

12. Williams JK, Carlson GW, Bostwick J, Bried JT, Mackay G. The effects of radiation treatment after TRAM flap breast reconstruction. *Plast Reconstr Surg.* 1997;100:1153–1160.

13. Carlson GW, Bostwock J, Styblo TM, et al. Skin-sparing mastectomy: oncologic and reconstructive considerations. *Ann Surg.* 1997;225:570–578.

14. Kroll SS, Ames F, Singletary SE, Schusterman MA. The oncologic risks of skin preservation at mastectomy with immediate breast reconstruction. *Surg Gynecol Obstet.* 1991;172:17–20.

15. Hartrampf CR Jr, Bennett GK. Autogenous tissue reconstruction in the mastectomy patient: a critical review of 300 patients. *Ann Surg.* 1987;205:508–518.

16. Kroll SS, Netscher DT. Complications of TRAM flap breast reconstruction in obese patients. *Plast Reconstr Surg.* 1989;86:886–892.

17. Holmstrom H. The free abdominoplasty flap and its use in breast reconstruction. *Scand J Plast Reconstr Surg.* 1979;13:423.

18. McGraw JB, Papp C, Edwards A, McMellin A. The autogenous latissimus breast reconstruction. *Clin Plast Surg.* 1994;21:279–288.

19. Kroll SS, Schusterman MA, Tadjalli HE, Singletary SE, Ames FC. Risk of recurrence after treatment of early breast cancer with skin-sparing mastectomy. *Ann Surg Oncol.* 1997;4:193–197.

20. Kroll SS, Miller MJ, Schusterman MA, Reece GP, Singletary SE, Ames F. The rationale for elective contralateral mastectomy with immediate bilateral reconstruction. *Ann Surg Oncol.* 1994;1:457–461.

5 | Delayed Breast Reconstruction

Role of Delayed Breast Reconstruction

Despite the many advantages of immediate reconstruction, there will always be a need for delayed breast reconstruction. Immediate reconstruction is not available in all medical centers, forcing many patients to seek delayed reconstruction even though they might have preferred that their reconstruction were immediate. Also, because of a change of mind or an improved prognosis, some patients who initially declined breast reconstruction may subsequently decide to seek it. In either scenario, patients will arrive in the plastic surgeon's office months or years after mastectomy requesting delayed breast reconstruction.

For the plastic surgeon, even though immediate reconstruction is preferable,[1] delayed breast reconstruction has some positive aspects. There is no need to schedule the operation jointly with a general surgeon, and the reconstruction can start at the beginning of the operating room day. Postoperative irradiation will not be required, and chemotherapy will not delay any needed revisions. Moreover, the patient will have lived with her mastectomy defect for a while and will perceive almost any type of result as an improvement. She is likely to be pleased with her outcome even if it is less than perfect, and unlikely to be critical of efforts the surgeon has made to help her.

Although delayed reconstruction is technically more difficult than immediate reconstruction, good results are nevertheless obtainable (Fig 5-1) and should be sought diligently. In this chapter, I will discuss ways in which that goal can be achieved.

Special Problems of Delayed Breast Reconstruction

Delayed breast reconstruction presents a number of special problems. Because no effort will have been made to spare uninvolved skin, much more tissue is usually missing in

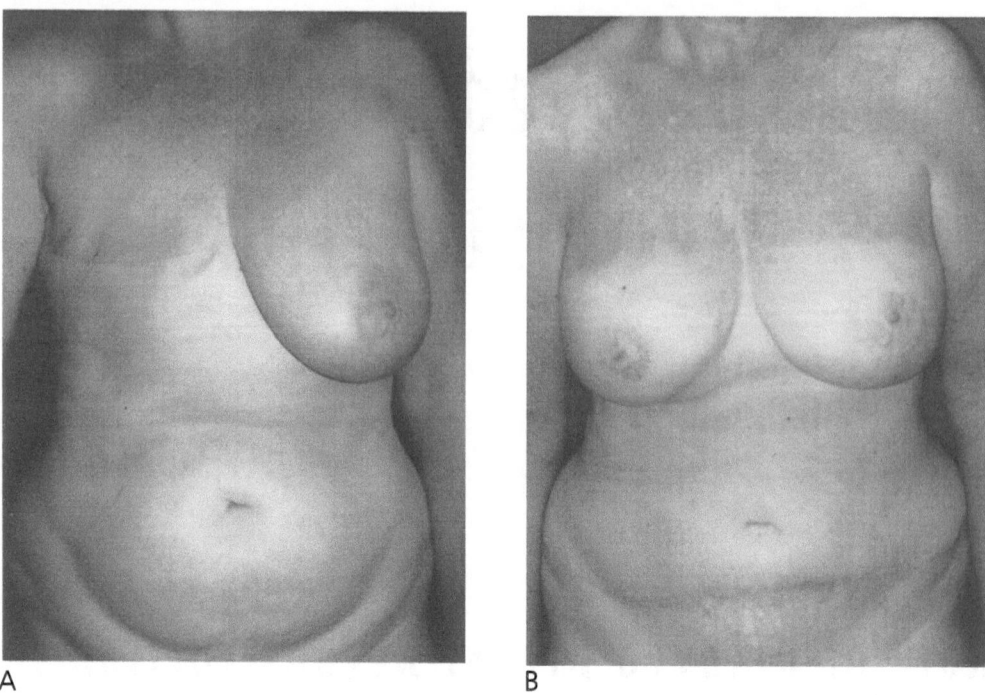

A   B

FIG. 5-1 (A) A 49-year-old patient after right mastectomy. (B) The same patient 1 year after delayed breast reconstruction with a pedicled TRAM flap. (From Kroll SS, Miller MJ, Schusterman MA, Reece GP, Singletary SA, Ames F. *Ann Surg Oncol.* 1994;1:457–461. Used with permission.) See color insert, p. I-8.

delayed reconstruction than would have been the case in immediate reconstruction, especially if a skin-sparing mastectomy[2,3] would have been used. More skin is usually required from the flap that has been selected to perform the reconstruction with, and more tissue volume as well. Finding enough skin to make an adequate breast is not usually a problem in transverse rectus abdominis myocutaneous (TRAM) flap[4–7] breast reconstruction, but it can be an obstacle when an alternative flap must be used. The surgeon needs to consider this preoperatively and plan the reconstruction so that sufficient skin will be available. It is helpful to measure the distance on the breast meridian from the clavicle to the inframammary fold, on both the mastectomy side and the contralateral breast (Fig 5-2). The difference between the two measurements is the width of flap skin paddle that will be required to achieve symmetry. To ensure having enough skin, a TRAM flap is usually the best choice. If a TRAM flap cannot be used or if there is not sufficient skin available from it or an alternative flap to create ptosis, a contralateral mastopexy or breast reduction may be required for symmetry.

Free Flap versus Pedicled Flap

At The University of Texas M. D. Anderson Cancer Center, free TRAM flaps are generally preferred[8] to pedicled TRAM flaps (because free flaps have a better blood supply

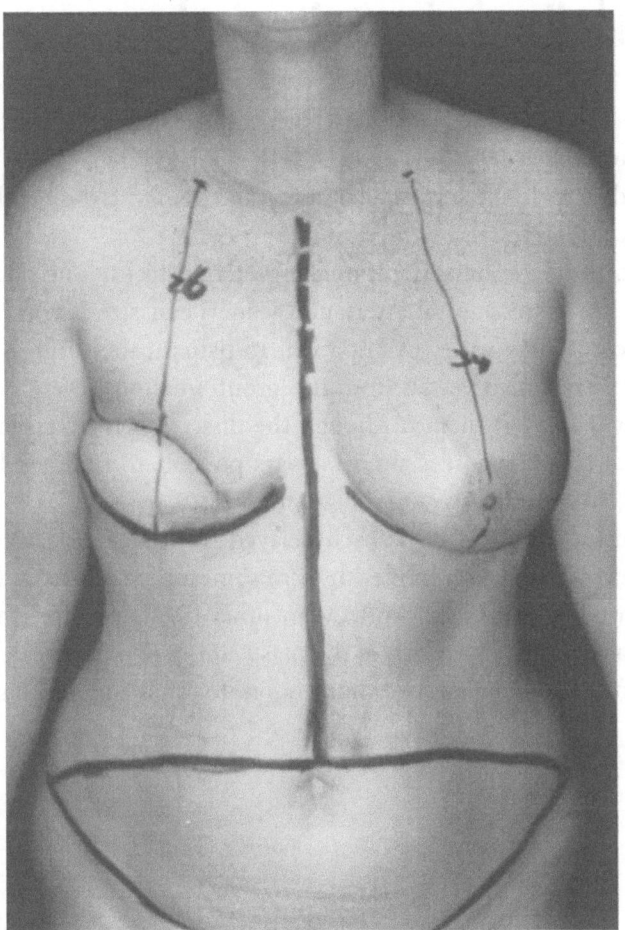

FIG. 5-2   Preoperative plan for delayed TRAM flap breast reconstruction. The difference between the distance from the clavicle to the inframammary fold on the mastectomy side and that on the normal side represents the width of skin paddle required to achieve symmetry without contralateral mastopexy.

and less donor site morbidity), but we are always prepared to perform a pedicled TRAM flap if the situation calls for it. The most common contraindication to a free TRAM flap is unsuitable blood vessels in the flap or recipient area, a problem that may not necessarily be apparent preoperatively. Unsuitable recipient vessels are more likely to be encountered in delayed reconstruction, when the previous surgery has caused scarring or vessel damage in the axilla. Before planning a free TRAM (or other) flap using the thoracodorsal vessels as recipients, the surgeon should check the patient for latissimus dorsi muscle function on the side of the mastectomy. If the latissimus dorsi muscle is functioning, the thoracodorsal artery and vein, which lie directly adjacent to the thoracodorsal nerve, are usually intact and patent. Even if they are intact preoperatively, however, they may be damaged during their dissection, so the surgeon needs to have an alternative plan ready. The backup plan could be a pedicled TRAM flap or use of the internal mammary vessels as an alternative recipient site.

Choice of Recipient Vessels

The choice of recipient vessels for free flap breast reconstruction is usually between the internal mammary vessels (Fig 5-3) and the subscapular system vessels in the axilla (Fig 5-4); these would include the subscapular artery and vein, the thoracodorsal vessels, and the circumflex scapular vessels.

In our institution we have traditionally preferred to use one of the vessels in the axilla, especially the thoracodorsal artery and vein. Their size is consistently adequate, and although the anatomy varies from patient to patient, the surgeon can find at least one suitable pair of recipient vessels from this group in almost every patient unless previous surgery has destroyed them. Although the dissection is occasionally complicated by the presence of scar tissue, it is almost always possible to find good recipient vessels in the axilla and successfully execute the anastomosis.

I have found it useful to begin each delayed free flap breast reconstruction with two teams whenever possible (even if each team sometimes consists only of a single surgeon). One team begins raising the TRAM or other free flap, while the other team reopens the old mastectomy scar, elevates the mastectomy flaps to create a pocket for the free flap, and explores the axilla. The thoracodorsal vessels should be sought inferiorly,

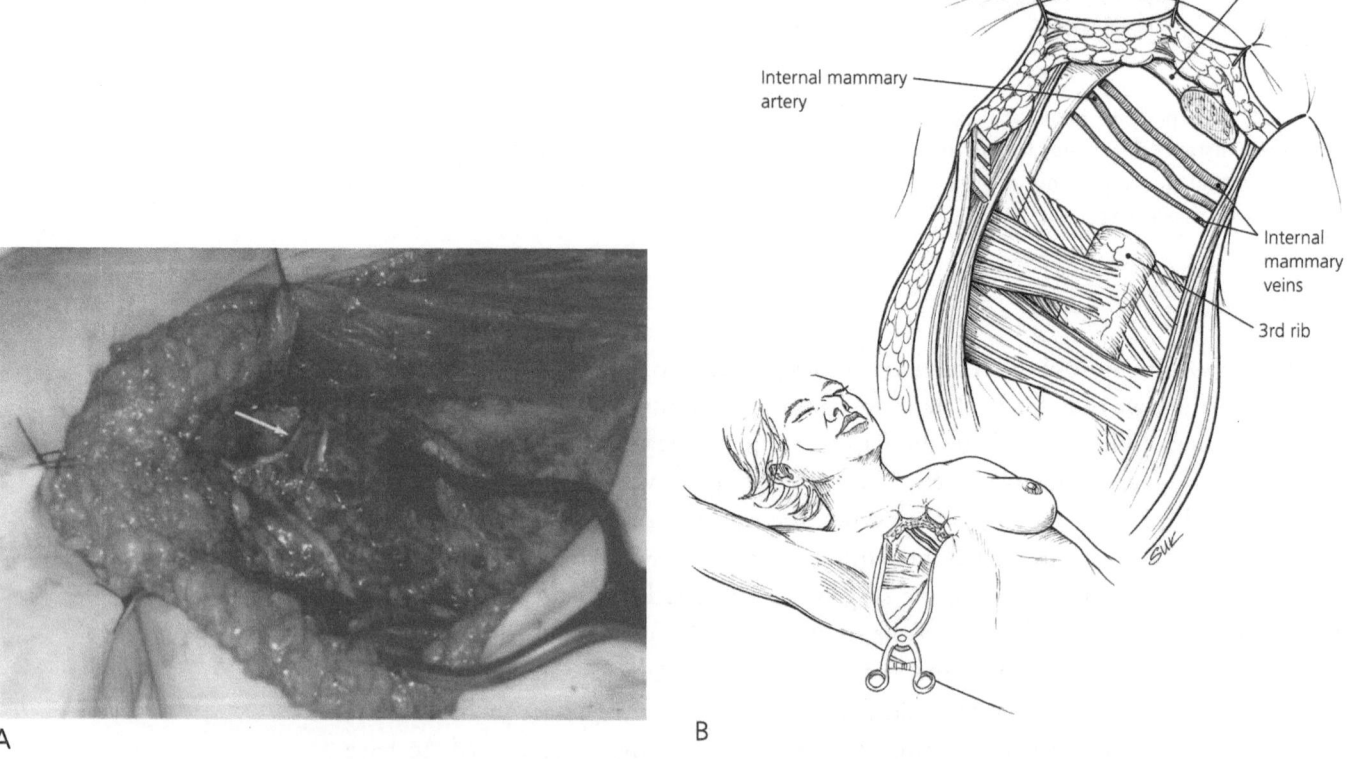

A   B

FIG. 5-3 The internal mammary vessels, after removal of the third costal cartilage. The artery is usually larger than the vein, but not always. (A) Photo (arrow points to internal mammary vessels). (B) Drawing of internal mammary vessels.

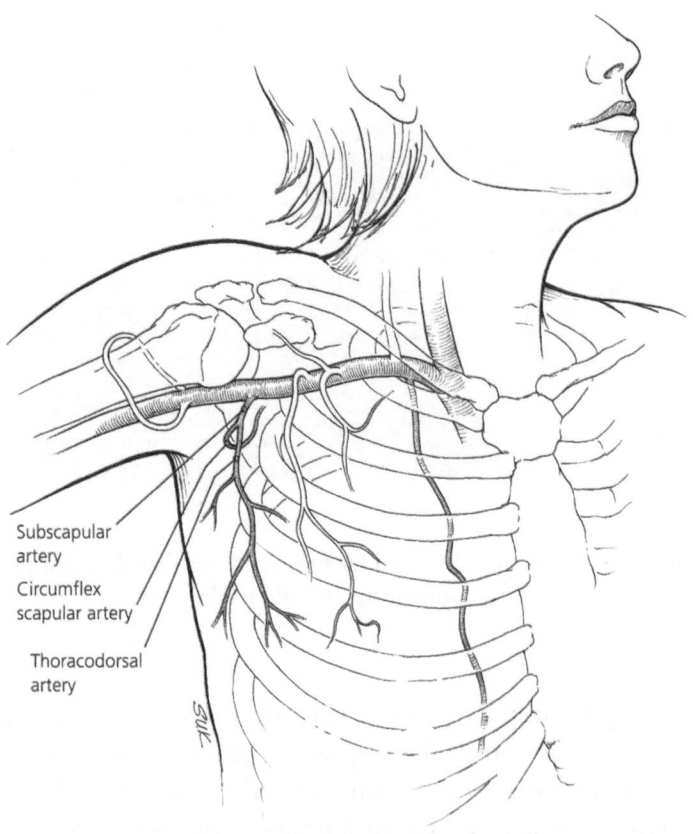

FIG. 5-4 The subscapular vascular system. The most commonly used recipient vessels are the thoracodorsals. If these are too small, the circumflex scapular or subscapular vessels may be suitable. See color insert, p. I-9.

just superficial to the latissimus dorsi muscle and sometimes more medial than would be the case were there no scarring from previous surgery. Usually there is scarring superficial to the vessels, but not deep to them, so the dissection is easier than might be expected. If the vessels are identified first inferiorly, below the point where the anastomoses will be performed, the chance for successful anastomoses will not be compromised if the vessels are injured during this initial identification.

Once the vessels are located, they are traced superiorly under loupe magnification (3.5 or 4.5 power). They should be freed up as far as possible superiorly, usually until either the circumflex scapular branch or the axillary vessels themselves are reached, so that the thoracodorsal vessels can be rotated anteriorly and the anastomoses performed as superficially (anteriorly) in the axilla as possible (Fig 5-5).

When the subscapular vessel system is adequately dissected in this way, there is almost always adequate pedicle length to allow comfortable anastomoses and proper positioning of the flap on the chest wall without vein grafts when a free TRAM flap, a Rubens fat pad free flap, or even a free inferior gluteal flap is used. If a superior gluteal flap is used, however, a vein graft will almost always be necessary.

Occasionally, the thoracodorsal vessels are unusually small and are unsuitable for use as recipients. In such cases, it is not unusual to find a larger-than-usual circumflex

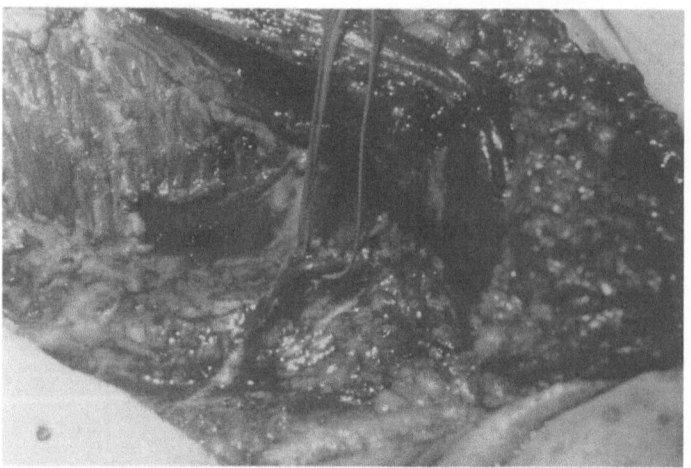

FIG. 5-5 The thoracodorsal vessels dissected far proximally so that they can be rotated anteriorly and the anastomoses can be performed superficially in the axilla.

scapular artery or an unusually long subscapular artery that can be used instead. When the thoracodorsal vessels are small, the surgeon should therefore expose and examine the circumflex scapular vessels. Before abandoning the thoracodorsal vessels, however, 2% papaverine solution should be applied liberally to the thoracodorsal vessels for 15 minutes to ensure that the apparent small size is not just temporary, and due to spasm induced by the dissection. This is especially important if there has been traction on the artery, which is very sensitive to even minor injury and easily goes into spasm.

Another alternative is the internal mammary vessels, which can be very satisfactory and in fact are preferred by many surgeons.[9–11] These vessels are almost always free of scarring from previous surgery and can be accessed by removing the third or fourth costal cartilage. Removing the fourth costal cartilage provides the easiest access and gives the best size match for end-to-end anastomosis of the artery, but sometimes the vein at that level is small. Using the third costal cartilage for access requires more skin retraction but provides a larger vein. The artery will also be slightly larger at that level. In the unlikely event that the artery is too large for an end-to-end anastomosis, an end-to-side anastomosis can be used. In the overwhelming majority of cases, however, an end-to-end anastomosis is practical and is the best choice. I find that the vessels are more likely to be of adequate size on the patient's right side, and am therefore more likely to choose the internal mammary vessels as recipients when it is the right breast that must be reconstructed.

The veins may vary in size, in distance from the sternum, and in number. One solution to the problem of variability in internal mammary vein size is to perform a color Doppler ultrasound examination of the vessels preoperatively.[9,10] This examination can determine the size, location, and number of veins—information that is very useful in deciding not only whether use of the internal mammary vessels would be appropriate, but which costal cartilage to resect for access to the vessels. In many cases, the vein branches somewhere between the second and fifth costal cartilage. If the cartilage resected for access is above the site of the branching, the vein will be single, larger, and easier to use as a recipient vessel.

I find dissection of the internal mammary vessels a bit more difficult than dissection of the subscapular system vessels, but perhaps that is only because I do it less often. Many very tiny and fragile venous branches supply the intercostal muscles, and these branches can cause troublesome bleeding during dissection through that tissue. This difficulty is compensated for, however, by a better position of the surgeon for the anastomosis. In delayed reconstruction, both of the patient's arms can be placed at her sides, rather than outstretched as they would have to be for an anastomosis in the axilla. This allows both the surgeon and the assistant to stand close to the anastomosis and in whatever position they find most comfortable, greatly facilitating the microsurgical portion of the procedure.

Movement of the operative field under the microscope with respiration can affect the surgeon's view of the anastomoses, but that is a relatively minor problem. If it is bothersome, the anesthesiologist can stop ventilating the patient for a few seconds while a suture is placed. One drawback to use of the internal mammary vessels is that if they are damaged during their dissection the surgeon may lose the option of performing an ipsilateral conventional TRAM flap as an alternative. This is not a significant problem in cases of unilateral breast reconstruction, but can be important when the reconstruction must be bilateral.

My own feeling about recipient sites is that the vessels in the axilla are very versatile and useful for most free flap breast reconstructions and are almost always the first choice for immediate reconstruction. For delayed reconstruction, the choice will vary from surgeon to surgeon. I generally prefer the thoracodorsal vessels if the axilla has relatively little scarring but believe that it is important to be able to use the internal mammary vessels should the situation require it. I do find that with increasing experience, I am using the internal mammary vessels more and more often, especially in cases where there has been previous irradiation and in patients who preoperative Doppler ultrasound examination indicates that the vascular anatomy is favorable.

Scar Tissue

Delayed breast reconstruction is always complicated by the presence of scar tissue. In addition to making dissection of axillary recipient vessels more difficult, scar tissue also can prevent the remaining breast skin from returning to its original position. To achieve a soft and aesthetically successful reconstruction, such scar tissue must be completely released. Usually there is a sheet of scar tissue deep to the mastectomy flaps, which must be aggressively released so that the mastectomy flaps can expand to their original dimensions. Only after this has been done can the missing tissue be accurately and successfully replaced.

Previous Irradiation

The previously irradiated chest wall presents the surgeon with special difficulties, some of which cannot be corrected. Radiation causes cellular injury that the body does not

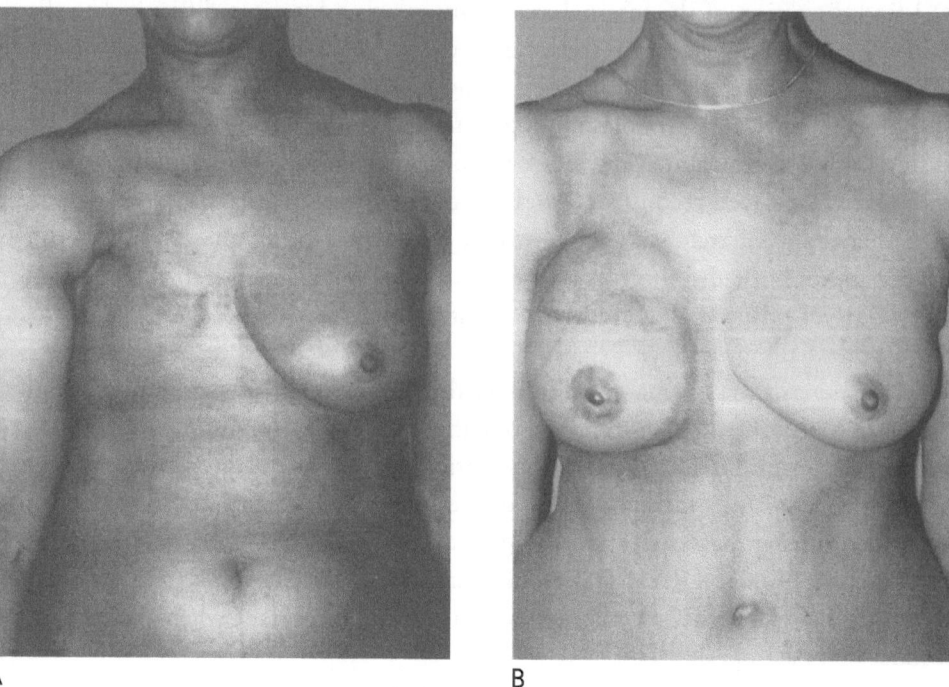

FIG. 5-6   (A) A patient after right near-radical mastectomy and heavy irradiation. (B) The same patient 3 years after TRAM flap breast reconstruction. The result is suboptimal, in part because the reconstructed breast is surrounded by radiation-damaged skin.

fully repair, so chronic radiation damage does not improve with time but instead deteriorates. Consequently, the irradiated tissues surrounding an autologous breast reconstruction will usually not blend into the tissues of the reconstruction as well as they would without irradiation. Often, irradiated skin will have to be sacrificed during the reconstruction, increasing the amount of skin required from the flap. The quality of result that can be obtained in a patient with previous irradiation (Fig 5-6) is therefore less optimal than that which can usually be achieved in a nonirradiated patient. To avoid disappointment, patients should be made aware of this prior to reconstruction.

In a previously irradiated patient, scar tissue is likely to be more dense and difficult to release than in a nonirradiated patient, and a vertical releasing incision in the lower mastectomy flap (Figs 5-7 and 5-8; also see chapter 17) is more likely to be required. Dissection of recipient vessels in the axilla may also be more difficult. The surgeon should be prepared for these challenges. Obviously, one way to solve the problem of a difficult dissection in a heavily scarred axilla is to use the internal mammary vessels as recipients; they may well have been irradiated but will not have had previous surgery.

Finally, the surgeon should remember that not all radiation is equal. The extent of injury depends on the dosage and the way the radiation was administered. Some irradiated patients will have heavy chest wall damage and need a chest wall reconstruction instead of, or in addition to, a reconstructed breast. Others will have had lower doses and have little or no perceptible injury to their chest wall skin (Fig 5-9). Each

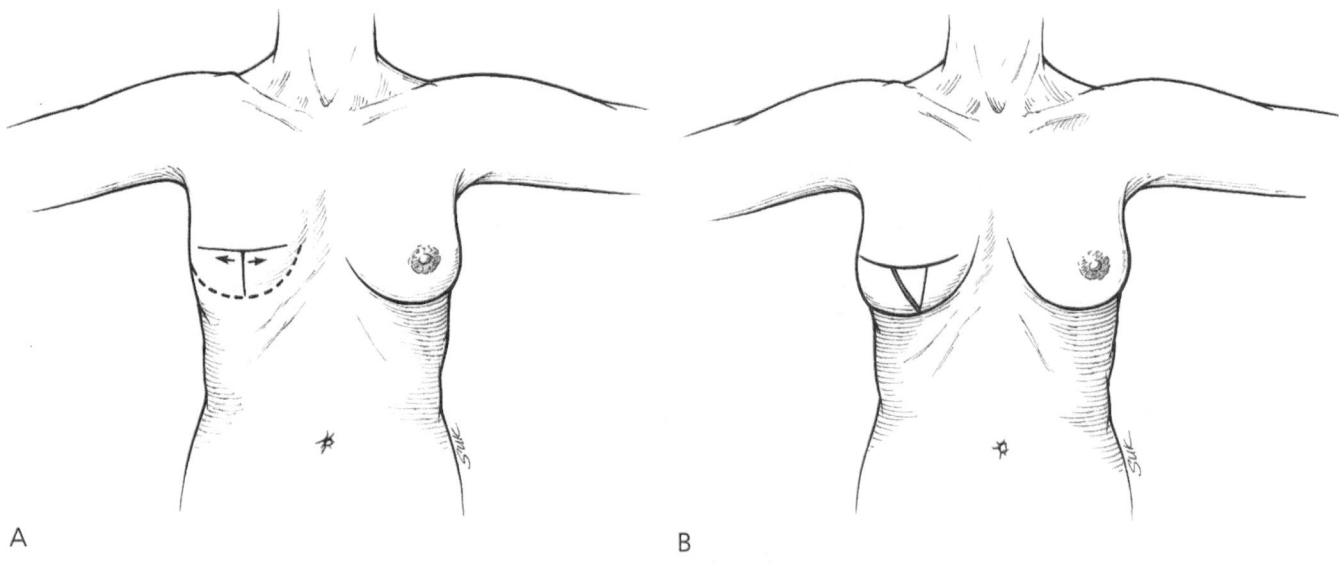

FIG. 5-7   (A) The vertical releasing incision for the inferior mastectomy flap. This is indicated when the skin is too tight to allow adequate expansion of the lower breast panel even after release of all scar tissue. (B) After the releasing incision, the lower breast skin brassiere expands to accommodate the volume of the flap.

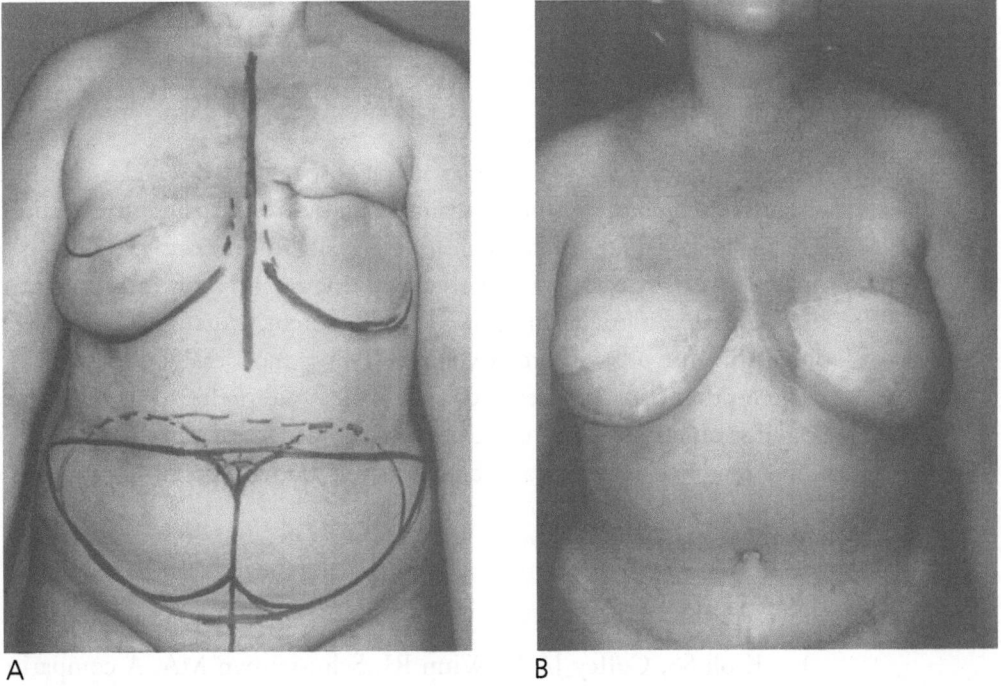

FIG. 5-8   (A) A patient after bilateral mastectomy and irradiation of the left side, with a plan for bilateral reconstruction. Note that a skin-sparing mastectomy had been done on the right, but not on the left. (B) The same patient after bilateral free TRAM flap breast reconstruction. A vertical releasing incision was required in the left inferior mastectomy flap.

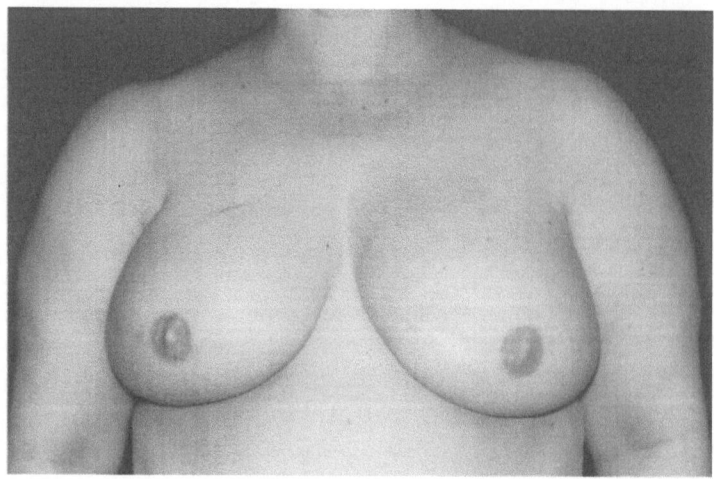

Fig. 5-9   A patient 4 years after bilateral free TRAM flap breast reconstruction. She had been treated previously with mastectomy and radiotherapy on the left side, but there is no apparent difference between the irradiated (left) and nonirradiated (right) sides. See color insert, p. I-10.

patient must be approached individually, and the surgical approach will vary with the circumstances.

Summary

Despite the advantages of immediate reconstruction, delayed breast reconstruction will always be required for some patients. Delayed reconstruction is technically more difficult than immediate reconstruction, especially in previously irradiated patients. All scar tissue must be released so that whatever original breast skin is present can expand into its original position, making the defect apparent. Missing skin must then be replaced, along with the missing breast volume. This is most easily done with a TRAM flap, although other flaps can be used successfully. We prefer to use free flaps with the subscapular vascular system, especially the thoracodorsal vessels, as recipients; but the internal mammary vessels can be used as well and are preferred by some surgeons.

References

1. Kroll SS, Coffey JA Jr, Winn RJ, Schusterman MA. A comparison of factors affecting aesthetic outcomes of TRAM flap breast reconstruction. *Plast Reconstr Surg.* 1995;96:860–864.

2. Carlson GW, Bostwick J, Styblo TM, et al. Skin-sparing mastectomy: oncologic and reconstructive considerations. *Ann Surg.* 1997;225:570–578.

3. Carlson GW. Skin sparing mastectomy: anatomic and technical considerations. *Am Surg.* 1996;62:151–155.

4. Hartrampf CR Jr, Scheflan M, Black PW. Breast reconstruction with a transverse abdominal island flap. *Plast Reconstr Surg.* 1982;69:216–224.

5. Elliott LF, Hartrampf CR Jr. Tailoring of the new breast using the transverse abdominal island flap. *Plast Reconstr Surg.* 1983;72:887–893.

6. Hartrampf CR Jr, Bennett GK. Autogenous tissue reconstruction in the mastectomy patient: a critical review of 300 patients. *Ann Surg.* 1987;205:508–518.

7. Grotting JC, Urist MM, Maddox WA, Vasconez LO. Conventional TRAM flap versus free microsurgical TRAM flap for immediate breast reconstruction. *Plast Reconstr Surg.* 1989;83:842–844.

8. Schusterman MA, Kroll SS, Weldon ME. Immediate breast reconstruction: why the free TRAM over the conventional TRAM flap? *Plast Reconstr Surg.* 1992;90:255–262.

9. Ninkovic M, Anderl H, Hefel A, Schwabegger A, Wechselberger G. Internal mammary vessels: a reliable recipient system for free flaps in breast reconstruction. *Br J Plast Surg.* 1995;48:533–539.

10. Hefel A, Schwabegger A, Ninkovic M, Moriggl B, Waldenberger P. Internal mammary vessels: anatomical and clinical considerations. *Br J Plast Surg.* 1995;48:527–532.

11. Arnez ZM, Valdatta MP, Tyler MP, Planinsek F. Anatomy of internal mammary vessels and their use in free TRAM flap breast reconstruction. *Br J Plast Surg.* 1995;48:540–545.

6 Bilateral Breast Reconstruction

Reconstruction of both breasts can be done either synchronously or asynchronously. Asynchronous reconstruction occurs when the two breasts are reconstructed at different times. When this happens, each breast is reconstructed separately, performing what is essentially two unilateral reconstructions. If a transverse rectus abdominis myocutaneous (TRAM) flap[1-4] was used for reconstruction of the first breast, another technique will have to be used for the second one because a TRAM flap can only be harvested once from each patient. In such a case, symmetry can be difficult to obtain. It is particularly difficult to match a TRAM flap reconstruction to a reconstruction performed with tissue expansion and an implant or any other technique that does not use autologous tissue (Fig 6-1). If the two reconstruction methods are more similar and only autologous tissue is used, symmetry can be much better (Fig 6-2). Only rarely, however, will it approach what can be achieved by reconstructing both breasts simultaneously using the same approach for the two sides (Fig 6-3). It is this simultaneous reconstruction of both breasts, using the same technique (most often TRAM flaps) for each side, that I will address in this chapter.

Advantages of Bilateral Reconstruction

Bilateral breast reconstruction has several advantages. It is usually relatively easy to achieve symmetry in bilateral breast reconstruction, provided that the mastectomies were performed in a similar way. Because one of the most important goals of breast reconstruction is symmetry, bilateral breast reconstruction is in many ways less challenging than unilateral reconstruction, and it often provides better aesthetic results.

Because fairly good symmetry is usually achieved in the initial breast mound reconstructions, revision surgery is required less often than after unilateral reconstruction and is of lesser magnitude (Fig 6-4). Another advantage of bilateral reconstruction is that the patient recovers from both right and left breast operations simultaneously. Con-

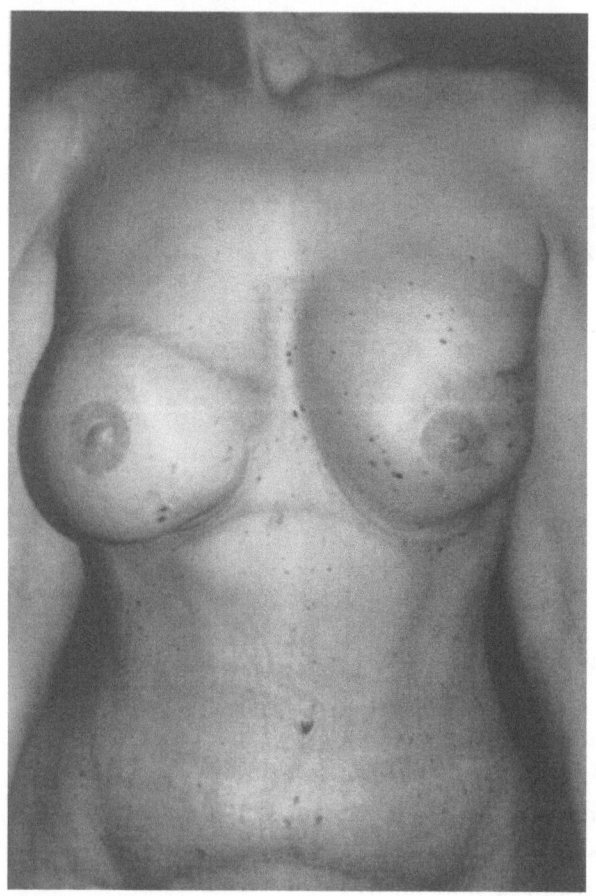

Fig. 6-1 Example of asymmetric bilateral breast reconstruction. The right breast was reconstructed with a pedicled TRAM flap, the left with tissue expansion and an implant. Although both breasts have acceptable shape, they do not match.

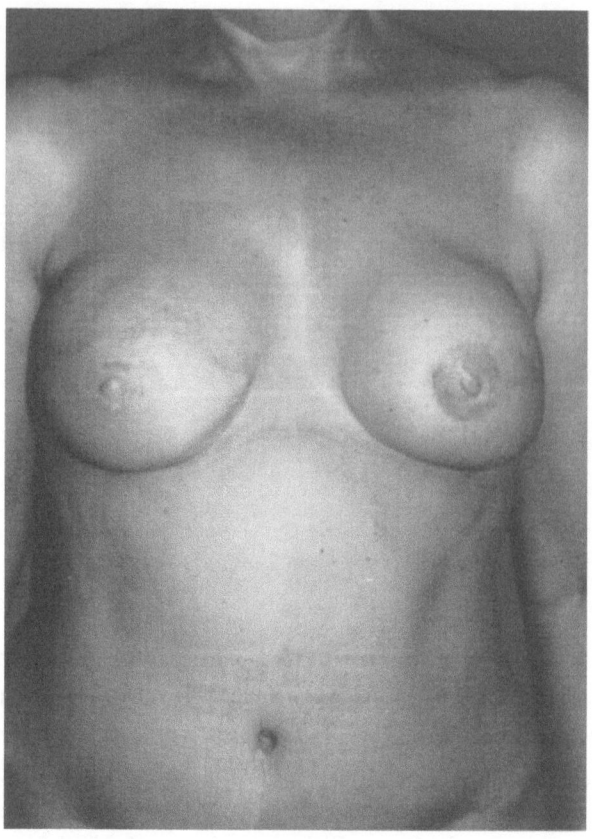

Fig. 6-2 Asymmetric bilateral breast reconstruction with two different autologous tissue techniques. The left breast was reconstructed with a TRAM flap and the right with a superior gluteal free flap. The symmetry is better than if an implant had been used for one side.

sequently, bilateral reconstruction is usually much less costly in terms of both patient effort and dollars than might be expected.[5,6] Moreover, bilateral reconstruction is more convenient for the patient than undergoing two separate reconstructions.

Disadvantages of Bilateral Reconstruction

In bilateral reconstruction, the initial reconstruction of the breast mounds, particularly if free flaps are used, can be long and tedious. Even when the surgery is uncomplicated, bilateral mastectomy with immediate bilateral free TRAM flap breast reconstruction can

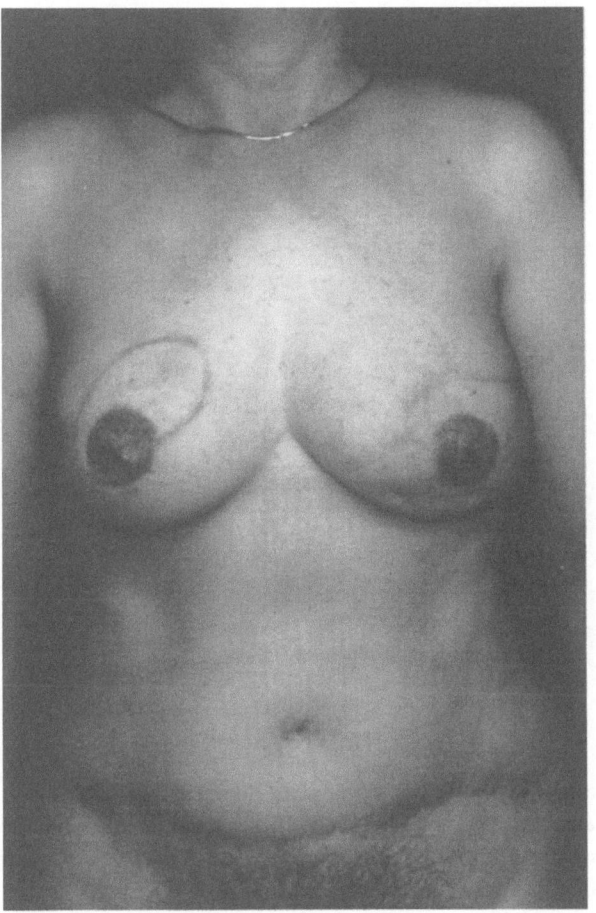

FIG. 6-3   Bilateral simultaneous breast reconstruction with free TRAM flaps. In this patient, who had bilateral breast cancer, the symmetry is good because the same technique was used for both sides. (From Kroll SS. *Clin Plast Surg.* 1998;25:251–259. Used with permission.) See color insert, p. I-11.

easily take 10 hours to complete. With obese patients, the required time and work are greatly increased. If experienced surgical assistance is available, the time can be reduced somewhat,[7] but the procedure is always long and exhausting. Should there be intraoperative complications, the surgery can be greatly prolonged, making the procedure stressful for the operative team.

If the surgical teams are not careful about hemostasis, blood loss can be significant and transfusion with all its attendant risks can be required. This problem, however, can usually be avoided or minimized. At our institution, most surgeons use electrocautery dissection; intraoperative blood loss is usually less than 500 ml and transfusions are ordinarily not required, even for bilateral reconstruction. Moreover, we encourage patients to donate a unit of blood several weeks preoperatively so that autologous blood is available if transfusion is required. These efforts do not eliminate the risk of a transfusion reaction, but they do reduce it considerably.

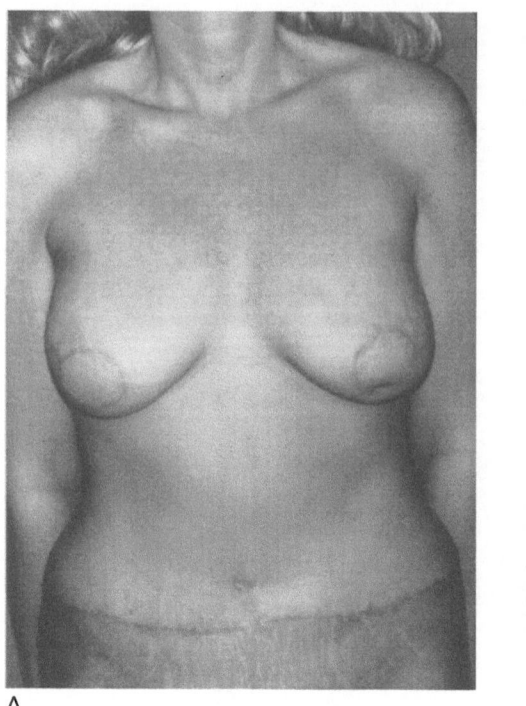
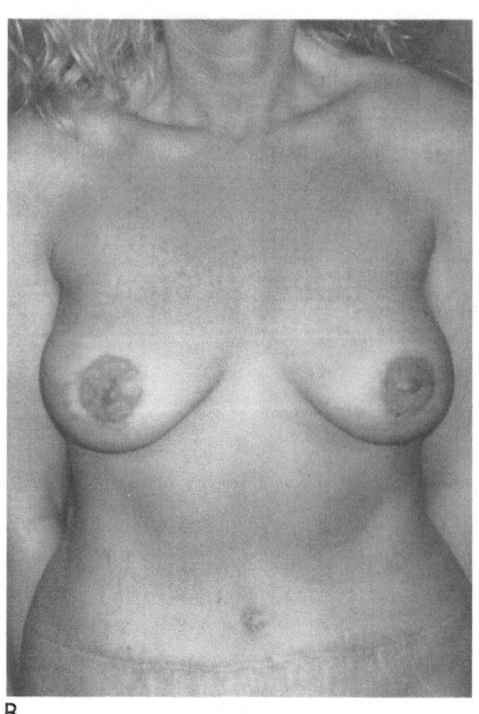

A   B

FIG. 6-4 (A) A patient 3 weeks after immediate bilateral free TRAM flap breast reconstruction. Without any revision, the symmetry is excellent. Minimal additional work was required to complete the reconstruction. (B) The same patient after one revision and followed by bilateral nipple reconstruction. (From Kroll SS. *Clin Plast Surg.* 1988;25:251–259. Used with permission.) See color insert, p. I-10.

Choice of Technique

At The University of Texas M. D. Anderson Cancer Center, the most popular technique for bilateral breast reconstruction is, by far, TRAM flaps.[8,9] The reasons for this popularity include the pliability of the transferred tissue, the ease with which the donor site can be hidden with normal clothing, and the flatter abdomen that usually is obtained as a result of the surgery. Virtually the entire procedure can be performed with the patient in the same position, sitting her upright for the final breast mound shaping. There is usually sufficient tissue to make two adequate breasts, even in very thin patients (see below), especially if free TRAM flaps are used.

Because of their reduced donor site morbidity, we prefer free TRAM flaps to conventional TRAM flaps. Because of the possibility that the recipient vessels could be small, absent, or injured, however, we tell all patients that despite our preference for the free flaps, pedicled TRAM flaps might have to be used instead. This is more likely to occur in delayed reconstruction, especially if previous radiotherapy has been administered, but even then is uncommon.

If a patient cannot have TRAM flaps because of a previous abdominoplasty or extreme obesity, a good second choice is the use of bilateral extended latissimus dorsi flaps.[10] This is a simpler operation and is especially appropriate if the patient is obese, if the skin of the back is especially lax, or if the size of the breasts required is very small. In our institution, extended latissimus dorsi flaps are a common method of breast reconstruction, second in popularity only to TRAM flaps.

If TRAM flaps are impossible and the patient cannot have (or refuses) bilateral extended latissimus dorsi flaps, the remaining choices are bilateral Rubens fat pad free flaps[11] or gluteal flaps.[12–15] These alternative flaps are more difficult than the previously described methods and require more time to perform. Because of this, we rarely use them for bilateral reconstruction, although they certainly are capable of providing excellent results.

It is worth noting that reconstruction with implants, while not ideal, is often less objectionable in the case of bilateral reconstruction than in unilateral reconstruction. Although the risk of capsular contracture is not avoided, the symmetry is likely to be better after bilateral implant-based reconstruction than when trying to match a natural breast with an implant-based mound. For patients who are not good candidates for autologous tissue reconstruction, bilateral implant-based reconstruction can sometimes be a good choice.

Rationale for the Use of Free Flaps in Bilateral Reconstruction

Pedicled TRAM flaps can be very effective for reconstructing the breast mounds in bilateral reconstruction, in many ways more so than in unilateral reconstruction. When a hemi-TRAM flap is used to reconstruct one breast mound, perfusion of tissue across the relatively avascular midline is not required. Consequently, partial flap loss is uncommon, and the advantage of better blood supply enjoyed by the free TRAM flap is less meaningful. For this reason, for the breast mounds themselves, the pedicled and free TRAM flaps are nearly equal, except perhaps in patients who are heavy smokers.

In the donor site, however, there is a vast difference between bilateral pedicled and free TRAM flaps. Bilateral pedicled TRAM flaps require sacrifice of much more muscle than do free flaps, and this muscle loss can significantly weaken the abdomen. After bilateral conventional TRAM flaps, only 26% of my patients have been able to do situps, compared to 75% after bilateral free TRAM flaps. The use of free TRAM flaps greatly reduces the amount of muscle sacrifice and thereby reduces donor site morbidity. It is for this reason, and not because of differences in the breast mounds, that we prefer free TRAM flaps for bilateral reconstruction in most patients.

Extended Free TRAM Flap in Thin Patients

Because of the excellent blood supply to free TRAM flaps, they can be manipulated in ways that conventional TRAM flaps cannot. In the case of very thin patients, the flap design can be extended as far laterally as the operating table will allow (Fig 6-5). When

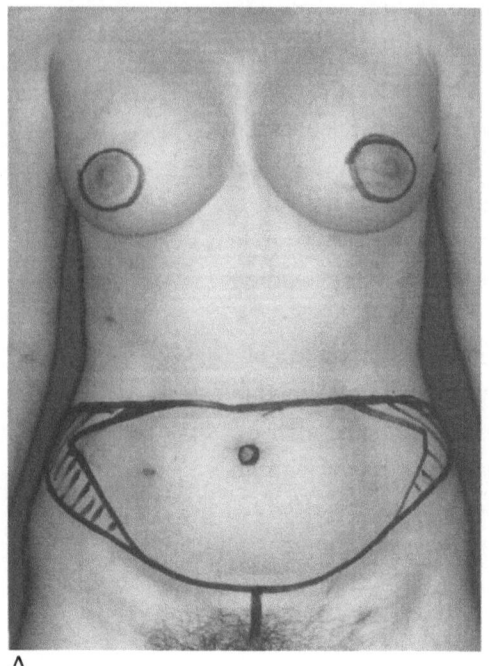
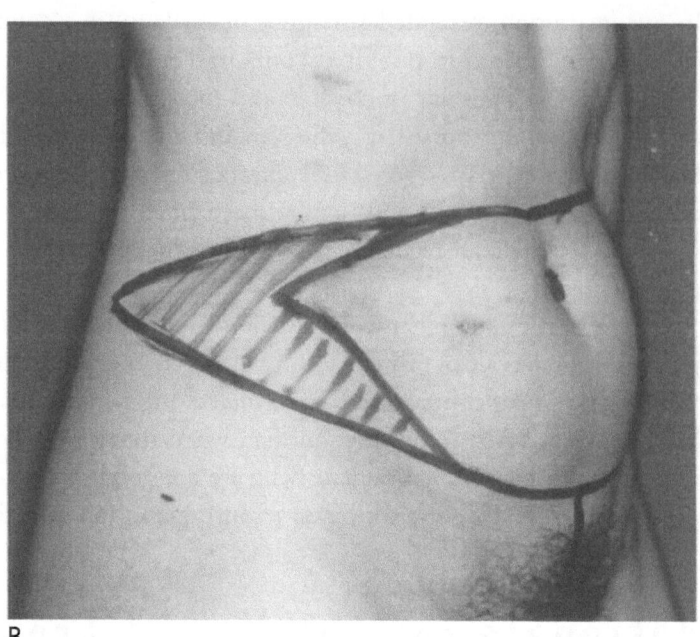

A   B

FIG. 6-5   (A, B) Design for extended free TRAM flaps for immediate bilateral breast reconstruction in a very thin patient. The flaps are extended laterally as far as the operating table will allow.

each flap is transferred to the contralateral breast, the extended lateral flap tail can be folded double (Fig 6-6) to increase breast mound volume and projection. This maneuver will allow reconstruction of breasts of reasonable size even in very thin patients (Fig 6-7). It will not permit the creation of very large breasts, but thin patients do not require large breasts; on such patients, large breasts usually look unnatural. The extended flap technique is especially useful for thin, small-breasted patients who have previously had breast augmentation. For these patients, by using extended bilateral free TRAM flaps, breasts of a size similar to their previous augmented ones can be obtained without having to resort to the use of implants.

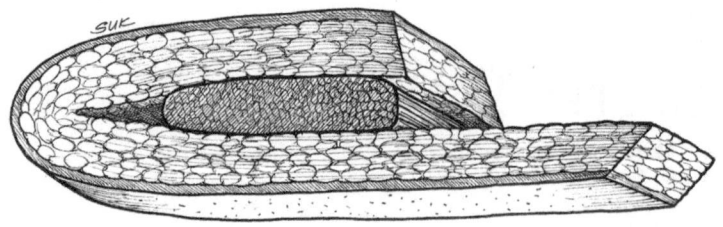

FIG. 6-6   Extended free TRAM flap folded double, to increase breast projection.

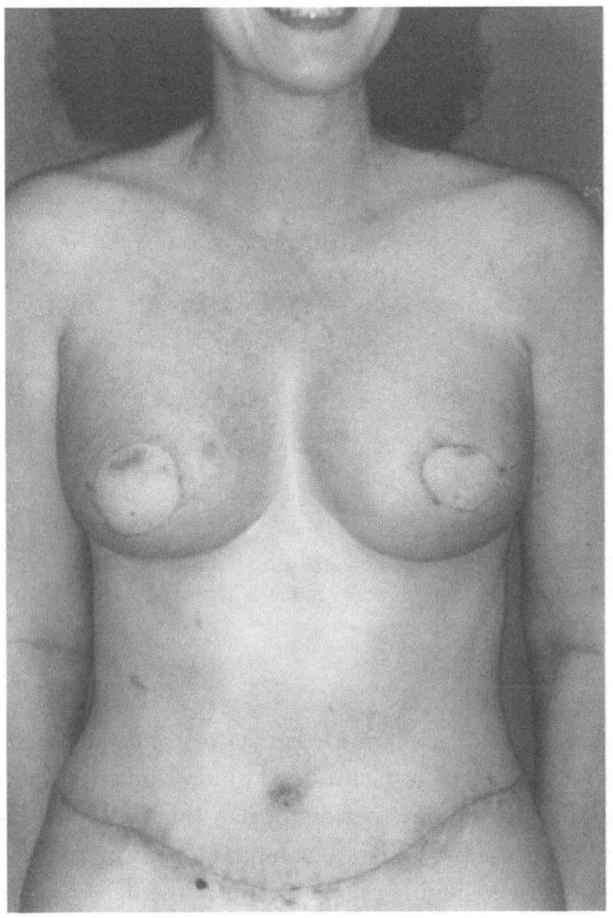

FIG. 6-7   Result of immediate bilateral breast reconstruction with extended free TRAM flaps (same patient as shown in Fig 6-9).

Repairing the Fascial Donor Site of Bilateral TRAM Flaps

Often, the most problematic part of any bilateral TRAM flap breast reconstruction is closure of the fascial donor site.[16],[17] In some cases, the difficulty of this closure can be significantly reduced by the technique used during flap elevation. Because tissue survival across the midline is not required, less flap perfusion is necessary than is the case in unilateral reconstruction. In raising the flaps, if the surgeon finds one lone vascular perforator entering a flap fairly laterally, it may be advisable to sacrifice that single perforator in order to preserve more abdominal fascia and facilitate the subsequent donor site closure—especially if the lateral perforator is relatively small. The decision of whether to sacrifice perforator(s) or fascia will depend on the vascular anatomy and the degree of abdominal laxity that is present.

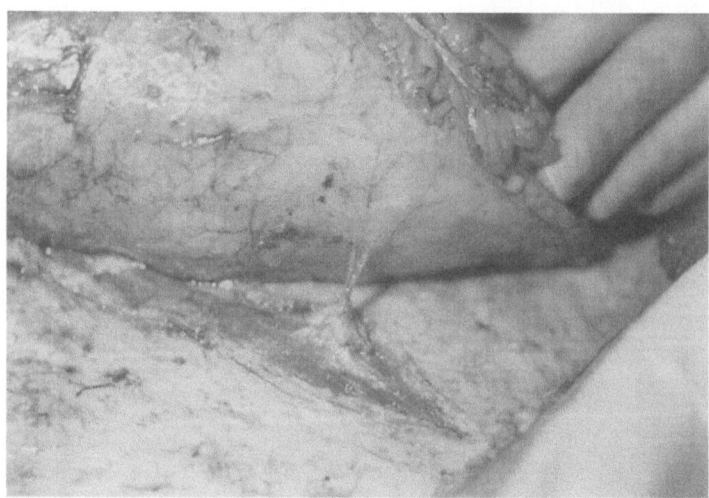

FIG. 6-8 Example of a perforator included with the flap but with preservation of almost all of the surrounding fascia. Only a small circle of fascia is removed with each perforator.

Alternatively, an isolated lateral or medial perforator can be preserved, but the fascia incised around it and preserved in situ in a fashion similar to the technique used in performing a deep inferior epigastric perforator flap (Fig 6-8). The muscle is harvested just as in any standard free TRAM flap, but more fascia is preserved. The small circular fascial defect created by including the perforator in the flap is connected to the main fascial defect by a horizontal fascial incision, and will be closed vertically (Fig 6-9) so that the closure does not add any lateral tension to the abdominal wall closure.

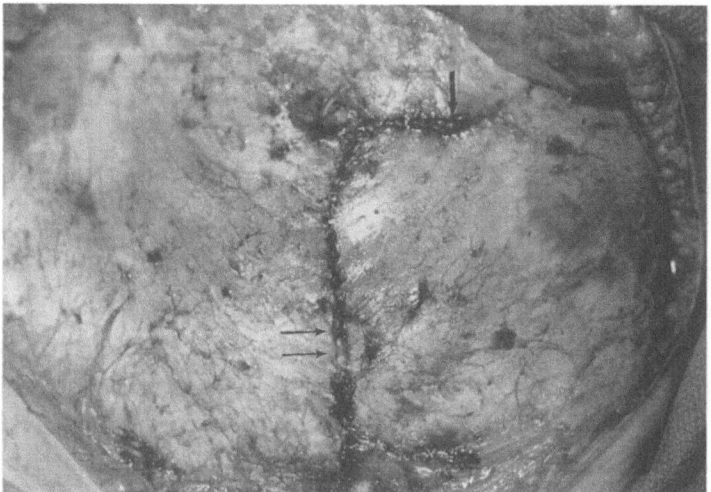

FIG. 6-9 The small circular fascial defect (arrow) was connected to the main fascial donor site defect (double arrows) with a horizontal incision. This was subsequently closed vertically to avoid adding lateral tension to the abdominal wall closure.

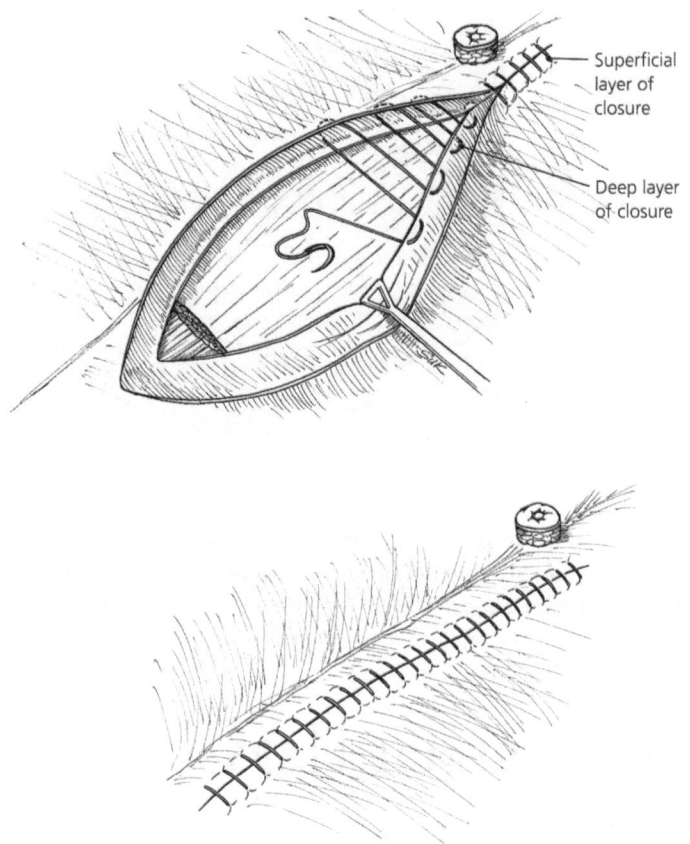

Superficial
layer of
closure

Deep layer
of closure

FIG. 6-10   Two-layer fascial closure at a TRAM flap donor site. In the deep layer, the internal oblique fascia is sutured to the midline fascia deep to the linea alba using a heavy (No. 1) permanent running suture.

After the flaps have been transferred, the two fascial donor sites are closed simultaneously, using running sutures so that the tension is widely distributed. Two deep running sutures are placed to attach the internal oblique fascia to the midline fascia (Fig 6-10) and then tightened together. If there is excessive tension and the donor sites resist closure, one side should be tightened and tied first. Then, on the other side, a row of figure-eight sutures of 2-0 Vicryl (polygalactin 910) should be placed without tension, then tightened all at once so that the tension is widely distributed. Each suture is then individually tied while the tension on the rest is maintained by an assistant (Fig 6-11).

If the closure has been unusually tight or if the sutures are tending to tear through the fascia, reinforcement of the abdominal wall with synthetic mesh may be advisable. I have found this necessary in only approximately 10% of bilateral TRAM flap patients. More recently, as I have harvested less and less fascia, I have used mesh even less frequently. Mesh should be used only to reinforce the fascia, however, never to replace it; the mesh can become infected and someday may need to be removed. The mesh should overlie the fascial closure, and be sutured to the abdominal wall circumferentially with 2-0 Vicryl or an equivalent (Fig 6-12). In that way, if the mesh ever needs to be removed, the abdominal wall beneath it should remain intact.

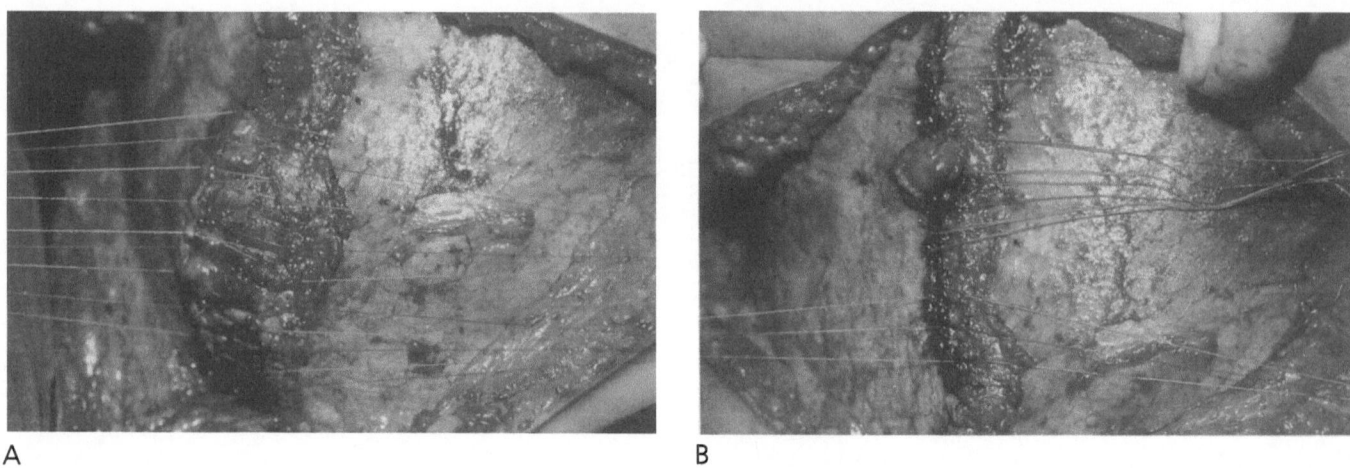

A   B

FIG. 6-11 (A) Multiple figure-eight sutures are used to close an overly tight wound. All the sutures are placed before any of them are tightened. The ends are then crossed. (B) The sutures are then all tightened simultaneously. The tension is maintained while each suture is individually tied. (From Kroll SS. *Ann Plast Surg.* 1989;23:104–111. Used with permission.)

Bilateral Perforator Flaps

A variation of the free TRAM flap, the deep inferior epigastric artery perforator (DIEP) flap,[18,19] can be useful in certain cases of bilateral autologous tissue breast reconstruction. In this technique, one or more perforating blood vessels entering the TRAM flaps from the rectus abdominis sheath are dissected from the surrounding muscle and followed as they join the deep inferior epigastric artery and vein. The dissection is continued to the origin of the deep inferior epigastric vessels, creating a long vascular pedicle that contains no muscle (Fig 6-13). Motor nerves are preserved when possible, and little or no muscle and fascia are sacrificed.

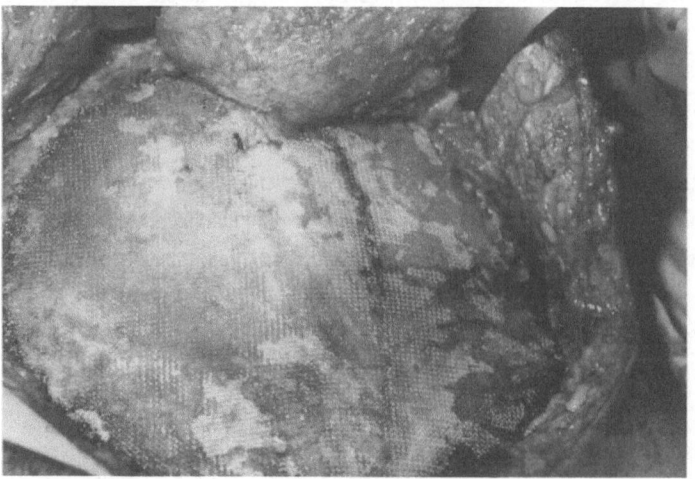

FIG. 6-12 Prolene mesh overlay to reinforce a donor site fascial closure.

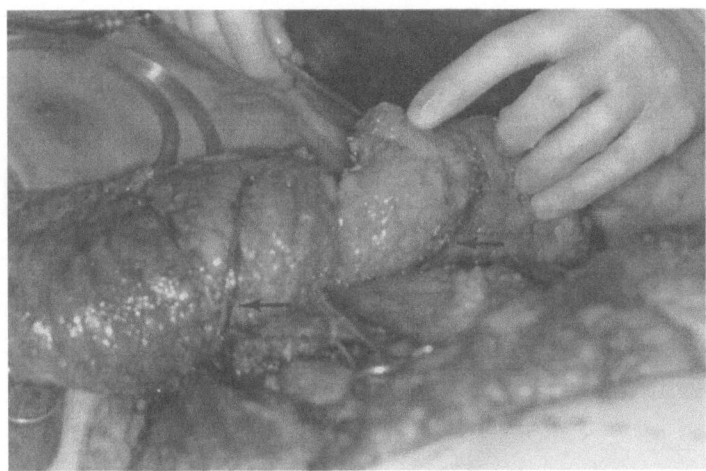

FIG. 6-13   Bilateral DIEP flaps (arrows point to the two pedicles). No muscle or fascia has been sacrificed.

The advantages of this technique are that abdominal closure is very easy and abdominal wall weakness or hernia is unlikely. The disadvantages of the technique are that it is time-consuming and that the blood supply to the flaps is less robust than that of standard free TRAM flaps. Bilateral DIEP flaps are usually not the technique of choice in heavy smokers, in whom reduction in flap blood supply would be undesirable. Because of the amount of time required, I would not ordinarily use this technique in an obese patient, in whom operating time is normally prolonged even when standard TRAM flaps are used. I tend to use this technique for bilateral reconstruction primarily in thin, athletic patients who are concerned about possible loss of rectus abdominis muscle function and who only require small breasts.

Latissimus Dorsi and Other Flaps

To perform bilateral breast reconstruction with latissimus dorsi flaps, the patient is first placed in the prone position with the arms outstretched (Fig 6-14). The flaps are raised and pockets created in the axillae; the dissection extends through the axillae and as far anteriorly as possible into the area that will be occupied by the flaps when they become breast mounds. Care is taken not to dissect below the planned inframammary fold. The flaps are tucked into these pockets, and the donor sites are closed securely over suction drains. The patient is then turned over into the supine position, reprepared, and redraped. The mastectomy incisions are reopened and the latissimus dorsi flaps identified. The breast pocket dissections are then extended to the desired boundaries of the new breasts. The latissimus dorsi flaps are withdrawn from their pockets and shaped into breast mounds (see chapters 16 through 18). After careful hemostasis is obtained, the wounds are then closed over a second pair

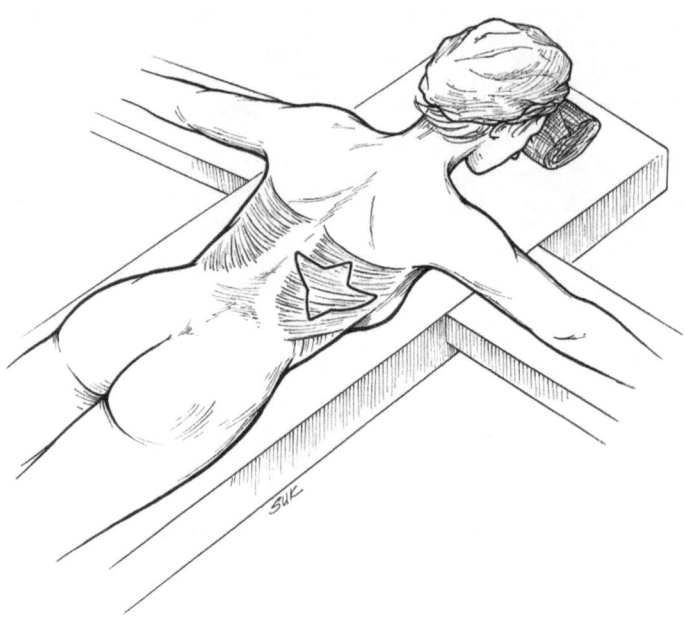

FIG. 6-14 Patient position for harvesting of bilateral latissimus dorsi flaps.

of suction drains, using the latissimus dorsi flaps to replace missing skin in the breasts.

    If bilateral flaps other than the latissimus dorsi or TRAM flaps must be used, I usually prefer to preform the two reconstructions separately to avoid a painfully long operative session. The advantage of bilateral simultaneous convalescence is lost, but symmetry can be achieved. Fortunately, bilateral reconstruction with such alternative flaps is rarely necessary.

Elective Contralateral Mastectomy with Bilateral Reconstruction

Because bilateral immediate breast reconstruction with TRAM flaps can be so successful, and because the risk of subsequently developing a second primary tumor in the opposite breast is significantly elevated in some patients with breast cancer, selected patients have elected to undergo prophylactic mastectomy on the side opposite their unilateral breast cancer.[20] This strategy allows them to benefit from the advantages of bilateral breast reconstruction, and reduces their risk of every having to undergo breast cancer treatment again. It also eliminates the need for follow-up mammography, although not the need for breast self-examination. This approach is aggressive and controversial, and will be more thoroughly discussed in a subsequent chapter. Here we will only say that it is capable of achieving outstanding results (Figs 6-15 and 6-16), and has been very popular with patients.

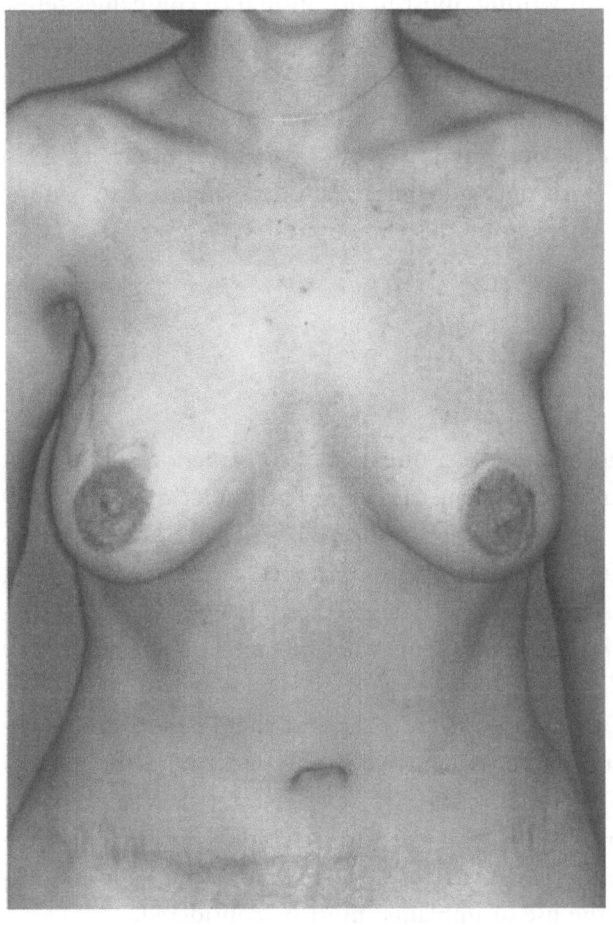 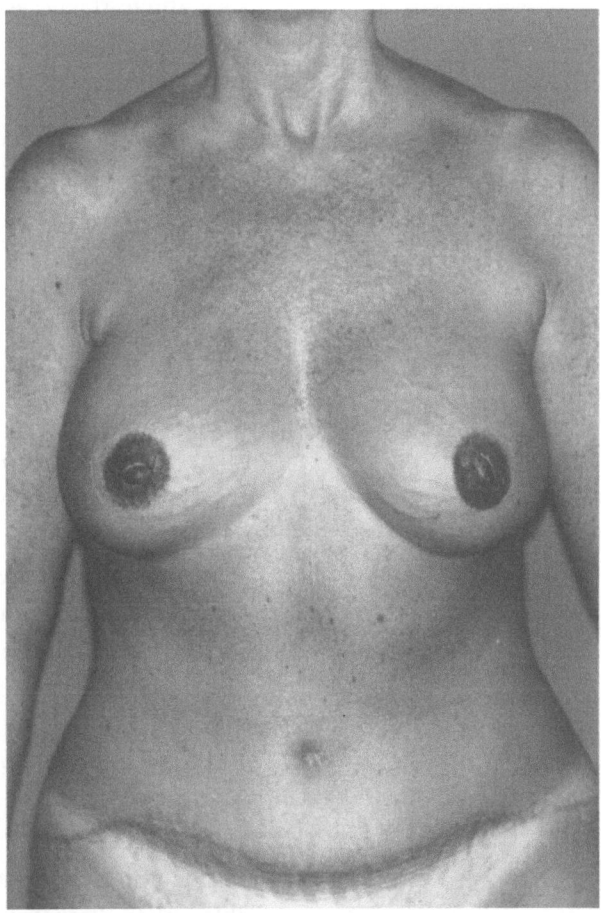

FIG. 6-15 Result of immediate bilateral free TRAM flap breast reconstruction.

FIG. 6-16 Result of immediate bilateral free TRAM flap breast reconstruction.

Costs of Bilateral Reconstruction

Because the patient can recover from the reconstruction of both breasts simultaneously and because good symmetry is usually obtained in the first operation and thus few revisions are necessary, the cost of providing bilateral mastectomy and breast reconstruction including reconstruction of both nipples is only approximately 5% more than that of providing a comparable unilateral mastectomy and reconstruction.[6] This is true even though the cost of the initial bilateral breast mound reconstruction is quite high. After the reconstruction has been completed, there are additional cost savings (for patients who undergo elective contralateral mastectomy) because the need for subsequent mammography of the contralateral breast is eliminated. Moreover, any costs associated with treatment of a second breast cancer (in those patients who would otherwise develop one) are eliminated. One could therefore argue that bilateral mastectomy with autologous tissue reconstruction is a very cost-effective way to manage unilateral breast cancer, if breast reconstruction is considered a routine part of that management.

Interestingly, at the time of this writing, most health insurance companies refuse to pay for prophylactic treatment of the contralateral breast, even though one could argue that it would be in their long-term financial interest to encourage women to undergo this form of therapy. Most patients who choose elective contralateral mastectomy must pay the costs of treatment of the opposite breast out of their own pockets. Even so, they are generally very satisfied with their outcomes and often volunteer to counsel other prospective patients who are considering the same option.

Summary

Bilateral reconstruction has many advantages over unilateral reconstruction and in most cases is preferable to two separate unilateral reconstructions. The results are usually very symmetric and consequently tend to be aesthetically superior to those of unilateral reconstructions. The free TRAM flap is the most commonly used technique, providing good results with minimal donor site morbidity. Bilateral free TRAM flap reconstruction has been sufficiently successful that some patients with unilateral breast cancer have chosen to undergo elective contralateral mastectomy and bilateral reconstruction. This approach can be very rewarding but has significant risks and should therefore be offered only by very experienced surgeons to patients who fully understand the hazards they are undertaking.

When TRAM flaps are impossible, bilateral extended latissimus dorsi flaps are often the next best choice. When neither TRAM flaps nor latissimus dorsi flaps are possible, other alternatives, including the use of implants, must be considered.

References

1. Hartrampf CR Jr, Scheflan M, Black PW. Breast reconstruction with a transverse abdominal island flap. *Plast Reconstr Surg.* 1982;69:216–224.
2. Elliott LF, Hartrampf CR Jr. Tailoring of the new breast using the transverse abdominal island flap. *Plast Reconstr Surg.* 1983;72:887–893.
3. Hartrampf CR Jr, Bennett GK. Autogenous tissue reconstruction in the mastectomy patient: a critical review of 300 patients. *Ann Surg.* 1987;205:508–518.
4. Grotting JC, Urist MM, Maddox WA, Vasconez LO. Conventional TRAM flap versus free microsurgical TRAM flap for immediate breast reconstruction. *Plast Reconstr Surg.* 1989;83:842–844.
5. Kroll SS, Evans GRD, Reece GP, et al. Comparison of resource costs between implant-based and TRAM flap breast reconstruction. *Plast Reconstr Surg.* 1996;97:364–372.
6. Kroll SS, Evans GRD, Reece GP, et al. Comparison of resource costs of free and conventional TRAM flap breast reconstruction. *Plast Reconstr Surg.* 1996;98:74–77.
7. Khouri RK, Ahn CY, Salzhauer MA, Scherff D, Shaw WW. Simultaneous bilateral breast reconstruction with the transverse rectus abdominis musculocutaneous free flap. *Ann Surg.* 1997;226:25–34.

8. Schusterman MA, Kroll SS, Miller MJ, et al. The free TRAM flap for breast reconstruction: a single center's experience with 211 consecutive cases. *Ann Plast Surg.* 1994;32:234–242.

9. Schusterman MA, Kroll SS, Weldon ME. Immediate breast reconstruction: why the free TRAM over the conventional TRAM flap? *Plast Reconstr Surg.* 1992;90:255–262.

10. McCraw JB, Papp C, Edwards A, McMellin A. The autogenous latissimus breast reconstruction. *Clin Plast Surg.* 1994;21:279–288.

11. Hartrampf CR Jr, Noel RT, Drazan L, Elliott LF, Bennett GK, Beegle PH. Rubens fat pad for breast reconstruction: a peri-iliac soft-tissue free flap. *Plast Reconstr Surg.* 1994;93:402–497.

12. Shaw WW. Breast reconstruction by superior gluteal microvascular free flaps without silicone implants. *Plast Reconstr Surg.* 1983;72:490.

13. Shaw WW. Microvascular free flap breast reconstruction. *Clin Plast Surg.* 1984;11:333–341.

14. Nahai F. Inferior gluteus maximus musculocutaneous flap for breast reconstruction. *Perspect Plast Surg.* 1992;6:65.

15. Codner MA, Nahai F. The gluteal free flap breast reconstruction: making it work. *Clin Plast Surg.* 1994;21:289–296.

16. Hartrampf CR Jr. In discussion: Drever JM, Hodson-Walker N. Closure of the donor defect for breast reconstruction with rectus abdominis myocutaneous flaps. *Plast Reconstr Surg.* 1985;76:563.

17. Kroll SS, Schusterman MA, Mistry D. The internal oblique repair of abdominal bulges secondary to TRAM flap breast reconstruction. *Plast Reconstr Surg.* 1995;96:100–104.

18. Allen RJ, Treece P. Deep inferior epigastric perforator flap for breast reconstruction. *Ann Plast Surg.* 1994;32:32–38.

19. Koshima I, Soeda S. Inferior epigastric artery skin flaps without rectus abdominis muscle. *Br J Plast Surg.* 1989;42:645–648.

20. Kroll SS, Miller MJ, Schusterman MA, Reece GP, Singletary SE, Ames F. The rationale for elective contralateral mastectomy with immediate bilateral reconstruction. *Ann Surg Oncol.* 1994;1:457–461.

7 Choice of Technique

A wide variety of techniques are currently available for postmastectomy breast reconstruction. The method that is best for any particular patient will depend on the patient, the surgeon, and the environment in which the reconstruction must be performed. No one technique is right for all patients. The surgeon must be familiar with the advantages and disadvantages of each technique and should not be rigidly committed to only one method of reconstruction. He or she should also be realistic about his or her own capabilities as well as those of the hospital and about the patient's physical limitations. Fortunately, there are enough techniques available that almost any patient can have successful reconstruction provided that the surgeon is flexible in his or her thinking and the patient is properly motivated.

Choosing Between Autologous Tissue and Implants

Although this is a book about autologous tissue breast reconstruction, there are some patients for whom implants remain the technique of choice. As discussed in chapter 2, implant-based reconstruction has certain short-term advantages that are offset by long-term disadvantages. For patients who are older than 65 years, who are in poor general health, or who have a poor tumor prognosis, the long-term disadvantages of breast implants may be of lesser importance than the short-term advantages of minimal surgery and rapid convalescence. Moreover, in patients undergoing bilateral reconstruction the difficulty of matching a natural breast with an implant is avoided, so implants can sometimes achieve acceptable results even when some degree of capsular contracture is present (Fig 7-1). This does not mean that implants are preferred for all bilateral reconstructions but only that, in a patient who is a marginal candidate for autologous tissue reconstruction, implants might be selected for some bilateral reconstructions when autologous tissues might have been chosen were the reconstruction unilateral.

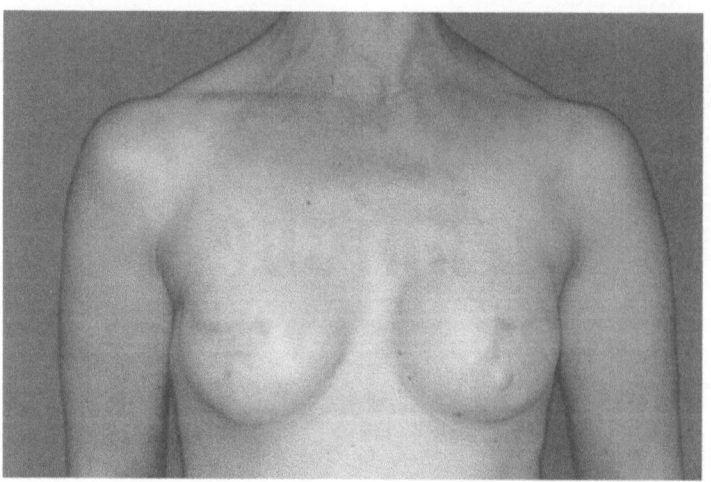

Fig. 7-1   Example of bilateral breast reconstruction performed with tissue expansion and saline-filled implants.

If implant-based reconstruction is selected, I prefer saline-filled implants because the incidence of capsular contracture is lower than that associated with silicone gel–filled implants. Capsular contracture is the most common problem associated with breast implants,[1-3] and its presence can easily outweigh any advantage gained by the more natural "feel" and lack of "rippling" associated with the silicone gel. Most patients who choose implant-based reconstruction are willing to accept some degree of a less natural feel or appearance as a trade-off for a softer and less troublesome breast. For these reasons, I avoid silicone gel–filled implants unless the patient insists on having them.

Choosing Between TRAM Flaps and Other Alternatives

For the overwhelming majority of patients, the transverse rectus abdominis myocutaneous (TRAM) flap[4,5] is the breast reconstruction method of choice. The TRAM flap is soft and easy to mold, has a good blood supply, and has a donor site scar that is relatively easily concealed. When closed properly, the donor site causes relatively little morbidity. The results of artistically successful TRAM flap reconstruction are outstanding and are rarely surpassed by those of any other technique (Figs 7-2 and 7-3). The TRAM flap is the most popular method of breast reconstruction in our institution and is the method of choice for almost all patients for whom it is not contraindicated.

Absolute contraindications to the TRAM flap include a previous TRAM flap, a previous abdominoplasty, extreme obesity,[6,7] and (usually) a potbelly habitus. Relative contraindications include poor general health, marked (but less-than-extreme) obesity, and unilateral reconstruction of a very small breast.

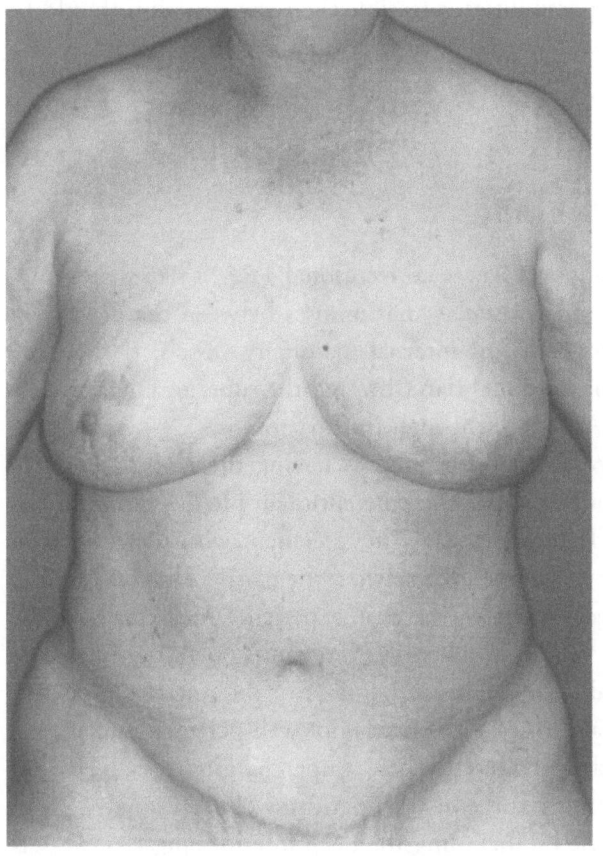

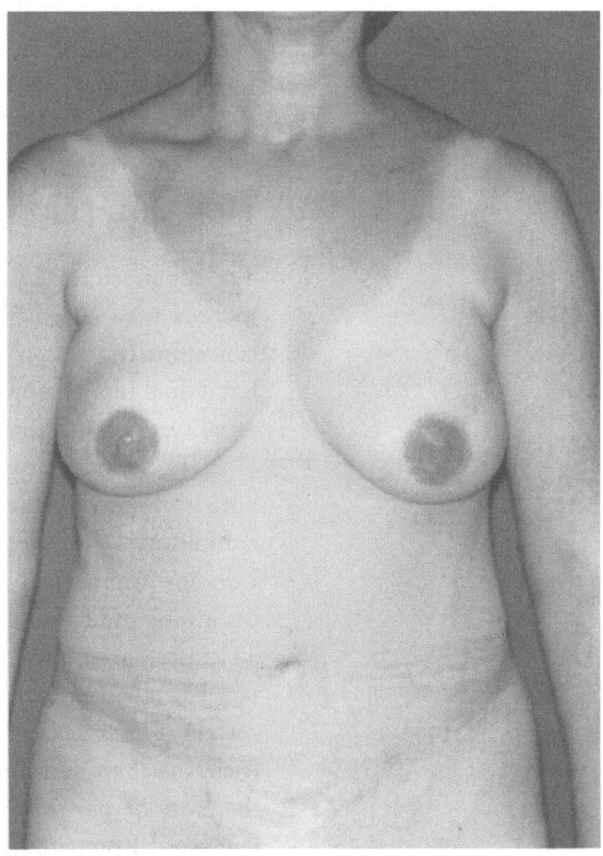

FIG. 7-2 Unilateral TRAM flap breast mound reconstruction. The breast is soft and matches the opposite breast very closely.

FIG. 7-3 Bilateral TRAM flap breast reconstruction. (From Kroll SS. *Clin Plast Surg.* 1998;25:135–143. Used with permission.)

Choosing the Free versus Conventional TRAM Flap

Both the free TRAM flap[8,9] and the conventional (pedicled) TRAM flap[4,5,10] are capable of achieving superb results. In my opinion, the free TRAM flap is superior because it has a better blood supply[11] and because it has less donor site morbidity (see chapter 9). For surgeons who are capable of performing the free TRAM flap and in environments where the necessary equipment and personnel are available, it is the procedure of choice unless there are no suitable recipient vessels. The conventional TRAM flap has no advantages that the free TRAM flap does not have, other than not requiring microvascular anastomoses.

    If the surgeon does not preform microvascular surgery, if the requisite equipment is lacking, or if no suitable recipient vessels are found, a conventional TRAM flap is the next best alternative. The conventional TRAM flap works well in the majority of patients who are otherwise suitable TRAM flap candidates and who do not smoke. In patients who do smoke, the blood supply of the conventional TRAM flap must be augmented either by using a double-pedicled technique[12] (which I almost never use anymore because I consider the donor site morbidity too severe), by delaying the flap,[13] or by supercharging it.[14] If none of these possibilities is feasible the reconstruction should be deferred until the circumstances have changed and the patient no longer smokes or a free TRAM flap can be performed.

The Supercharged TRAM Flap

The supercharged TRAM flap[14] is a hybrid flap, a conventional TRAM flap that is augmented with one or more auxiliary microvascular anastomoses between the deep inferior epigastric vessels and the thoracodorsal or internal mammary vessels. It therefore has a dual blood supply: that of a conventional flap (through the superior epigastric arterial system) and that of a free TRAM flap (through the anastomoses).

The supercharged TRAM flap is often criticized as having the worst aspects of both techniques—the donor site morbidity of the conventional TRAM flap and the complexity of the free TRAM flap. I am not entirely in agreement with that criticism. I do not recommend it as a primary technique except when the plastic surgeon is at the beginning of his or her career and seeks a safe way to gain experience in performing the anastomoses required for free TRAM flaps, or when the surgeon is operating in an unfamiliar environment where the quality of the instruments or of the microscope is uncertain. For salvage of a conventional TRAM flap that is not well perfused after transfer to the chest wall, however, supercharging has no equal. Supercharging, ideally, would therefore be part of the repertoire of any surgeon who performs conventional TRAM flaps, and I prepare for its possible use by including the deep inferior epigastric vessels with every conventional TRAM flap that I elevate.

The Perforator Flap

The deep inferior epigastric perforator (DIEP) flap[15–17] (Fig 7-4) is a variation of the free TRAM flap in which the surgeon harvests only the blood vessels that supply the flap from the abdominal wall (see chapter 10). All of the rectus abdominis muscle, which is dissected away from the perforating vessels, is left in situ. In raising this flap, all but two or three perforators to the flap itself must be sacrificed, so the blood supply to the flap is less robust than that of a standard free TRAM flap.

The DIEP flap may be especially useful for unilateral reconstruction in patients with very small breasts. In such situations the reduced blood supply to the flap is not important since only a small amount of tissue will be required to make the breast. It is also a possible choice for patients with a minimal amount of a potbelly habitus, since the DIEP flap weakens the abdominal wall much less than a standard free TRAM flap (although such patients are far from ideal candidates for any type of TRAM flap and might be better candidates for extended latissimus dorsi flaps or other techniques).

Because the DIEP flap has so little donor site morbidity, it should also be considered in many cases of bilateral reconstruction. The reduced donor site morbidity, however, is offset by the length and complexity of the procedure and by the fact that reducing the number of perforators to the flap reduces the flap's blood supply, increasing the risks of partial flap loss and fat necrosis. At the time of this writing, my own pref-

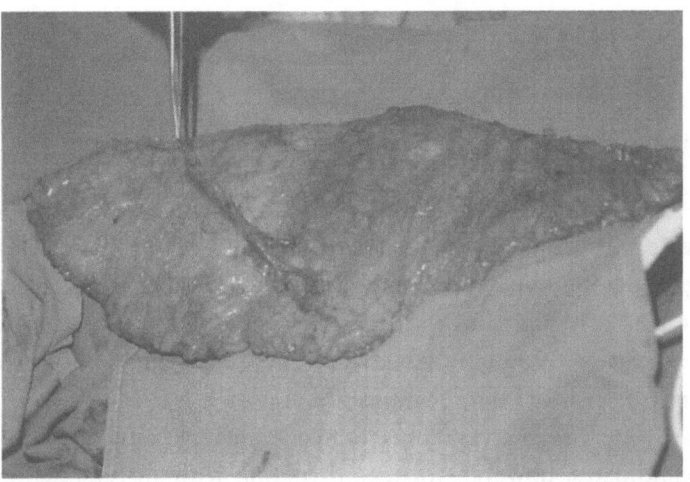

FIG. 7-4   DIEP flap.

erence is to consider the DIEP flap for bilateral reconstruction only in athletic patients who are especially concerned about maintaining a strong abdomen. In such patients, I examine the anatomic distribution of the perforating blood vessels as I elevate the flaps (Fig 7-5). If on each side there is one very large dominant perforator or a distinct lateral row of two large perforators, I will probably perform bilateral perforator flaps. If the perforators are all grouped together medially, standard free TRAM flaps will leave a donor site that is easily closed, even bilaterally, and remains the preferred alternative. In most cases, bilateral free TRAM flaps are still the best choice since they are technically easier than the perforator flaps and the operating time is so much shorter.

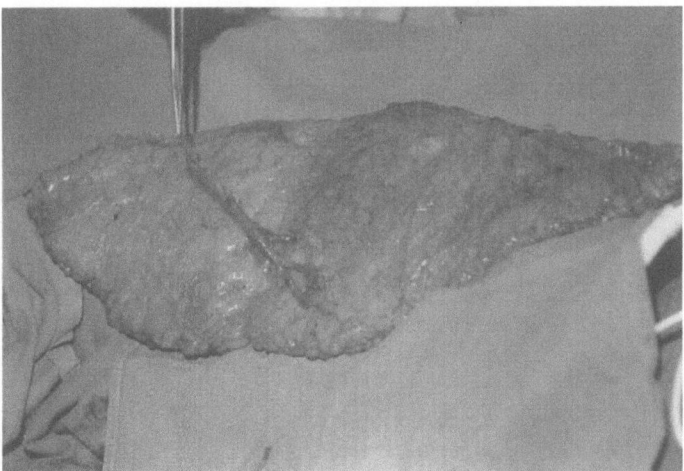

FIG. 7-5   Perforating blood vessels entering a TRAM flap from the rectus abdominis sheath. In some patients, these can be easily exposed with careful dissection, facilitating selection of the technique to be used based on the vascular anatomy.

Special Situations

Obese Patients

Patients who are extremely obese (those with a weight/height index—body weight in kilograms divided by height in meters—greater than 54, or those who have a large, overhanging panniculus adiposus) should not have a TRAM flap because the incidence of complications is very high and the aesthetic results that can be obtained are usually limited by the patient's overall poor body appearance. The length of time required for the surgery and the risk of complications are almost linear functions of the degree of obesity[7] and are therefore unacceptably elevated in such patients. Patients who are obese can be good candidates, however, for reconstruction with an extended latissimus dorsi myocutaneous flap.[18] In obese patients there is usually abundant subcutaneous tissue in the back, allowing reconstruction of a reasonably large breast. Although the size of the breast achieved in this way may not reach the proportions of its opposite counterpart (Fig 7-6), the opposite breast is often overly large and will benefit from any breast reduction that is required to achieve symmetry.

Although the TRAM flap is contraindicated in extremely obese patients, moderately obese patients can get quite good results from a TRAM flap if the surgeon is willing to perform the additional work that is required (Figs 7-7 and 7-8). The surgical procedure itself is more lengthy in obese patients because of the effort required to dissect through thick layers of fat and because the anatomy is obscured by adipose tissue surrounding the blood vessels and other structures—tissues that must be retracted or removed during the dissection. Transferring and shaping the flap are also more difficult because the flap is heavier and more unwieldy, and cannot be folded. Complications are more frequent and revisions are necessary more often. If a free TRAM flap is used, the risk of flap loss is higher than it is in thinner patients. Nevertheless, excellent results can be obtained in moderately obese patients if the patient is motivated and the surgeon perseveres.

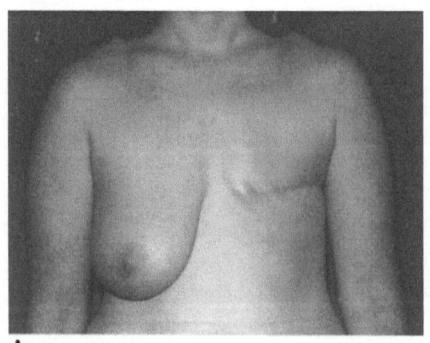 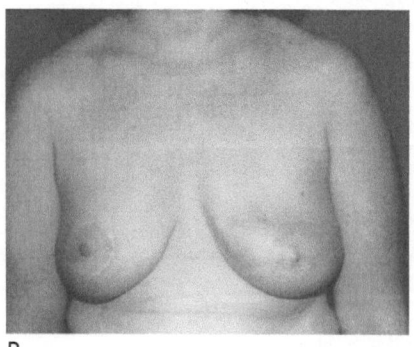 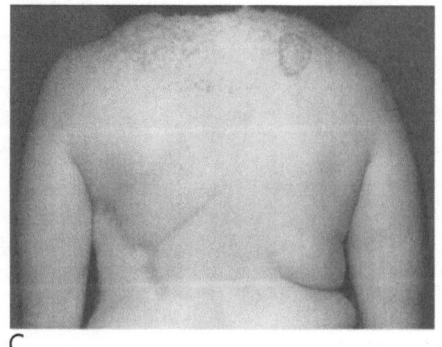

A B C

FIG. 7-6 Patient before (A) and after (B) delayed breast reconstruction with an extended latissimus dorsi flap. A reduction mammaplasty was performed on the opposite side. (C) The donor site scar.

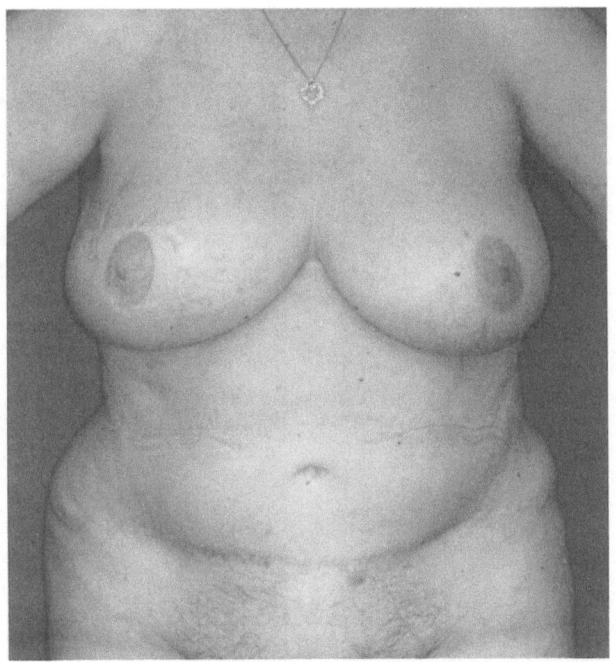

FIG. 7-7   Result of an immediate free TRAM flap breast reconstruction in an obese patient.

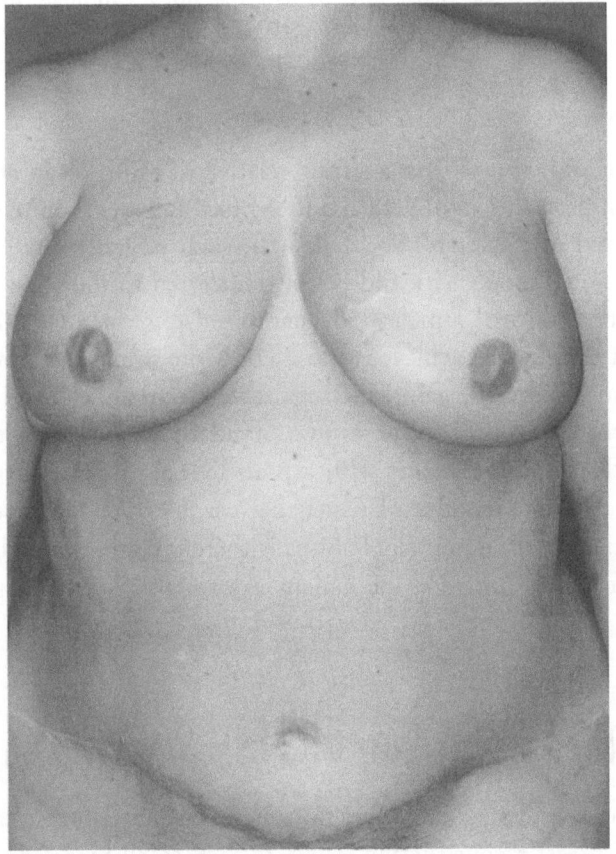

FIG. 7-8   Result of bilateral free TRAM flap breast reconstruction in an obese patient.

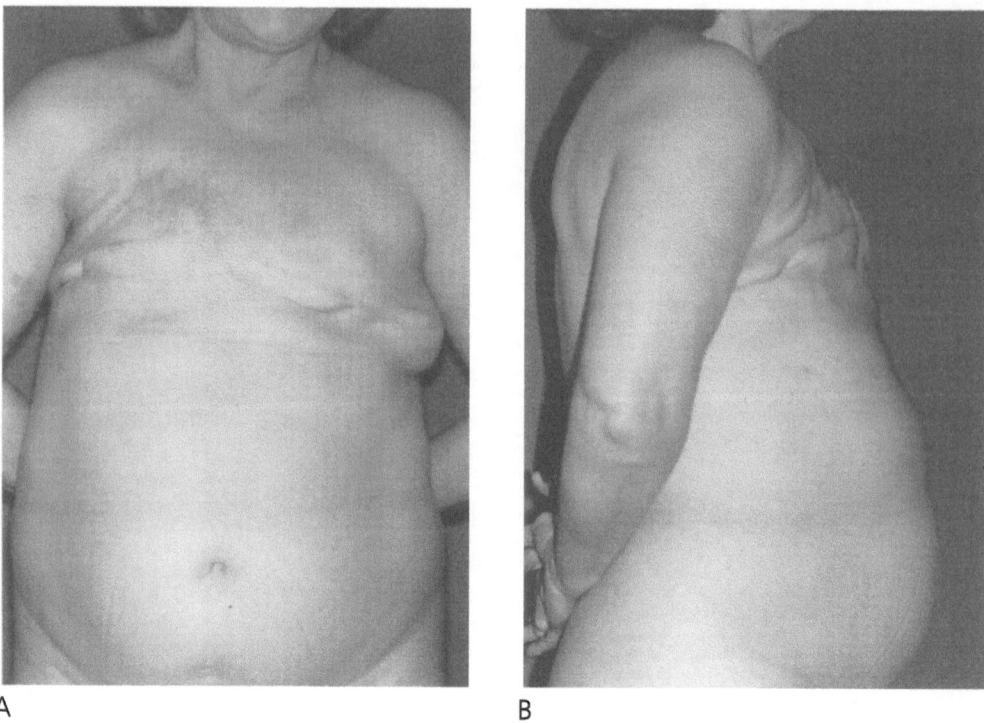

A   B

FIG. 7-9 (A, B) Patient with a potbelly habitus who subsequently underwent delayed bilateral breast reconstruction with DIEP flaps. This patient was not a candidate for bilateral TRAM flaps. (From Reece GP, Kroll SS. *Clin Plast Surg.* 1998;25:235–249. Used with permission.)

A potbelly habitus (Fig 7-9) is a strong relative (if mild) or an absolute (if severe in degree) contraindication to a unilateral TRAM flap and an absolute contraindication to a double-pedicled or bilateral TRAM flap. In such patients, the excess fat is contained within the abdominal cavity and is not transferred to the chest wall as it would be in patients with a normal female body habitus. Consequently, the size of the reconstructed breast that can be achieved is limited. More important, the excess intraabdominal fat will push outward against the repaired abdominal wall and can lead to hernia formation if the fascia is not very strong. Standard TRAM flaps should therefore be avoided in such patients. Patients with a potbelly habitus can have reconstruction with a DIEP flap, but the amount of tissue that can be obtained is still limited. The best option in patients with a potbelly habitus is therefore an extended latissimus dorsi flap or a gluteal free flap, provided the patient is a suitable candidate for those procedures.

Unilateral Reconstruction of Very Small Breasts

Patients who require unilateral reconstruction of a very small breast can certainly undergo TRAM flap breast reconstruction safely. In fact, small-breasted patients are usually also thin patients—patients who are excellent surgical candidates, recover rapidly from surgery, and have unusually low complication rates.

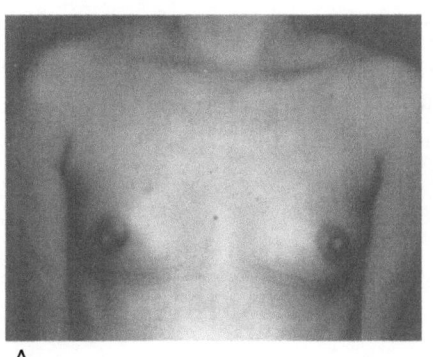 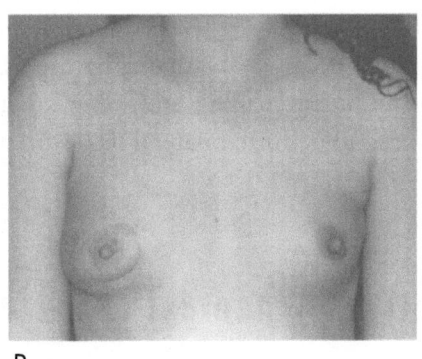 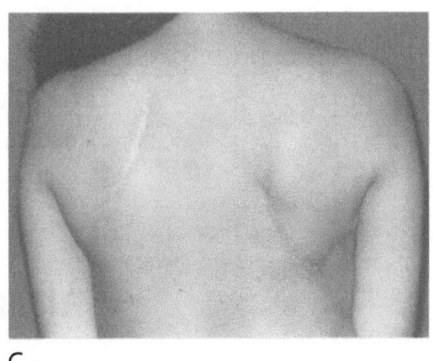

A   B   C

FIG. 7-10   (A) Patient with very small breasts presented for immediate unilateral reconstruction. (B) Result of right breast reconstruction with an extended latissimus dorsi flap. (C) The donor site scar.

Nevertheless, patients with very small breasts are not always ideal candidates for unilateral reconstruction with TRAM flaps. With a TRAM flap, it is difficult to make the reconstructed breast mound very small. Multiple revisions are often necessary to achieve symmetry (unless the reconstruction is bilateral, in which case symmetry is easily achieved and the size of the breast is not an issue) or the patient chooses to undergo augmentation of the opposite breast. Often the surgeon has the impression that a TRAM flap in such patients is a "long run for a short slide," requiring a large effort to create a breast mound only to end up having to throw most of it away.

One good solution to this problem is to use an extended latissimus dorsi flap. Even in thin patients, this technique us capable of creating a breast that is large enough to match a very small breast. This is usually possible without requiring a fleur-de-lis pattern, so only a linear scar is created on the back (Fig 7-10). The extended latissimus dorsi flap requires a simpler and shorter operation than the TRAM flap, has less operative risk, and requires a shorter hospital stay. For many patients, this is a good compromise that will create an adequate breast without resorting to the use of an implant.

Another solution to the problem of reconstructing a very small breast in a patient who will not accept a donor site scar on the back is a DIEP flap. Although this is not a simpler operation, it does have less donor site morbidity than the standard TRAM flap. Also, because there is no muscle included with the flap and because the location of the vascular supply is precisely known, reducing the volume of a perforator flap is easier than with a standard free TRAM flap. For a small-breasted patient who does not desire contralateral augmentation, and who refuses the extended latissimus dorsi flap, a DIEP flap may well be the technique of choice.

Bilateral Breast Reconstruction

Bilateral breast reconstruction can be performed with conventional TRAM flaps, free TRAM flaps, DIEP flaps, or extended latissimus dorsi flaps. All of these can be performed bilaterally in one operation. Free gluteal flaps[19–21] or Rubens fat pad flaps[22] can also be performed bilaterally in one operation, but the time required can be excessively long; since these operations (unlike the TRAM flap) can be performed on each side independently, I would prefer to do them in two operative sessions. In this way, the surgical team is not excessively fatigued by the tissue transfer, and sufficient attention can be paid to the breast shaping and other artistic aspects of the reconstruction. Fortunately, the need to perform bilateral reconstruction with alternative flaps arises only very rarely.

Alternatives When a TRAM Flap Is Not Possible

If the patient has had a previous TRAM flap or abdominoplasty or if a TRAM flap is contraindicated for other reasons, another technique must be selected. The simplest alternative, for patients who do not object to a donor site scar on the back, is an extended latissimus dorsi flap.[18] If the patient objects to that scar or if there is insufficient tissue or laxity in the back, a gluteal free flap[19,20] or the Rubens fat pad free flap[22] should be considered. These operations (described in other chapters) are more technically difficult than the TRAM flap, but the donor site scars are acceptable and excellent results can be obtained.

When a TRAM flap is not possible, I prefer to examine the patient to see if one of these three alternatives is particularly appropriate. For example, some patients have unusually large buttocks and are therefore especially good candidates for a gluteal flap, while others have lax dorsal skin that lends itself to use in an extended latissimus dorsi flap. If there is no clear preference for one method based on the patient's individual anatomy, I let the patient decide for herself which donor site she would prefer.

Although some surgeons have reported good results from lateral thigh flaps, I believe that in the majority of cases the donor site scar is unacceptable; therefore, I do not use this technique. Similarly, although excellent results can be obtained with the superior gluteal free flap[21] (see chapter 13), this flap requires a vein graft in most cases and therefore I no longer use it. The donor site and flap characteristics are similar to those of the inferior gluteal flap, which usually does not require a vein graft. I will, however, consider using a superior gluteal artery perforator flap, since this usually does not require a vein graft.

Algorithms for Choosing the Most Appropriate Technique

Each surgeon has different abilities, and each hospital has different attributes. Just as no one technique is best for all patients, no algorithm is right for every surgeon or every environment. The algorithms that are presented here (Figs 7-11 and 7-12) work well for me at The University of Texas M. D. Anderson Cancer Center but might not be appropriate for other surgeons in other situations. These algorithms are therefore presented only as a rough guide, to be modified as necessary to fit individual circumstances.

If the patient who requests breast reconstruction is physiologically older than 65 years, is in poor health, or has a dismal tumor prognosis, she is considered a candidate for implant-based reconstruction (or for no reconstruction at all). If she refuses recon-

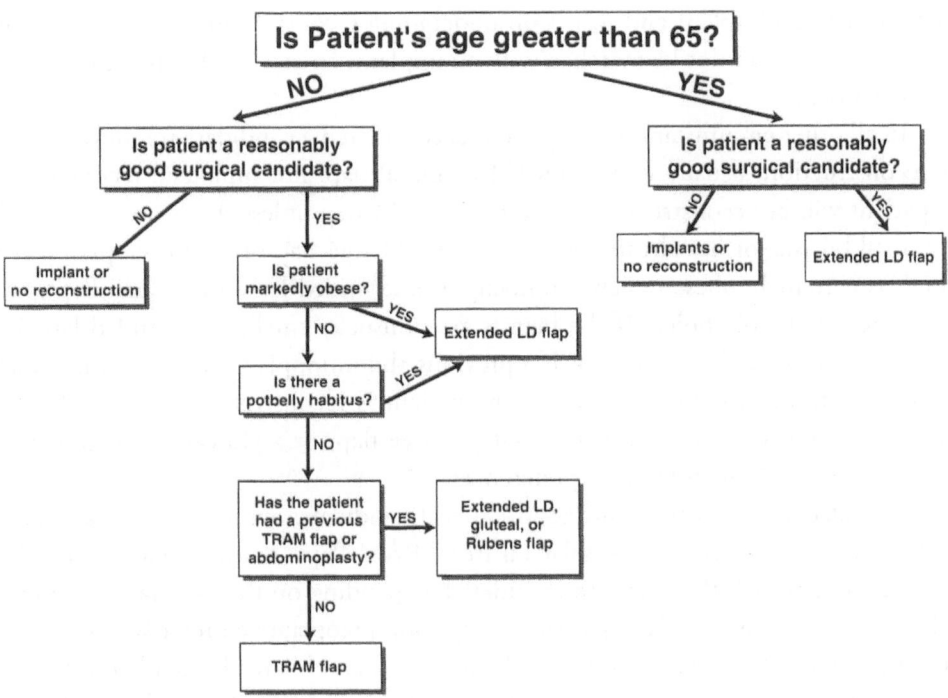

FIG. 7-11   Algorithm for choosing a technique for unilateral breast reconstruction. This algorithm may have to be modified for each surgeon based on his or her individual circumstances.

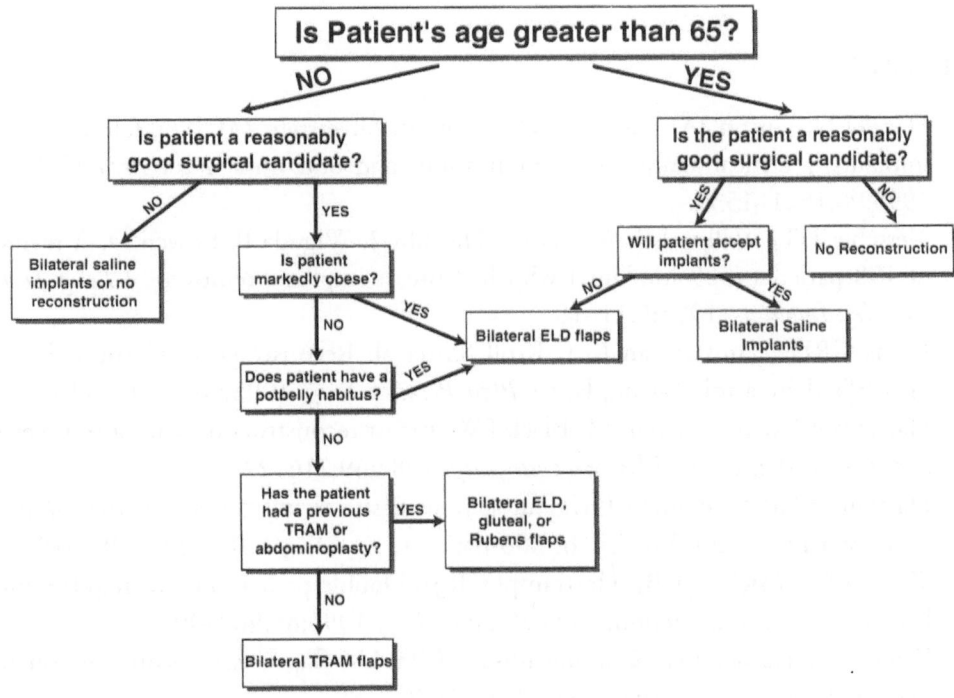

FIG. 7-12   Algorithm for choosing a technique for bilateral breast reconstruction. This algorithm may have to be modified for each surgeon based on his or her individual circumstances.

struction with an implant and insists on undergoing reconstruction, or has a contralateral breast that could not be matched with an implant, an extended latissimus dorsi flap may be chosen.

In all other circumstances, the patient is considered a candidate for autologous tissue reconstruction, usually with a TRAM or DIEP flap. For unilateral reconstruction, the patient will be reconstructed with a free TRAM flap unless she is overly obese, has very small breasts, or has already had a previous TRAM flap or abdominoplasty. If the patient is extremely obese or has a potbelly, the extended latissimus dorsi flap is usually the technique of choice. If the breasts are unusually small, an extended latissimus dorsi flap or a DIEP flap is chosen. If a previous abdominoplasty or TRAM flap makes TRAM flap reconstruction impossible, the patient is reconstructed either with an extended latissimus dorsi flap, a Rubens fat pad free flap, or a gluteal free flap, depending on the patient's anatomy and preferences.

For bilateral reconstruction, good surgical candidates who are moderately obese usually have reconstruction with bilateral free TRAM flaps. If the patient is not obese, free TRAM flaps or DIEP flaps are considered, depending on the vascular anatomy and individual circumstances. If the patient is very thin, preoperative breast size is irrelevant (since the original breasts do not have to be matched) and bilateral extended free TRAM flaps (see chapters 6 and 9) are used. If the patient is very obese, bilateral extended latissimus dorsi flaps are used to avoid an overly prolonged operation and the very high complication rates associated with TRAM flaps in such patients. If the patient is a marginal candidate for autologous tissue reconstruction, bilateral implant-based reconstruction may be selected in some circumstances, since moderate degrees of capsular contracture are likely to be symmetric and a natural ptotic breast does not have to be matched.

References

1. Handel N, Jenson JA, Black Q, Waisman JR, Silverstein MJ. The fate of breast implants: a critical analysis of complications and outcomes. *Plast Reconstr Surg.* 1995;96:1521–1533.

2. Netscher DT, Walker LE, Weizer G, Thornby J, Wigoda P, Bowen D. A review of 198 patients (389 implants) who had breast implants removed. *J Long-Term Eff Med Implants.* 1995;5:11–18.

3. Evans GRD, Schusterman MA, Kroll SS, et al. Reconstruction in the radiated breast: is there a role for implants? *Plast Reconstr Surg.* 1995;96:1111–1115.

4. Hartrampf CR Jr, Scheflan M, Black PW. Breast reconstruction with a transverse abdominal island flap. *Plast Reconstr Surg.* 1982;69:216–224.

5. Hartrampf CR Jr, Bennett GK. Autogenous tissue reconstruction in the mastectomy patient: a critical review of 300 patients. *Ann Surg.* 1987;205:508–518.

6. Wagner DS, Michelow BJ, Hartrampf CR Jr. Double-pedicle TRAM flap for unilateral breast reconstruction. *Plast Reconstr Surg.* 1991;88:987–997.

7. Kroll SS, Netscher DT. Complications of TRAM flap breast reconstruction in obese patients. *Plast Reconstr Surg.* 1989;86:886–892.

8. Schusterman MA, Kroll SS, Weldon ME. Immediate breast reconstruction: why the free TRAM over the conventional TRAM flap? *Plast Reconstr Surg.* 1992;90:255–262.

9. Grotting JC, Urist MM, Maddox WA, Vasconez LO. Conventional TRAM flap versus free microsurgical TRAM flap for immediate breast reconstruction. *Plast Reconstr Surg.* 1989;83:842–844.

10. Elliott LF, Hartrampf CR Jr. Tailoring of the new breast using the transverse abdominal island flap. *Plast Reconstr Surg.* 1983;72:887–893.

11. Boyd JB, Taylor GI, Corlett R. The vascular territories of the superior epigastric and the deep inferior epigastric systems. *Plast Reconstr Surg.* 1984;73:1–14.

12. Ishii CH, Bostwick J, Raine TJ, Coleman JJ, Hester TR. Double-pedicle transverse rectus abdominis myocutaneous flap for unilateral breast and chest-wall reconstruction. *Plast Reconstr Surg.* 1985;76:901–907.

13. Codner MA, Bostwick J, Nahai F, Bried JT, Eaves FF. TRAM flap vascular delay for high-risk breast reconstruction. *Plast Reconstr Surg.* 1995;96:1615–1622.

14. Harashina T, Sone K, Inoue T, et al. Augmentation of circulation of pedicled transverse rectus abdominis musculocutaneous flaps by microvascular surgery. *Br J Plast Surg.* 1987;40:367–370.

15. Koshima I, Soeda S. Inferior epigastric artery skin flaps without rectus abdominis muscle. *Br J Plast Surg.* 1989;42:645–648.

16. Allen RJ, Treece P. Deep inferior epigastric perforator flap for breast reconstruction. *Ann Plast Surg.* 1994;32:32–38.

17. Blondeel N, Boeckx WD. Refinements in free flap breast reconstruction: the free bilateral deep inferior epigastric perforator flap anastomosed to the internal mammary artery. *Br J Plast Surg.* 1994;47:495–501.

18. McCraw JB, Papp C, Edwards A, McMellin A. The autogenous latissimus breast reconstruction. *Clin Plast Surg.* 1994;21:279–288.

19. Nahai F. Inferior gluteus maximus musculocutaneous flap for breast reconstruction. *Perspect Plast Surg.* 1992;6:65.

20. Codner MA, Nahai F. The gluteal free flap breast reconstruction: making it work. *Clin Plast Surg.* 1994;21:289–296.

21. Shaw WW. Breast reconstruction by superior gluteal microvascular free flaps without silicone implants. *Plast Reconstr Surg.* 1983;72:490.

22. Hartrampf CR Jr, Noel RT, Drazan L, Elliott LF, Bennett GK, Beegle PH. Rubens fat pad for breast reconstruction: a peri-iliac soft-tissue free flap. *Plast Reconstr Surg.* 1994;93:402–407.

8 Conventional (Pedicled) TRAM Flap

Advantages of the Conventional TRAM Flap

The conventional (pedicled) transverse rectus abdominis myocutaneous (CTRAM) flap was the first truly effective method of autologous tissue breast reconstruction,[1-3] and even today it remains the most commonly used technique of autologous tissue breast reconstruction in the world. Unlike the free TRAM flap, the CTRAM flap does not require microsurgical training or equipment and therefore can be performed in almost any hospital capable of major surgery. The technique does not require the presence of recipient blood vessels, so it is not hindered by scarring from previous surgery in the axilla. With proper patient selection, it has a high success rate and is capable of achieving excellent results (Figs 8-1 and 8-2), although the percentage of cases in which excellent results are achieved is slightly lower than that obtainable with the free TRAM flap.[4]

The CTRAM flap takes slightly less time to perform than the free TRAM flap and is slightly less expensive.[5] Intensive postoperative flap monitoring is not required, so postoperative care is easier. All in all, the CTRAM flap is easier and simpler than the free TRAM flap.

Disadvantages of the Conventional TRAM Flap

The CTRAM flap also has several disadvantages. It does not have as good a blood supply as does the free TRAM flap.[6] The CTRAM flap therefore does not work as well in patients who smoke unless the blood supply of the flap is augmented by "supercharg-

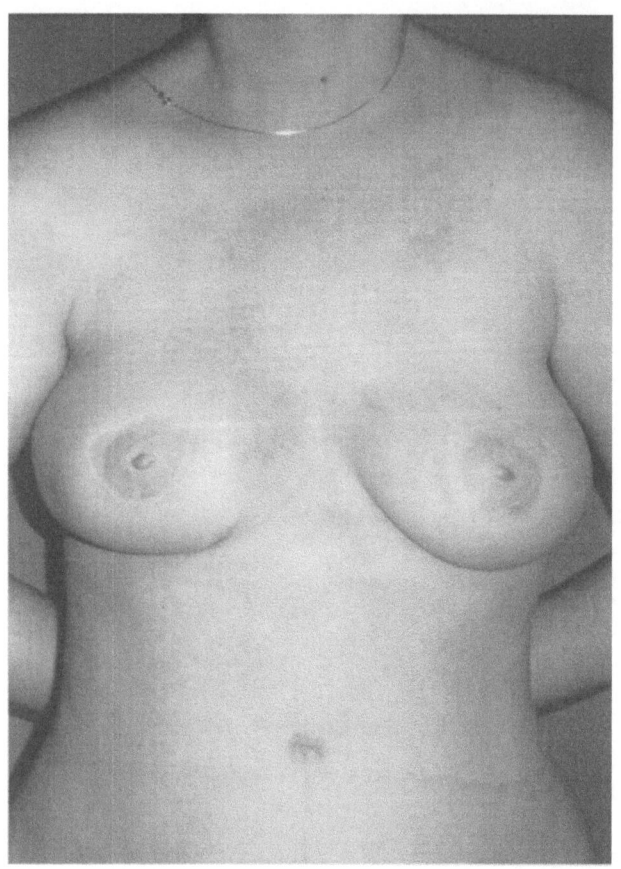

FIG. 8-1   Result of immediate breast reconstruction with a conventional TRAM flap.

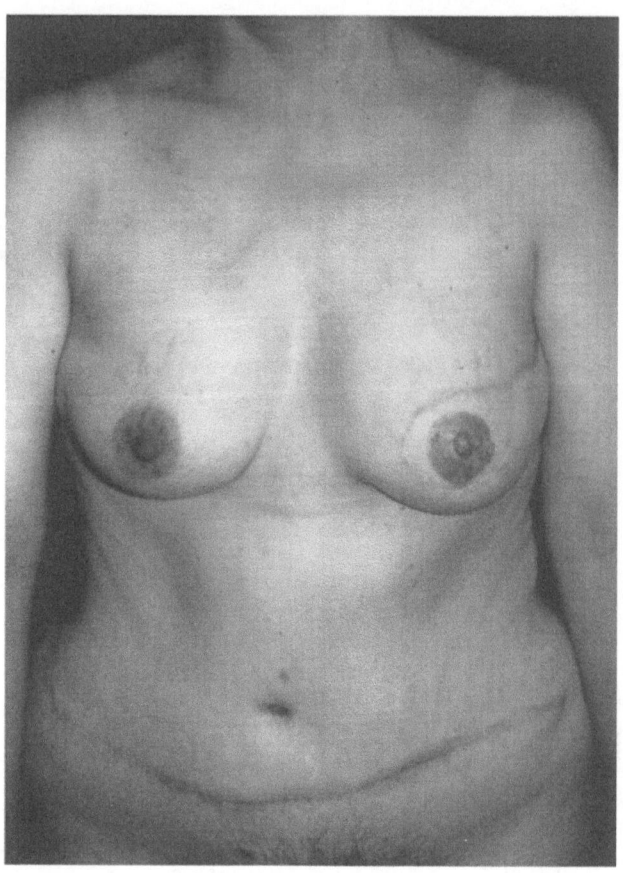

FIG. 8-2   Result of bilateral immediate breast reconstruction with conventional TRAM flaps. (From Kroll SS. *Plast Reconstr Surg.* 1994;94:637. Used with permission.)

ing" the flap[7] (performing an auxiliary microvascular anastomosis to supplement its blood supply), delaying it[8] (by performing a flap delay procedure), or using a double-pedicle technique.[9,10] Because of the CTRAM flap's less robust blood supply, partial flap necrosis and fat necrosis are more common than after a free TRAM flap. Because of partial flap loss and because the CTRAM flap cannot be manipulated as freely as a free flap, the aesthetic results tend not to be quite as good as those attainable with the free TRAM flap.[4]

The CTRAM flap requires sacrifice of much more muscle than the free TRAM flap does.[11] Consequently, postoperative pain is greater, and recovery from the surgery is slower. After recovery, patients who have had CTRAM flaps (especially bilateral ones) have a weaker abdomen than do those who have had free TRAM flaps and are less likely to be able to perform situps.[12] Also, a previous cholecystectomy or splenectomy may have divided the upper rectus abdominis muscle, precluding elevation of a CTRAM flap on that side.

In general, the free TRAM flap (discussed in detail in chapter 9) is more versatile and is preferable for most patients, provided the surgeon has the requisite equipment, help, and experience. Nevertheless, it must be clearly understood that the differences between the two methods are not great. The CTRAM flap remains an excellent technique and is capable of achieving outstanding results in properly selected patients.

Double-Pedicled TRAM Flap

For unilateral breast reconstruction, one way of improving a CTRAM flap's blood supply is to use two pedicles[9,10] (Fig 8-3). When both rectus abdominis muscles are used for one flap, the blood supply to that flap is essentially doubled. This modification reduces the incidence of partial flap and fat necrosis and facilitates successful breast reconstruction in patients who smoke.

Unfortunately, harvesting both rectus abdominis muscles in this way also greatly increases the donor site morbidity. Because twice as much muscle is sacrificed, the abdominal wall is significantly weakened. Only 27% of patients are subsequently able to perform situps. Because more fascia must be harvested, the abdominal closure is tighter and patients have more postoperative pain. Recovery from the surgery is more difficult and takes longer than after a single-pedicled flap. The use of synthetic mesh for reinforcement of the abdominal wall is more likely to be necessary, and postoperative hernias are more difficult to repair.

For these reasons, the double-pedicled CTRAM flap is no longer as popular as it once was and, in our institution, it is rarely, if ever, considered the method of choice.

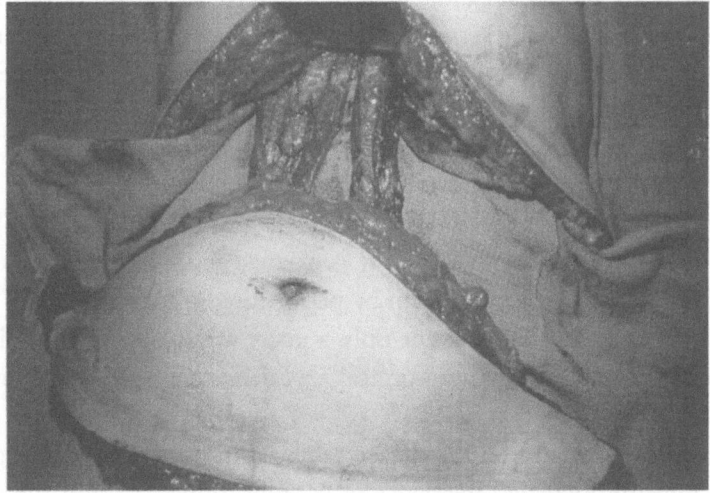

FIG. 8-3 Double-pedicled TRAM flap. Both rectus abdominis muscles are mobilized (and sacrificed), weakening the abdominal wall.

Delayed TRAM Flap

Another way to improve the blood supply to a CTRAM flap is to perform a flap delay.[8] By partially elevating the flap and by dividing the deep inferior epigastric artery and vein, blood flow through the superior epigastric vessels is increased. After 7 to 14 days, the TRAM flap can be elevated and transferred with a much reduced risk of partial flap loss.

Use of the delayed TRAM flap has the advantage of extending the usefulness of the CTRAM flap to patients who smoke. It has the disadvantage, however, of requiring an extra surgical procedure under general anesthesia. The flap delay also increases the duration of hospital stay, and increases expense. Finally, it destroys the option of "supercharging" the flap, should that prove to be necessary. For this reason, flap delay is not particularly popular with surgeons who have the capability of performing microvascular surgery, and I do not use it. It is an attractive option, however, for surgeons who rarely perform free flaps. For those surgeons, flap delay is believed to be a useful and effective strategy for improving the blood supply of the CTRAM flap.

Patient Selection

Patient selection is very important to the success of breast reconstruction with CTRAM flaps. The ideal patient is not obese but has sufficient abdominal fat to allow breast reconstruction without extending or folding the flap. She does not smoke[10] and has not smoked in the past. She has no upper abdominal scars that would interfere with flap elevation and no midline scars to prevent use of tissue across the midline. Patients who meet these criteria usually do quite well with a single-pedicled CTRAM flap, with good results obtained in most cases.

Patients who are not ideal candidates can also have successful reconstruction with CTRAM flaps, but it may be necessary to modify the technique. For current or former smokers, delaying the flap or supercharging can be very effective. For surgeons who are trained in microsurgery, supercharging the flap can be an ideal option. The surgeon raises the CTRAM flap in the usual way except that the deep inferior epigastric vessels are harvested with the flap (see following chapter). If after flap transfer the flap appears to have a good blood supply, the auxiliary pedicle is not used and the CTRAM flap is completed as usual. If the flap blood supply is deemed inadequate, however, the auxiliary pedicle can be used to rescue the flap by performing anastomoses with one or both of the thoracodorsal vessels. This is not only a good way to avoid complications, but also for surgeons without much microsurgical experience a way to learn how to do free TRAM flaps.

Although very successful results can be achieved in obese patients (Fig 8-4), these patients have a greatly increased incidence of complications,[10,13] and the time and effort required from the surgeon are increased. Consequently, extremely obese patients are not good candidates for TRAM flap breast reconstruction. Fortunately, such patients can be excellent candidates for extended latissimus dorsi flaps[14] (see chapter 12). The patient's obesity can be assessed by dividing the patient's weight in kilograms by

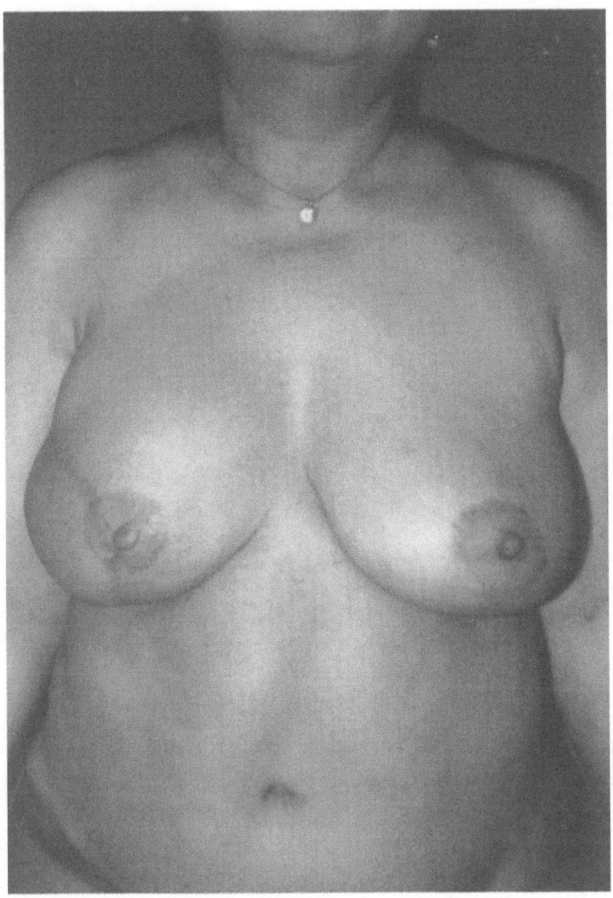

FIG. 8-4   Result of immediate conventional TRAM flap breast reconstruction in an obese patient. Despite the obesity, the result is good.

her height in meters to obtain a weight/height index. If this index is less than 50, the patient is usually accepted for a TRAM flap at our institution. If the index is greater than 54, the patient is rejected or advised to lose weight before a TRAM flap is considered. If the index falls between these two numbers, other considerations such as previous surgery, smoking, age, and general health are considered before a decision is made.

If the patient is unusually thin and does not have enough subcutaneous tissue to reconstruct a breast with a standard CTRAM flap, she may be considered for an extended free TRAM flap (see chapters 6 and 9).

Designing the Flap

The flap is designed with the patient in the standing position. The surgeon attempts to make the two sides of the flap symmetric. If possible, the lateral tips of the flap are placed adjacent to concavities in the patient's contour (Fig 8-5) to minimize postoperative formation of "dog-ears."

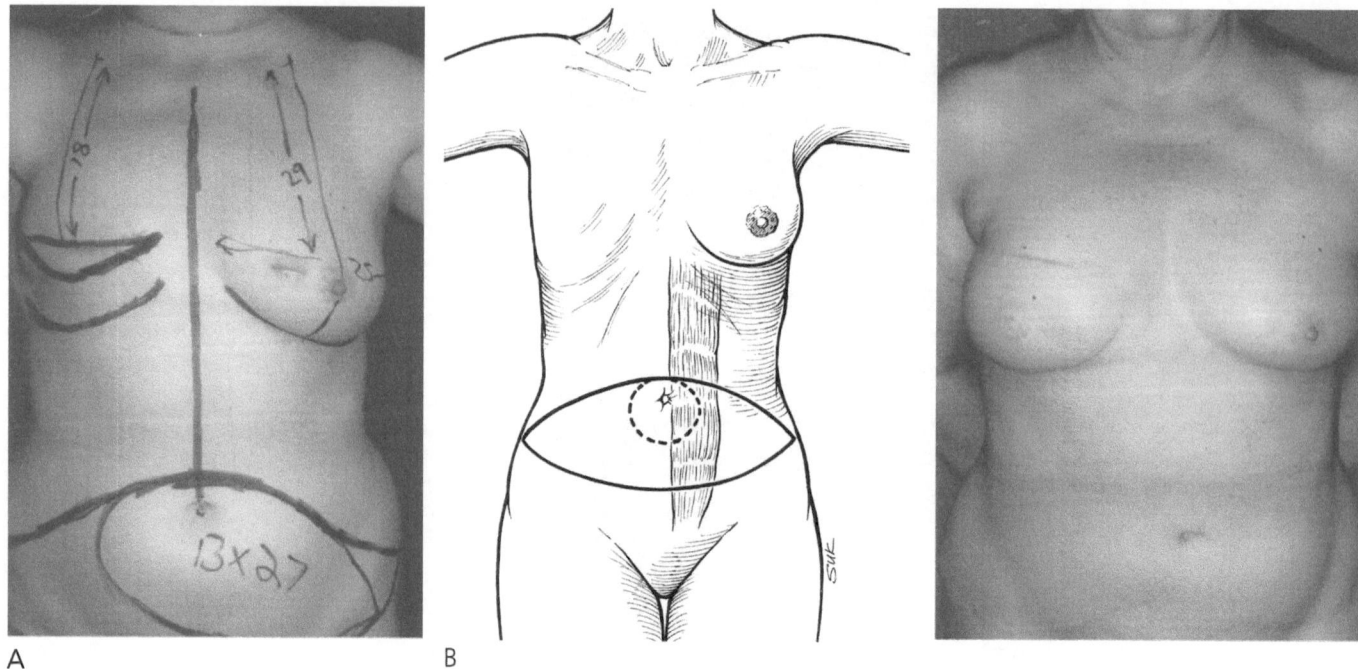

A   B

FIG. 8-5 (A) Design of conventional TRAM flap to be used for delayed breast reconstruction. (B) Dotted circle shows where the most important perforators are located. (C) Result of the reconstruction.

The flap pattern should maximally capture the "perforator area" near the umbilicus (surrounded by a dotted line in Fig 8-5B) where most perforating vessels from the rectus abdominis muscle enter the flap. For this reason, the upper border of the flap should be located just above the umbilicus. This creates a defect in the flap where the umbilicus was but reduces the amount of tissue inferiorly where blood supply is more precarious.

In a delayed breast reconstruction, because skin that overlies the "tunnel" in the epigastric region will be pulled inferiorly when the TRAM flap donor site is closed, the inframammary fold should be designed 2.5 cm higher than that of the contralateral breast. In an immediate reconstruction, the inframammary fold is not designed by the plastic surgeon, so this aspect of flap design is ignored.

Elevating the Abdominoplasty Flap

The first step in raising the TRAM flap is to dissect an abdominoplasty-type flap superiorly, exposing the rectus sheaths bilaterally and setting the stage for dissection of the tunnel that will connect the abdominal and chest wall dissections. In elevating this abdominoplasty flap, the surgeon must remember that its blood supply will come from lateral perforating vessels; therefore, if the dissection is too wide, abdominoplasty flap edge necrosis can occur in the midline. It is best to limit the initial dissection to only that portion of the flap overlying the rectus abdominis muscles (Fig 8-6). During skin

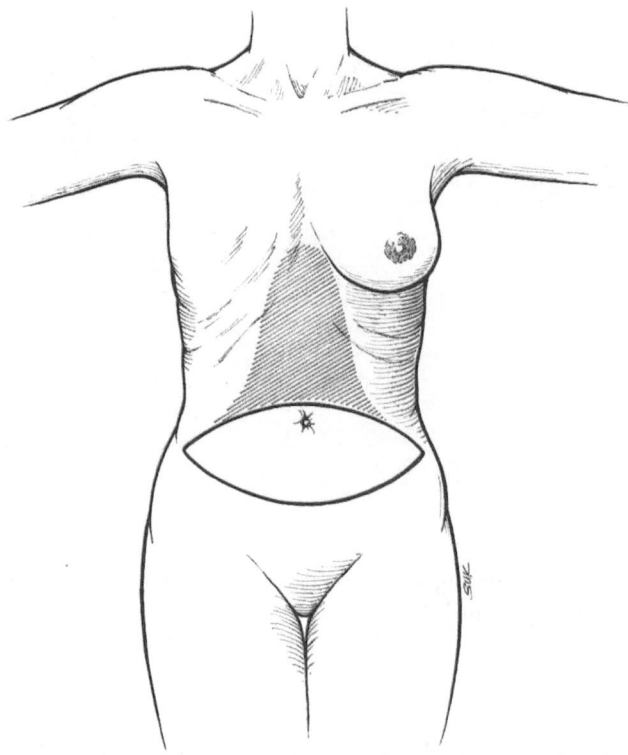

FIG. 8-6 In developing the abdominoplasty flap, only the shaded area (overlying the two rectus abdominis sheaths) should be undermined.

closure, provided that good capillary refill is present in the lower midline flap skin, additional dissection can be performed if necessary to facilitate the closure. It is not necessary, however, to release all abdominal tension lines by wide undermining since they will usually disappear spontaneously over time.

The flap should be raised in the plane between the subcutaneous fat and the fascia to allow good visualization of the fascia and facilitate its later repair. If fat is left on the fascia in an attempt to protect the rectus abdominis sheath from injury, subsequent repair will be more difficult and may be inaccurate, leading to possible errors and formation of a bulge or hernia.

Elevating the TRAM Flap

The TRAM flap is elevated on each side from lateral to medial, with the surgeon looking for the lateral row of perforating vessels entering the flap from the rectus abdominis sheath. I prefer to perform this dissection with electrocautery, which allows better visualization of the anatomy. Usually, a V-shaped split in the fascia (Fig 8-7) will be visible just lateral to each perforating vessel, allowing the vessels to be located without injuring them.

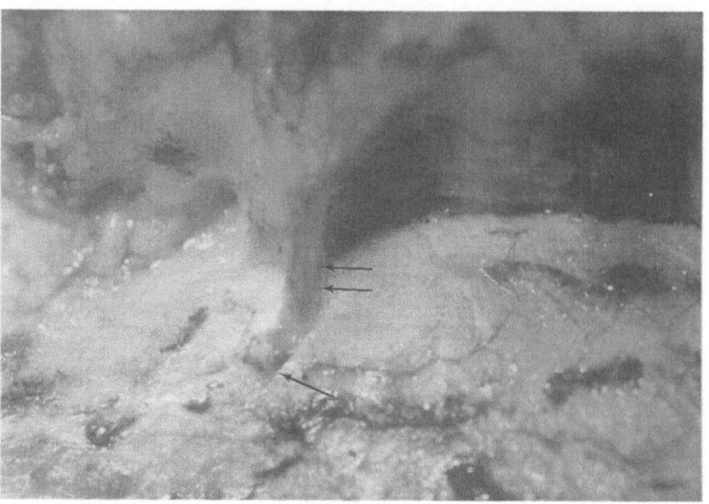

FIG. 8-7   Close-up of a perforating vessel (double arrows), showing the V-shaped split in the fascia (arrow) that is often present laterally.

The perforating lateral vessels almost always form a neat vertical row that curves medially as it progresses inferiorly (Fig 8-8). This relationship facilitates identification of all the perforators once the first one is located. In the CTRAM flap, all the perforators are generally included to maximize flap perfusion, although the most inferior one is actually expendable since it usually is not directly connected to the epigastric vascular system.

The rectus abdominis sheath is incised 2 or 3 mm lateral to the row of perforators on the side chosen to form the pedicle, and the fascia is reflected laterally to ex-

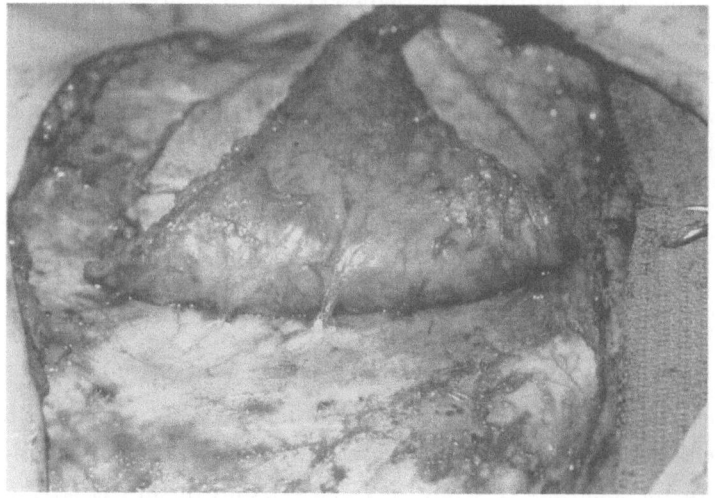

FIG. 8-8   Lateral row of perforators. This row is almost always present and forms a gently curved line.

pose the underlying muscle. The muscle is then harvested in its entirety or split, according to the preferences of the surgeon.

Splitting the Muscle

Harvesting the entire width of the rectus abdominis muscle is the easiest way to elevate a TRAM flap and provides the maximum blood supply to the flap. To do this, the surgeon simply dissects around the lateral border of the muscle, ligating and dividing the intercostal vessels and nerves as they enter the muscle laterally while the dissection proceeds superiorly.

It is possible, however, to leave much of the rectus abdominis muscle in situ, splitting the muscle and using only the central part of it to carry blood to the flap. Although there are no data to prove this, many surgeons (including myself) believe that this approach is less harmful to the donor site.

To split the muscle, I like to penetrate it with a hemostat approximately 1.5 cm lateral to the row of perforators and several centimeters below the umbilicus, gently spreading the hemostat and looking for blood vessels or underlying fascia (Fig 8-9). If blood vessels are encountered just beneath the tips of the hemostat, it is withdrawn and another try made more laterally. If fascia is seen, the muscle is grasped with a Babcock clamp (which is relatively atraumatic) on either side of the penetration. The muscle is then lifted up and a careful examination made of the area beneath it, looking for the deep inferior epigastric vessels. Palpation of the muscle between its deep and superficial surfaces can be useful in locating the deep inferior epigastric artery if it is not immediately visible.

Once the vessels are located, a decision about where to split the muscle is made. If a site different from the existing penetration is desired, a new penetration is made

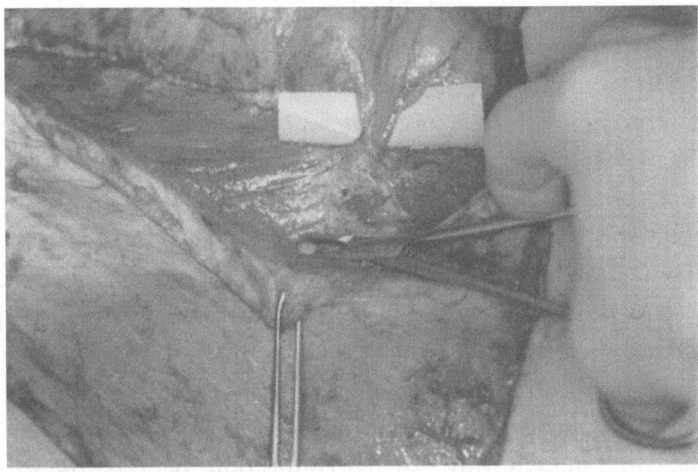

FIG. 8-9   Penetrating the muscle with a hemostat lateral to the perforators. This must be done gently to avoid bleeding.

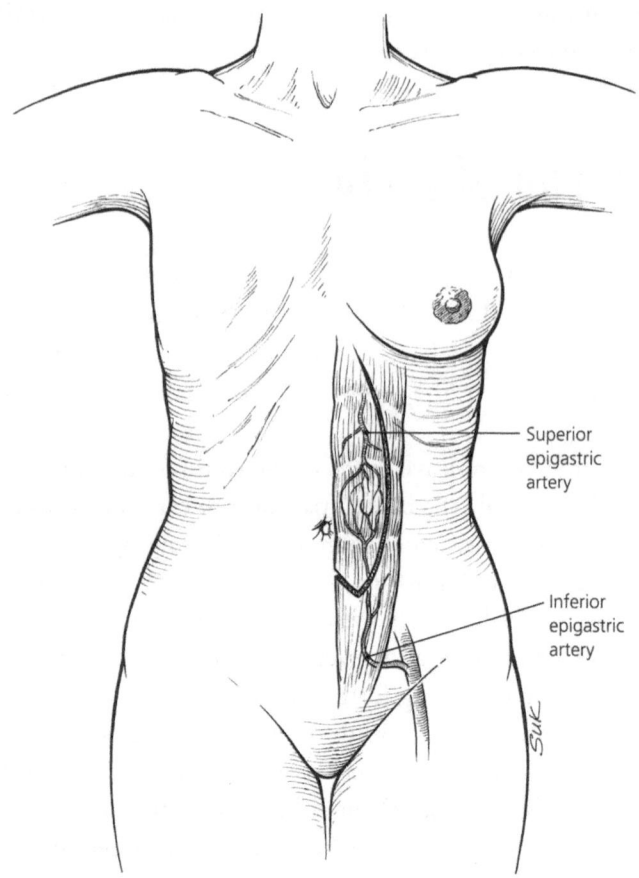

FIG. 8-10 Muscle-splitting incision. The muscle pedicle should be widest at the "choke area" just above the umbilicus, where the connections between the inferior and superior epigastric systems can consist only of capillaries.

with a hemostat. Otherwise, the existing opening is enlarged superiorly and inferiorly, obtaining meticulous hemostasis with bipolar electrocautery.

I prefer to dissect the deep inferior epigastric vessels all the way to their origin (as for a free TRAM flap; see chapter 9), harvesting them with the flap so that it can be "supercharged" if necessary. Other surgeons, especially those who do not perform microsurgery, may prefer to ligate and divide the vessels when they are first seen.

The muscle-splitting incision should curve laterally to widen the muscle pedicle almost to the full width of the muscle near the umbilicus, including more arteriolar connections between the inferior and superior epigastric systems (Fig. 8-10). Once this "choke area" is passed, the muscle pedicle can be narrowed again as it approaches the costal margin. After the dissection passes the costal margin, the muscular pedicle can be narrowed radically to minimize the epigastric bulge that would otherwise be present. The superior epigastric vessels should be identified where they exit between the xiphoid and the costal margin. Any vascular connections between the superior epigastric vessels and the costal marginal vessels must be divided if they interfere in any way with flap rotation, and visualizing the superior epigastric vessels makes that much easier and safer.

The preservation of muscle medially is of debatable benefit, since any preserved muscle will be denervated and nonfunctional. Nevertheless, many surgeons (including myself) do it. Before preserving muscle medially, however, the surgeon should locate the superior epigastric artery (by palpation with a finger or with a hand-held Doppler). A medial muscle-splitting incision should be made only after the vessels have been positively identified, because the benefits of medial preservation are questionable and justify only the most minimal of risks.

Creating the Tunnel

The surgeon must create a tunnel that is wide enough to allow free passage of the flap but is narrow enough to distort the inframammary fold only minimally. This can be accomplished by directing the tunnel more medially (in part under the opposite breast) and entering the pocket left by removal of the breast from the medial direction (Fig 8-11). A good rule of thumb is that the tunnel should be wide enough to allow passage of the surgeon's fist. If the flap is unusually large and a wider tunnel must be created that destroys the inframammary fold, the fold can be partially restored with sutures after the flap has been transferred. The tunnel should be left wide enough, however, to prevent any pinching or kinking of the flap pedicle.

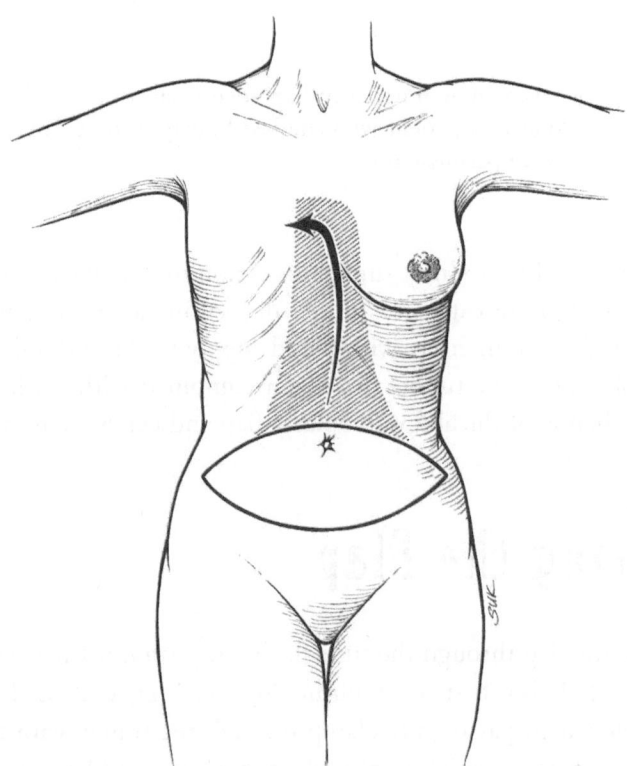

FIG. 8-11   Tunnel between the abdominal and breast pocket dissections. The tunnel should be central and should enter the breast pocket from the medial direction to avoid excessively disturbing the inframammary fold.

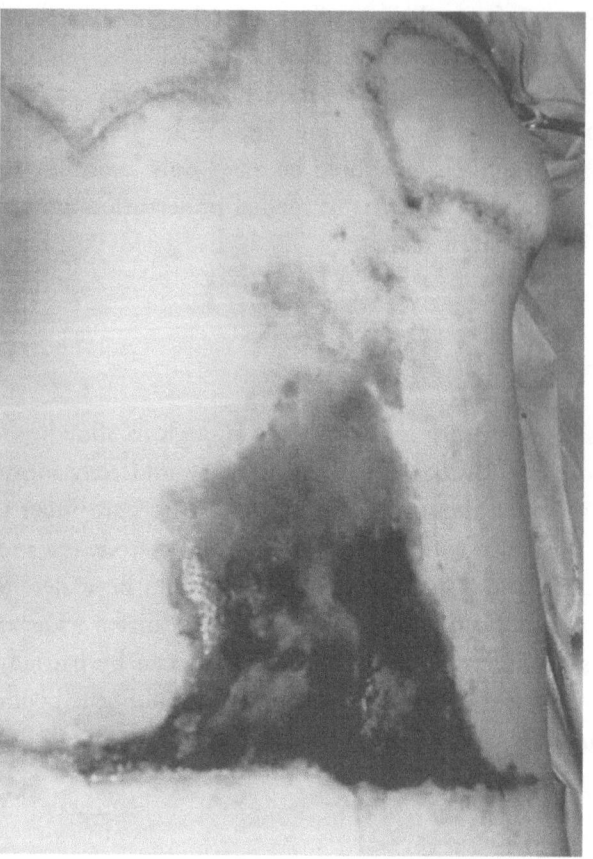

FIG. 8-12 Example of severe abdominoplasty flap edge necrosis after bilateral conventional TRAM breast reconstruction in a patient who smoked heavily. (From Kroll SS. *Plast Reconstr Surg.* 1994;94:637. Used with permission.)

The surgeon should try to limit tunnel dissection to only what is required for safe passage of the flap. A more extensive tunnel dissection not only deforms the inframammary fold but also can interfere with blood supply to the abdominoplasty flap. In patients who smoke, extensive tunnel dissection combined with a wide lateral dissection can lead to ischemia of the abdominoplasty flap and extensive necrosis (Fig 8-12).

Transferring the Flap

When transferring the flap through the tunnel, the surgeon must make certain that the pedicle is not twisted. This is best accomplished by attaching an Allis clamp to the contralateral flap tip and then passing the clamp through the tunnel with the flap trailing behind it. The surgeon uses a mixture of pulling, pushing, and back-and-forth rocking to pass the flap through. The clamp serves to orient the flap so that it is not inadvertently twisted and provides a handle for pulling the flap through the tunnel. If the tunnel is too tight, the flap is withdrawn and the tunnel enlarged before another attempt at flap transfer is made.

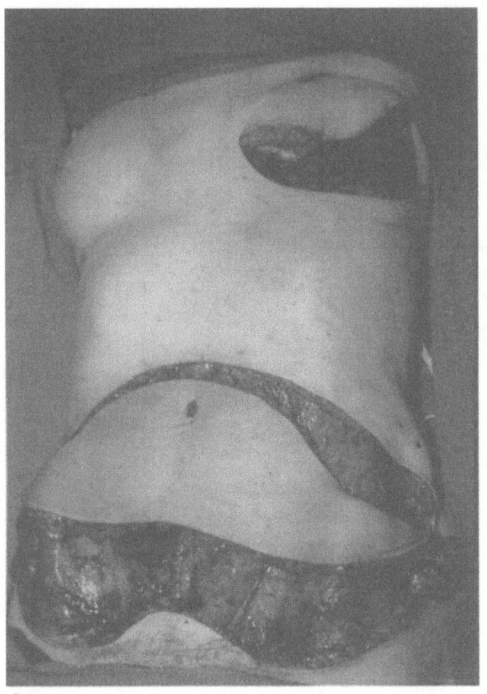 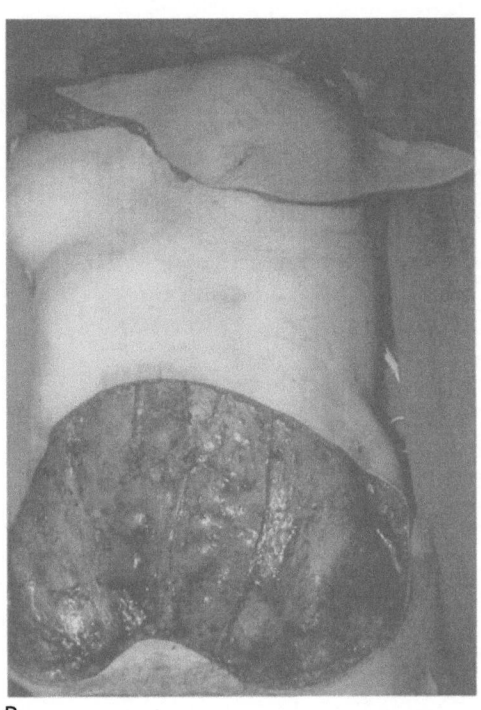

A   B

FIG. 8-13   (A) Double-pedicled CTRAM flap just prior to transfer. (C) The flap immediately after transfer through the tunnel between the abdomen and the breast.

After the flap has been transferred (Fig 8-13), the pedicle should be examined to make sure it is not kinked or otherwise impeded. If a vessel branch is restricting or kinking the pedicle, the branch should be clipped and divided.

Closing the Donor Site Defect

After the flap has been transferred, the next step is closure of the fascial donor site defect. This step is performed immediately after flap transfer to give the flap time to adjust to its new position before assessing its viability. Viability should be assessed after the donor site is repaired because a tight donor site closure can affect the pedicle and blood supply of the flap.

Fascial donor site repair is one of the most important parts of the TRAM flap operation. If the repair is performed incorrectly, an abdominal bulge or hernia will occur.[15] The key to a successful repair is to attach strong lateral fascia (internal oblique fascia) to strong media fascia (midline fascia deep to the linea alba) with strong sutures. Any fascial repair technique that does this will be successful.[16]

I prefer to attach the internal oblique fascia to the midline fascia with a running suture of No. 1 Novafil (polyethylene) (Fig 8-14). It is essential to make sure that each suture does in fact contain the fascia that is required. Laterally, the internal oblique fascia is visible, and the surgeon needs merely to identify it and include it in each stitch. Medially, to include the midline fascia deep to the linea alba, the point of the needle is in-

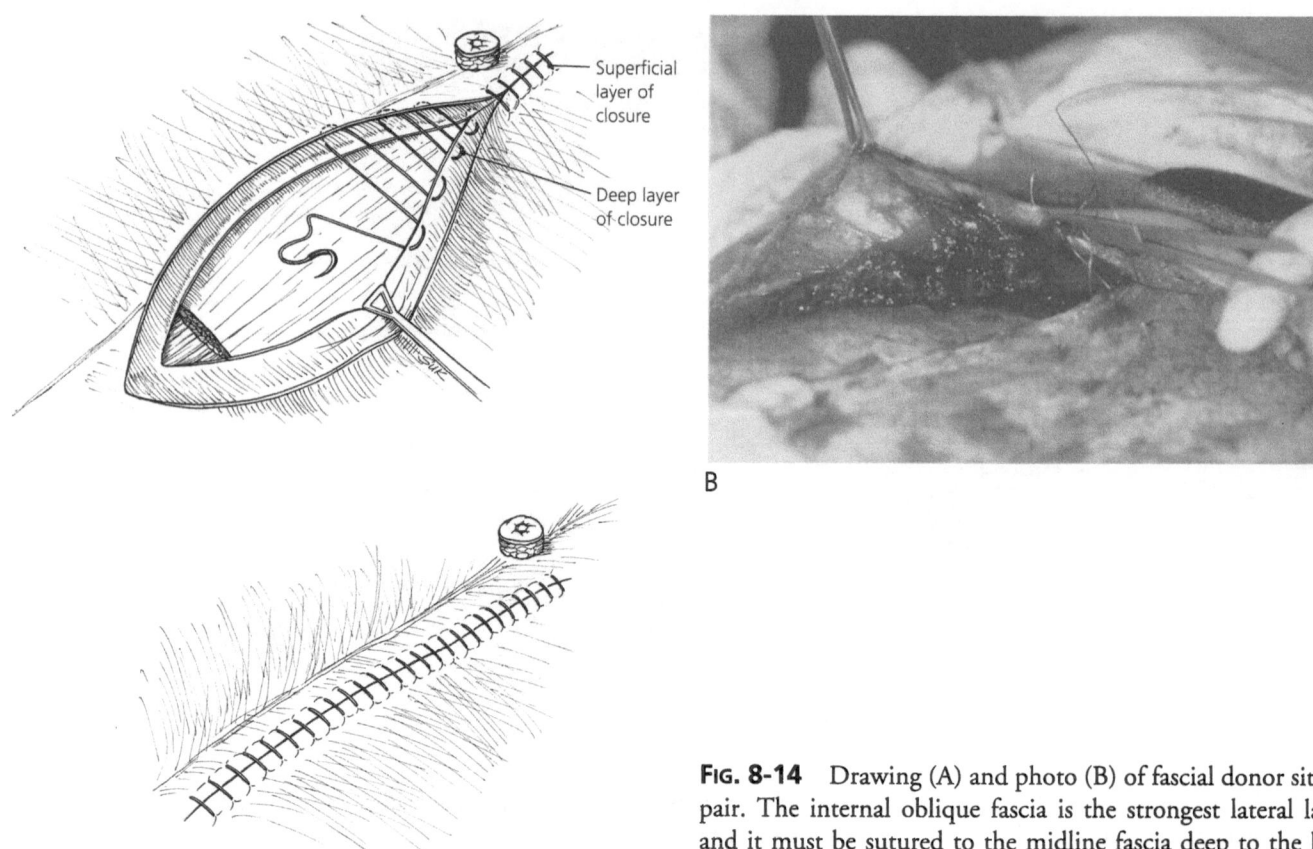

FIG. 8-14   Drawing (A) and photo (B) of fascial donor site repair. The internal oblique fascia is the strongest lateral layer, and it must be sutured to the midline fascia deep to the linea alba.

serted into the posterior rectus sheath close to its medial border and then exits from the anterior sheath. In that way, the medial reflection and the midline fascia should always be included. Even so, the quality of each suture bite should be tested for strength and security by tugging on the needle while it remains in the tissue. The fascial closure is continued superiorly until 1 or 2 cm below the xiphoid. The remaining anterior rectus abdominis sheath is then left open to allow unimpeded passage of the vascular pedicle.

After the running suture has been securely tied and the knot buried so that it will not be palpable through the skin, a second layer of No. 1 Novafil encompassing all layers of the rectus abdominis sheath is placed to reinforce the closure. A similar running suture is used on the contralateral side to plicate the fascia and move the umbilicus closer to the midline (Fig 8-15). Again, the knots should be buried.

After the fascial donor site defect has been closed, a suction drain is inserted in the abdomen and passed out through a small stab wound in the mons pubis. The table is then flexed and towel clips are used to close the abdominal wound temporarily.

For reconstruction of the navel, the umbilicus is located by palpation, and a new horizontal opening is made in the skin for it. It is best to limit this horizontal opening to 1.5 cm or less, to keep the reconstructed umbilicus inconspicuous. The towel clips are then released, and some fat is removed from the area under the new opening for the umbilicus. If the patient is at all obese, the fat in the midline is thinned with scissors to simulate the presence of a median raphe. Hemostasis is then obtained with electrocautery. Next, the umbilicus is tacked over to the midline with a 3-0 Vicryl (poly-

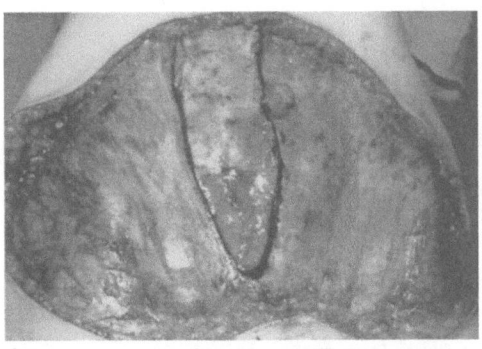

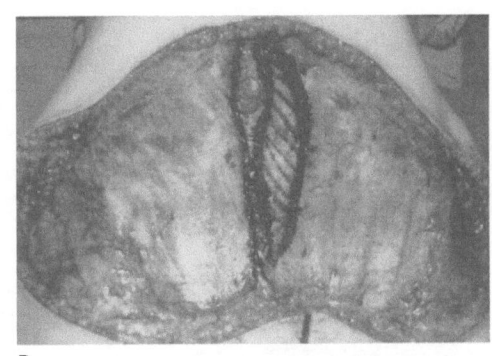

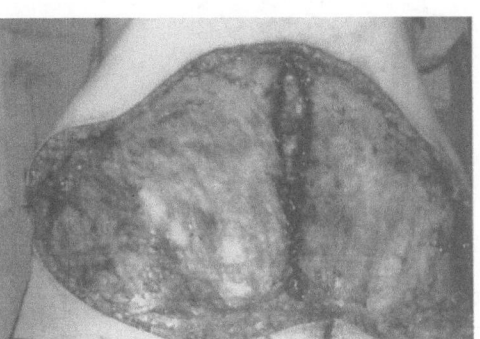

FIG. 8-15 (A) Fascial defect from a single-pedicled CTRAM flap. (B) After closure of the fascial defect, a plan for plication of the contralateral side is drawn with methylene blue dye. The plication should extend superiorly as far as the xiphoid. (C) After the plication, the umbilicus has been brought back almost to the midline.

galactin 910) suture, and three sutures are placed to attach the umbilicus to the deep fascia and to the skin (Fig 8-16). These sutures, when they are eventually tied, will invert the umbilicus, making it less conspicuous and giving it an illusion of normalcy.

With the table still flexed, excess fat is trimmed and Scarpa's fascia is then repaired with interrupted sutures of 2-0 Vicryl. As in an abdominoplasty, the abdominal flap may need to be advanced medially to reduce the lateral dog-ears. If dog-ears are present despite this, the incisions are extended laterally, and additional skin is removed until the dog-ears are fully corrected. It is important to correct the dog-ears completely because this is far easier to do in the operating room than it will be later on in the clinic and because despite wishful thinking, the dog-ears rarely will disappear spontaneously.

The skin is then closed with buried dermal sutures of 3-0 Vicryl and with running subcuticular sutures of 3-0 Prolene (polypropylene). The previously placed umbilical sutures are tied, and the remaining umbilical wound is repaired with 4-0 chromic sutures.

Trimming the Flap

After the flap is transferred, it is trimmed to the approximate size required. It is then loosely inset, and additional trimming is performed until the volume of the opposite breast is matched as closely as possible. For the flap to remain viable, the surgeon should see bright red bleeding from all flap edges immediately after they are trimmed. If only dark blood is seen initially, even if the bleeding turns a brighter red later, the flap will

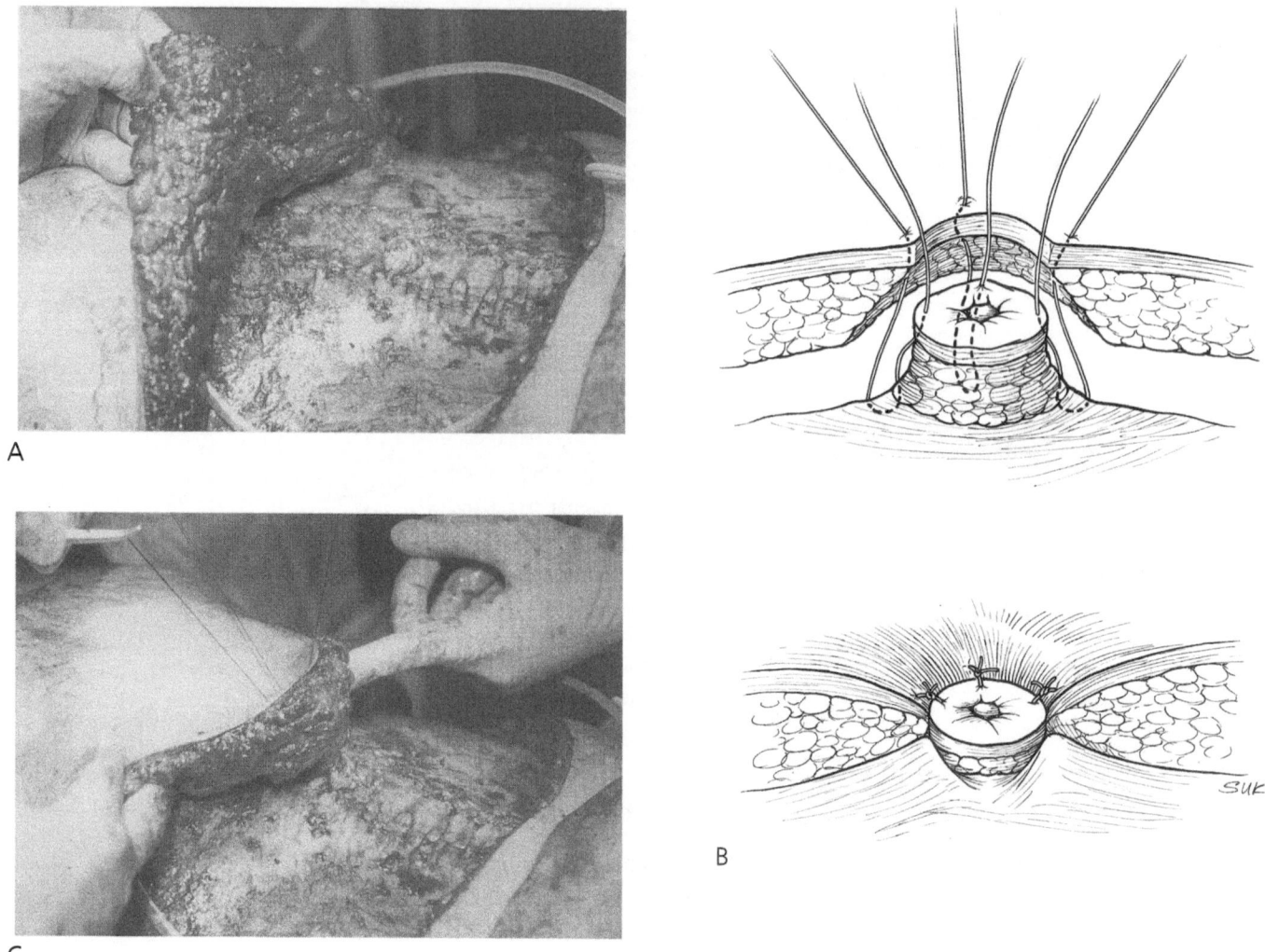

FIG. 8-16 (A) Umbilical tacking sutures are used to invert the umbilicus and attach it to the deep fascia to make it less conspicuous. (B) Sutures have been placed but not tightened. (C) As the sutures are tightened, the abdominal skin surrounding the umbilicus is drawn down to the fascia.

probably not survive in its entirety and supercharging will be necessary to achieve a successful outcome.

Supercharging the Flap

"Supercharging" of the TRAM flap is here defined as augmenting the flap's blood supply by performing auxiliary microvascular anastomoses[7] between the deep inferior epigastric vessels and either the internal mammary vessels or branches of the subscapular vascular system (see chapter 9). Supercharging is possible only if the deep inferior epigastric vessels have been elevated with the flap. In my practice, I routinely harvest these vessels whenever I perform a CTRAM flap because I have found it impossible to predict preoperatively which flaps will need to be supercharged.

Supercharging is effective in salvaging a poorly perfusing CTRAM flap and is also good training for surgeons who wish to progress to the use of the free TRAM flap. It is not always necessary to perform anastomoses of both the artery and the vein. If only a venous recipient vessel is available (a situation that may occur after a radical mastectomy, when the only available recipient vessel may be the axillary vein), a venous anastomosis may be enough to effectively rescue the flap. Success in this situation can be gauged by a return to normal color and bright red bleeding from the flap edges after the venous anastomosis has been completed. If both a recipient artery and vein are available, however, I generally perform an anastomosis to each vessel, since the microscope and instruments have already been mobilized and the extra time required to perform the second anastomosis is therefore minimal.

Since I began performing free TRAM flaps, I have found that my tolerance for marginally adequate flap perfusion has decreased, and I find myself supercharging most of the (few) CTRAM flaps that I still do. I have never been sorry that I supercharged a CTRAM flap but there are several flaps that I did not supercharge that I wish I had.

Insetting the Flap

Once the flap has been successfully transferred and the blood supply has been deemed adequate, the flap is shaped and sutured to the edges of the surrounding defect as described in chapters 16 through 18. The tunnel should then be checked to make sure that the pedicle is not twisted or pinched. If the inframammary fold has been excessively released, sutures are placed to restore it medially, with care taken to avoid compromising the flap pedicle. A suction drain is then placed in the axilla. I close the skin with buried dermal 3-0 Vicryl sutures, and then a running subcuticular 3-0 prolene suture; but any suitable skin closure technique can be used.

The most important points in finishing the CTRAM flap are to achieve the proper shape and volume and to be sure that the flap perfusion is adequate. If the surgeon suspects that the flap perfusion is insufficient, flap supercharging should be performed if at all possible to minimize the risk of flap necrosis and to avoid compromising the result.

Summary

The CTRAM flap was the first truly successful method of autologous tissue breast reconstruction and remains a very acceptable alternative for patients who are in good health, do not smoke, and are not excessively obese. It is the best choice for surgeons who do not perform microvascular surgery or who are in environments where the free TRAM flap is not practical. For patients who smoke, the CTRAM flap should be augmented in some way to increase flap blood supply—either by delaying the flap, using two pedicles, or supercharging it.

The CTRAM flap can be highly successful in creating a soft, natural-looking breast mound. All the good that results, however, can be spoiled if an unrepairable abdominal wall hernia occurs. Prevention is the best cure. Only the fascia that is required to maintain flap blood supply should be harvested, and no more. A secure repair that attaches the internal oblique fascia to the strong midline fascia deep to the linea alba should be performed with a heavy (No. 1) permanent running suture. If this is done, abdominal wall hernias will be rare and can be easily corrected when they do occur, and unfortunate outcomes of TRAM flap surgery will be uncommon.

References

1. Hartrampf CR Jr, Scheflan M, Black PW. Breast reconstruction with a transverse abdominal island flap. *Plast Reconstr Surg.* 1982;69:216–224.
2. Elliott LF, Hartrampf CR Jr. Tailoring of the new breast using the transverse abdominal island flap. *Plast Reconstr Surg.* 1983;72:887–893.
3. Hartrampf CR Jr, Bennett GK. Autogenous tissue reconstruction in the mastectomy patient: a critical review of 300 patients. *Ann Surg.* 1987;205:508–518.
4. Kroll SS, Coffey JA Jr, Winn RJ, Schusterman MA. A comparison of factors affecting aesthetic outcomes of TRAM flap breast reconstruction. *Plast Reconstr Surg.* 1995;96:860–864.
5. Kroll SS, Evans GRD, Reece GP, et al. Comparison of resource costs of free and conventional TRAM flap breast reconstruction. *Plast Reconstr Surg.* 1996;98:74–77.
6. Boyd JB, Taylor GI, Corlett R. The vascular territories of the superior epigastric and the deep inferior epigastric systems. *Plast Reconstr Surg.* 1984;73:1–14.
7. Harashina T, Sone K, Inoue T, et al. Augmentation of circulation of pedicled transverse rectus abdominis musculocutaneous flaps by microvascular surgery. *Br J Plast Surg.* 1987;40:367–370.
8. Codner MA, Bostwick J, Nahai F, Bried JT, Eaves FF. TRAM flap vascular delay for high-risk breast reconstruction. *Plast Reconstr Surg.* 1995;96:1615–1622.
9. Ishii CH, Bostwick J, Raine TJ, Coleman JJ, Hester TR. Double-pedicle transverse abdominis myocutaneous flap for unilateral breast and chest-wall reconstruction. *Plast Reconstr Surg.* 1985;76:901–907.
10. Wagner DS, Michelow BJ, Hartrampf CR Jr. Double-pedicle TRAM flap for unilateral breast reconstruction. *Plast Reconstr Surg.* 1991;88:987–997.
11. Grotting JC, Urist MM, Maddox WA, Vasconez LO. Conventional TRAM flap versus free microsurgical TRAM flap for immediate breast reconstruction. *Plast Reconstr Surg.* 1989;83:842–844.
12. Kroll SS, Schusterman MA, Reece GP, Miller MJ, Robb GL, Evans GRD. Abdominal wall strength, bulging, and hernia after TRAM flap breast reconstruction. *Plast Reconstr Surg.* 1995;96:616–619.
13. Kroll SS, Netscher DT. Complications of TRAM flap breast reconstruction in obese patients. *Plast Reconstr Surg.* 1989;86:886–892.
14. McCraw JB, Papp C, Edwards A, McMellin A. The autogenous latissimus breast reconstruction. *Clin Plast Surg.* 1994;21:279–288.
15. Hartrampf CR Jr. In discussion: Drever JM, Hodson-Walker N. Closure of the donor effect for breast reconstruction with rectus abdominis myocutaneous flaps (discussion). *Plast Reconstr Surg.* 1985;76:563.
16. Kroll SS, Marchi M. Comparison of strategies for preventing abdominal-wall weakness after TRAM flap breast reconstruction. *Plast Reconstr Surg.* 1992;889:1045–1053.

9 Free TRAM Flap

Advantages of the Free TRAM Flap

Since 1991, the free transverse rectus abdominis myocutaneous (TRAM) flap has become the most popular method of breast reconstruction at The University of Texas M. D. Anderson Cancer Center because it has a low failure rate and minimal donor site morbidity, and achieves aesthetically successful results in a high proportion of cases.[1,2] Compared with some of the alternative autologous tissue flaps, the free TRAM flap is technically simple and can be executed fairly quickly. It can be used in the overwhelming majority of patients, and for patients who are suitable candidates, the free TRAM flap is almost always the first choice.

Compared to the conventional TRAM (CTRAM) flap,[3,4] the free TRAM flap requires less sacrifice of donor site muscle (Fig 9-1) and therefore weakens the abdomen less. It does not require sacrifice of any muscle from the upper abdomen, so donor site pain is reduced and recovery is easier and more rapid. Patients return to work earlier and are more likely to be able to do abdominal exercises when their convalescence has been completed.

The free TRAM flap has a better blood supply than the CTRAM flap[5] and is less likely to suffer from partial flap loss or fat necrosis. Because of the better blood supply, the surgeon can be more aggressive about folding, trimming, or otherwise shaping the free TRAM flap. Moreover, secondary revision is easier because the main blood supply to the flap comes from above so that standard breast reduction techniques can be used to reshape the breast mound. Consequently, the aesthetic results tend to be better with the free TRAM flap, although the results of CTRAM flap breast reconstruction in selected patients can be quite good.

Disadvantages of the Free TRAM Flap

The free TRAM flap also has some disadvantages. It does require microvascular anastomoses, with all the requirements for adequate training, experience, and equipment that entails. If an anastomosis fails, the blood supply to the flap is lost and unless the

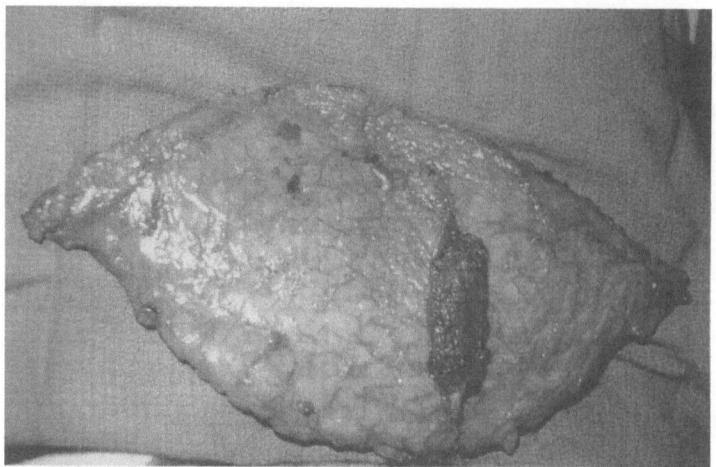

FIG. 9-1   Pedicle of a free TRAM flap. Only a minimal amount of muscle tissue has been sacrificed. (From Kroll SS. *Clin Plast Surg.* 1998;25:251–259. Used with permission.)

problem is quickly corrected, the flap will not survive. Emergent exploration of the pedicle of a free TRAM flap is therefore occasionally necessary, sometimes (inconveniently) in the middle of the night. Despite salvage attempts total loss of the flap can occur and is more common with the free TRAm flap (1%)[6] than with a CTRAM flap (0.5%) (unpublished results).

To maintain high success rates, the free TRAM flap should be monitored postoperatively, which requires effort and expense. When flaps must be returned to the operating room for salvage, additional expense is incurred. Because of this, the free TRAM flap is more expensive in resource costs than the CTRAM flap,[7] although the difference is not great (less than 5%).

Patient Selection

Virtually all patients who are candidates for any type of TRAM flap are candidates for free TRAM flap breast reconstruction. Because of the flap's excellent blood supply, a history of smoking is not by itself a contraindication to a free TRAM flap. Although patients who smoke have a higher incidence of necrosis of secondary flaps (such as the umbilicus or the abdominoplasty and mastectomy flaps),[8] the necrosis is usually minor and generally heals without additional surgery. Abdominoplasty flap necrosis after a free TRAM flap is less common (as well as of lesser degree) than after a CTRAM flap, probably because there is no need to dissect a tunnel to connect the abdominal and breast pocket dissections, a tunnel that is particularly wide and potentially troublesome in bilateral CTRAM flap reconstruction.

The only patients who should not have a free TRAM flap are (a) those who are so obese that any type of TRAM flap is contraindicated (those whose weight in kilograms divided by height in meters [weight/height index] is greater than 54),[9] (b) those

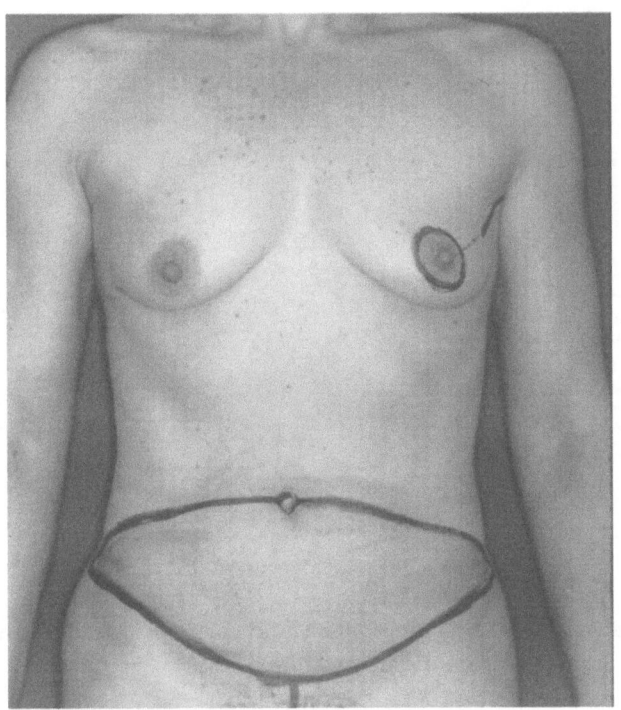

FIG. 9-2   Design of a free TRAM flap breast reconstruction. The surgeon tries to hide the lateral dog-ear in a concavity, if possible.

with a potbelly habitus, and (c) those who have had previous TRAM flap or abdominoplasty and therefore lack the requisite tissue for harvest of a TRAM flap.

Designing the Flap

The design of the free TRAM flap is virtually identical to that of a CTRAM flap. The surgeon tries to hide any lateral dog-ear that will be present after closure of the flap donor site in a concavity, if one is present (Fig 9-2). As in the CTRAM flap, the contralateral muscle is ordinarily used as the pedicle, giving the flap the transverse orientation on the chest wall (Fig 9-3) that best mimics the shape of a normal mature breast.

If a vertical infraumbilical midline scar is present, the flap should be designed approximately 6 cm higher than the usual pattern to include some unscarred midline skin above the umbilicus. This will usually allow sufficient perfusion across the midline to allow most of the flap to survive, permitting a successful reconstruction (Fig 9-4). The resulting abdominal donor site scar will be higher and more difficult to conceal, but most patients consider this an acceptable price for achieving a symmetrical breast mound reconstruction.

If the patient has had a previous abdominoplasty, TRAM flap breast reconstruction is precluded. If she has had only a "miniabdominoplasty," however, reconstruction with a TRAM flap may still be possible. Review of the previous operative note should

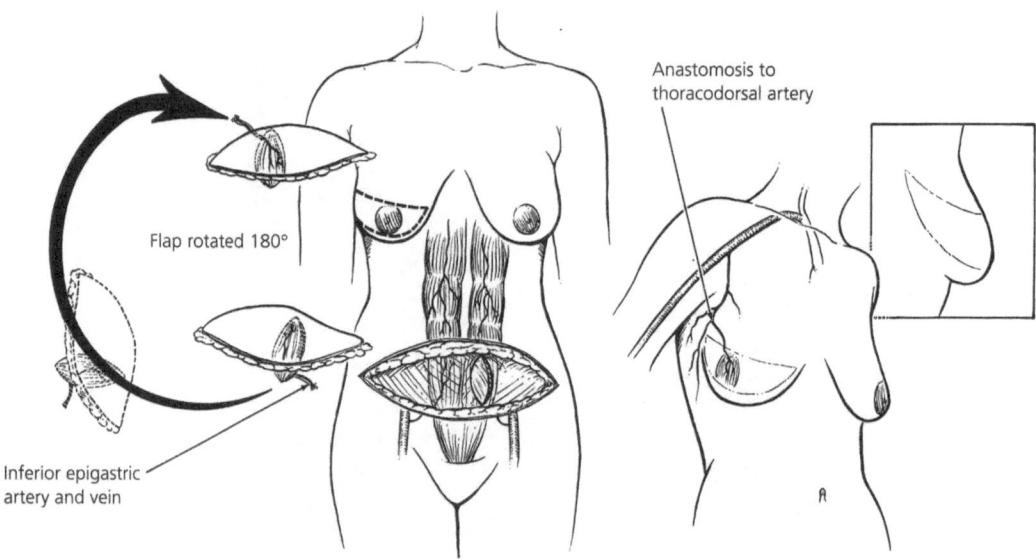

FIG. 9-3 The contralateral rectus abdominis muscle is used as a pedicle. This gives the flap a horizontal orientation that mimics the contour of a mature breast.

be performed to ensure that perforating blood vessels have not been transected above the umbilicus. The flap must be harvested from the midabdominal region, and careful preoperative evaluation for the presence of perforators should be performed. If perforators are found, however, the reconstruction can be successful (Fig 9-5). Again, the abdominal donor site scar will be higher than usual, and the patient must be made aware of that preoperatively.

Elevating the Abdominoplasty Flap

The first step in raising the free TRAM flap is to dissect an abdominoplasty-type flap superiorly, in a fashion similar to that used in the CTRAM flap but stopping just short of the xiphoid. As in the CTRAM flap, the dissection should be confined to the area overlying the rectus abdominis muscles (Fig 9-6) to avoid compromising the blood supply to the abdominoplasty flap. During skin closure, provided that good capillary refill is present in the lower midline flap skin, additional dissection can be performed if necessary to facilitate the closure. It is not necessary, however, to release all abdominal tension lines by wide undermining since they will usually disappear spontaneously over time.

In more obese patients, beveling of the incision at the superior edge of the TRAM flap is useful not only to increase flap volume but also to improve the match in thickness between the normally thicker abdominoplasty flap and the abdominal layer at the inferior edge of the donor site (Fig 9-7). As in the CTRAM flap, the dissection should be in the plane between the subcutaneous fat and the fascia to allow good visualization of the fascia and facilitate its later repair.

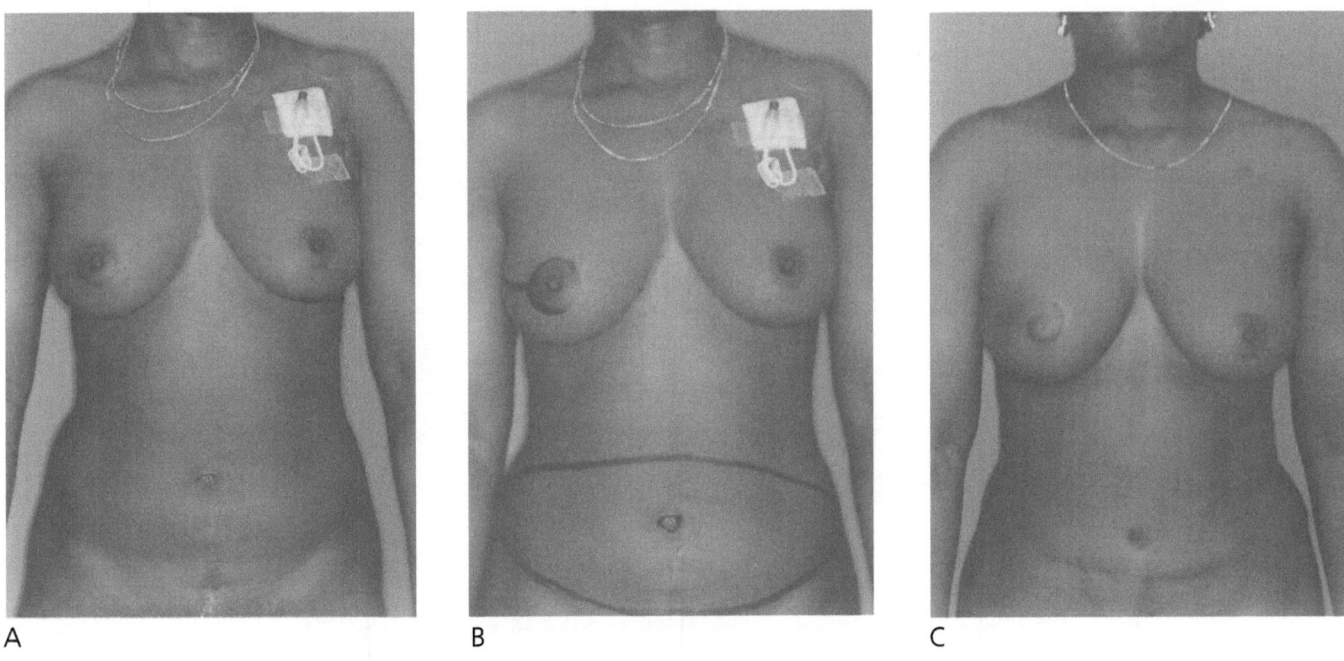

A   B   C

FIG. 9-4   (A) Patient with a vertical midline infraumbilical scar requesting immediate breast reconstruction. (B) Plan for a TRAM flap designed higher than usual to include unscarred midline skin above the umbilicus, which will improve flap perfusion across the midline. (C) Result of free TRAM flap reconstruction and one revision, prior to areolar tatooing.

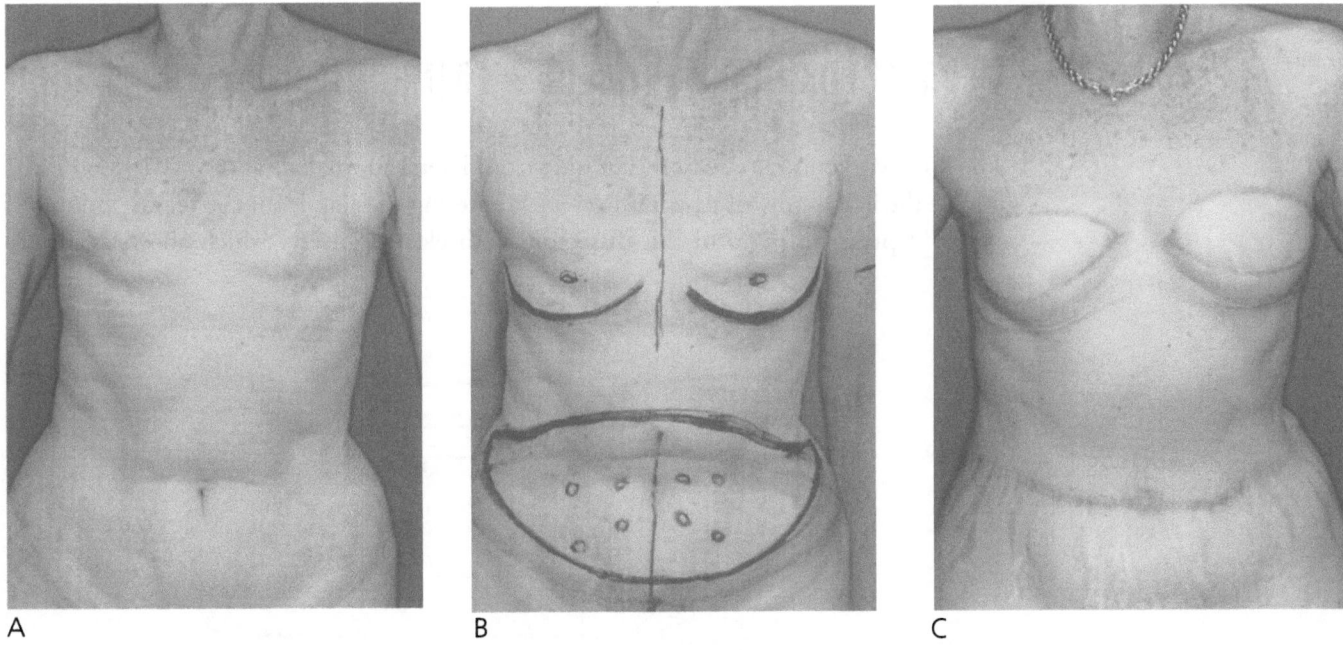

A   B   C

FIG. 9-5   (A) Patient who has had a previous miniabdominoplasty. The perforators normally used for nourishing a TRAM flap have been destroyed. (B) Plan for the TRAM flap. Perforators have been located and mapped out, and the flap has been designed at a higher level. (C) The early result, before any revision or nipple reconstruction. Flap transfer was successful and there was no fat necrosis.

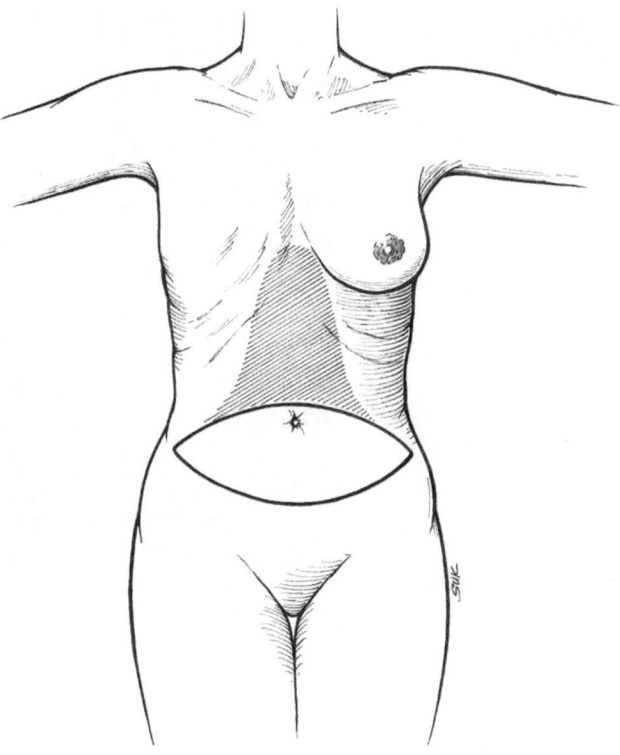

FIG. 9-6 The abdominoplasty flap dissection should be confined to the area overlying the rectus abdominis muscles, to avoid interrupting lateral perforators and reducing its blood supply.

Elevating the TRAM Flap

The TRAM flap is elevated on each side from lateral to medial, with the surgeon looking for the lateral row of perforating vessels entering the flap from the rectus abdominis sheath. I prefer to perform this dissection with electrocautery, which allows better vi-

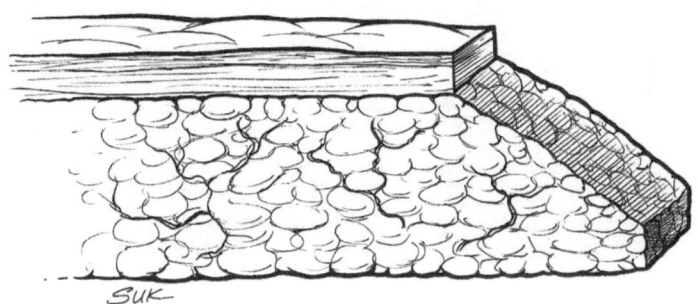

FIG. 9-7 Drawing of the superior edge of the TRAM flap incision (cephalad is to the right). In all but thin patients, the superior TRAM flap incision should be beveled to increase the tissue volume of the TRAM flap and to better match the abdominoplasty flap to the lower abdominal wall skin.

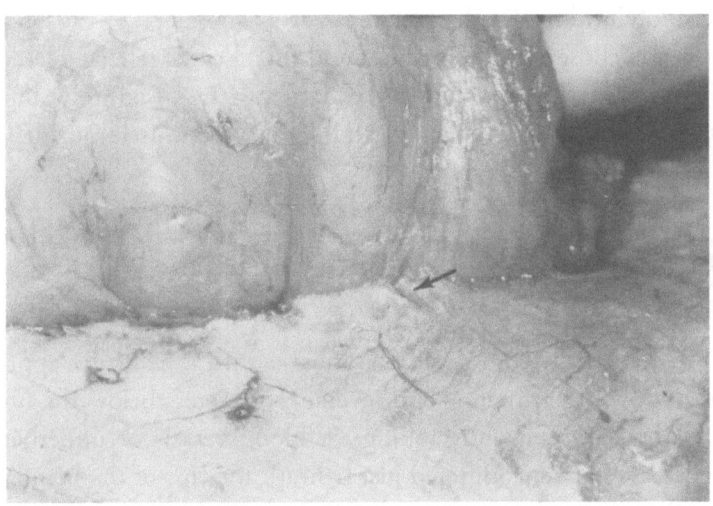

FIG. 9-8   A V-shaped split (arrow) is often present in the fascia just lateral to the perforators, helping to identify them.

sualization of the anatomy. Usually, a V-shaped split in the fascia (Fig 9-8) will be visible just lateral to each perforating vessel, allowing the vessels to be located without injuring them.

The perforating lateral vessels almost always form a neat vertical row that curves medially as the row progresses inferiorly (Fig 9-9). The relationship facilitates identification of all the perforators once the first one is located. In a unilateral free TRAM flap, all the perforators are generally included to maximize flap perfusion, although the most inferior one is expendable since it usually does not connect with the inferior epigastric vascular system.

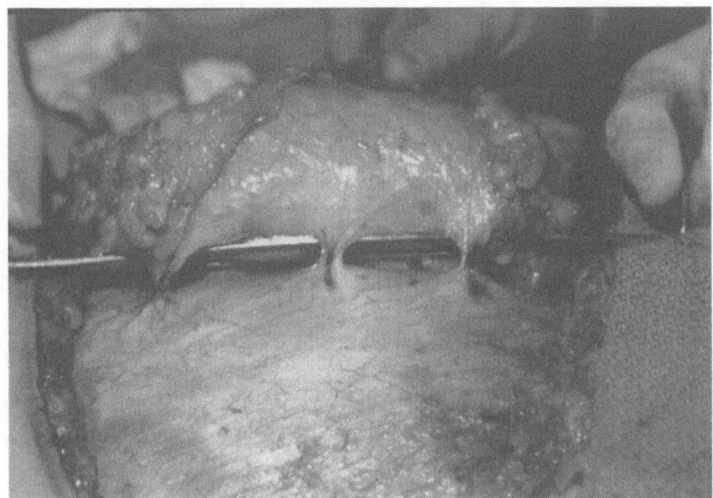

FIG. 9-9   Usually, the lateral perforators form a vertical row that gently curves medially toward the inferior part of the flap.

The rectus abdominis sheath is incised 2 or 3 mm lateral to the lateral row of perforators on the side chosen for the pedicle, and the fascia is reflected laterally to expose the underlying muscle. The muscle can be harvested in its entirety, but my personal preference is to split it (at least laterally) and leave some muscle in situ.

Splitting the Muscle

As in the CTRAM flap, I like to split the muscle with a hemostat approximately 1.5 cm lateral to the row of perforators and several centimeters below the umbilicus, carefully spreading the hemostat and looking for blood vessels or underlying fascia (Fig 9-10). If blood vessels are encountered just beneath the tips of the hemostat, it is withdrawn and another try made more laterally. If fascia is seen, the muscle is grasped with a Babcock clamp (which is less traumatic than an Allis clamp) on either side of the penetration. The muscle is then lifted up and a careful examination made of the area beneath it, looking for the deep inferior epigastric vessels. Palpation of the muscle between its deep and superficial surfaces can be useful in locating the deep inferior epigastric artery if it is not visible.

Once the vessels are located, a decision is made about where to split the muscle. If a site different from the existing penetration is desired, a new penetration is made with a hemostat. Otherwise, the existing opening is enlarged superiorly and inferiorly, obtaining meticulous hemostasis with bipolar electrocautery.

I prefer to dissect the deep inferior epigastric vessels all the way to their origin, making the pedicle as long as possible. This makes the anastomoses easier because the longer pedicle makes it easier for the surgeon to orient the vessels in a way that makes performance of the anastomoses comfortable. The additional length also facilitates sub-

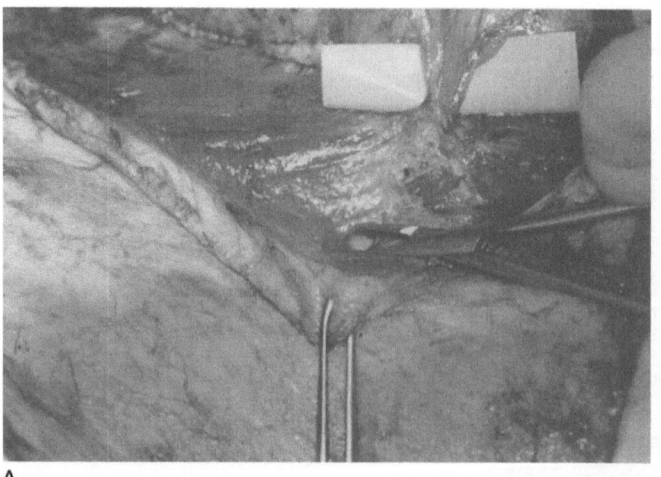
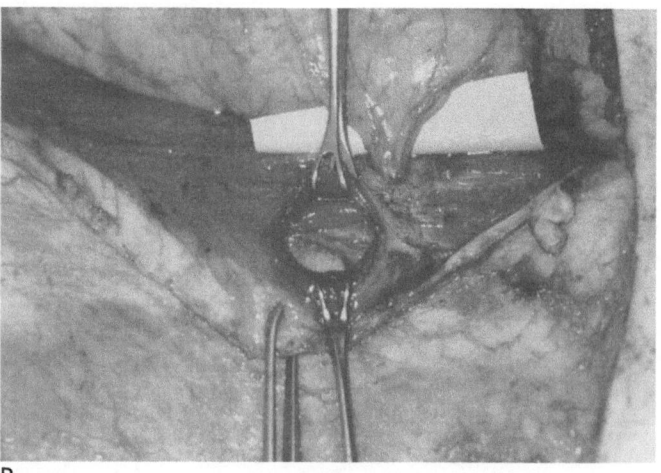

A   B

FIG. 9-10   (A) Gently splitting the rectus abdominis muscle vertically with a hemostat, the surgeon looks for the white fascia beneath the muscle. If blood vessels are encountered instead, the hemostat is withdrawn and another try made more laterally. (B) The muscle is grasped with Babcock clamps and lifted and separated so that the blood vessels can be identified.

sequent positioning of the flap on the chest wall as medially as necessary to get the best possible aesthetic result. Moreover, when the deep inferior epigastric vessels are dissected more inferiorly, they get larger as well as longer, providing larger caliber vessels for easier anastomoses.

Once the vascular dissection has been completed and the surgeon is certain that the pedicle is intact, the flap is elevated on the contralateral side. I prefer to wait until the vascular pedicle has been safely dissected before elevating the opposite side of the flap, because if the flap's pedicle is injured during its dissection the opposite side can then still be used in its stead. Elevating the contralateral side of the flap prior to pedicle dissection makes the pedicle dissection technically easier, but eliminates any chance of using the opposite deep inferior epigastric vessels to perform the free tissue transfer should that be necessary.

After the opposite side of the flap has been elevated, but before dividing the rectus abdominis muscle above the flap, the recipient vessels in the axilla or on the chest wall are exposed (see below) and examined. If they are adequate, a decision is made to proceed with free transfer of the flap. If they are not adequate, the flap can still be converted at this point to a CTRAM flap and the operation completed as described in chapter 8.

Committing to a Free Tissue Transfer

After the donor and recipient vessels have been examined and found adequate, the rectus abdominis muscle is divided above the flap in its middle third, eliminating the possibility of conversion to a CTRAM flap. The opposite side of the TRAM flap is then dissected off the deep abdominal fascia past the midline, exposing the most medial ipsilateral perforating vessels. This dissection must be done very carefully because these medial perforators are more difficult to visualize than the lateral ones and injury to them is more likely. The rectus abdominis sheath is then incised just medial to the most medial of the larger perforators (smaller ones are ignored), exposing the muscle beneath. A small amount of this medial fascia should be preserved if possible to facilitate subsequent closure of the fascial defect. If desired, a large amount of the fascia can be preserved as was described in chapter 8. Doing so will reduce the tension on the fascial closure and significantly reduce postoperative pain, but is dependent on the use of the anterior rectus abdominis sheath close to the midline, where it is weaker, in the closure.

The muscle is separated from the deep surface of the rectus abdominis sheath and the distribution of blood vessels on its undersurface examined. If the vessels all enter the muscle in its middle third and if there are no significant medial perforators along the medial edge of the muscle, some of the medial muscle can be preserved. This is especially likely to be possible if relatively large perforators are present in the lateral row. Medial muscle preservation should have a low priority, however, since the muscle will almost certainly be denervated and therefore nonfunctional. Muscle should be preserved medially only if the surgeon is fairly certain that blood supply to the flap will not be significantly compromised as a result.

Once the flap has been elevated sufficiently that the only remaining attachment is the vascular pedicle (Fig 9-11), the flap is secured to the surrounding tissue with staples (so that inadvertent traction will not be applied to the vascular pedicle) and is left to perfuse in situ while attention is turned to the recipient site.

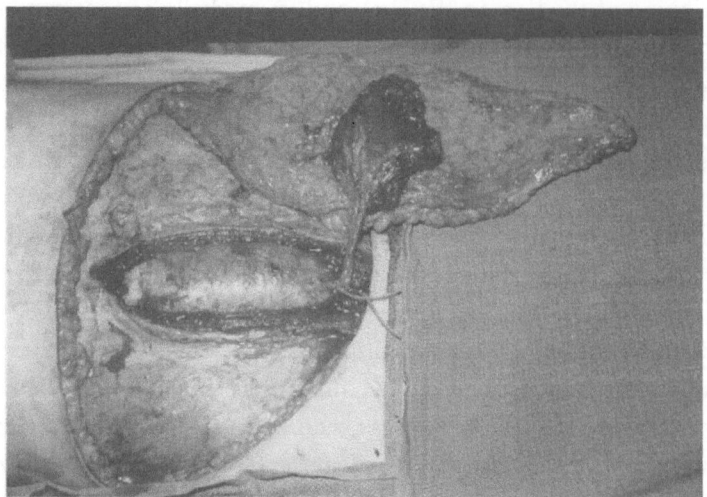

FIG. 9-11 Flap attached to the abdomen only by the deep inferior epigastric vessels, where it is left to perfuse in situ.

Choosing and Preparing the Recipient Vessels

At M. D. Anderson Cancer Center, the most commonly used recipient vessels for free TRAM flap breast reconstruction are the thoracodorsal artery and vein. In immediate reconstruction, they are the obvious choice because they are usually exposed by the oncologic surgeon during the course of an axillary dissection (Fig 9-12). In delayed breast reconstruction, the thoracodorsal vessels must be dissected out of the surrounding scar tissue, which sometimes can be difficult. Nevertheless, because of our familiarity with these vessels and because they are almost always satisfactory, we often use them.

Subscapular Vascular System

Anatomic details vary from patient to patient, but every patient has a subscapular artery and vein, which usually give off the circumflex scapular vessels and continue as the thoracodorsal vessels (Fig 9-13). The thoracodorsal vessels, in turn, each give off a large serratus branch; after this, they usually become too small to use for anastomosis to the deep inferior epigastric vessels.

In most patients, the best place to perform an anastomosis is on the thoracodorsal vessels just above the serratus branch. Here, the vessels are still of adequate size and yet long enough to allow a comfortable anastomosis and a pedicle that is not under tension when the flap is positioned on the chest wall. In some patients, the thoracodorsal vessels will be unusually small and not suitable for connection with the deep inferior epigastric vessels. In that situation, there may be a more suitable circumflex scapular branch that can be used instead. The surgeon should be flexible, and use whichever ves-

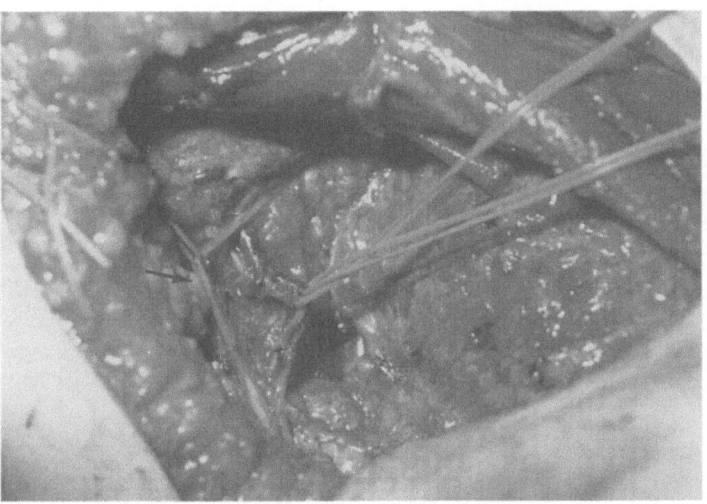

FIG. 9-12.   Axilla after axillary dissection, with the thoracodorsal vessels exposed. Placing a vessel loop around the thoracodorsal nerve (arrow) and displacing it away from the vessels greatly facilitates the vascular dissection.

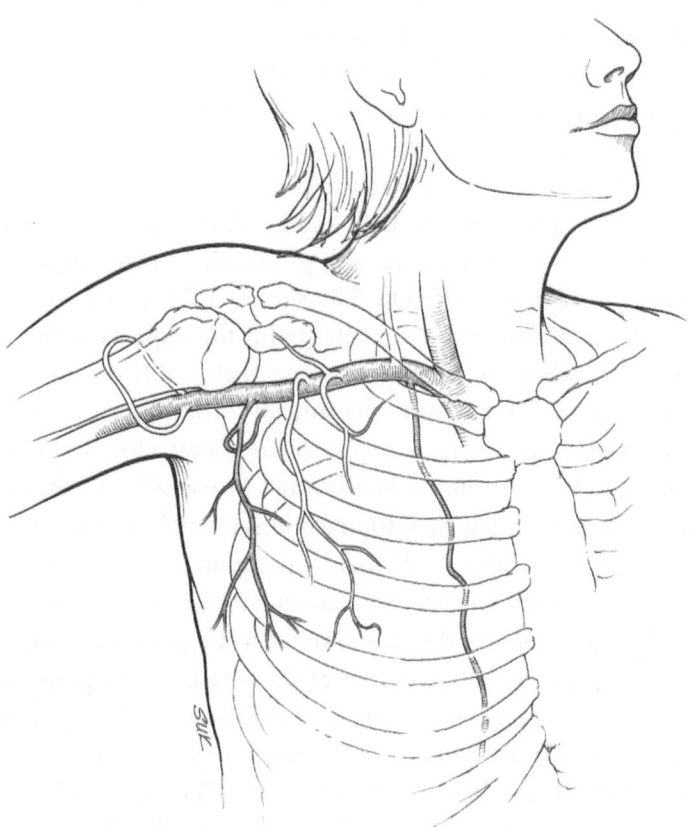

FIG. 9-13.   Anatomy of the subscapular vascular system.

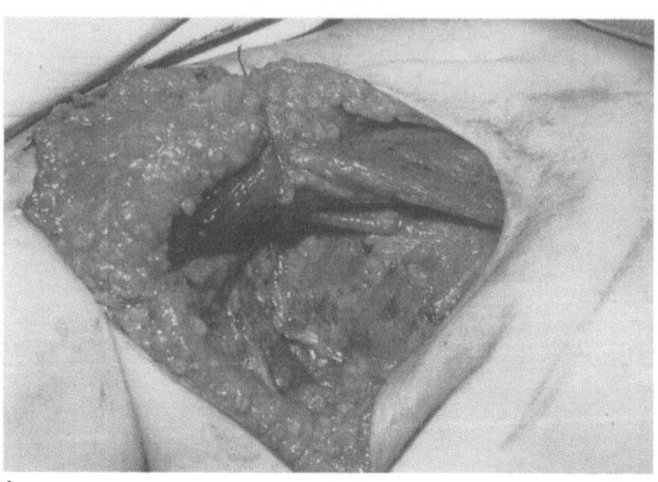
A

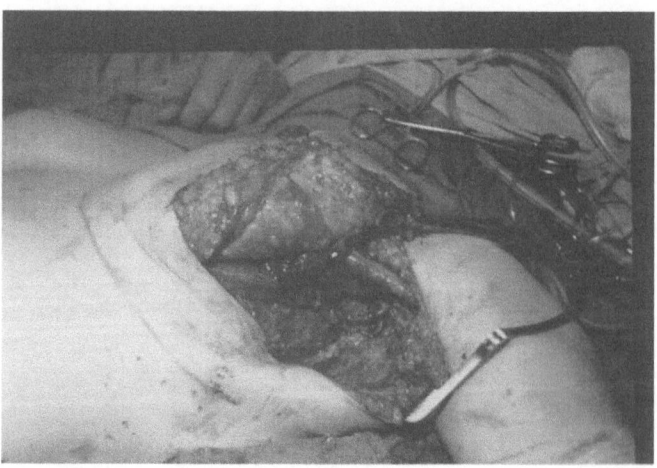
B

FIG. 9-14   (A) Retracting sutures hold the skin and pectoralis major muscle out of the way without interposing a metal retractor between the surgeon and the anastomotic site. (B) An Adson-Beckman retractor provides excellent exposure of the thoracodorsal vessels, but can interfere with anastomosis, so I rarely use it.

sels seem to be most appropriate. It is important to remember, however, that the vessels are usually in spasm after their dissection and may appear to be much smaller than they truly are. Before making a decision about which vessels to use as recipients, the surgeon should apply a few drops of 2% papaverine solution to the surface of the vessels. After 15 minutes, they will often increase dramatically in size as the spasm is released, and thus become suitable for their intended use.

The first step in dissection of the subscapular system vessels is to place retracting sutures of 2-0 Vicryl (polygalactin 910) in the pectoralis major muscle and the skin (Fig 9-14A). This provides exposure of the field and minimizes the need for mechanical retractors (Fig 9-14B), which can interfere with positioning of the surgeon's hands, making the anastomosis itself more difficult. The sutures that retract the pectoralis major muscle medially and superiorly are especially useful for improving the view of the assistant, who will be standing on the opposite side of the table during the anastomoses. Because of the importance of exposure, the surgeon should place as many of these sutures as are necessary to gain adequate access to the thoracodorsal vessels.

The thoracodorsal vessels should be dissected proximally at least as far as the circumflex scapular branches so that they (thoracodorsal vessels) can be rotated anteriorly. This part of the dissection is often facilitated by (temporary) placement of a Whitlander retractor to spread the tissues immediately adjacent to the vessels (Fig 9-15). The anterior rotation of the vessels allows the anastomoses to be performed superficially in the axilla, rather than deep in a hole. Dissection of the vessels is best performed with loupe magnification (I use 4.5 power) and is facilitated by placing vessel loops around the artery, vein, and nerve to retract and separate them. Avoiding all but the most minimal traction on the artery will reduce the problem of spasm. Hemostasis is accomplished with bipolar electrocautery, small hemoclips, and ligatures of 4-0 silk. When the dissection has been completed, a folded moist gauze sponge forms a platform for the anastomosis, along with a piece of colored plastic material to serve as a background (Fig 9-16).

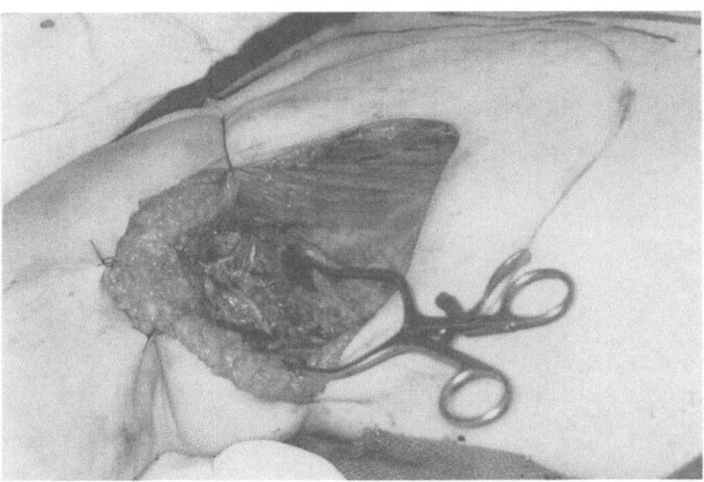

FIG. 9-15   A Whitlander retractor can be helpful in dissecting the vessels. Before beginning the anastomosis, however, the retractor is removed.

Once the dissection of the recipient site is completed, the vessels are tied off just above the serratus branch, placed in temporary atraumatic microvascular (Ackland) clamps, and divided. The operating microscope is brought into the field, and the vessel ends are prepared for anastomosis by removing the distal adventitia. The operating table is tilted away from the surgeon and toward the surgical assistant (Fig 9-17), improving the assistant's view of the axilla. If additional retraction sutures are required to pull the pectoralis major muscle more medially, they are placed at this time.

Removal of the adventitia is useful for several reasons. First, this vessel preparation allows the surgeon to position (and reposition) the microscope and other equip-

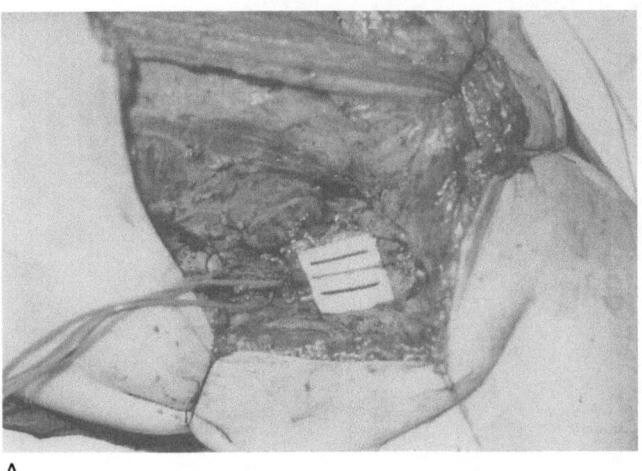

A

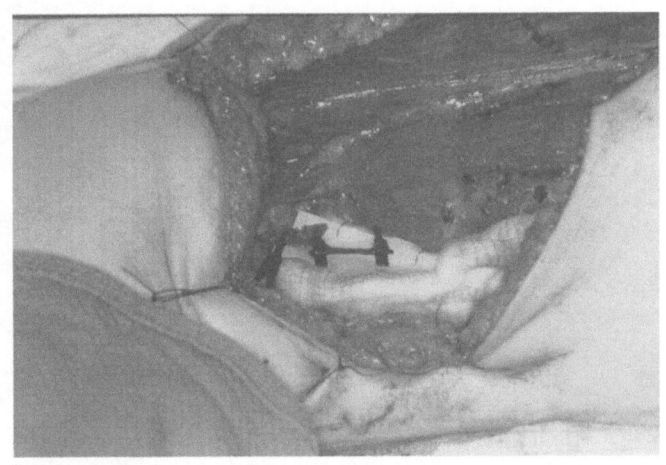

B

FIG. 9-16   (A) A neurosurgical cottonoid sponge soaked with 2% papaverine has been placed over the recipient vessels. After 15 minutes, all traces of vascular spasm are usually resolved. (B) A folded gauze sponge forms a platform for the vessels so that the anastomosis can be performed more superficially. A piece of colored plastic forms a good background.

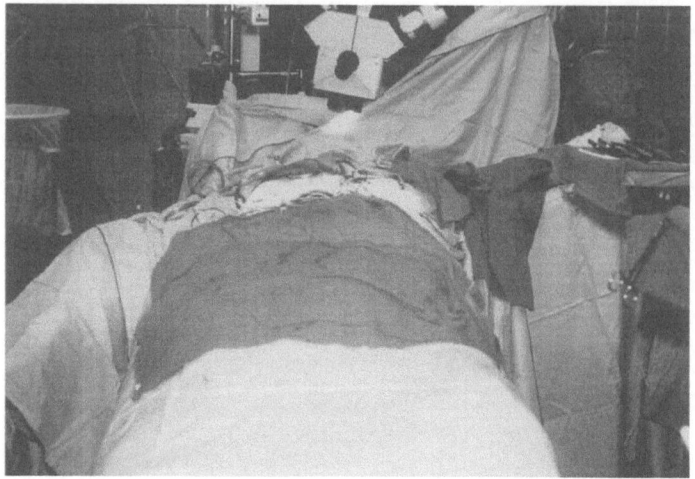

FIG. 9-17   The operating table is tilted away from the surgeon so that the assistant, who stands across the table between the patient's shoulder and head, can see into the axilla.

ment to achieve a comfortable arrangement while the flap is not yet ischemic and there is therefore no urgency to complete the anastomosis. During this exercise, towels are placed to support the surgeon's forearms and hands (Fig 9-18), and the microscope head direction is adjusted until the most comfortable arrangement is found.

Second, removal of the adventitia near the anastomosis facilitates identification of tiny cut or avulsed vascular branches that are constricted and may not bleed immediately following the anastomosis but can cause serious trouble later. These small branches, if not identified and closed off with sutures, can lead not only to subsequent hematomas but also to vascular spasm and eventual thrombosis.

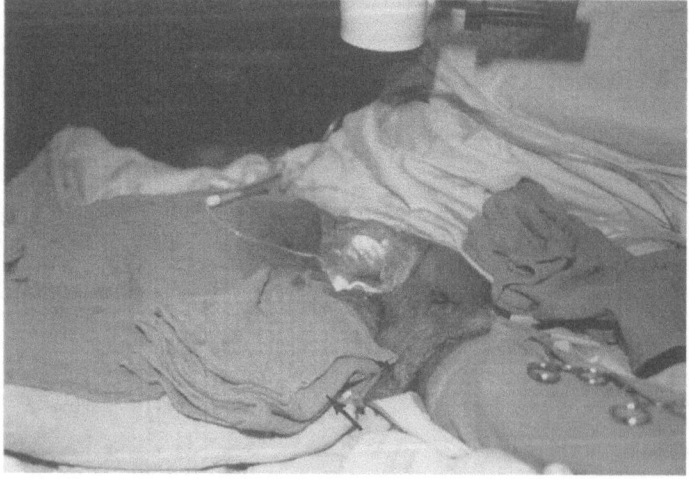

FIG. 9-18   Sterile cloth towels (arrow) are placed below the axilla to support the surgeon's forearms and wrists. This improves precision and reduces tremor. (The flap is in the axilla, to the right of the towels.)

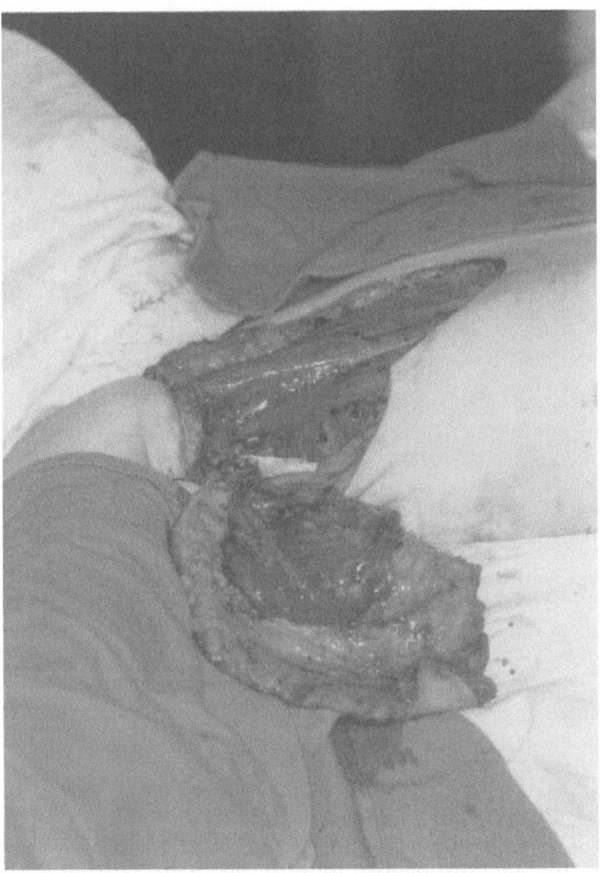

FIG. 9-19   The flap is brought into the axilla and fixed to the patient or the drapes with towel clips.

Finally, removal of the adventitia makes tying the knots in the microvascular sutures easier and avoids the possibility of adventitia getting trapped inside the lumen of the vessel during the anastomosis.

After preparation of the recipient vessels, the flap is harvested by ligating the deep inferior epigastric vessels at their origin with 2-0 silk. The flap is then brought into the axilla and fixed to the patient or to the drapes with towel clips in preparation for the anastomoses (Fig 9-19). The vein is examined to make sure that it is not twisted, and the anastomoses are performed as described below.

Internal Mammary Vessels

An alternative to the thoracodorsal vessels is the internal mammary vessels, which are preferred by some surgeons[10–15] and can be especially useful when irradiated scar tissue in the axilla makes dissection of the subscapular vascular system difficult. The internal mammary vessels are usually unaffected by previous surgery and therefore are free of surrounding scar. They also have the advantage of placing the flap more medially, where the most well vascularized portion of the flap can be used to form the breast (Fig

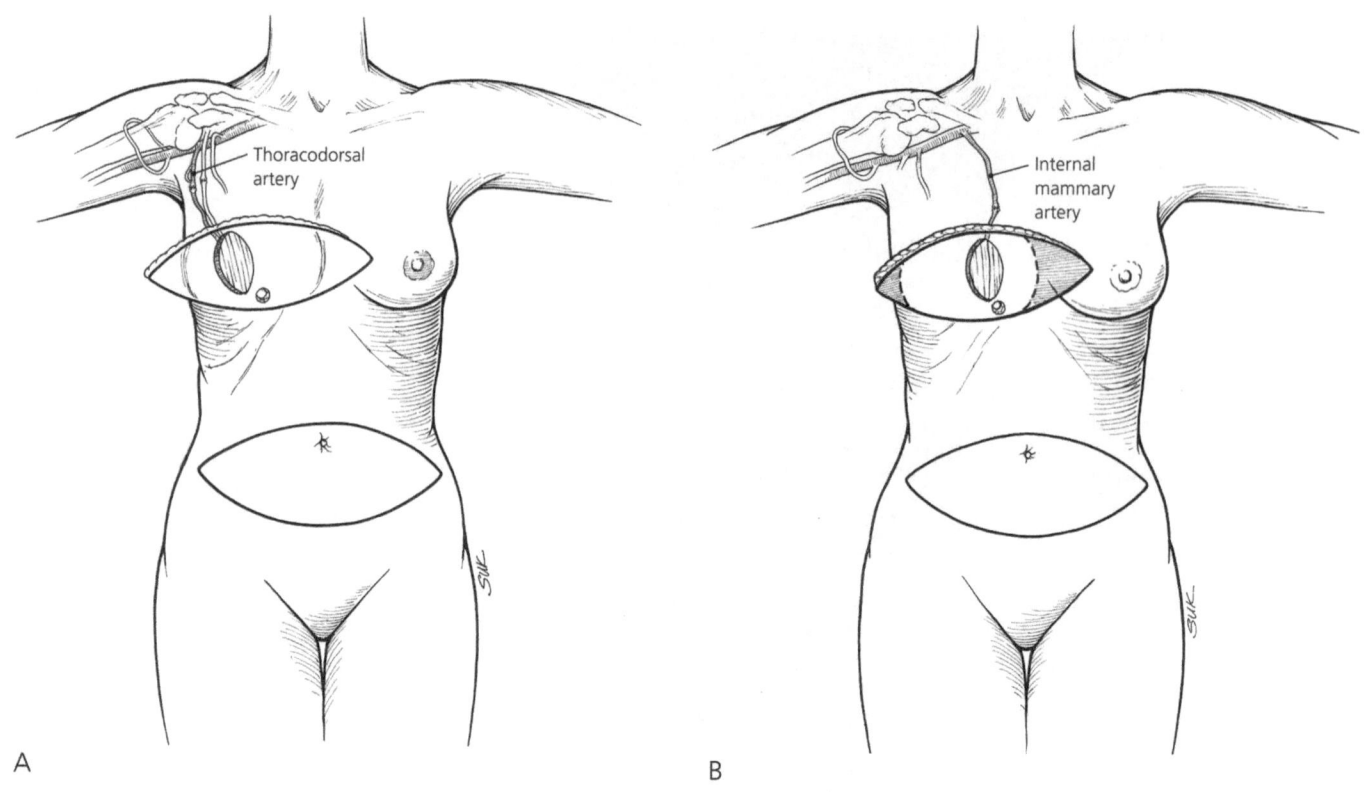

A   B

FIG. 9-20   (A) When the thoracodorsal vessels are used as recipients, the most well vascularized portion of the flap is somewhat lateral, so that the less well vascularized tissue across the midline must be used to form the medial portion of the breast. (B) When the internal mammary vessels are used as recipients, the most well vascularized part of the flap can be used to form the central and medial portions of the breast.

9-20). They can be approached by removal of the third or fourth costal cartilage and are usually of adequate size to match the deep inferior epigastric vessels accurately. The artery is usually quite large and provides strong blood flow, but the vein is sometimes small, especially on the patient's left side.

The first step in dissection of the internal mammary vessels is placement of retracting sutures in the skin. Next, the costal cartilage of the third or fourth rib is removed with periosteal elevators medially up to its junction with the sternum to achieve the required exposure (Fig 9-21). Some surgeons advocate removal of the fourth costal cartilage because that provides a better size match for the artery and more pedicle length; others (including myself) prefer removing the third costal cartilage in most cases because the vein will be larger. A preoperative color Doppler ultrasound examination is extremely helpful for predicting the location and size of the vein or veins, and can help the surgeon to decide which costal cartilage to remove for best access to the vessels.[10] In either case, if the internal mammary vein proves to be too small, the costal cartilage of the rib above (including the second rib, if necessary) can be removed and the vessels exposed more superiorly.

Using loupe magnification, the vessels are identified and separated from one another. Soft flexible plastic "vessel loops" placed around the vessels will aid in their dissection (Fig 9-22). The vessels should be dissected into the intercostal muscles both dis-

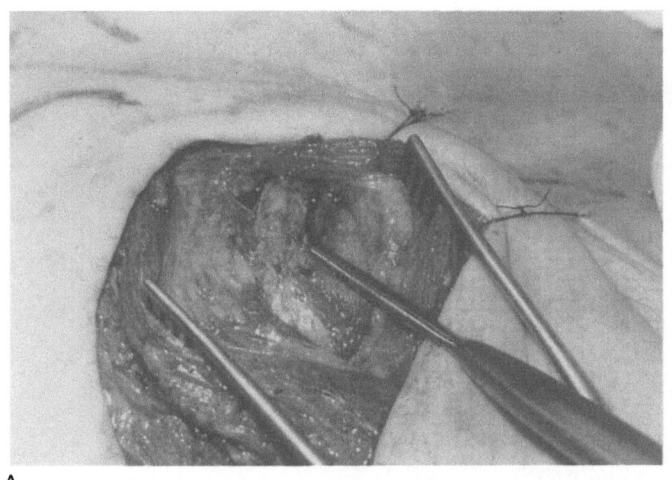

A

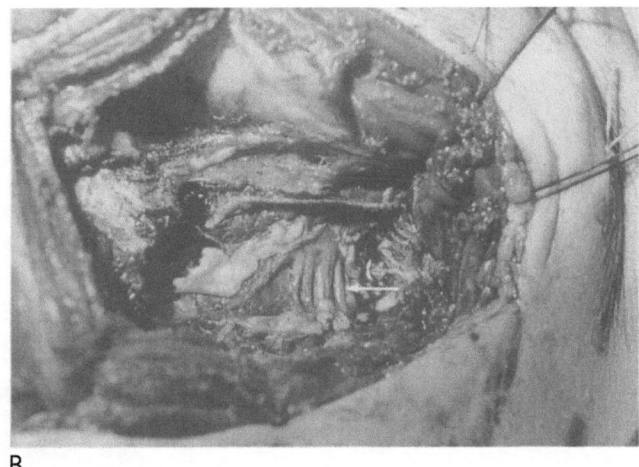

B

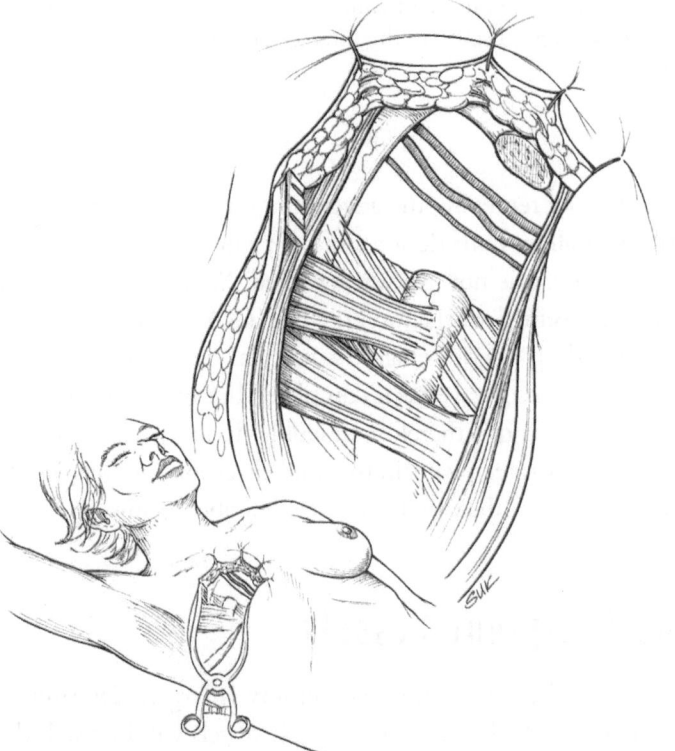

C

FIG. 9-21 (A) The third costal cartilage is completely removed using a periosteal elevator. The perchondrium is then removed to expose the internal mammary vessels. (B) Internal mammary vessels (arrow). The artery is usually larger than the deep inferior epigastric artery, but the vein is usually smaller. (C) Drawing of the internal mammary vessels.

tally and proximally to gain length so that the anastomoses can be performed in a more accessible location. This part of the dissection must be done carefully because many fragile branches enter the intercostal muscles (especially from the vein) and can cause significant bleeding. Actual removal of part of the intercostal muscle superficial to the vessels is helpful in achieving better exposure and mobilization and is therefore advocated.

Once the vessels are sufficiently mobilized, they are ligated distally, placed in atraumatic microvascular clamps, and divided. The operating microscope is brought into the

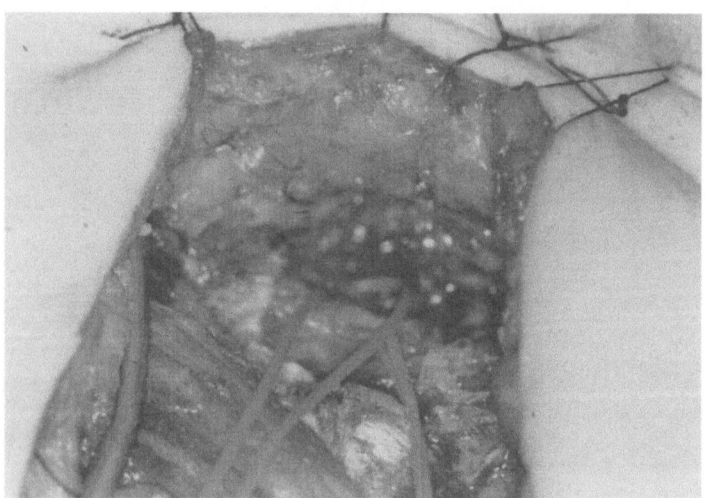

Fig. 9-22 Vessel loops are placed around the internal mammary vessels to aid in their dissection. The vessels are dissected proximally and distally in the intercostal muscles, to obtain more length and facilitate anastomosis.

field and the vessel ends are prepared by removing the adventitia. Orienting the vessels so that they are parallel to the ribs will allow both donor and recipient vessels to be at the same level, ensuring that the anastomosis is not awkwardly tilted. When the vessels are ready and the microscope position is deemed satisfactory, the free TRAM flap is harvested and brought up to the chest. A long deep inferior epigastric vascular pedicle is not necessary for flap placement once the anastomoses have been completed but makes positioning of the flap during the anastomosis easier and is therefore desirable. It also permits switching to the use of the thoracodorsal vessels as recipients in the unlikely event that that should prove to be necessary. The anastomoses are then performed as described below.

Arm Positioning and Recipient Vessels

The position of the patient's arm on the side of the mastectomy is largely determined by the surgeon's choice of recipient vessels. If the thoracodorsal vessels will be used, the arm must be positioned at 85 to 90 degrees to the chest wall to permit access to the axilla (Fig 9-23). The arm should be abducted no more than 90 degrees to avoid excessive traction on the brachial plexus traction that could otherwise lead to nerve dysfunction in the hand. Flexing the elbow slightly by placing some towels or foam under the patient's hand and wrist also relieves tension on the brachial plexus and helps to avoid these injuries, which usually resolve spontaneously but can temporarily be most distressing to both the patient and the surgeon. The surgeon should also take care, when the patient is positioned on the operating table, that the arm board does not extend inferiorly significantly farther than the patient's arm. Otherwise, the arm board will interfere with the surgeon's ability to stand close enough to the axilla to be comfortable during the anastomoses. If the arm board was placed too inferiorly, the surgeon should slide it cephalad (without further abducting the arm) until he or she can get into a more

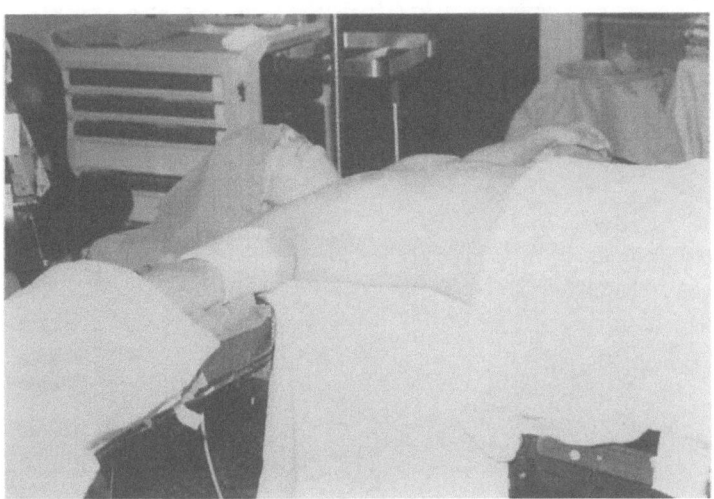

FIG. 9-23   Patient with arm outstretched, in preparation for a free TRAM flap using the thoracodorsal vessels as recipients. The arm should be abducted no more than 90 degrees (preferably less), but the arm boards should be sufficiently cephalad that it does not interfere with the surgeon's ability to stand close to the axilla. The elbow can also be flexed slightly to reduce tension on the brachial plexus.

correct and comfortable position. This maneuver is very important, because it can be very difficult to perform an anastomosis when the surgeon is in an uncomfortable position. Obviously, it is much easier to correct this problem before the patient has been prepared and draped than during the operation, when repositioning of the arm board may be difficult or even impossible.

If the internal mammary vessels are to be used as recipients, and if access to the axilla for lymph node dissection will not be required, the arm can be tucked in at the patient's side (Fig 9-24). The elbow should be placed slightly akimbo, or lateral, to allow better access to the most lateral part of the breast. Protective foam padding must be placed under the elbow, and the position of the hand should be checked to make sure it will not be injured when the patient's back is raised into the sitting position. Without interference from an outstretched arm, the surgeon can stand wherever he or she is most comfortable during the anastomoses. An arm board or sled should not be used, as these will interfere with the surgeon's ability to stand close to the patient, and defeat the purpose of tucking the arms. Positioning the arms at the side in this way greatly facilitates the anastomoses, and is one of the major advantages of using the internal mammary vessels as recipients. It can make access to intravenous lines more complicated for the anesthetist, but with proper equipment and preparation this difficulty can be overcome.

I prefer to position the arms symmetrically, either both arms outstretched or both tucked in at the sides. In this way, when the patient is placed in the near-sitting position she is more likely to be symmetrical, facilitating comparison of the two breasts. Care should be taken during the draping to be sure that the tops of the shoulders remain visible so that the patient's symmetry can be properly evaluated when she is placed in the sitting position, and the surgeon can tell if she is leaning off to one side.

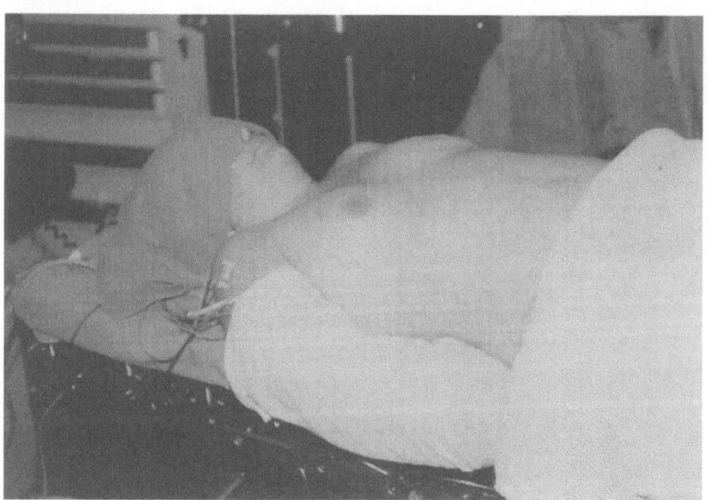

FIG. 9-24   Patient with arm tucked in at her side, in preparation for a free TRAM flap using the internal mammary vessels as recipients. The elbows should be slightly akimbo to allow free access to the lateral part of the breast. This arm position greatly facilitates the anastomosis by permitting the surgeon to stand wherever he or she is most comfortable.

Performing the Anastomoses

Some surgeons prefer a running suture for the arterial anastomosis and interrupted sutures for the venous anastomosis, while others (including myself) prefer the reverse. It probably makes no difference provided that the anastomoses are technically correct. Any combination of running and/or interrupted sutures can be successful.

Venous Anastomosis

I prefer to perform the venous anastomosis first so that when it is finished, it can be released without any need to reapply a clamp while the other anastomosis (the artery) is being completed. The donor and recipient veins are placed in a medium-sized double-approximating clamp. It is essential that the vein not be twisted, because such twists are by far the most common cause of a venous thrombosis.

After the adventitia is cleaned from the donor vein, 9-0 nylon sutures are placed and tied laterally, 180 degrees apart. In my technique, the needles are left attached and the suture ends left long so that they can be used for retraction. The vein is sutured under tension so that the back wall will pull away and is less likely to be inadvertently included in the front wall stitches. An interrupted suture is placed through the anterior walls of the two veins, at the midpoint between the two lateral sutures. One tail of this suture is left long, to be used for traction (Fig 9-25).

One of the two long sutures with needles attached is then used to perform a running closure of the front wall of the venous anastomosis. An assistant places traction simultaneously on the middle traction stitch and the running suture to pull the vein edges that are being sutured away from the back wall (Fig 9-26). During placement of the first stitch (the most lateral one), the back wall should be inspected visually because it is close by and can be inadvertently included in this stitch (Fig 9-27). For subsequent sutures, the traction makes inclusion of the back wall unlikely.

When the closure approaches the middle traction stitch, the assistant lets that one go and pulls instead on the tail of the more lateral stitch (the one with the other needle attached). The surgeon then pulls upward on the middle traction suture, drawing the vein edges away from the back wall and making suture placement very easy (Fig 9-28). After the middle stitch is passed, the tension is continued using the running and lateral sutures. During the last stitch (the most lateral one), the back wall is again visually inspected. The running suture is then tied to the suture tail that the assistant has been using for traction.

The double-approximating clamp is then flipped over, exposing the repaired back wall. A middle traction suture is placed, just as on the first side. The long suture with the remaining needle is untangled from the clamp and the back wall closed, again with a running suture.

Because the back wall is most vulnerable to being included in the suture at the lateral extremes of the repair, a useful trick is to have the assistant put tension on the two middle traction sutures, while the surgeon pulls upward (toward himself or herself) with the running suture. This effectively converts the stitch placement from a lateral (and vul-

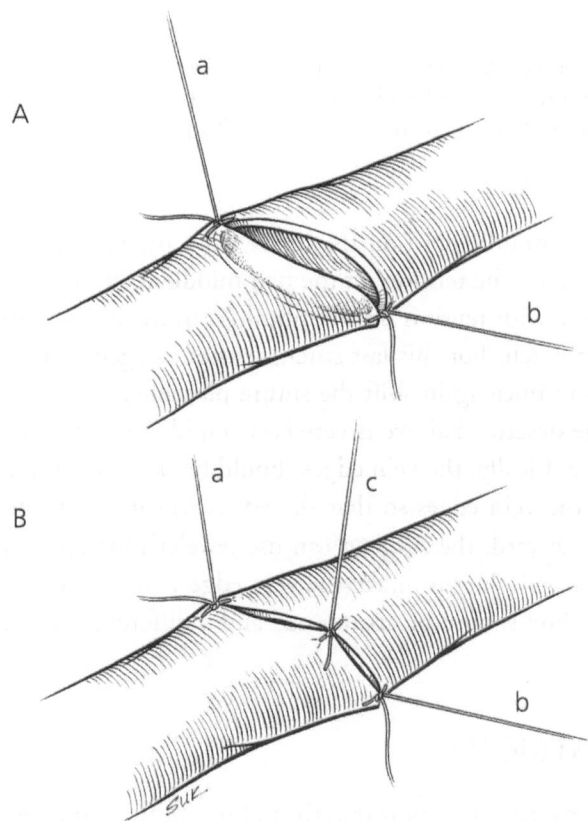

FIG. 9-25 (A) Sutures "a" and "b" are placed connecting the two vein ends 180 degrees apart. (B) A suture "c" is then placed midway along the venous anastomosis, to be used for traction.

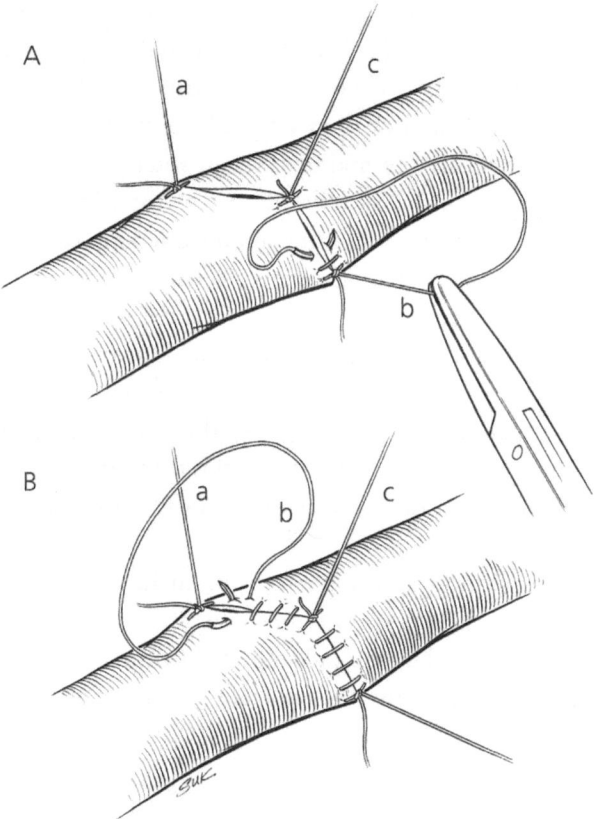

FIG. 9-26 (A) During venous anastomosis, the sutures are placed close to the vein edges, using both the running suture "b" and middle traction suture "c" to pull the vein edges away from the back wall. (B) Suture "a" is tied to the loose end of suture "b."

nerable) position to a middle position that is far from the back wall and therefore safe. After one or two stitches, the tension on the two middle traction sutures is released, and the normal technique with tension on the running suture and one middle suture is resumed until the last stitch. For this last stitch, tension is again applied to the two middle traction sutures to once again shift the suture placement to a safe, central position.

The technique described above is very easy, rapid, and safe provided that the two vein edges are visible. Ideally, the vein edges should be slightly everted. The needle bites should be close to the vein edges so that the edges will not roll inward. If one of the vein edges does roll inward, the surgeon can use jeweler's forceps in the hand opposite that holding the needle-holder to make the vein edge visible. If this is not possible, the above-described method should be abandoned and a different suturing technique used.

Arterial Anastomosis

Although many microsurgeons report that thrombosis of the venous anastomosis is more common than arterial thrombosis, in my own practice I have had the opposite experience. I find arteries to be more temperamental, developing spasm and occasionally thrombosis in the anastomosis when veins (as long as they are not twisted) rarely do.

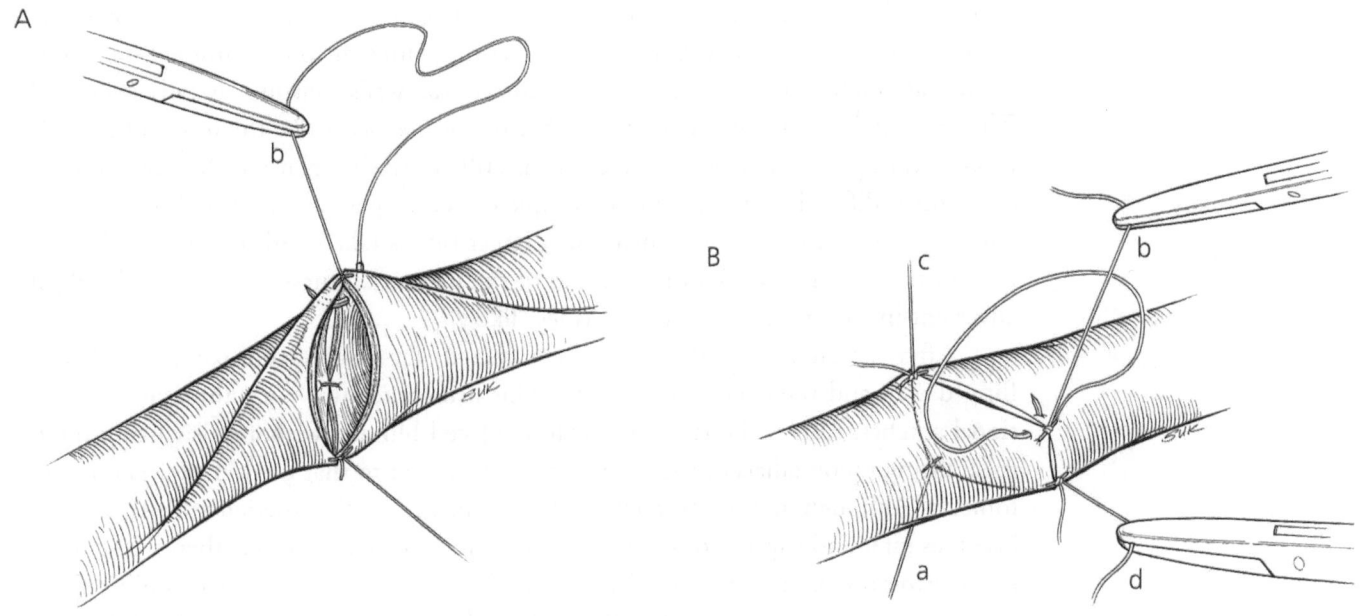

FIG. 9-27 (A) The first, most lateral stitch of the venous anastomosis should be visually inspected by pulling suture "b" across the vein; this is the one stitch most likely to inadvertently include the back wall. (B) Alternatively, an interrupted middle traction stitch can be placed in the back wall ("d") to pull the back wall away and make suture placement safe.

For that reason, I prefer to use interrupted sutures, which are more precise than running sutures, for my arterial anastomoses.

First, the arteries are placed in a double-approximating (Ackland) clamp, bringing the vessels' ends close together so that the repair will be performed without tension.

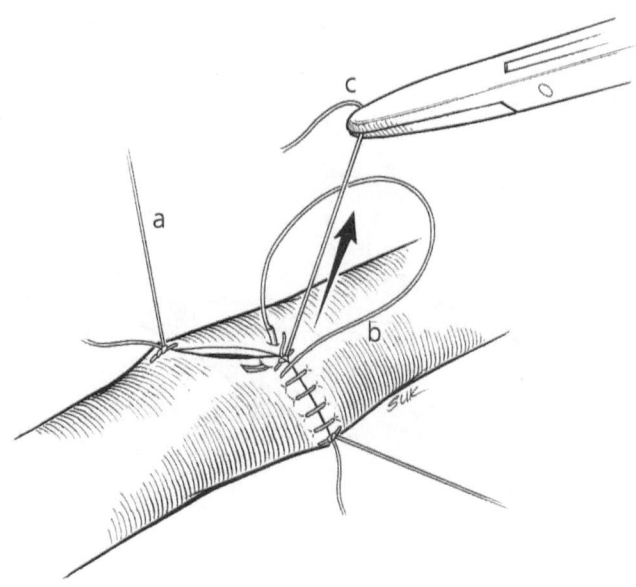

FIG. 9-28 During venous anastomosis, pulling up on the middle traction suture makes placement of stitches in that area very easy and safe.

Next, two lateral sutures of 9-0 nylon are placed, 180 degrees apart, leaving one tail of each suture long to serve as a handle for traction. Three or four additional interrupted sutures are then placed through the anterior arterial walls, starting laterally (Fig 9-29). The first stitch should always be whichever one is deemed to be the most difficult, because suturing is easiest when the artery is still relatively open and becomes progressively more difficult as the closure is completed. Having an assistant pull on one of the lateral traction sutures is often helpful. A larger bite is taken with the needle than that used in the venous anastomosis. Because of the relative stiffness of the arterial wall, inadvertent inclusion of the back wall is less likely.

After the anterior wall closure is completed, the double-approximating clamp is flipped over and the back wall repaired. This usually requires only three or four additional stitches. Often, the last stitch will be placed blindly, without visualizing the lumen, lifting up on adjacent sutures in a fashion similar to that used in the venous anastomosis. Although not recommended for beginners, with experience this maneuver becomes safer and capture of the back wall is unlikely. The clamp is then released, and the anastomosis is inspected for leakage. If there is significant leakage, additional sutures are placed as necessary. Small side branches, in particular, should be closed off with a suture, even if they are not bleeding at the time.

After the anastomosis, there is usually some arterial spasm where the vessel had been clamped. Application of 2% papaverine solution and a suitable waiting period will often induce this contraction to release. Localized adventitial removal can also be effective in relieving spasm, but the manipulation may lead to additional spasm in a different location. Unless the spasm is very localized, treatment with papaverine alone is usually the best course.

After the anastomosis has been completed, the rectus abdominis fascia on the flap is sutured to the pectoralis muscle on the chest wall with 2-0 Vicryl, to stabilize the flap and prevent tension on the pedicle (Fig 9-30). The flap is shaped into a rough ap-

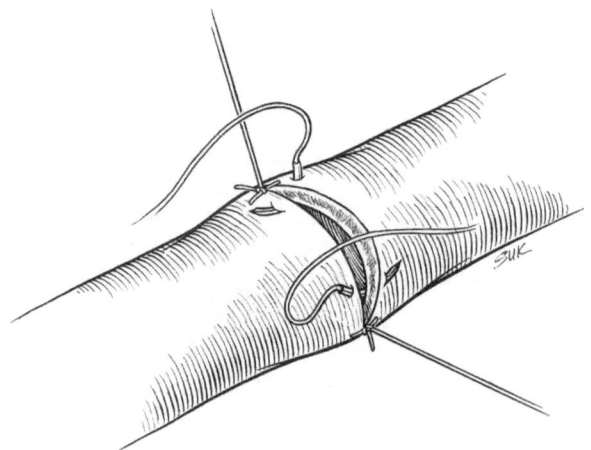

FIG. 9-29   The arterial anastomosis is made with interrupted sutures, starting laterally and saving the easiest (more central) ones for the end. Some suture ends are left long for traction if needed.

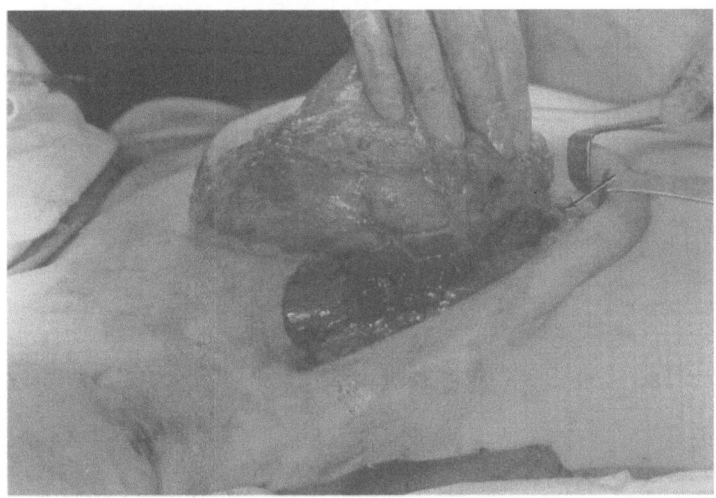

FIG. 9-30   Once the anastomoses have been completed, the fascia of the anterior rectus abdominis sheath is attached to the pectoralis major muscle with a 2-0 Vicryl suture (arrow) to stabilize the flap and prevent traction on the pedicle.

proximation of the desired breast shape and sutured to the medial edge of the mastectomy defect for additional stability. It is then left to perfuse on the chest wall while the donor site is being closed, allowing time for any vascular spasm to be released.

Closing the Donor Site Defect

As in the CTRAM flap operation, fascial donor site repair is one of the most important parts of the procedure. The main difference is that after the free TRAM procedure, the fascial donor defect is smaller and therefore easier to close. If the repair is performed incorrectly, however, an abdominal bulge or hernia can still disable the patient and ruin an otherwise successful operation.[16] The key to a successful repair is to attach the internal oblique fascia laterally to the strong midline fascia (deep to the linea alba) with a heavy running suture.[17] Any fascial repair technique that does this will be successful.

If the needed fascial edge is anywhere near the midline, I generally repair the fascial defect in two layers. First, I attach the internal oblique fascia to the midline fascia with a running suture of No. 1 Novafil (polyethylene) (Fig 9-31). It is essential to make sure that each bite of suture does in fact contain this strong fascia. Laterally, the internal oblique fascia is visible, and the surgeon needs merely to identify it for each stitch. Medially, to include the midline fascia deep to the linea alba, the point of the needle is inserted into the posterior rectus abdominis sheath close to its medial border and then exits from the anterior sheath. In that way, the medial reflection and the midline fascia are always included. Even so, the quality of each suture bite should be tested for strength and security by tugging on the needle after each stitch. The fascial closure is

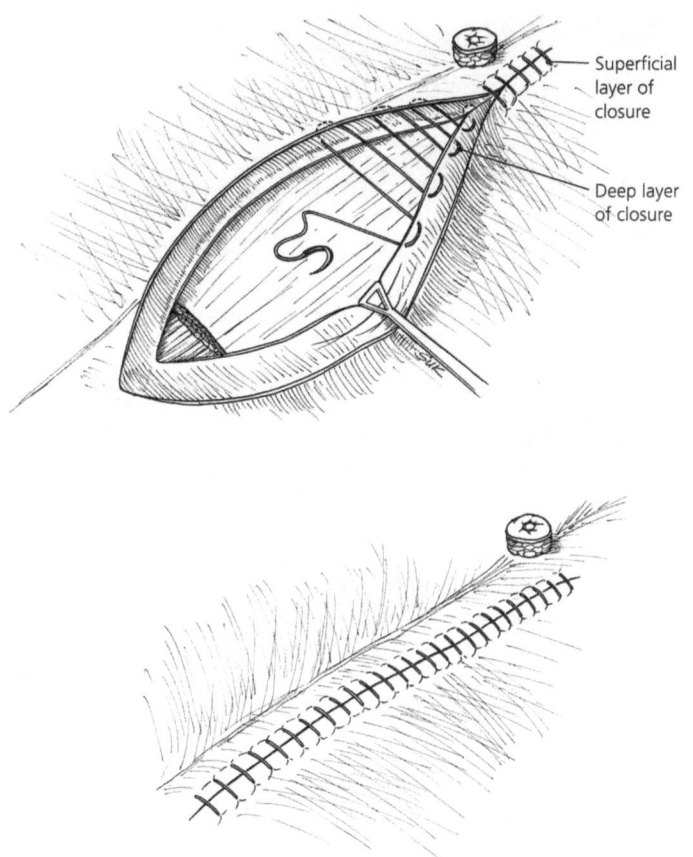

Superficial
layer of
closure

Deep layer
of closure

Fig. 9-31 Closure of the fascial donor site is performed in two layers, using running heavy (No. 1) monofilament suture.

continued superiorly until the wound is closed. The suture is then tied so that the end is buried.

If the medial fascia edge is not near the midline, I generally close the fascial defect in a single layer with Number 1 Prolene (polypropylene) running suture. The internal oblique layer must still be included securely in each stitch. If the tension is not excessive, a single-layered closure may suffice. If the sutures do not seem to be securely holding in the medial fascia (which is usually weaker than its lateral counterpart), however, the midline fascia should be included in the repair as in the two-layered closure.

After the first layer has been completed, a plan for superior fascial plication to avoid a dog-ear and make the fascial tightening symmetric (Fig 9-32) is drawn with methylene blue. A second layer of No. 1 Novafil or Prolene (polypropylene) sutures is then placed, using horizontal running mattress sutures where the fascia must be plicated and a simple running suture inferiorly where only reinforcement of the first layer is required. If only a single-layered closure is being performed, the reinforcement of the previously closed portion of the wound is omitted. Another running horizontal mattress suture is used on the contralateral side to plicate the fascia and move the umbilicus back toward the midline. Again, all knots should be buried so they will not be palpable through the skin. In most cases of unilateral reconstruction, it is also necessary to tack

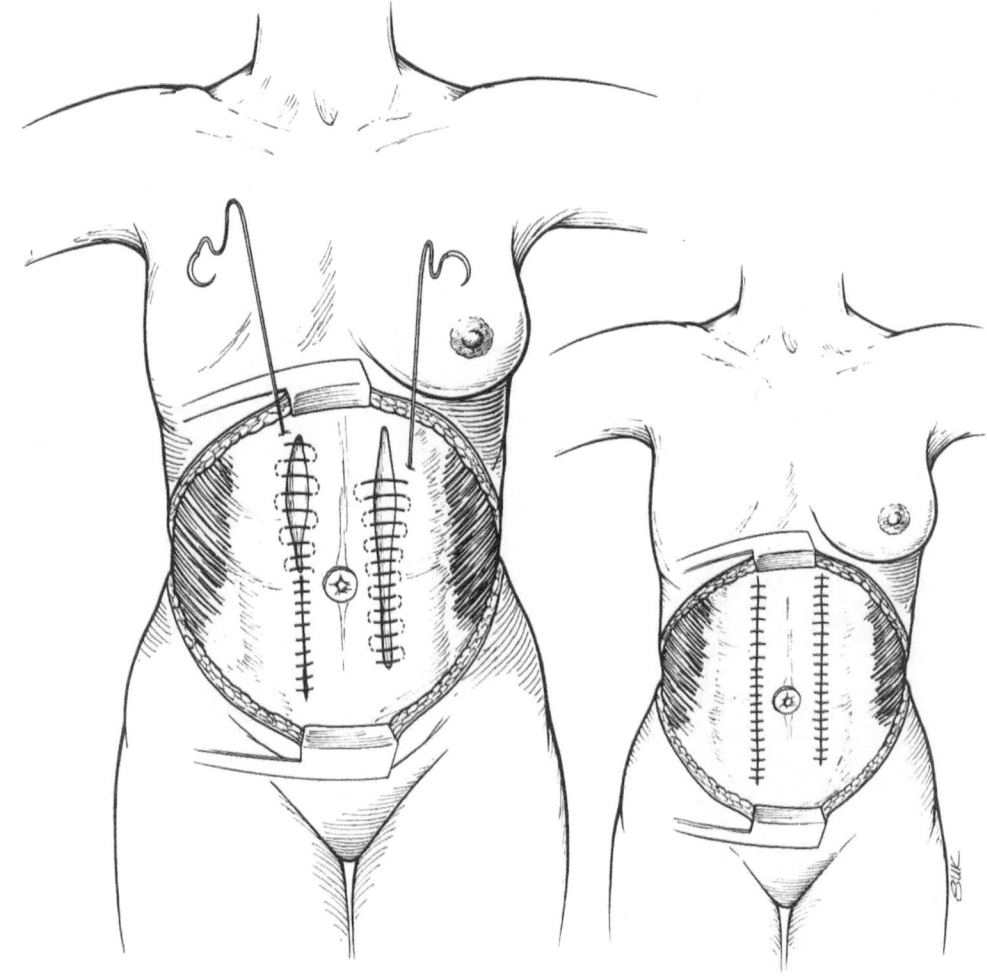

FIG. 9-32   Plan for plication of the upper abdominal and contralateral abdominal fascia.

the umbilicus to the midline with a single suture of 3-0 Vicryl, to truly bring it back to the center.

After the fascial donor site defect has been closed, a suction drain is inserted in the abdomen and led out through a small stab wound in the mons pubis. The table is then flexed, and towel clips are used to close the abdominal wound temporarily.

For reconstruction of the navel, the umbilicus is located by palpation, and a new horizontal opening is made in the skin for it. It is best to limit this horizontal opening to 1.5 cm or less, to keep the reconstructed umbilicus inconspicuous. The smaller and less conspicuous the umbilicus, the better the aesthetic result will be. The towel clips are then released, and some fat is removed from the area under the new opening for the umbilicus. If the patient is at all obese, the fat in the midline is thinned with scissors to simulate the presence of a median raphe. Hemostasis is then obtained with electrocautery. Next, the umbilicus is tacked over to the midline with a 3-0 Vicryl suture, and three sutures are placed to attach the umbilicus to the deep fascia and to the skin

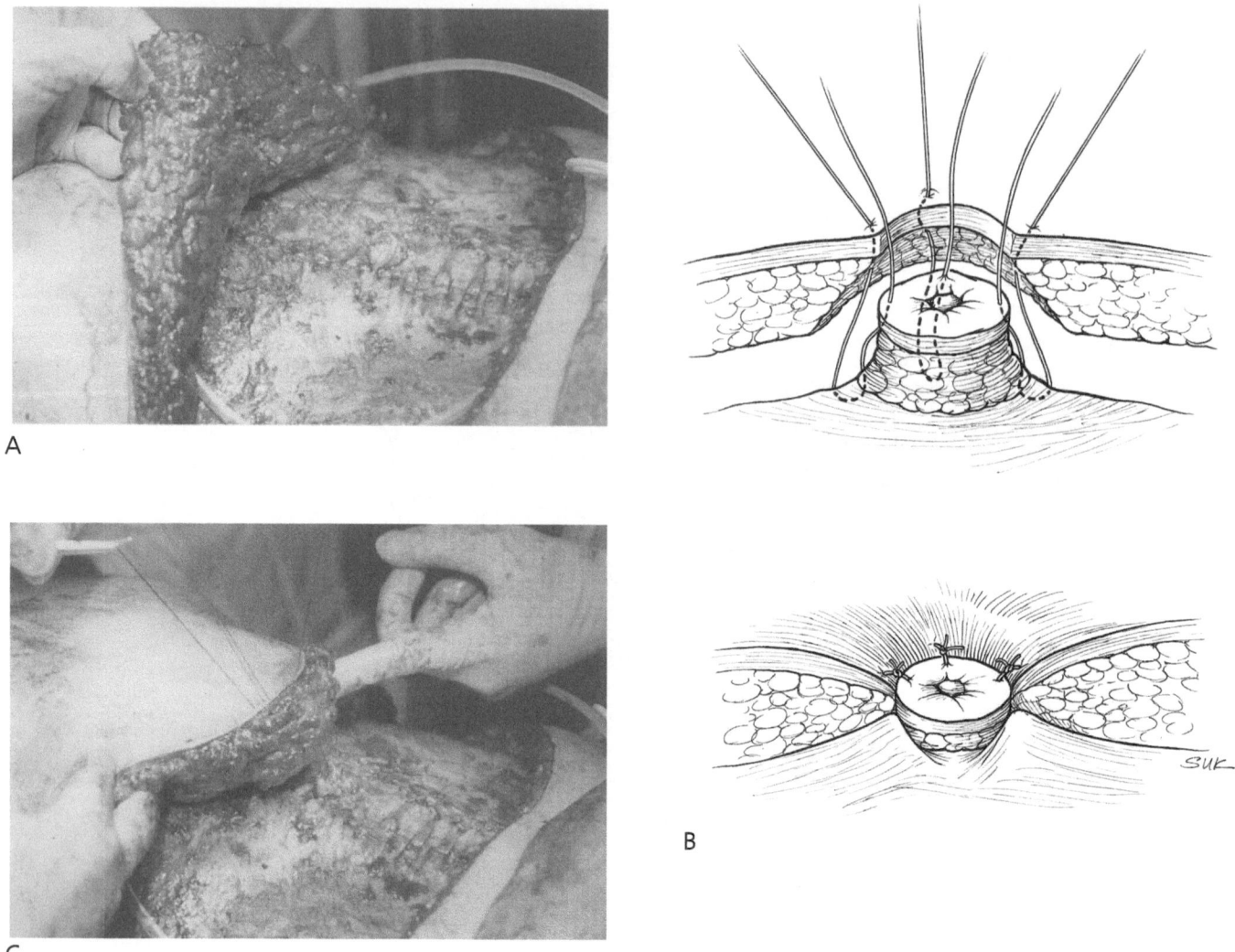

FIG. 9-33 (A) Umbilical tacking sutures are used to invert the umbilicus and attach it to the deep fascia to make it less conspicuous. (B) Sutures have been placed but not tightened. (C) As the sutures are tightened the abdominal skin surrounding the umilicus is drawn down to the fascia.

(Fig 9-33). These sutures, when they are eventually tied, will invert the umbilicus, making it less conspicuous and giving it an illusion of normalcy.

With the table still flexed, Scarpa's fascia is then repaired with interrupted sutures of 2-0 Vicryl. As in an abdominoplasty, the abdominal flap may need to be advanced medially to reduce the lateral dog-ears. If dog-ears are present despite this, the incisions are extended laterally, and additional skin is removed until the dog-ears are fully corrected. It is important to correct the dog-ears completely because this is far easier to do in the operating room than it will be later on in the clinic and because, despite wishful thinking, the dog-ears will rarely disappear spontaneously.

The skin is then closed with buried dermal sutures of 3-0 Vicryl and with running subcuticular sutures of 3-0 Prolene. The previously placed umbilical sutures are tied, and the remaining umbilical wound repaired with 4-0 chromic sutures.

Trimming the Flap

Once the flap has been successfully transferred and the blood supply has been deemed adequate, the flap is shaped and sutured to the edges of the surrounding defect as described in chapters 16 through 18. The medial edge of the flap, which is normally the part farthest from the pedicle, is trimmed until bright red bleeding is seen coming from the cut edges. Hemostasis is achieved, and the medial edge of the flap is sutured to the edges of the mastectomy defect. The breast pocket is completed (see chapters 16 and 17) and the volume adjusted as necessary. Tissue should be removed from the side ipsilateral to the pedicle only when the viability of the tissue across the midline has been positively established by seeing adequate bleeding from the flap edges.

Preparing for Flap Monitoring

The portion of the flap that will remain exposed is determined by replacing the mastectomy flaps and appropriate marking with a surgical pen. The mastectomy flaps are checked for viability to determine how much TRAM flap skin will need to remain exposed. A sterile hand-held ultrasonic Doppler pencil probe is then used to locate an audible signal on the exposed skin paddle. This site is marked with a suture of 6-0 Prolene to facilitate postoperative flap monitoring. Monitoring with this method is very simple: if an arterial signal is heard, one can be sure that the arterial anastomosis is patent. A nurse should check this signal every hour for the first 3 postoperative days, calling the surgeon if the signal disappears. Often a venous signal can be heard as well. A venous obstruction, however, is usually also accompanied by a sudden change in the flap's color.

If a pencil Doppler signal cannot be located on the exposed skin paddle intraoperatively, the surgeon can search for an alternative signal on the skin nearby. If one is found, it may be possible to reposition the flap so that the Doppler signal is exposed. If not, the surgeon can leave open a window in the native breast skin to expose the Doppler signal temporarily (Fig 9-34). This window can then be closed 1 week later, using local anesthesia, when flap monitoring is no longer required.

If no signal at all can be fond with a pencil Doppler probe and yet the flap is obviously viable, monitoring can be performed with a laser Doppler unit. This alternative allows continuous monitoring, signaling possible pedicle thrombosis by a sudden drop in the laser Doppler reading. Although this method works well in theory, we have found that in practice false alarms occur commonly when the probe is inadvertently loosened by the patient. Also, the decrease in the laser Doppler reading is not always sudden, making the signal at times difficult to interpret. I therefore prefer the simplicity of the hand-held pencil Doppler probe.

Often, a pencil Doppler signal that is weak or absent in the operating room will become stronger (or present, if there was none previously) when the general anesthesia is terminated. For this reason, if no signal could be found in the operating room, it is worth checking the flap again in the recovery room once the patient is awake. If a pen-

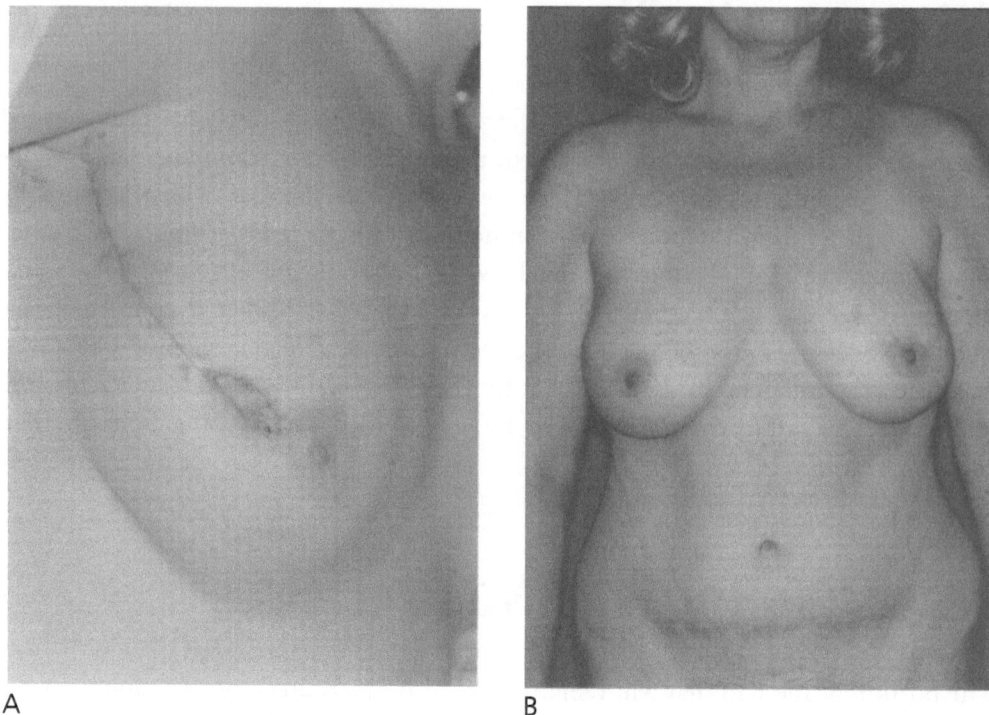

A   B

FIG. 9-34   (A) A temporary window can be created to allow direct monitoring of the flap. The exposed flap skin is removed and the window closed 1 week later. (B) After healing is completed, no visible traces of the window remain.

cil Doppler signal can be found, I always use pencil Doppler monitoring in preference to any other method, even when arrangements had previously been made to monitor the flap with a laser Doppler or other unit.

One other method we use (less commonly) to monitor our free TRAM flaps is a buried 20 MHz Doppler probe.[18] This method provides a continuous signal and therefore can detect a thrombosis very quickly. The disadvantages of this approach are the time that is required to place the probe, a tendency for false alarms when the probe is displaced, and the need to leave the wires in place for 3 weeks after the free flap procedure.

Summary

The free TRAM flap is reliable, has minimal donor site morbidity, and provides consistently good results. It has therefore become our breast reconstruction method of choice for most patients. Key points for successful performance of the free TRAM flap include adequately exposing the recipient vessels, dissecting an adequate pedicle length, and making sure that the vein in the pedicle is not twisted. Only the fascia required to maintain flap viability should be harvested, and the repair of the donor site must be secure, with care taken to close the internal oblique fascia securely to the midline fascia deep to the linea alba with heavy permanent sutures. When properly executed, the free TRAM flap can provide outstanding results with a low rate of failure.

References

1. Schusterman MA, Kroll SS, Weldon ME. Immediate breast reconstruction: why the free TRAM over the conventional TRAM flap? *Plast Reconstr Surg.* 1992;90: 255–262.
2. Schusterman MA, Kroll SS, Miller MJ, et al. The free TRAM flap for breast reconstruction: a single center's experience with 211 consecutive cases. *Ann Plast Surg.* 1994;32:234–242.
3. Hartrampf CR Jr, Scheflan M, Black PW. Breast reconstruction with a transverse abdominal island flap. *Plast Reconstr Surg.* 1982;69:216–224.
4. Hartrampf CR Jr, Bennett GK. Autogenous tissue reconstruction in the mastectomy patient: a critical review of 300 patients. *Ann Surg.* 1987;205:508–518.
5. Boyd JB, Taylor GI, Corlett R. The vascular territories of the superior epigastric and the deep inferior epigastric systems. *Plast Reconstr Surg.* 1984;73:1–14.
6. Kroll SS, Schusterman MA, Reece GP, et al. Choice of flap and incidence of free flap success. *Plast Reconstr Surg.* 1996;98:459–463.
7. Kroll SS, Evans GRD, Reece GP, et al. Comparison of resource costs of free and conventional TRAM flap breast reconstruction. *Plast Reconstr Surg.* 1996;98: 74–77.
8. Kroll SS. Necrosis of abdominoplasty and other secondary flaps after TRAM flap breast reconstruction. *Plast Reconstr Surg.* 1994;94:637–643.
9. Kroll SS, Netscher DT. Complications of TRAM flap breast reconstruction in obese patients. *Plast Reconstr Surg.* 1989;86:886–892.
10. Ninkovic M, Anderl H, Hefel A, Schwabegger A, Wechselberger G. Internal mammary vessels: a reliable recipient system for free flaps in breast reconstruction. *Br J Plast Surg.* 1995;48:533–539.
11. Hefel A, Schwabegger A, Ninkovic M, Moriggl B, Waldenberger P. Internal mammary vessels: anatomical and clinical considerations. *Br J Plast Surg.* 1995;48: 527–532.
12. Arnez ZM, Valdatta MP, Tyler MP, Planinsek F. Anatomy of internal mammary vessels and their use in free TRAM flap breast reconstruction. *Br J Plast Surg.* 1995;48:540–545.
13. Dupin CL, Allen RJ, Glass CA, Bunch R. The internal mammary artery and vein as a recipient site for free-flap breast reconstruction: a report of 110 consecutive cases. *Plast Reconstr Surg.* 1996;98:685–689.
14. Feng LW. Recipient vessels in free-flap breast reconstruction: a study of the internal mammary and thoracodorsal vessels. *Plast Reconstr Surg.* 1997;99:405–416.
15. Clark CP, Rohrich RJ, Copit S, Pittman CE, Robinson J. An anatomic study of the internal mammary veins: clinical implications for free-tissue transfer. *Plast Reconstr Surg.* 1997;99:400–404.

16. Hartrampf CR Jr. Closure of the donor defect for breast reconstruction with rectus abdominis myocutaneous flaps (discussion). *Plast Reconstr Surg.* 1985;76:563.

17. Kroll SS, Marchi M. Comparison of strategies for preventing abdominal-wall weakness after TRAM flap breast reconstruction. *Plast Reconstr Surg.* 1992;89:1045–1053.

18. Swartz WM, Izquierdo R, Miller MJ. Implantable venous Doppler microvascular monitoring: laboratory investigation and clinical results. *Plast Reconstr Surg.* 1994;93:152–163.

10 Deep Inferior Epigastric Perforator Flap

The deep inferior epigastric perforator (DIEP) flap is a variation of the free transverse rectus abdominis myocutaneous (TRAM) flap in which one or more perforating branches of the deep inferior epigastric artery and accompanying veins are dissected out of the rectus abdominis muscle so that only the blood vessels, and no muscle tissue, are harvested with the flap (Fig 10-1).[1–4] Moreover, little or no fascia is sacrificed, making closure of the donor site much easier, theoretically a particularly useful feature in bilateral cases. Despite the fragile appearance of the pedicle the flap is usually adequately vascularized, although usually not as well as in the standard free TRAM flap.

Advantages of the DIEP Flap

The advantage of the DIEP flap is that donor site morbidity is reduced to the absolute minimum. Little or no muscle is sacrificed and, whenever possible, the nerve supply of the muscle is maintained. Postoperative pain and abdominal wall weakness are therefore reduced, and the umbilicus remains centered in the abdomen. The abdominal fascial closure is easily accomplished even in bilateral cases, and postoperative bulges or hernias are very rare.

Disadvantages of the DIEP Flap

The disadvantages of the DIEP flap include a somewhat reduced flap blood supply, so fat necrosis and partial flap loss are more common (Figs 10-2 and 10-3). This is especially true when unilateral reconstruction is performed and if part of "Zone IV" (the contralateral end of the flap farthest from the blood supply) must be used. Also, raising this flap takes more time than raising a free TRAM flap and can be somewhat tedious. The perforating blood vessels are exposed and are more vulnerable to traction injury than they are in a free TRAM flap, when they are surrounded and protected by

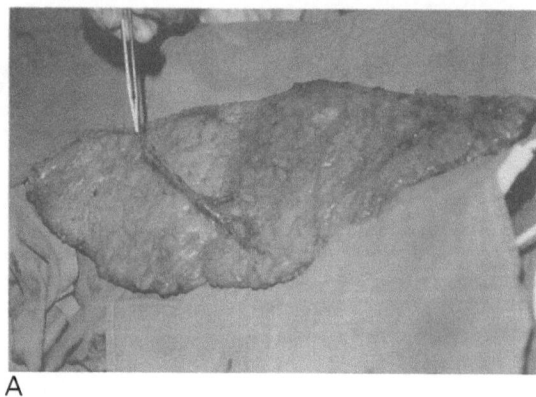
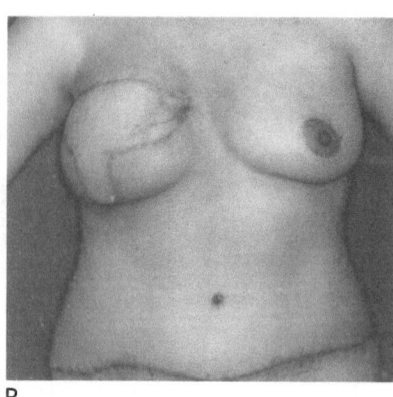

A   B

FIG. 10-1 (A) DIEP flap. No muscle is included in the flap. (B) Early result of reconstruction. There was some ischemia of the medial tip of the flap, but it resolved after treatment.

muscle in their more distal, smaller, and more vulnerable segments. Finally, although the entire rectus abdominis muscle may be preserved, much of the muscle may be denervated and/or devascularized and may therefore not be functional.

Surgical Technique

The flap is elevated from lateral to medial just as in a free TRAM flap, identifying the lateral row of perforating vessels that enter the flap from the rectus abdominis sheath (Fig 10-4). It can be helpful to separate the flap widely from the deep abdominal fas-

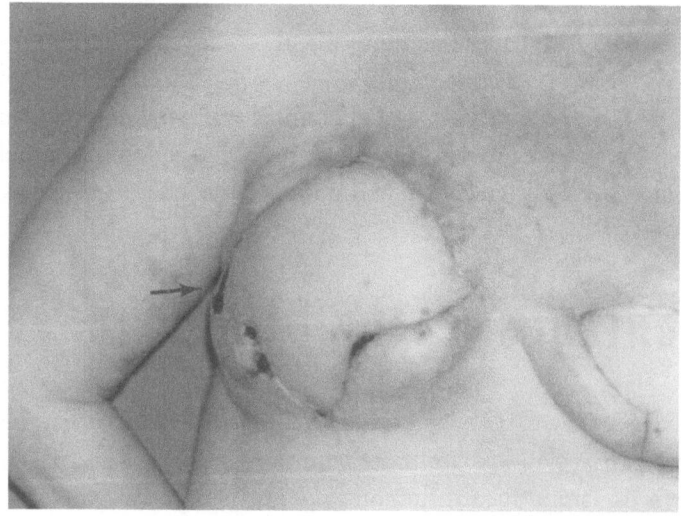

FIG. 10-2 Patient with partial flap necrosis (arrow) after bilateral DIEP flap breast reconstruction. Partial flap necrosis is rare in bilateral free TRAM flaps. The patient was a smoker and also had some mastectomy flap edge necrosis. She also had previous irradiation on the right side.

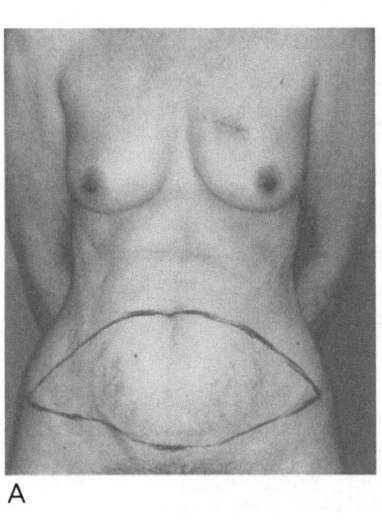

A

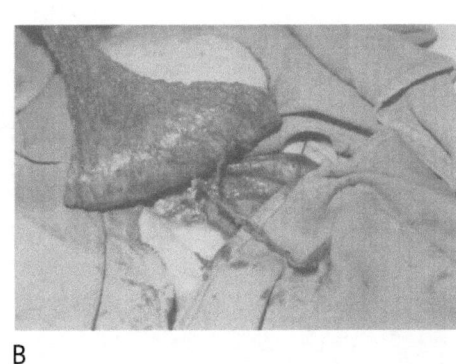

B

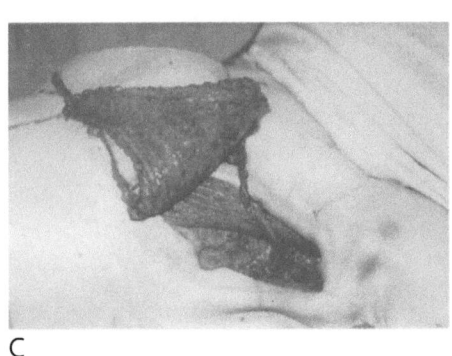

C

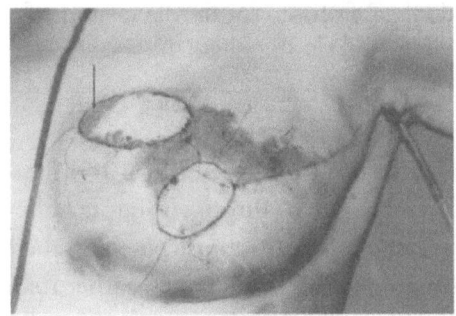

D

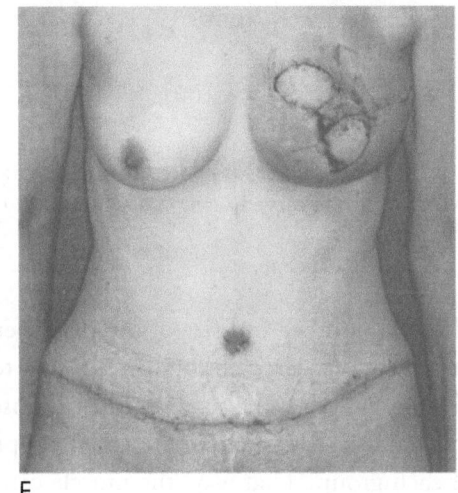

E

FIG. 10-3 (A) Patient with plan for immediate reconstruction of the left breast using a DIEP flap. The patient was a nonsmoker, and the tumor was in the upper inner quadrant. (B) The DIEP flap, just prior to the anastomoses. (C) After the anastomoses, showing the long pedicle of the flap. (D) Four days later, the patient has signs of mastectomy flap necrosis and, more significantly, partial loss of the underlying flap (arrow). (E) The patient was explored, and most of the flap was viable. There is, however, some fat necrosis in the medial portion of the breast mound.

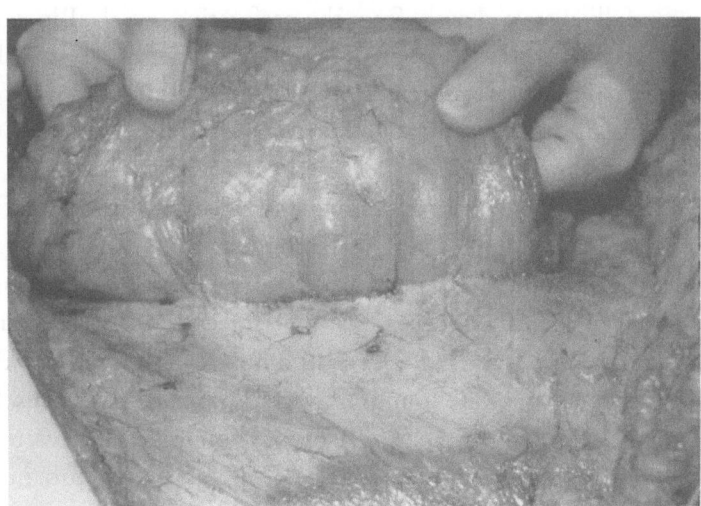

FIG. 10-4   Lateral row of TRAM flap perforators, which can usually be identified without injury.

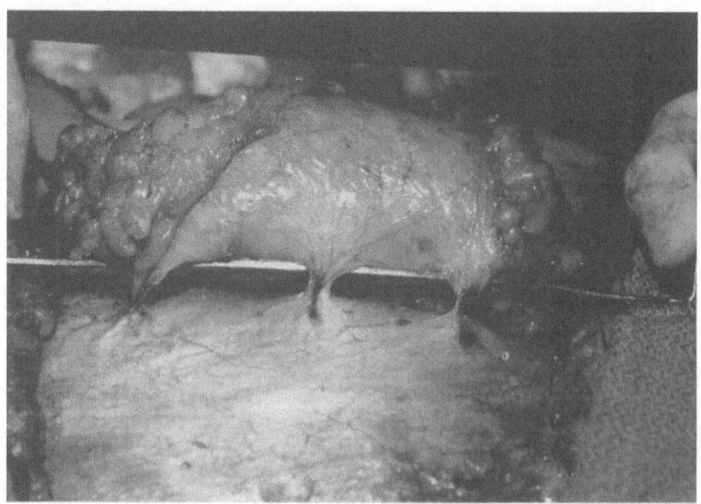

Fig. 10-5   TRAM flap separated from the deep abdominal fascia except for the major perforators, which were preserved using a combination of blunt and electrocautery dissection.

cia so that the number and size of the main perforators can be assessed (Fig 10-5). Unless there is one very large perforator, it is best to preserve two or three perforators rather than rely only on one. The surgeon must choose which perforators to use based on their size and location. It is better to use all lateral perforators or all medial ones, rather than some of each group. That way, the muscle can be split longitudinally, which causes far less donor site injury than would be caused by cutting across it horizontally. In the overwhelming majority of cases, the lateral row of perforators is used unless one very large medial perforator is identified that would be capable of nourishing the entire flap by itself, or unless the lateral row of perforators is judged to be excessively small.

The fascia is incised around the chosen perforators, and the incisions are connected. The fascia is then reflected laterally. Under loupe magnification, the muscle is carefully dissected away from the perforating vessels. Bipolar electrocautery or small vascular clips are used to obtain hemostasis when small vascular branches (of which there are many) are encountered. One or more fishhook retractors attached to rubber bands are useful for retracting the muscle away from the vessels during this stage of the dissection (Fig 10-6).

If only medial perforators are used, and if those perforators quickly pass deep to the muscle without a long intramuscular course, the nerve supply to the muscle can be easy to maintain. If lateral perforators are used (as is usually the case), care must be taken to identify and preserve the larger motor nerve branches as they cross over the perforating vessels (Fig 10-7). If no motor nerve branches that are large enough to warrant preservation are found, however, some degree of muscle denervation is likely. Motor nerves that cross between two perforators will have to be divided to extricate the flap from the donor site. These nerves can be reapproximated after the flap has been harvested, using one or two sutures of 10-0 nylon, to facilitate reinnervation of the muscle.

If an adequately sized lateral row of perforators is found, the muscle can be split longitudinally and will probably remain adequately vascularized. If both medial and lat-

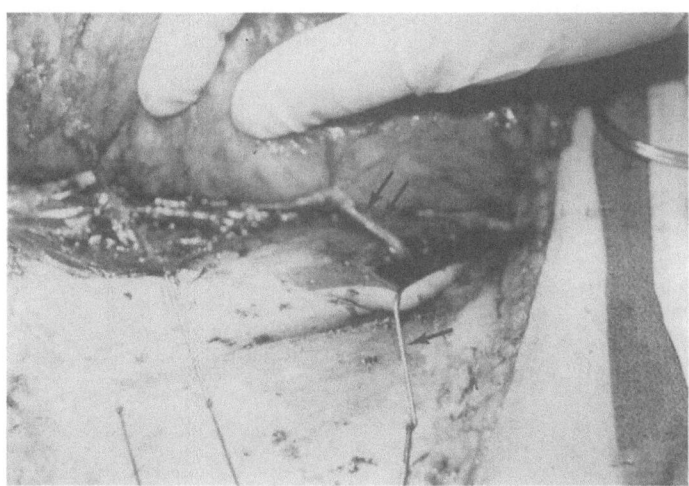

FIG. 10-6 Fishhook retractors (arrow) attached to rubber bands are helpful in retracting the muscle away from the perforators (double arrows).

eral perforators must be harvested, however, the muscle must be cut transversely and the intramuscular blood supply disturbed more widely. In that case, some of the muscle may end up being devascularized and, although preserved in situ, nonviable. This negates much of the advantage of using the DIEP flap, so in most cases only the lateral or medial row of perforators should be used, but not both.

Once the intramuscular dissection has been completed, the remaining dissection is identical to that of a free TRAM flap. I prefer to dissect the deep inferior epigastric vessels all the way to their origin, making the pedicle as long as possible. As in the free TRAM flap, the flap is then left attached by its blood vessels to perfuse in the abdomen

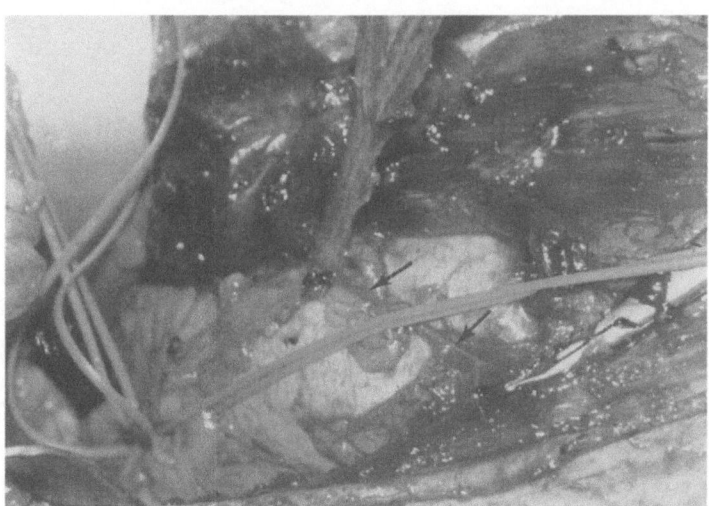

FIG. 10-7 Large motor nerve branch (arrows) crossing over a perforating blood vessel. Using loupe magnification, these branches can be dissected away from the vessels and preserved.

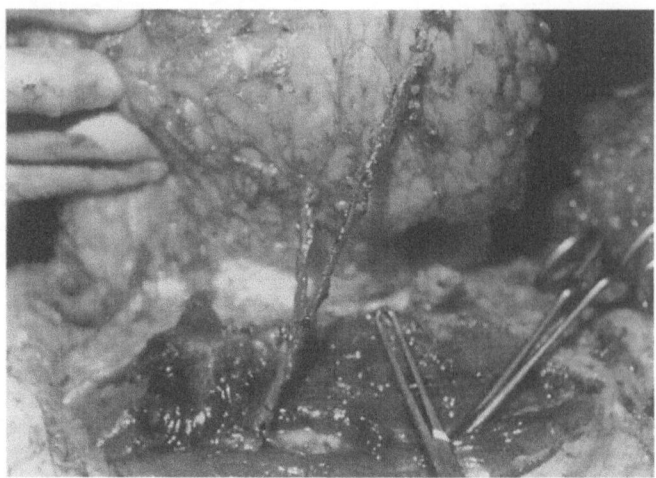

FIG. 10-8   DIEP flap perfusing in situ. It is still attached to the abdomen by the deep inferior epigastric vessels.

until the recipient vessels have been prepared for the transfer (Figs 10-8 and 10-9). From this point onward, the operation proceeds just as any free TRAM flap would. Because the pedicle is longer than that of the standard free TRAM flap, extreme care must be taken to avoid twisting of the vein. As long as the vein is not twisted, however, the additional pedicle length is not a disadvantage. It can, in fact, make the anastomoses technically easier, allowing the flap to be positioned where it does not interfere with placement of the surgeon's hands close to the blood vessels. This is advantageous even when the internal mammary vessels are used as the recipient site, when a long pedicle would not otherwise be necessary to reach the recipient vessels.

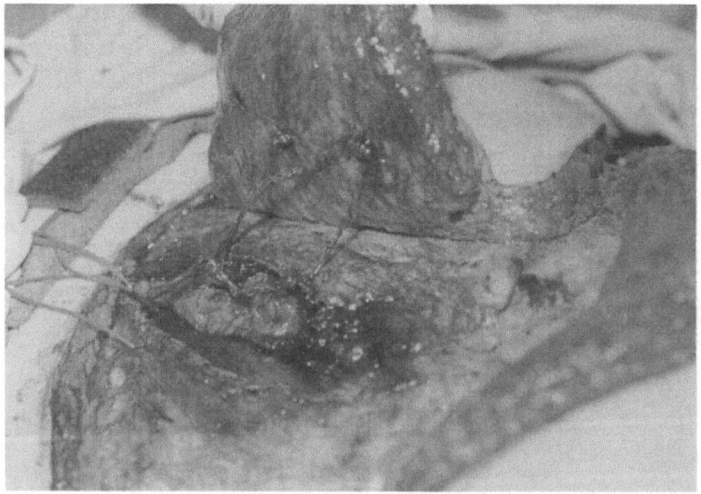

FIG. 10-9   Another DIEP flap still attached to the abdomen, awaiting transfer. This flap had three perforators that were preserved to nourish the flap.

The DIEP flap can be performed with use of either the internal mammary or thoracodorsal vessels as recipients. Most surgeons who perform many DIEP flaps prefer to use the internal mammary vessels, in part because this does not require use of the contralateral part of the flap to create the medial portion of the breast mound. By using mainly the ipsilateral half of the flap, and positioning the entrance of the pedicle into the flap near the breast meridian (which is easily reached if the internal mammary vessels have been used as recipients), the surgeon partially avoids the problem of reduced blood supply to the DIEP flap (compared to that of the standard free TRAM flap), and fat necrosis is minimized. This strategy works best, however, when only a small breast must be reconstructed, and when use of the majority of the flap to achieve adequate breast volume is not required.

Because practically no fascia is sacrificed, closure of the donor site is easy, even in bilateral cases. The umbilicus does not need to be recentered, and the risk of developing a bulge or hernia is minimal. Closure of the fascial donor site can therefore be delegated to a junior member of the surgical team and be performed simultaneous with the shaping of the breast, saving considerable time.

Indications

The DIEP flap is indicated whenever the surgeon believes that the advantages of minimal sacrifice of fascia and muscle outweigh the disadvantages of reduced blood supply and longer operative time. This situation is most likely when only 65 or 70% of the flap will be required (to make a relatively small breast), in which case reduced flap blood supply is less important, or in bilateral reconstruction when the surgeon believes that the extended time required for bilateral perforator flaps will be outweighed by reduced donor site morbidity and ease of abdominal fascial closure. Bilateral perforator flaps are rarely appropriate for obese patients, however, for whom the operative times are already extremely long even when using simpler techniques. I also strongly consider performing a DIEP flap whenever I find a lateral row of perforators that is located more laterally than usual, so that performance of a standard TRAM flap would require a sacrifice of more than the usual amount of muscle and fascia. I also consider it in any patient where large perforators are found during the free TRAM flap dissection.

Contraindications

The only absolute contraindications to performance of a DIEP flap are a previous TRAM flap or abdominoplasty, in which case the necessary perforators do not exist. In my opinion, relative contraindications would include a pronounced potbelly habitus (because there is usually insufficient subcutaneous tissue present to make an adequate breast), and the need to use most of the TRAM flap to make an adequately sized breast (because the DIEP flap usually has less robust perfusion than the standard TRAM flap). I also consider the intraoperative finding of only comparatively small perforators to be a relative contraindication to proceeding with a DIEP flap. Although most patients have large enough perforators to allow the selection of two or three that will adequately nourish the flap, some patients have only a larger number of relatively smaller ones. In that situation, I prefer to convert the procedure to a standard free TRAM flap rather than attempt to dissect many very tiny perforators from the muscle.

Influence of the DIEP Flap on the Free TRAM Flap

Because donor site morbidity is very acceptable with the standard free TRAM flap,[5,6] because the DIEP flap requires much more time than a free TRAM flap to perform, because the tedious dissection entails some risk of injury to the blood vessels, and because sacrifice of some of the perforators inevitably reduces blood supply to the flap, the DIEP flap has not yet been widely adopted by surgeons who perform free flap breast reconstruction. It has, however, influenced my performance of the standard free TRAM flap. Particularly in bilateral cases, even if I am not planning a perforator flap I find that I often will separate the flap from the abdominal fascia and look at the perforating blood vessels, as if I were going to perform a perforator flap. I may then decide to sacrifice a lateral perforator to reduce the width of the fascial donor site defect, provided that adequate other, more medial perforators are present. In this way, donor site closure is facilitated and postoperative pain reduced without performing bilateral perforator flaps and unduly prolonging the operative time.

Alternatively, a single laterally positioned perforator can be included with the flap without sacrificing the surrounding fascia (Fig 10-10). Under loupe magnification, the fascia is incised 1 mm around the perforator (or dissected away from the vessel without including a rim of fascia), just as it would be in performing a perforator flap. The small hole in the fascia is then connected to the main fascial incision that encompasses the remaining perforators. The result is a fascial defect that is similar in size to what would have been present had the lateral perforator been sacrificed. This approach is especially useful in unilateral breast reconstruction, when sacrifice of a lateral perforator may be unwise (since perfusion across the flap's midline is necessary and therefore any reduction in flap perfusion is best avoided) but at the same time, a large fascial defect that would pull the umbilicus off the midline and mandate a wide plication of the opposite side (for symmetry) would be undesirable.

Conclusions

At the time of this writing, the place of the DIEP flap in breast reconstruction is still evolving. In my opinion, it is a useful and interesting technique. It appeals to me because it causes only minimal donor site morbidity, something that the standard TRAM flap does not always do. If my first priority were always to minimize donor site morbidity rather than to create the best possible breast mound, I would perform DIEP flaps in most of my patients. Because my first priority is to achieve the best possible

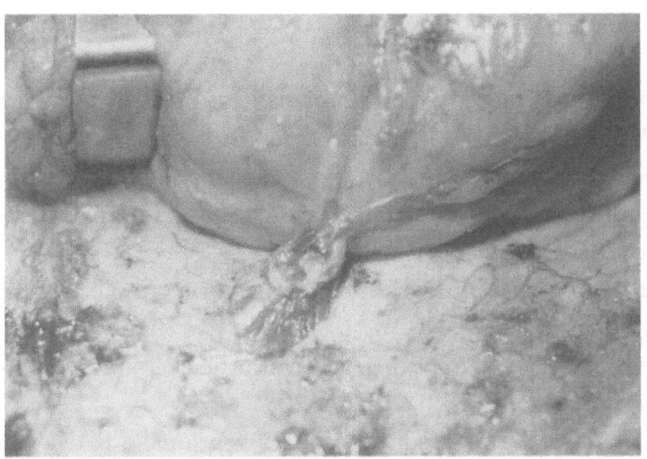 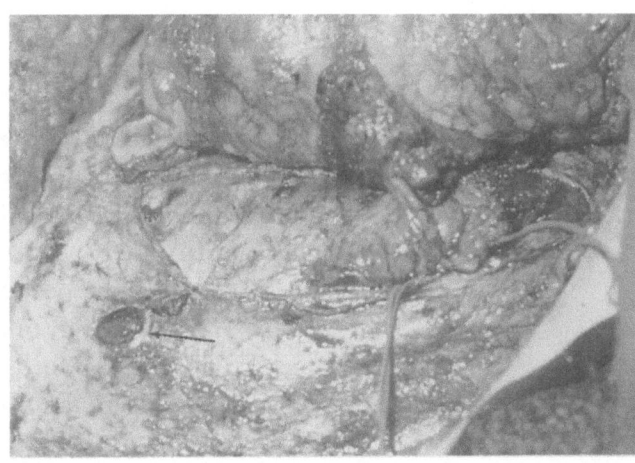

A   B

Fig. 10-10   (A) A lateral perforator has been isolated and a fascial incision made around it. (B) The small defect left by removal of this perforator (arrow) was connected to the main fascial incision, and continued elevation of the free TRAM flap performed in the usual way. The incision connecting the two defects has been temporarily closed with a few sutures. It will be permanently closed in an almost horizontal direction once the flap has been harvesting, thus not increasing tension on the main fascial defect closure.

aesthetic results in the breast, because I believe that the DIEP flap has a higher risk of fat necrosis and partial flap loss than the standard free TRAM flap does, and because the morbidity of the standard free TRAM flap is usually low anyway, I am currently using the DIEP flap only in selected patients. These would include patients who require only a relatively small part of their flap to make an adequately sized breast (including some patients undergoing bilateral reconstruction), and very athletic patients who wish to minimize donor site muscle loss even if the breast must be smaller than I would prefer. Most other patients, I believe, are better served with a standard free TRAM flap.

I believe that the DIEP flap is elegant, but is technically demanding. It is not for all patients, and not for all surgeons. Nevertheless, it is an exciting development and bears considerable further study.

Summary

The DIEP flap is a modification of the free TRAM flap in which one or more perforating blood vessels are dissected away from the rectus abdominis muscle so that no muscle need be included in the flap. This technique has the advantage of reduced donor site morbidity but requires more time for flap elevation and results in a less robust flap blood supply than the standard free TRAM flap. At the time of this writing, the DIEP flap remains relatively new, and its final status in autologous tissue breast reconstruction has not yet been clearly defined. It is an important new development in the field of autologous tissue breast reconstruction, however, and clearly deserves further attention.

References

1. Allen RJ, Treece P. Deep inferior epigastric perforator flap for breast reconstruction. *Ann Plast Surg.* 1994;32:32–38.

2. Blondeel N, Boeckx WD. Refinements in free flap breast reconstruction: the free bilateral deep inferior epigastric perforator flap anastomosed to the internal mammary artery. *Br J Plast Surg.* 1994;47:495–501.

3. Koshima I, Soeda S. Inferior epigastric artery skin flaps without rectus abdominis muscle. *Br J Plast Surg.* 1989;42:645–648.

4. Guzzetti T, Morris R, Webster MHC. Early experience with the deep inferior epigastric perforator flap. *Eur J Plast Surg.* 1997;20:205–208.

5. Grotting JC, Urist MM, Maddox WA, Vasconez LO. Conventional TRAM flap versus free microsurgical TRAM flap for immediate breast reconstruction. *Plast Reconstr Surg.* 1989;83:842–844.

6. Kroll SS, Schusterman MA, Reece GP, Miller MJ, Robb GL, Evans GRD. Abdominal wall strength, bulging, and hernia after TRAM flap breast reconstruction. *Plast Reconstr Surg.* 1995;96:616–619.

11 TRAM Flap Postoperative Care and Complications

ostoperative care of patients after breast reconstruction with the conventional transverse rectus abdominis myocutaneous (TRAM) flap, the free TRAM flap, and the deep inferior epigastric perforator (DIEP) flap is similar. TRAM flap breast reconstruction is major surgery, lasting many hours. Patients therefore require careful postoperative evaluation of their fluid balance and hematocrit, as well as monitoring of the flap. Despite the magnitude of the surgery, however, most patients recover rapidly and uneventfully provided that preventive measures are taken to avoid gastric dilatation, hypovolemia, and atelectasis.

Gastric Dilatation and the Nasogastric Tube

Harvesting a TRAM flap ordinarily tightens the abdominal wall, reducing its compliance and making respiration more difficult. If this interference with respiratory mechanics is aggravated by postoperative gastric dilatation,[1] respiratory failure can occur rapidly, with life-threatening consequences. Postoperative gastric dilatation can easily be prevented by a nasogastric tube. A nasogastric tube should always be in place during the TRAM flap procedure, because it facilitates closure of the abdominal donor site. Although some of my colleagues believe it unnecessary, I prefer to leave the tube in place overnight in most cases. I do this because the consequences of gastric dilatation can be so serious. If the patient has no nausea the following morning and has relatively normal pulmonary function, the nasogastric tube is removed and a slow advance from clear liquids to a regular diet is begun. If there is nausea or reason to suspect poor pulmonary function, however, the nasogastric tube is left in place until bowel sounds or flatus are present.

Urine Output

A Foley catheter is helpful in the early postoperative period both to avoid bladder distention and to monitor urine output. A urine output of less than 35 ml/h is usually due to hypovolemia, which should be corrected to keep the blood pressure from dropping and possibly reducing flap blood flow. Most TRAM flap patients (especially the younger ones) are not at serious risk for congestive heart failure and are better off getting too much fluid than too little. They should receive intravenous fluids at a high enough rate to prevent hypovolemia; my practice is to give dextrose 5% in half-strength normal saline with 20 meq/L potassium at 125 to 150 ml/h, depending on the patient's size. If the hourly urine output falls below 35 ml/h for 2 consecutive hours, an additional fluid bolus is given unless signs of fluid overload are present.

The Foley catheter is usually left in place for approximately 2 days, both for patient comfort and to monitor urine output. Once the patient is able to go to the bathroom without assistance, however, the catheter is discontinued.

Pain Management

Most patients receive pain medication intravenously via a patient-controlled analgesia (PCA) pump. Our standard dose is a basal rate of 1 to 2 mg/h of morphine sulphate, with additional morphine doses (1 mg every 15 minutes) given as needed. If the patient cannot tolerate morphine, therapeutically equivalent doses of meperidine (Demerol) or hydromorphone (Dilaudid) can be used instead. Patients are advised that the narcotic will reduce their pain but will increase nausea and cause constipation, so they are encouraged to use only what they need. Each day, the basal rate is reduced as the patient's pain diminishes. Usually the basal rate has been eliminated by the fourth day and the patient started on oral pain medication (hydrocodone with acetaminophen [Vicodin or Lortabs] or oxycodone with acetaminophen [Percocet] 1 to 2 tablets every 3 hours). As soon as the patient is comfortable without the PCA pump, it is eliminated and the oral dose of pain medication gradually reduced.

Intravenous ketorelac (Toradol)[2] is useful in the first few days because it potentiates the effects of the narcotics without increasing their side effects. We have not found it to significantly increase our incidence of hematoma. Because intravenous Toradol is expensive, once the patient is taking oral medication the Toradol is discontinued and replaced with oral ibuprofen 200 mg every 3 hours as needed.

Avoiding Constipation

Because all narcotics are constipating and because abdominal straining should be avoided to protect the abdominal repair, patients are started on stool softeners (docusate [Colace, Surfak] or equivalent, 1 tablet twice daily) as soon as they have progressed to a regular diet. The stool softeners should be continued for at least 1 month following discharge from the hospital. Suppositories (bisacodyl [Dulcolax] or equivalent) are also used to avoid constipation and are preferable to oral laxatives, which are best avoided.

Prevention of Atelectasis

Some degree of atelectasis is inevitable after TRAM flap surgery and must be countered by efforts to reexpand the patient's lungs. Patients are encouraged to perform breathing exercises with an incentive spirometer every hour during the first 2 days. In most cases they also get out of bed after noon on the first postoperative day, ambulating and sitting in a chair at least three times per day afterwards. As soon as they are able to walk to the bathroom without difficulty (usually on the second or third day), the Foley catheter is removed. In this way, the patient is encouraged to get out of bed more often, which helps to reduce atelectasis.

Free Flap Monitoring

Pencil Doppler Monitoring

If a free flap has been performed, it should be monitored at hourly intervals for a full 3 days.[3] The easiest way to monitor the arterial blood flow to the flap is with a pencil ultrasonic Doppler probe over the exposed skin paddle, provided that an adequate signal was located intraoperatively and marked with a 6-0 Prolene (polypropylene) suture (Fig 11-1). Usually an arterial signal can be heard clearly, and sometimes a venous signal can be identified as well. This, combined with observation of skin color (to monitor venous return) and capillary refill, is reliable and straightforward. If the Doppler signal disappears, or the skin color turns dark or blue (suggesting venous pedicle obstruction), the patient should be returned immediately to the operating room so that the problem can be identified and corrected (Fig 11-2).

Laser Doppler Monitoring

If a pencil Doppler signal could not be identified intraoperatively, laser Doppler monitoring can be taped to the skin as an alternative.[4–7] This technique depends on the correct functioning of the laser Doppler probe and unit. The surgeon follows the laser Doppler reading, looking for changes. A sudden decrease in the reading suggests pedicle obstruction and requires flap exploration. Unfortunately, a sudden decrease in the laser Doppler reading can also be caused by a loose or dislodged probe. Also, the magnitude of the signal tends to vary spontaneously, making the laser Doppler less straightforward and more difficult to interpret than monitoring with a hand-held pencil Doppler unit.

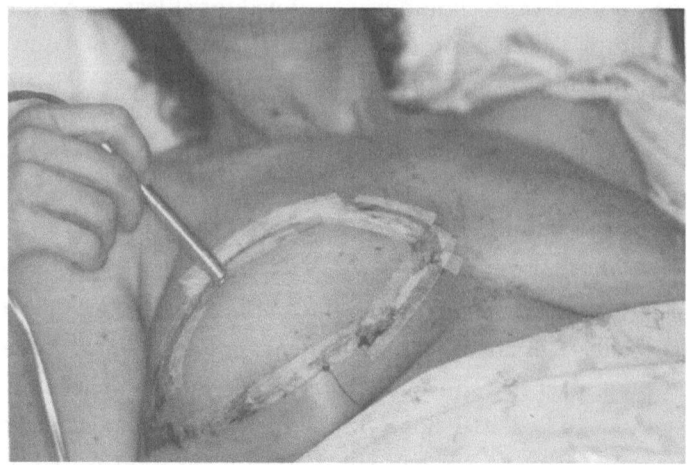

FIG. 11-1 Monitoring the flap with a hand-held pencil Doppler probe. This is the simplest method of flap monitoring and is therefore preferred if a signal can be located. See color insert, p. I-11.

Buried 20 MHz Probe

Another method of flap monitoring that can be useful when no signal is identifiable with the pencil Doppler probe is the buried 20 MHz Doppler probe[8] (Fig 11-3). The probe is connected to a unit that monitors the Doppler signal continuously. If the probe is placed over the deep inferior epigastric artery, the sound of the pulse is loud, unambiguous, and very easy to follow; but a venous obstruction may not be detected. If the probe is placed over the vein, the signal may be ambiguous and more difficult to interpret. If visible flap skin is present, a reasonable approach can be to monitor the arterial signal with the buried Doppler and to use the skin color and capillary refill to monitor the vein.

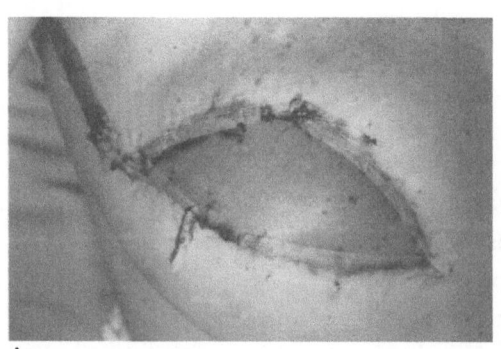
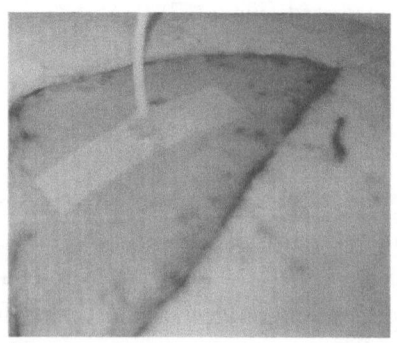
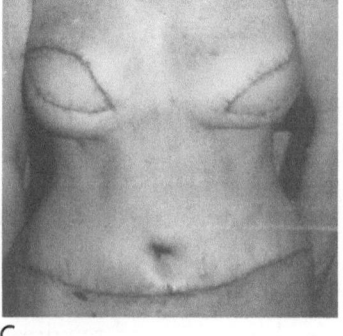

A B C

FIG. 11-2 (A) Free TRAM flap compromised by venous obstruction. The flap is blue. See color insert, p. I-12. (B) Laser Doppler probe subsequently used to monitor the flap. (C) Six days after revision of the venous anastomosis, the flap is viable. See color insert, p. I-12.

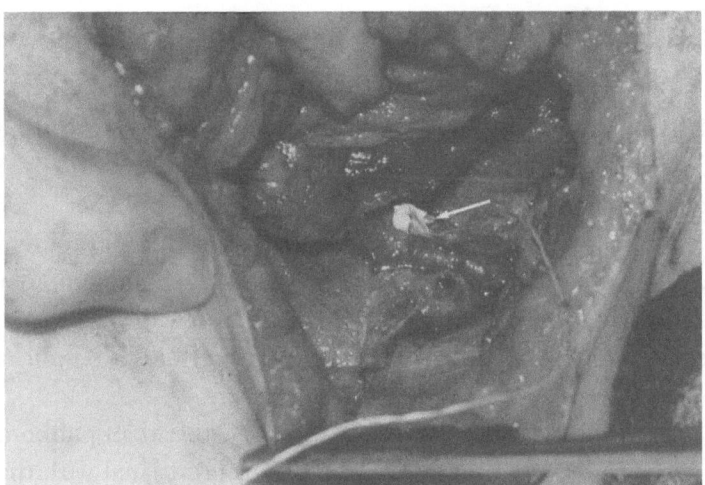

FIG. 11-3   A 20 MHz Doppler probe attached by a weak silicone glue to a Teflon sleeve (arrow), which is sutured around the flap's pedicle. This is a useful way to monitor a buried flap. The probe is pulled out 3 weeks after the surgery.

Early Exploration

Whatever method of flap monitoring is selected, it is necessary to be ready to move quickly to explore the pedicle if there is any suggestion of possible obstruction.[9] Once a pedicle has become obstructed, there is only a limited time during which the flap can be salvaged before irreversible changes occur. It is far better to return to the operating theater for a false alarm than to miss an opportunity to save a failing flap, so the surgeon should have no hesitation about exploring any pedicle that is questionable. After 3 days of hourly flap monitoring, the monitoring is decreased to every 4 hours until the patient leaves the hospital.

Anticoagulants

The value of anticoagulants after free flaps remains unproven. We have found that low-dose heparin (an intraoperative bolus of 2000 to 3000 U followed by 100 to 300 U/h for 5 days) does no harm, increasing the risk of hematoma only from 5% to 6%,[10] and probably reduces the risk of deep venous thrombosis and pulmonary embolism. In cases in which the donor or recipient vessels appear diseased or if intraoperative thrombosis has occurred, I generally use therapeutic doses of heparin, administering a bolus of 5000 to 6000 U (depending on the patient's weight) and titrating the dose to achieve a partial thromboplastin time of 1.5 times normal. This treatment is usually maintained for 1 week and seems to be effective, but carries the risk of a 20% incidence of hematoma. If systemic anticoagulation has been used, I often will prescribe 1 aspirin tablet daily after the patient leaves the hospital. Again, the benefit is unproven but the intervention seems to do no harm.

Postoperative Fever

Most TRAM flap patients will have some temperature elevation during the evening of the second or third postoperative day. This is almost always due to atelectasis and normally does not require a chest X-ray, blood cultures, or other extensive workup unless special circumstances are present. The treatment for this problem in the overwhelming majority of patients is deep breathing, coughing, and ambulation. The patient's tongue should also be examined because often it will be very dry, suggesting that the patient is hypovolemic. In that case, increased fluids are indicated to correct the deficit.

If fever persists for more than a few days, causes other than pulmonary should be looked for. These can include urinary tract infections (associated with the use of a Foley catheter), sepsis caused by a central intravenous catheter (if one is present), and thrombophlebitis. A very rare cause of postoperative fever is abdominal sepsis caused by inadvertent inclusion of the bowel in a stitch used to close the fascial donor site. Although this is very uncommon, it can be fatal if not diagnosed and aggressively treated early in its course, so it should be considered whenever unexplained fever is present. If abdominal sepsis is suspected, immediate consultation with a general surgeon should be requested.

Another possible cause of an elevated temperature can be partial flap necrosis. If partial flap necrosis is present, early debridement and reshaping of the breast may cause the temperature to return to normal (see below). This diagnosis should be considered secure only when the other common causes of fever have been ruled out, but should be considered whenever fever is accompanied by partial flap loss, since effective treatment (debridement) is available.

Management of Early Postoperative Problems

Respiratory Difficulty

All TRAM flap patients have some decrease in pulmonary function because the abdominal wall has been tightened and its compliance reduced. Fortunately, most properly selected TRAM flap patients are healthy and tolerate this without difficulty. If respiratory problems arise, however, the decreased pulmonary excursion can make things worse than they otherwise would be.

If the patient develops sudden respiratory difficulty in the early postoperative period, the possibility of gastric dilatation should be considered immediately. If a nasogastric tube is in place, it should be checked to make sure it is functioning properly. If there is no nasogastric tube, one should be inserted; this may correct the problem immediately, preventing further deterioration and making extensive diagnostic testing unnecessary. Speed is essential because respiratory difficulty caused by gastric dilatation can progress rapidly to respiratory arrest, making an already serious problem much more dangerous.

If gastric dilatation is not the problem, fluid overload or pulmonary embolus should be considered and the appropriate tests ordered without delay. In our institution, leg compression boots are routinely used for patients undergoing TRAM flaps, making deep venous thrombophlebitis and pulmonary embolus unusual. If low-dose heparin is being administered, pulmonary embolus is even more unlikely. Still, it must always be considered and, if present, treated immediately with therapeutic doses of intravenous heparin.

Partial Flap Loss

Loss of more than a very small part of a TRAM flap should be treated aggressively by early debridement (within the first 5 days).[11] Early and aggressive management is recommended for three reasons. First, a large volume of necrotic tissue is somewhat toxic and can cause fever and malaise, which are relieved by debridement. The debridement will not only make the patient feel better but may shorten hospitalization and hasten recovery as well. Second, if the necrotic tissue is not debrided it will drain for many weeks, causing patient anxiety and discomfort. Third, once the patient leaves the hospital she may not return for the needed correction, even though it might be in her best interest to do so.

If the area of necrosis is small, it may not need surgical correction. If it is large, however, it may require a second flap to salvage the reconstruction (Fig 11-4). If a second major flap is required, it is best to get it over with and do it before the patient leaves the hospital; this avoids arguments with the patient's insurance company and quickly resolves the problem. In general, if the reconstruction is ultimately successful, the patient will be happy and satisfied even when a second flap was unexpectedly required.

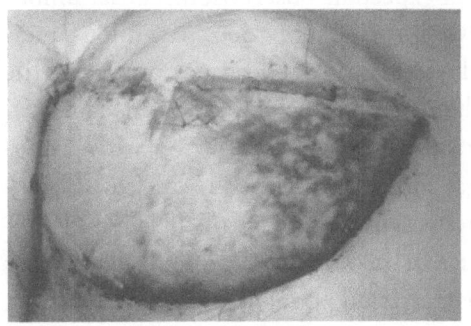 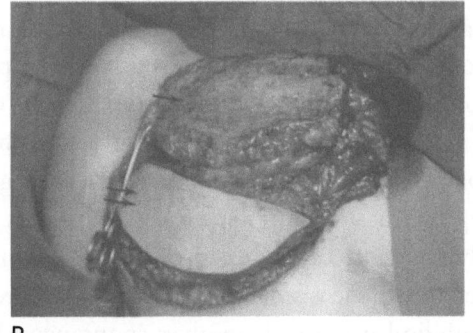 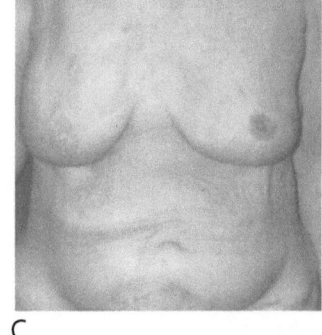

A   B   C

FIG. 11-4 (A) Patient with partial flap necrosis after a pedicled TRAM flap. The patient was a heavy smoker. (B) The necrotic tissue was debrided acutely, and the remaining TRAM flap (arrow) was covered with a latissimus dorsi flap (double arrows). (C) The final result, after contralateral breast reduction, was reasonably acceptable. (From Kroll SS, Freeman P. *Ann Plast Surg.* 1989;22:58–64. Used with permission.)

Care After Discharge from the Hospital

All TRAM flap patients have suction drains in the abdominal donor site and under the reconstructed breast. It is far better to leave the drains in too long than to remove them too early. If the drains are still in place when the patient leaves the hospital (as is often the case), I instruct her to empty the drains once each day and record the output. The patient returns to the clinic when any of the drains has produced less than 25 ml/d for 2 days in a row; at that time, that drain is removed. Even following this conservative regimen, however, some patients will subsequently develop seromas that require aspiration with a syringe or insertion of a new drain.

Patients should not stress their abdominal wall during the healing process. They should take a stool softener twice daily for at least 30 days, and they are advised to avoid lifting anything heavier than 10 pounds for 6 to 12 weeks. They are instructed not to attempt situps until 6 months after the surgery, and then only if they have no abdominal wall problems.

In my patients, running subcuticular sutures are used for the skin, and the sutures are removed only after 3 weeks. The sutures are left in that long in an attempt to support the healing wound and reduce the scar widening that typically occurs in the abdominal donor site.

Complications

Umbilical, Mastectomy Flap, and Abdominoplasty Flap Necrosis

Partial umbilical necrosis is common, especially in patients who smoke.[12] While inconvenient for the patient, it causes little or no permanent morbidity. It should be treated by cleaning the affected area with cotton-tipped applicators and hydrogen peroxide, local debridement where appropriate, and expectant observation. Partial umbilical necrosis may take up to 2 months to resolve, but ordinarily does so without additional surgery. Unless there is underlying prosthetic mesh, umbilical necrosis is of little consequence and has only minimal effect on the patient's final appearance (Fig 11-5).

Mastectomy flap necrosis is also common, especially in conjunction with a skin-sparing mastectomy by an inexperienced general surgeon. It is usually caused by making the mastectomy flaps excessively thin, thereby depriving them of their blood supply. In most cases, because the underlying TRAM flap is viable and the volume of necrotic tissue is small, mastectomy flap necrosis causes no permanent problem. As with umbilical necrosis, it resolves spontaneously over a period of 8 to 10 weeks and often has minimal or no effect on the final result (Fig 11-6).

Abdominoplasty flap necrosis is more common in patients who smoke, and can be caused by excessively wide undermining of the abdominoplasty flaps.[12] Because of the need to dissect a tunnel between the abdominal dissection and the defect in the breast, it is more common after conventional TRAM flaps than after free TRAM flaps. It is also more common, and likely to be more severe, after a bilateral reconstruction.

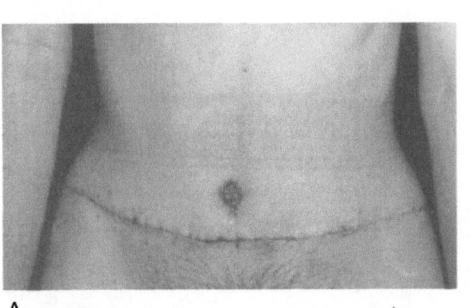
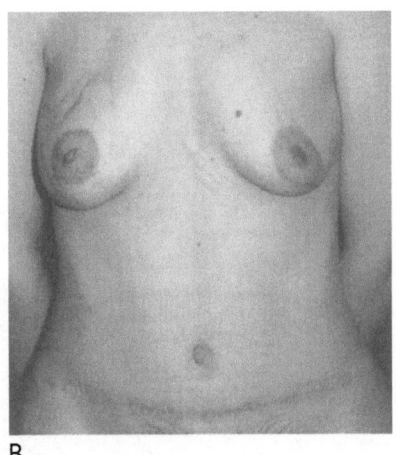
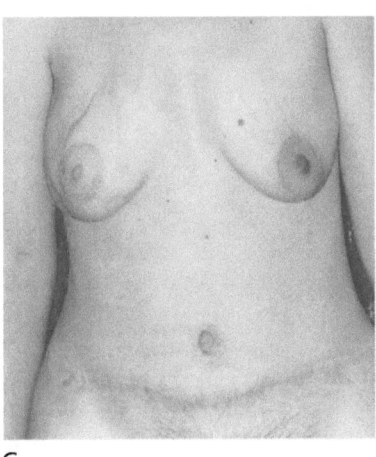

A   B   C

FIG. 11-5 (A) Umbilical necrosis after a TRAM flap. (B) One year later, the final outcome was not significantly compromised. (C) Subsequently, the patient had a successful full-term pregnancy, which left stretch marks but was otherwise uneventful.

Abdominoplasty flap necrosis can range in severity from trivial to devastating (Figs 11-7 and 11-8). In minor cases, it can sometimes be excised and the wound closed primarily. In more severe cases, debridement, dressing changes, and healing by secondary intention provide the best course. In the worst cases, skin grafting followed by late corrective surgery may be necessary. By far the best strategy is prevention by avoiding wide undermining of the abdominoplasty flap in the first place.

If prosthetic mesh has been used to reinforce the fascial closure, exposure caused by abdominoplasty flap necrosis can resolve spontaneously, with healing by secondary intention occurring around the exposed mesh. Unfortunately, this technique of events does not occur invariably, and the mesh can become infected, ultimately requiring removal. For this reason, prosthetic mesh should never be used to replace rectus abdo-

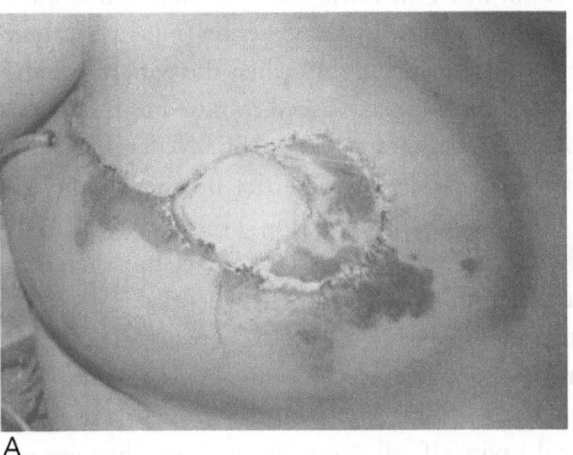
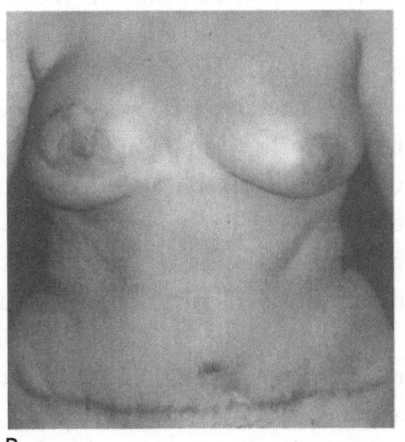

A   B

FIG. 11-6 (A) Early appearance of mastectomy flap necrosis. The underlying TRAM flap was well perfused. (B) The same patient, after healing by secondary intention and scar revision.

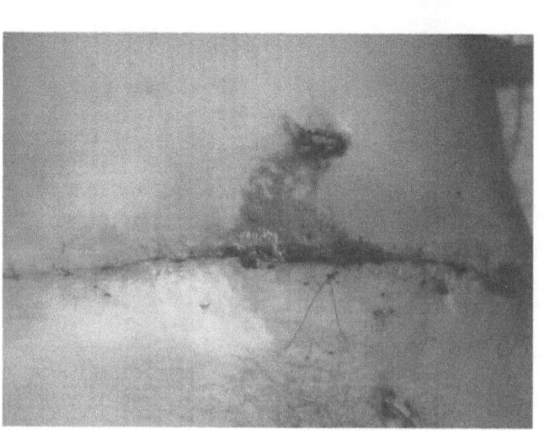
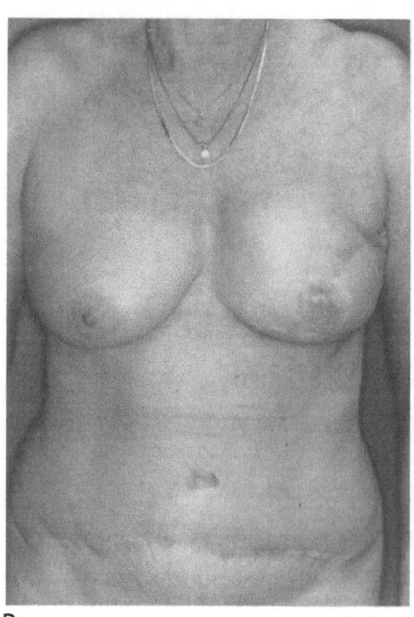

A   B

FIG. 11-7   (A) Abdominoplasty flap necrosis. This is most common in patients who smoke. (B) The final outcome, which was not significantly compromised by the abdominoplasty flap necrosis, although the breast shape was not ideal.

minis sheath fascia, only to reinforce it.[13,14] In that way, should the mesh need to be removed, the patient will not be left with abdominal wall incompetence.

Abdominal Bulging, Weakness, and Hernia

Abdominal wall bulges and hernias are uncommon when the fascia has been correctly repaired,[15,16] but they can occur even in experienced hands. Bulges and hernias are far more common after bilateral reconstruction, when the fascia has been subjected to more tension than is present after unilateral reconstruction. In a true hernia (Fig 11-9), there is a defect of the abdominal fascia that forms a palpable ring when the patient is lying supine. The hernia becomes apparent when the patient is asked to raise her head or to raise both legs simultaneously. In a bulge (sometimes called a "TRAM flap hernia"), there is no palpable defect, but diffuse (and usually asymmetric) bulging of the abdominal wall is obvious when the patient stands upright (Fig 11-10). In the overwhelming majority of these bulges, the external oblique fascia is intact but there is a defect of the internal oblique fascia, resulting in a partial-thickness hernia.

For both hernia and bulge, the treatment consists of surgical repair.[17] The repair requires general anesthesia with deep relaxation to reduce abdominal wall tension. The abdominal fascia is widely exposed, and a vertical incision is made through it over the bulge or hernia, entering the abdominal cavity. If adhesions are present, they are released. In a true hernia, the abdominal wall is simply repaired with a heavy running suture. If a bulge is present, the inner surface of the abdominal wall is inspected for the presence of a "shelf" formed by the retracted internal oblique fascia (Fig 11-11). If

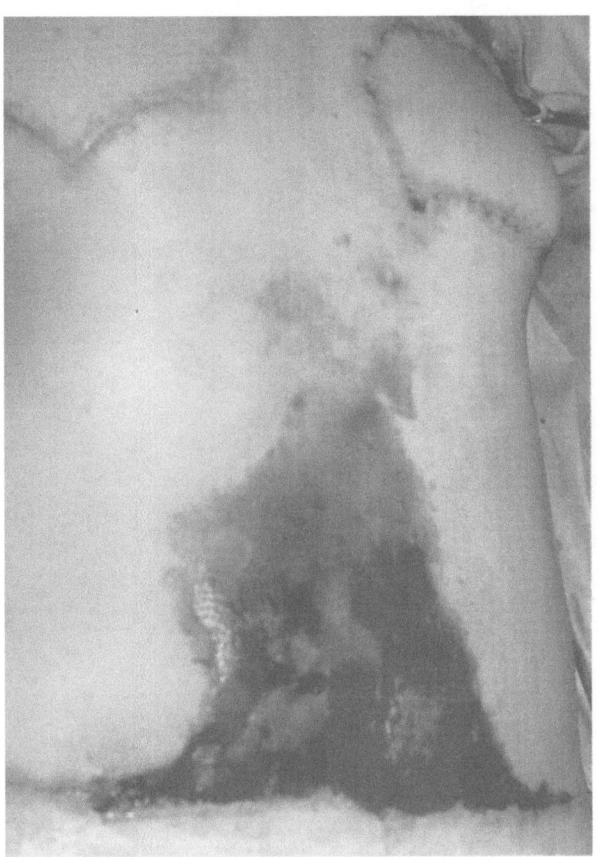

FIG. 11-8 Severe abdominoplasty flap necrosis after bilateral conventional TRAM flap breast reconstruction (performed elsewhere) in a heavy smoker. This complication is difficult to treat, and can be avoided by not undermining the abdominoplasty flap too widely. (From Kroll SS. *Plast Reconstr Surg.* 1994;94:637–643. Used with permission.)

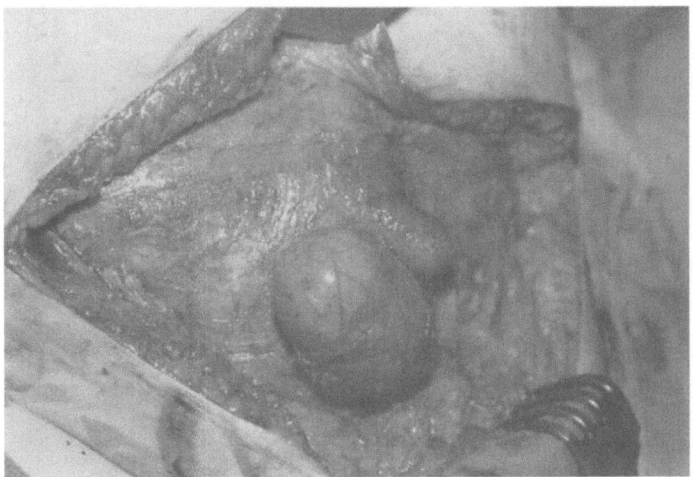

FIG. 11-9 True hernia following a TRAM flap. A distinct defect was palpable in the abdominal wall. (From Kroll SS. *Clin Plast Surg.* 1998;25:35–143. Used with permission.)

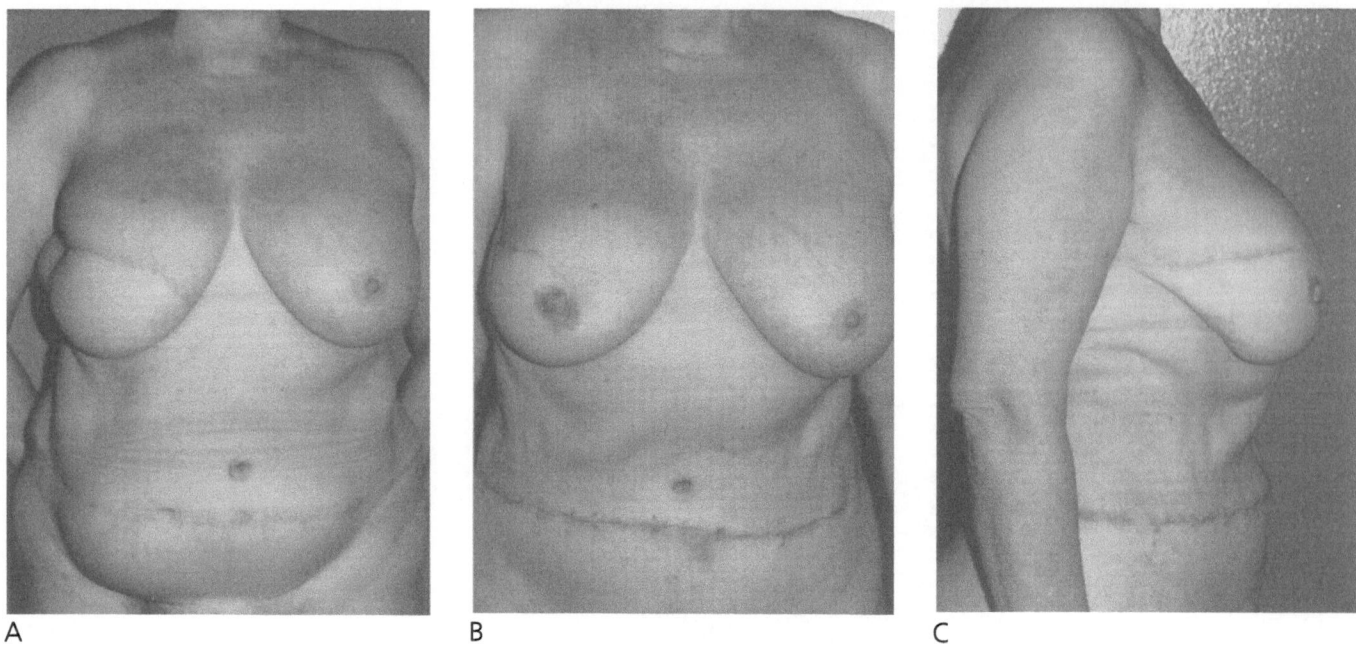

A B C

FIG. 11-10 (A) TRAM flap "bulge." Although not a true hernia, this can be very disabling. (B,C) After repair of the bulge and revision of the reconstructed breast.

found, this shelf is grasped by Allis forceps and pulled medially (Fig 11-12). This layer is then sutured to the midline fascia deep to the linea alba with a heavy running suture, just as in a correctly performed original repair. If the fascia was not properly repaired at the initial surgery, this may be all that is required. If the surgeon knows that the fascia was repaired correctly in the original closure or if there is any doubt at all

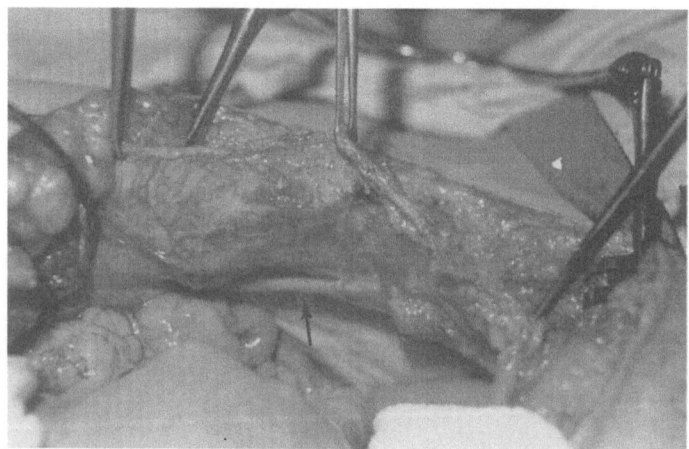

FIG. 11-11 Intra-abdominal "shelf" (arrow) formed by the retracted internal oblique fascia. To repair the bulge, it is necessary to suture this fascia securely to the midline fascia deep to the linea alba.

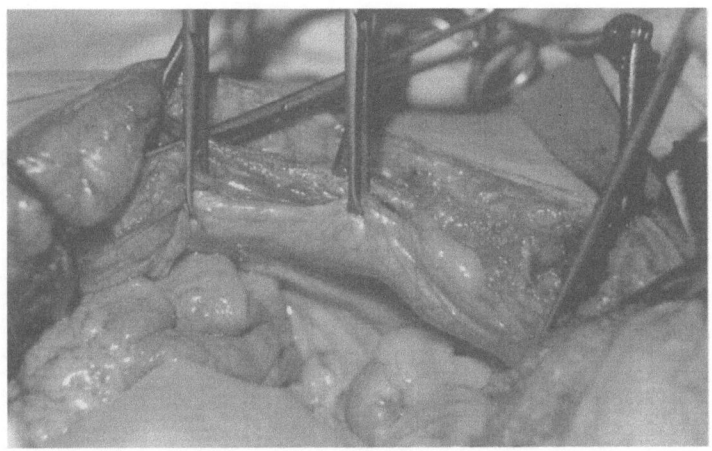

FIG. 11-12   The repair is facilitated by grasping the internal oblique fascia with Allis forceps.

about the strength of the current repair, however, reinforcement with prosthetic mesh is indicated for added security. If mesh is required, I prefer Prolene mesh to Marlex even though I am not aware of any firm evidence that supports that view.

In some cases, patients who appear to have no abdominal wall defect on physical examination will complain of persisting localized weakness and discomfort. In certain of these patients, surgical exploration has revealed the presence of small dehiscences of the internal oblique layer. Repair of these dehiscences has led to disappearance of the symptoms. The surgeon should therefore have a high index of suspicion, especially in bilateral cases, and seek and repair possible internal oblique separations whenever credible symptoms of weakness persist for more than 6 months (Fig 11-13).

TRAM flap breast reconstruction is a wonderful operation that can restore normal form to patients after mastectomy. It can lead to long-lasting and natural results that closely mimic natural breasts and can be highly satisfactory. When abdominal bulging or hernia occurs, however, the disability that results can effectively destroy the patient's ability to live a normal life and nullify any benefit of reconstruction that the surgeon has achieved. It is therefore essential to prevent abdominal hernias and bulges by performing donor site closure correctly in the first place. When hernias and bulges do occur, they must be properly repaired. Only by keeping these unfortunate complications to the lowest possible level can TRAM flap breast reconstruction remain popular and successful.

Keloids

Keloids can occur in susceptible patients and can be troublesome (Fig 11-14). The best management is avoidance, by not performing elective surgery on patients who form keloids. Keloids should not be confused with hypertrophic scars, however, which will often resolve spontaneously in time without specific treatment. Many patients who believe themselves to be keloid formers, because of hypertrophic vertical abdominal scars

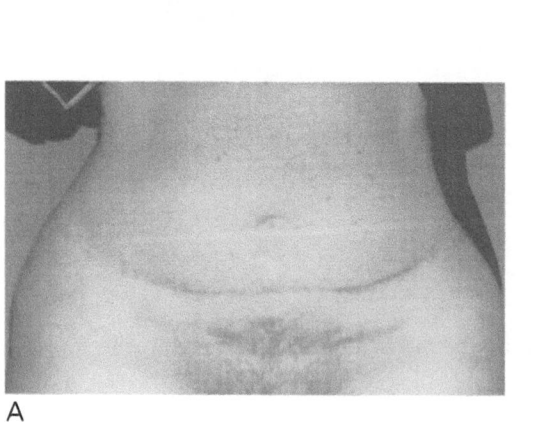
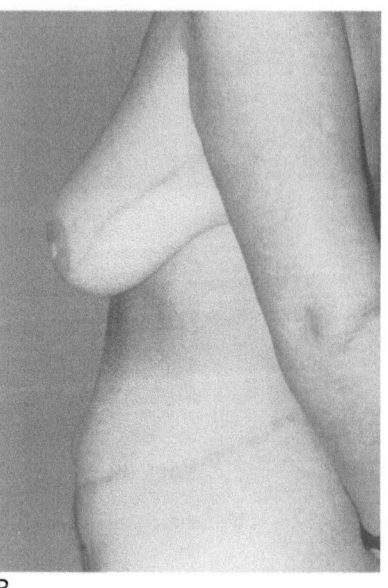

A

B

Fig. 11-13   (A, B) Patient who developed increasing abdominal weakness 1 year after bilateral free TRAM flap breast reconstruction. Although on physical examination there were no clear signs of a bulge or hernia, surgical exploration revealed a dehiscence of the internal oblique layer. Repairing that dehiscence, and overlying the repair with mesh, relieved all symptoms.

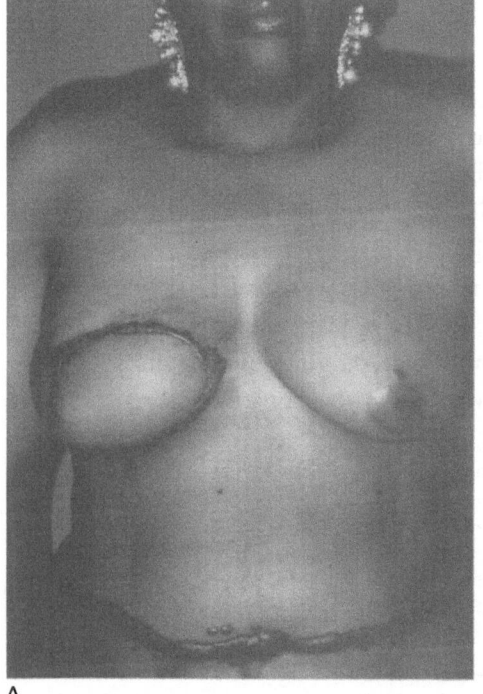
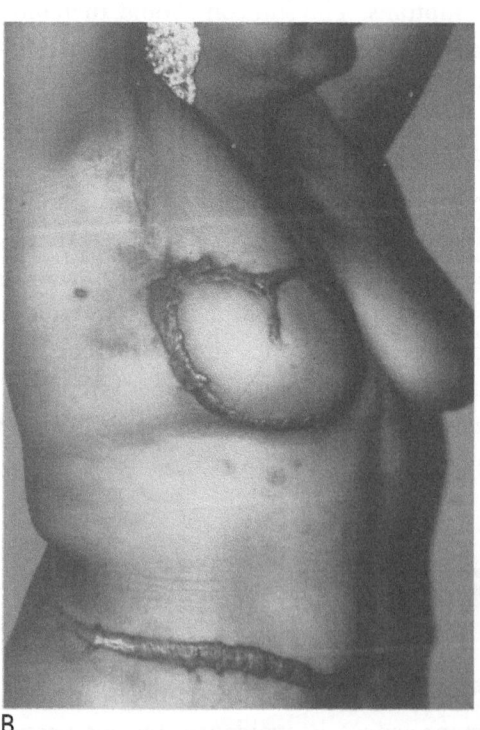

A

B

Fig. 11-14   (A, B) Patient with keloids following a TRAM flap breast reconstruction.

or prominent scars on the shoulder, are not. A useful test is to examine the patient's earlobes. If the patient has pierced ears but has not developed keloids in the earlobes, she is probably not a keloid former. If the patient is a true keloid former, TRAM flaps or any other form of autologous tissue breast reconstruction is contraindicated. If true keloids do develop, scar revision followed by early low-dose radiotherapy is appropriate treatment.

Infection

Infections are common in the presence of ischemic partial flap loss. These infections, however, are usually caused by the presence of necrotic tissue rather than by aggressive bacterial invasion. The proper treatment for these opportunistic infections is debridement, with antibiotics playing only a very secondary role. Infection may also occur around prosthetic mesh used to reinforce the abdominal wall, usually following overlying abdominoplasty flap necrosis. If the infection does not resolve with debridement and antibiotic treatment, the mesh may ultimately have to be removed. If necessary, the mesh can be replaced 6 months later provided that the tissues are well vascularized and remain free of infection.

Infections that are not related to tissue ischemia or to foreign bodies are rare but can occur. I have seen one patient who developed a widespread low-grade infection with an atypical mycobacterium (Fig 11-15). This infection resisted control with ordinary antibiotics and was impossible to treat until special mycobacterial cultures were performed and the appropriate antibiotics identified.

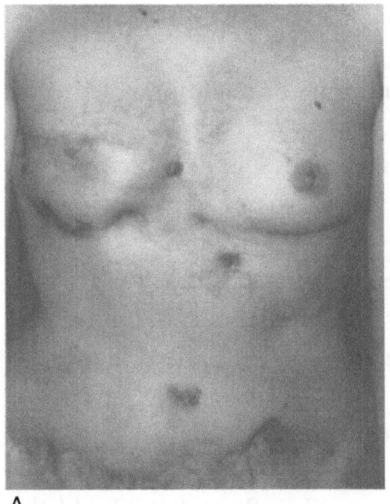 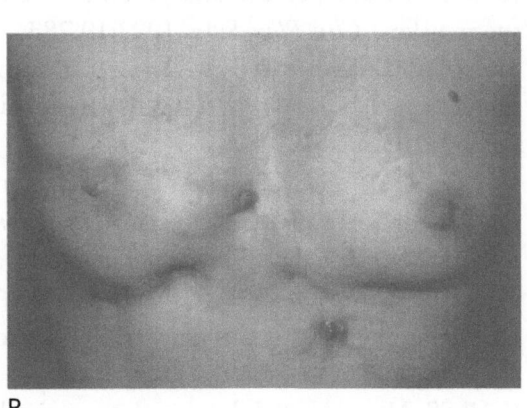 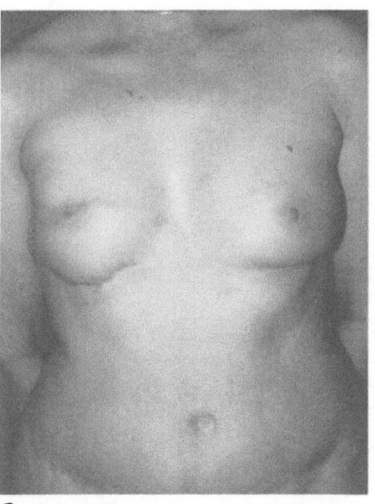

A   B   C

FIG. 11-15   (A, B) Patient 1 year after a TRAM flap breast reconstruction, showing multiple cutaneous abscesses that resisted treatment with ordinary antibiotics. (C) After specific treatment of a typical mycobacterial infection, the problem resolved.

Summary

TRAM flap breast reconstruction is major surgery and requires careful postoperative management of fluids and pulmonary function. Dehydration and atelectasis should be prevented or treated, as should gastric dilatation. If a free flap has been performed, postoperative flap monitoring is performed hourly for 3 days. If significant partial flap loss occurs, it should be treated aggressively with early debridement and, if necessary, tissue replacement. Abdominal bulges and hernias should be prevented by meticulous and secure closure of the fascial donor site (or sites). If they occur despite all efforts, they should be repaired aggressively by exposing the dehiscent internal oblique layer and attaching it securely to the midline fascia with heavy permanent running suture, often (especially in bilateral cases) adding reinforcement with synthetic mesh.

References

1. Jambor CR, Steedman DJ. Acute gastric dilatation after trauma. *J R Coll Surg Edinb.* 1991;36:29–31.
2. Strom BL, Berlin JA, Kinman JL, et al. Parenteral ketorolac and risk of gastrointestinal and operative site bleeding. A postmarket surveillance study. *JAMA.* 1996;275:376–382.
3. Kroll SS, Schusterman MA, Reece GP, et al. Timing of pedicle thrombosis and flap loss after free tissue transfer. *Plast Reconstr Surg.* 1996;98:1230–1233.
4. Machens HG, Mailaender P, Rieck B, Berger A. Techniques of blood flow monitoring after free tissue transfer: an overview. *Microsurgery.* 1994;15:778–786.
5. Bornmyr S, Arner M, Svensson H. Laser Doppler imaging of finger skin blood flow in patients after microvascular repair of the ulnar artery at the wrist. *J Hand Surg [Br]* 1994;19:295–300.
6. Tuominen HP, Asko-Seljavaara S, Svartling NE, Harma MA. Cutaneous blood flow in the TRAM flap. *Br J Plast Surg.* 1992;45:261–269.
7. Jones NF. Intraoperative and postoperative monitoring of microsurgical free tissue transfers. *Clin Plast Surg.* 1992;19:783–797.
8. Swartz WM, Izquierdo R, Miller MJ. Implantable venous Doppler microvascular monitoring: laboratory investigation and clinical results. *Plast Reconstr Surg.* 1994; 93:152–163.
9. Hidalgo DA, Jones CS. The role of emergent exploration in free-tissue transfer: a review of 150 consecutive cases. *Plast Reconstr Surg.* 1990;86:492–498.
10. Kroll SS, Miller MJ, Reece GP, et al. Anticoagulants and hematomas in free flap surgery. *Plast Reconstr Surg.* 1995;96:643–647.
11. Kroll SS. The early management of flap necrosis in breast reconstruction. *Plast Reconstr Surg.* 1991;87:893–901.
12. Kroll SS. Necrosis of abdominoplasty and other secondary flaps after TRAM flap breast reconstruction. *Plast Reconstr Surg.* 1994;94:637–643.
13. Hartrampf CR Jr. In discussion: Drever JM, Hodson-Walker M. Closure of the donor defect for breast reconstruction with rectus abdominis myocutaneous flaps. *Plast Reconstr Surg.* 1985;76:563.

14. Kroll SS, Marchi M. Comparison of strategies for preventing abdominal-wall weakness after TRAM flap breast reconstruction. *Plast Reconstr Surg.* 1992;89:1045–1053.

15. Mizgala CL, Hartrampf CR Jr, Bennett GK. Assessment of the abdominal wall after pedicled TRAM flap surgery: 5- to 7-year follow-up of 150 consecutive patients. *Plast Reconstr Surg.* 1994;93:988–1002.

16. Chen L, Hartrampf CR Jr, Bennett GK. Successful pregnancies following TRAM flap surgery. *Plast Reconstr Surg.* 1993;91:69–71.

17. Kroll SS, Schusterman MA, Mistry D. The internal oblique repair of abdominal bulges secondary to TRAM flap breast reconstruction. *Plast Reconstr Surg.* 1995;96:100–104.

The Extended Latissimus Dorsi Myocutaneous Flap

12

The standard latissimus dorsi myocutaneous flap[1-4] was one of the first methods of breast reconstruction ever described and in fact was used as early as 1898 by the Italian surgeon Tansini.[5] When used over a silicone gel– or saline-filled implant (which replaces the missing breast volume), the latissimus dorsi flap restores breast shape by replacing missing skin. This technique is well known to all plastic surgeons. Its chief disadvantage is the frequent development of capsular contracture and other problems associated with breast implants (Fig 12-1).

The extended latissimus dorsi (ELD) flap,[6,7] a modification of the standard latissimus dorsi flap, transports additional tissue from the back so that a breast implant is not required. This avoids all problems associated with implants, most importantly the almost inevitable eventual development of capsular contracture.

Advantages of the Extended Latissimus Dorsi Flap

The chief advantage of the ELD flap is that it does not require use of a breast implant. Consequently, the reconstructed breast is soft, moves like a real breast, and usually develops some degree of sensibility. As in all breast reconstructions with autologous tissue, the quality of the result tends to improve with time, as the scars soften and fade (Fig 12-2).

Compared with the transverse rectus abdominus myocutaneous (TRAM) flap, the ELD flap has the advantage of relative simplicity. It requires a shorter operative time than the TRAM flap, and recovery is easier. There is no microvascular anastomosis, so returns to the operating room for exploration of the pedicle are rare. The ELD flap is therefore appropriate for some patients who are less than ideal surgical candidates, especially those who are denied TRAM flap reconstruction because of obesity or advanced age, or because of a previous abdominoplasty or TRAM flap (Fig 12-3).

Finally, the ELD flap has the potential for bilateral use without requiring that both breasts be reconstructed simultaneously. A patient who has had unilateral breast recon-

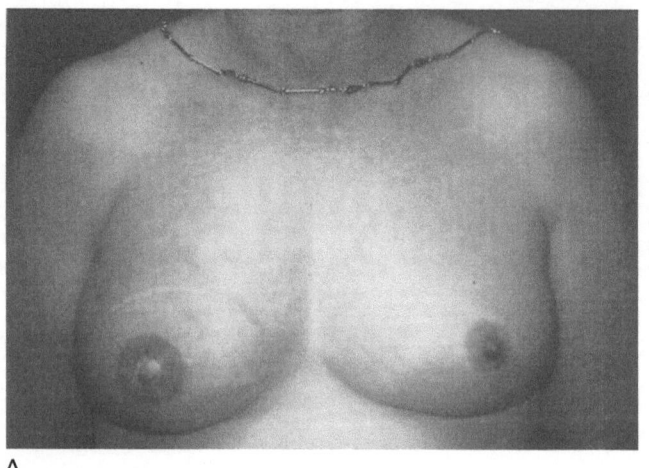

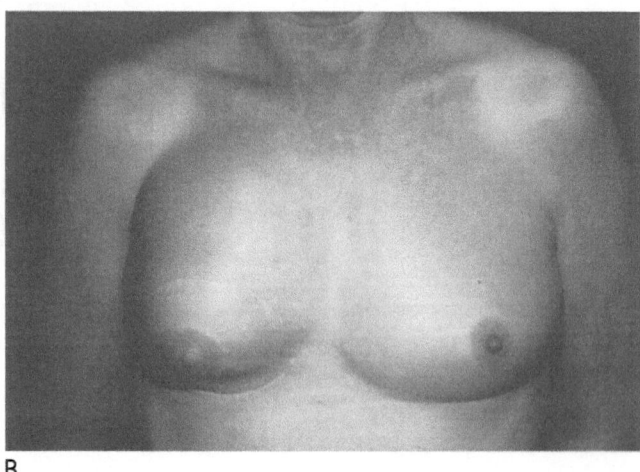

FIG. 12-1   (A) Result of a delayed breast reconstruction using a standard latissimus dorsi flap over a silicone gel breast implant. (B) Two years later, showing significant capsular contracture.

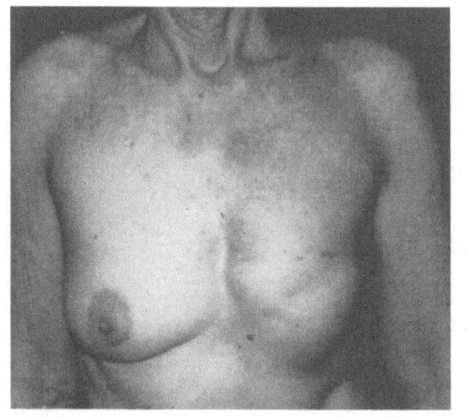

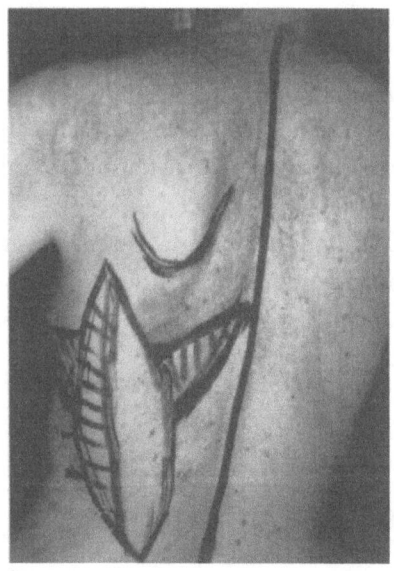

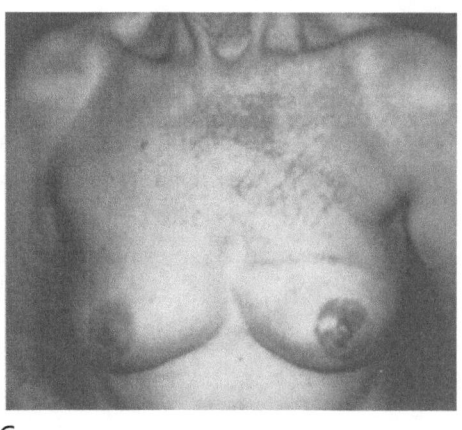

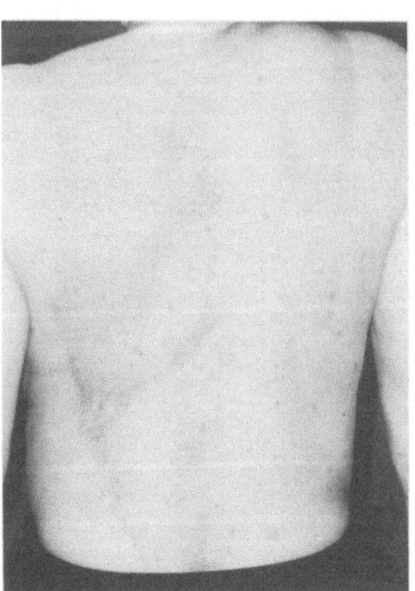

FIG. 12-2   (A) Patient after an unsuccessful attempt at breast reconstruction using tissue expansion. (B) Plan for reconstruction using a star pattern ELD flap. (C) Result 2 years later. See color insert, p. I-13. (D) Donor site. (From Kroll SS. *Clin Plast Surg*. 1998;25:135–143. Used with permission.)

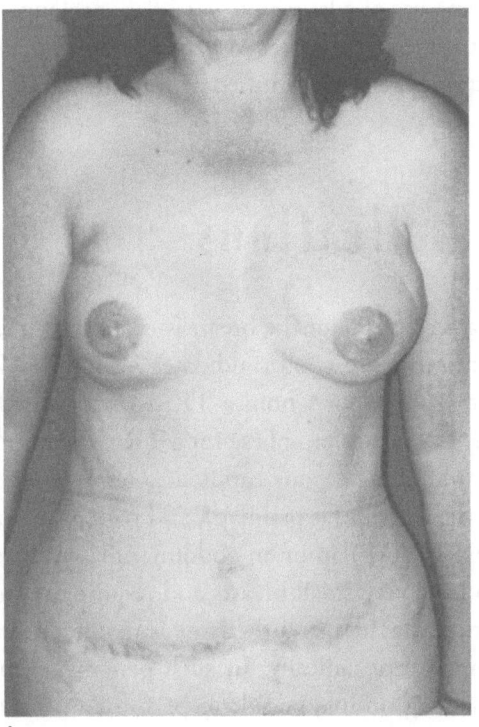 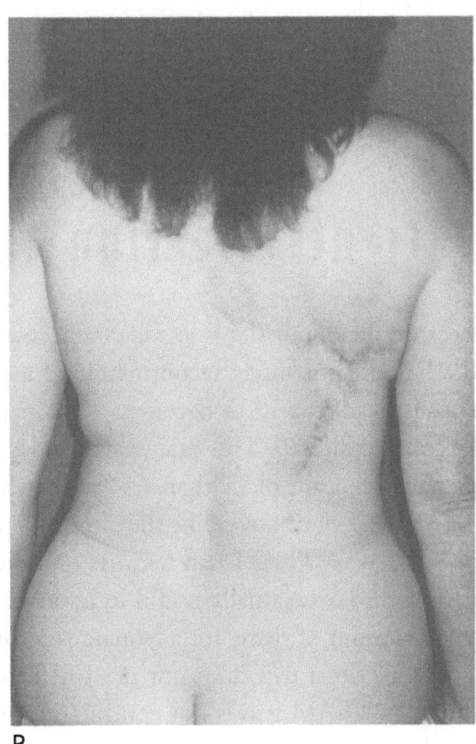

A   B

FIG. 12-3   (A) Patient with a TRAM flap breast reconstruction on the right, and an ELD flap reconstruction on the left. (B) Donor site on the back, which is not attractive.

struction with an ELD flap, therefore, can undergo reconstruction of the opposite breast with the same technique at some future time, should that become necessary. This can be an advantage if the patient is at high risk for development of a second primary contralateral breast cancer but does not choose to undergo prophylactic contralateral mastectomy with bilateral TRAM flap reconstruction at the time of her initial surgical treatment.

Disadvantages of the Extended Latissimus Dorsi Flap

The most important disadvantage of the ELD flap is the donor site scarring, which is more extensive than that of a standard latissimus dorsi flap. In extreme cases, the back can be robbed of so much tissue that it has an unattractive "skeletal" appearance. Also, the scars are more difficult to conceal with clothing than those of other techniques like the TRAM flap.

Breast shaping is more difficult with an ELD flap than with a TRAM flap. This is because the ELD flap contains a larger proportion of dermis, and much less pliable fat. What fat is present is attached to the dermis and is therefore more difficult to mold into the desired form. There is less available tissue in many patients, so the filling of the breast pocket can occasionally be inadequate and the breast shape irregular.

Finally, as in any surgical procedure involving use of a latissimus dorsi flap, prolonged drainage and seroma formation are not rare. Patients should expect to have a drain in their donor site for many weeks, especially if the dissection has been performed with electrocautery.

Patient Selection and Indications

Because the donor site is less favorable and because shaping of the breast is more difficult, the ELD flap is rarely recommended for patients who are good candidates for a TRAM flap. Instead, the ELD flap is used primarily in patients for whom a TRAM flap would be contraindicated. This category includes patients who are too obese for a TRAM flap,[8,9] patients who are older than 65 years (who would also be poor candidates for complex TRAM flap alternatives like the gluteal flaps or the Rubens fat pad flap), and patients who cannot have a TRAM flap because of a previous TRAM flap or an abdominoplasty. The ELD is also occasionally useful in patients who have very small breasts and require only a small amount of tissue for adequate reconstruction. Because so little tissue is required, the latissimus dorsi flap does not need to be extended very radically. In such patients, even though a TRAM flap is not contraindicated, the surgeon may decide to perform an ELD flap because it is simpler, takes less time, and has less potential morbidity.

Obese Patients

An excellent indication for an ELD flap is a patient who desires autologous reconstruction but is too obese for a TRAM flap. Although it is technically possible to perform TRAM flaps on such patients, the risk of complications increases in direct proportion to the patient's obesity.[9] Moreover, in very heavy patients the effort required to perform a TRAM flap, the operating time, and the risk of failure are all increased. For these reasons, patients with a weight/height index (weight in kilograms divided by height in meters) greater than 55 are usually rejected as candidates for a TRAM flap.

Fortunately, such patients often make excellent candidates for breast reconstruction with an ELD flap (Figs 12-4 and 12-5). Because of their obesity, there is often a thick layer of dorsal subcutaneous fat that can be used to construct an adequate breast. Although contralateral breast reduction may be required to achieve symmetry and the aesthetic results are usually less perfect than those that can be achieved in thinner patients, the results can be very satisfying for the patients.

Older Patients

Age is not an absolute contraindication to a TRAM flap. Nevertheless, many surgeons (including myself) are reluctant to recommend a complex elective operation to most patients older than 65 years. Obviously, each patient must be judged as an individual, and some older patients can obtain excellent results from TRAM flap breast recon-

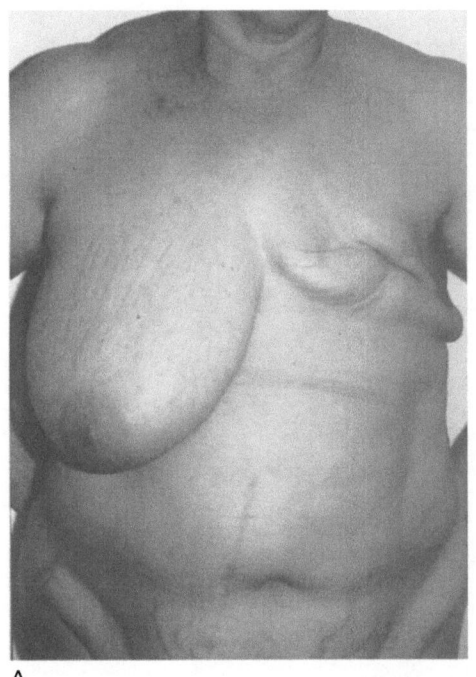
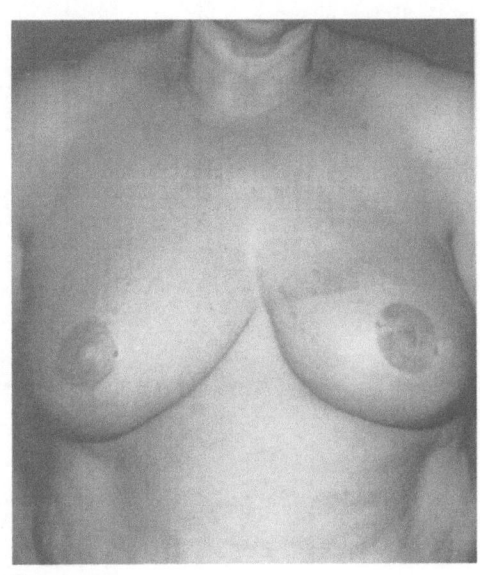

A   B

FIG. 12-4   (A) Obese patient who requested delayed breast reconstruction. Because of her obesity, she was not a candidate for a TRAM flap. (B) Result after reconstruction with an ELD flap and contralateral breast reduction.

struction. In general, however, I am reluctant to perform TRAM flaps on patients who are older than 65 unless they are unusually fit and healthy.

For patients who are older than 65 but who insist on having breast reconstruction, an ELD flap can be a good choice. The ELD flap combines the advantages of autologous tissue reconstruction with those of a simpler and safer procedure. The patient's objective is usually a normal appearance in clothing, with a minimum risk of requiring additional surgery. The ELD flap usually achieves those goals without difficulty (Fig 12-6). Moreover, older patients tend to be less concerned about the appearance of the donor site scars on the back. For these reasons, the ELD flap is often my first choice for breast reconstruction in older patients.

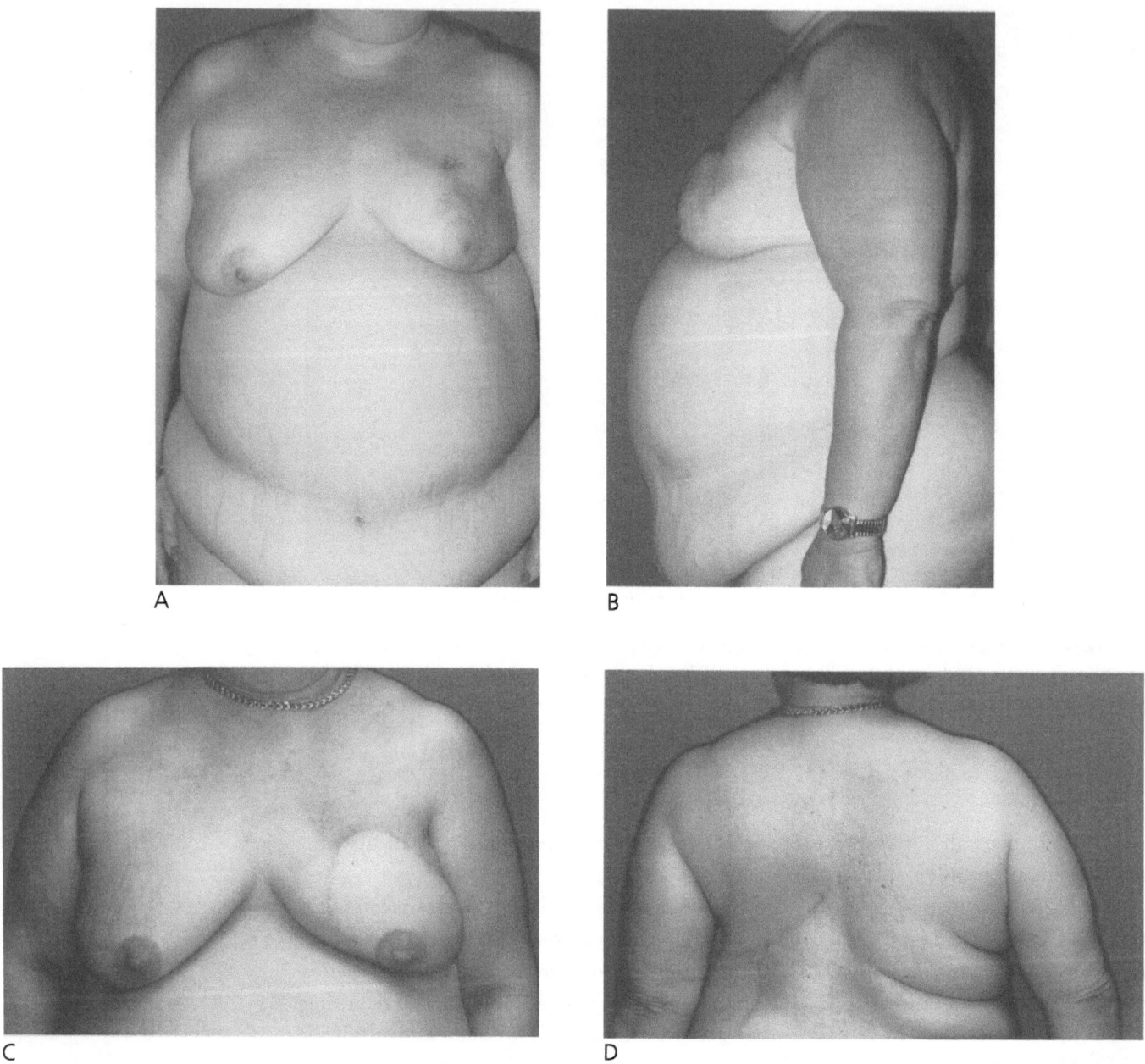

FIG. 12-5   (A, B) Very obese patient who desired autologous tissue breast reconstruction. (C) Result of reconstruction with an ELD flap. (D) Donor site.

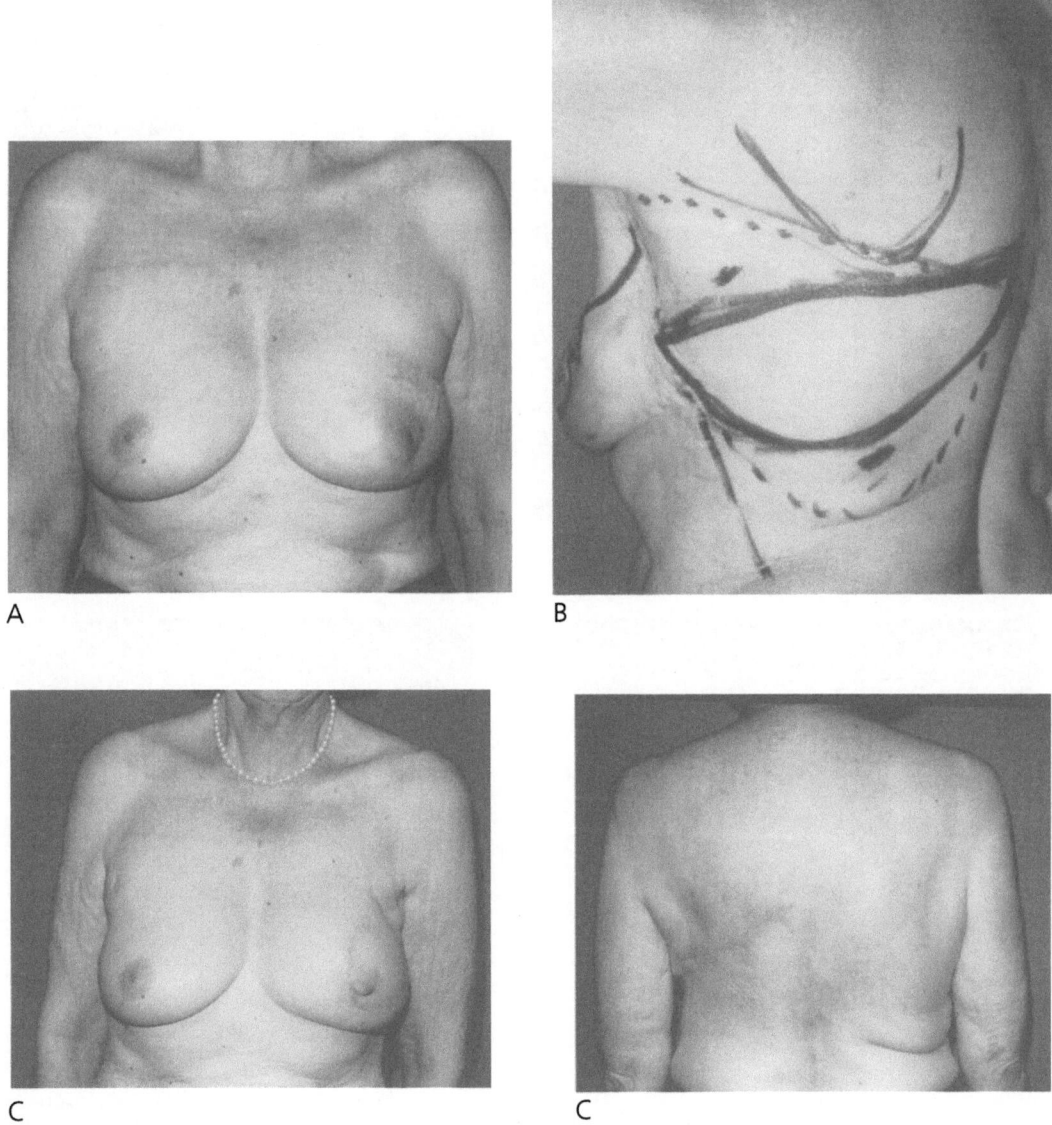

FIG. 12-6 (A) A 68-year-old woman who requested immediate breast reconstruction. (B) Plan for an ELD flap with a horizontal skin pattern. (C) Result 1 year after reconstruction. (D) Donor site.

Patients with Very Small Breasts

Patients with very small breasts, who are usually small and thin, are ideal surgical candidates and can almost always have technically successful TRAM flap breast reconstruction without difficulty. Nevertheless, in such patients, it is often difficult to achieve breast symmetry unless the patient desires augmentation of the opposite side. Even after multiple revisions, the reconstructed breast may remain larger than the natural one. Moreover, it seems unreasonable to work so hard to transfer a TRAM flap to the patient's chest only to have to throw most of it away.

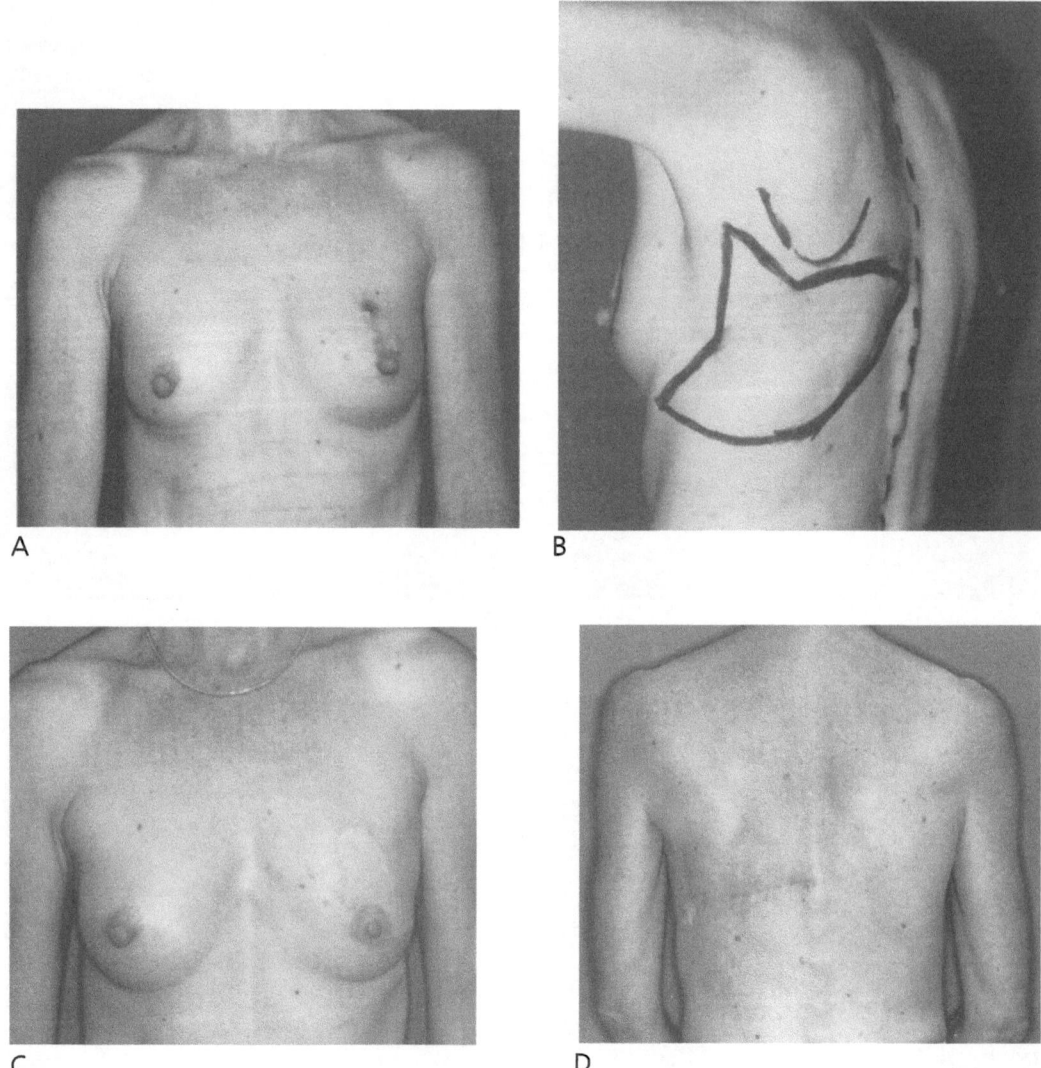

FIG. 12-7 (A) Thin patient with small breasts who desired immediate breast reconstruction with autologous tissue. (B) Plan for an ELD flap. (C) Result 2 years later. Note that there is some irregularity medially due to a slight insufficiency of tissue there. (D) Donor site.

For such patients, an ELD flap can be a good compromise (Figs 12-7 and 12-8). Because only a small amount of tissue must be transferred, the ELD flap can often be smaller than usual, so donor site morbidity is minimal. The size of the ELD flap is better matched to the desired breast mount than a TRAM flap would be, and the operative time, hospital stay, and need for revisions are all kept to a minimum. The donor site scar is less attractive and more difficult to conceal than that of a TRAM flap, however. For patients who find this scar objectionable, a deep inferior epigastric perforator flap may prove to be a more acceptable alternative.

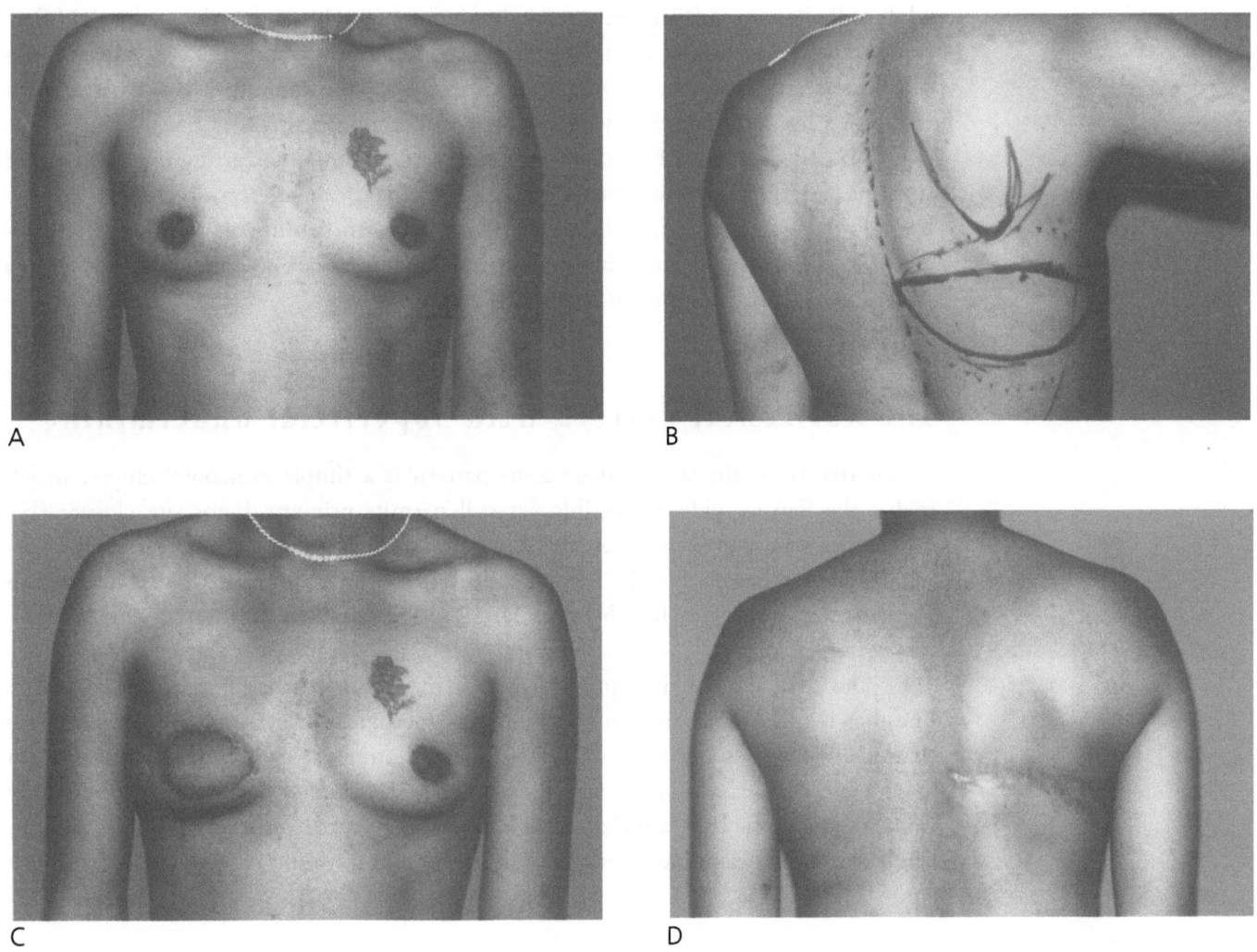

FIG. 12-8 (A) Patient with small breasts who requires a right modified radical mastectomy. (B) Plan for an ELD flap using a horizontal elliptical pattern. (C) Result of the ELD flap reconstruction. (D) Donor site.

Designing the Flap

The amount of tissue transferred with the latissimus dorsi flap can be increased in three ways. One way is simply to increase the amount of skin harvested by using a fleur-de-lis or star pattern. A second approach is the transfer of additional subcutaneous fat overlying the muscle, in addition to that carried with overlying skin. The third approach is to harvest the flap from lower in the back, where there is more fat.

The Fleur-De-Lis or Star Pattern

As originally described, the ELD flap used a variation of the three-pointed fleur-de-lis pattern;[6,10] a superior extension increased the amount of skin harvested with the flap while still allowing primary closure of the donor site. This approach, or the modification that uses a four-pointed star pattern (Fig 12-2), significantly increases the amount of transferred skin and underlying fat. In most cases, the amount of tissue is sufficient to create a mound that will adequately match the opposite breast.

The disadvantage of this approach is that the donor site scarring is extensive and (if a star pattern is used) may include a junction of vertical and horizontal scars. Wound breakdown at this point is not rare (Fig 12-8) and can be difficult to manage postoperatively. Even when primary healing occurs, the donor scars are often visible when the patient wears a bathing suit or a low-backed gown.

The Horizontal Pattern with Superficial Undermining

An alternative to the star or fleur-de-lis pattern is a simple horizontal ellipse, which makes the flap as wide as possible yet still permits primary donor site closure (Fig 12-6). The skin above and below the skin paddle is undermined at the level of the dorsal analogue of Scarpa's fascia, leaving subcutaneous fat deep to that fascia attached to the latissimus dorsi muscle. This deep fascia and fat are then transferred with the flap, increasing its volume.

The advantage of this approach is that the donor scar is limited to a transverse line that is more easily hidden by clothing. The disadvantages include the possibility that insufficient tissue may be transferred, necessitating use of a small implant to form a symmetrical breast mound, and the risk that the skin of the back may be overly thinned, giving the back a skeletonized look. Moreover, excessive thinning of back skin can lead to insufficient blood supply, skin necrosis, and wound breakdown at the donor site.

Low Horizontal Elliptical Pattern

In this approach, advocated by Professor Neven Olivari, the flap is harvested from lower in the back where the layer of fat is thicker (Fig 12-9). There is also more laxity and, if the flap is extended anteriorly, the fat is similar to that found in the TRAM flap and is therefore easier to shape. The advantages of this technique are that there is more available tissue and the donor site scar is less visible. The disadvantages are that a separate incision is required for access to the pedicle of the flap in the axilla and that the blood supply of the flap (situated farther from the pedicle) may be less reliable.

Which Design Is Best?

I generally prefer the fleur-de-lis pattern for most patients because it provides more tissue and is likely to permit adequate reconstruction without using an implant. This design also provides better exposure of the flap's pedicle. When only a small breast is required, however, I use a simple horizontal ellipse since it leaves a more aesthetic donor site scar. I generally leave some subcutaneous fat attached to the muscle above and below the skin paddle, but I am not radical about this undermining because I want to

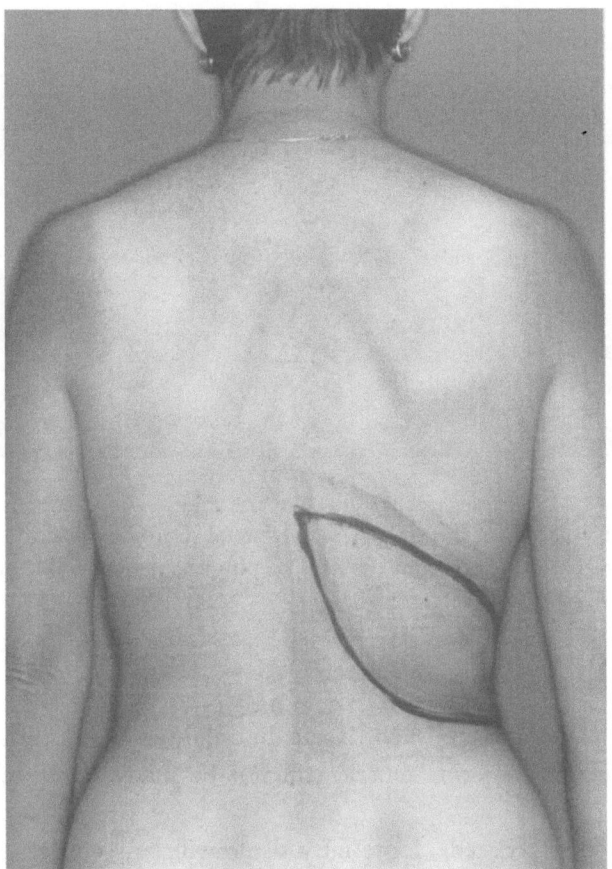

Fig. 12-9   Design for an ELD flap using the low horizontal skin pattern. This provides more tissue and a less visible scar, but somewhat reduced blood supply to the flap.

avoid skeletonizing the back. I have not personally used the low elliptical pattern enough times to judge it fairly but have seen good results from it and plan to use it again.

Elevating and Transferring the Flap

After the flap is designed, the patient is placed on the operating table in the lateral decubitus position on a beanbag, to prevent shifting (Fig 12-10). The skin above and below the flap is undermined at the level of the dorsal analogue of Scarpa's fascia (Fig 12-11), or deeper. The back flaps should be left sufficiently thick that vascularity is not compromised. When the superior and lateral edges of the muscle are reached, the dissection is deepened, exposing the muscle borders.

The latissimus dorsi muscle is then separated from the underlying tissue, beginning superomedially near the lower edge of the scapula. Blunt dissection with a finger is often helpful in safely creating a plane between the latissimus muscle and the rib cage superior to the serratus anterior muscle, just inferior to the pedicle (Fig 12-12). The blunt dissection is continued to the lateral border of the muscle, to establish the proper

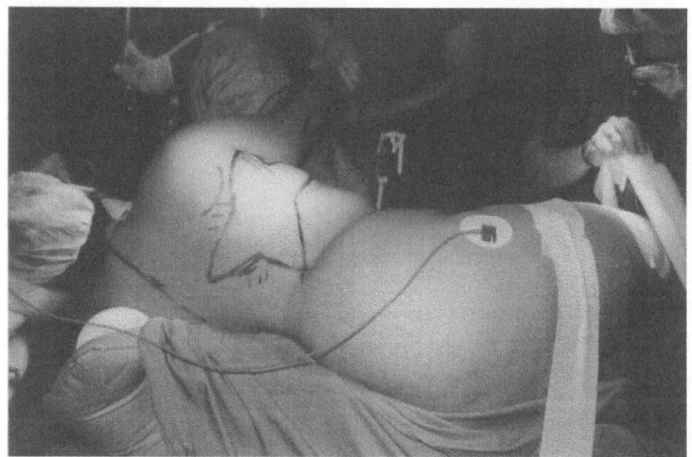

FIG. 12-10   Patient placed on a beanbag, in the lateral decubitus position. The beanbag becomes rigid after evacuation of air from the bag, keeping the patient stable even when the table is rotated.

plane. Once this plane is established, it can be followed inferiorly and laterally, ensuring that the serratus anterior muscle will not be inadvertently elevated with the ELD flap.

As the dissection proceeds, loose fatty tissue will be seen deep to the latissimus dorsi muscle, attached to its fascial connections with the serratus anterior muscle. At this level, the blood supply to the latissimus dorsi muscle is quite good. Much of this fat can therefore be left attached to the flap, increasing its volume (although at the price of increasing the skeletonization of the back).

As the dissection proceeds distally, the blood supply to the latissimus dorsi muscles becomes less robust. At the lower edge of the latissimus dorsi muscle, flap perfu-

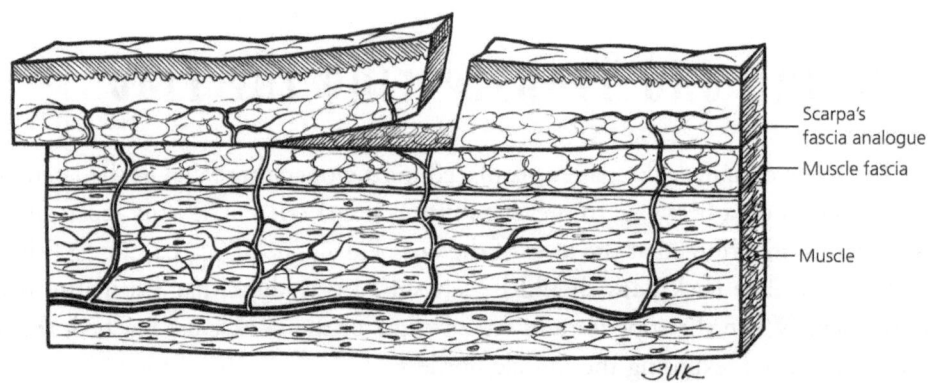

FIG. 12-11   Undermining the skin at the level of a fascial layer similar to that of Scarpa. The layer is always present but not always obvious. It is better to undermine in a plane that is too deep than to risk making the back flaps excessively thin.

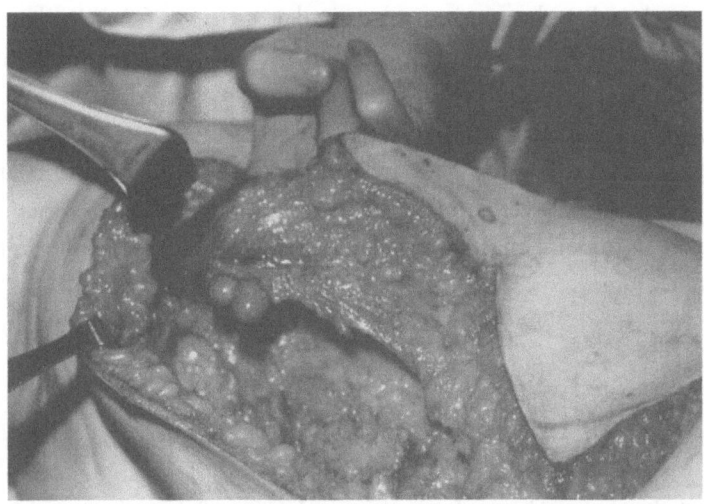

FIG. 12-12 Blunt dissection with a finger is useful to identify a safe plane of dissection deep to the latissimus dorsi muscle. This is best done just above the level of the scapular tip.

sion may be poor. Although abundant subcutaneous fat surrounds the distal muscle at this location, its transportability is uncertain. The amount of inferior fat left attached to the muscle should therefore be limited, especially in patients who smoke.

Once the flap is freed up inferiorly, the thoracodorsal vessels are identified, and the latissimus insertion divided above them, superior to where the pedicle joins the muscle. A tunnel is then created high in the anterior axilla to join the pedicle dissection and the breast pocket on the anterior chest. This breast pocket is dissected just superficial to the pectoral muscles, re-creating the defect of the original mastectomy by reopening the original mastectomy scars. The dissection is facilitated by rotating the table so that the patient is almost supine. The limit of this dissection is the mirror image of the borders of the opposite breast, which will have previously been determined with the patient standing upright.

Once the breast pocket is created, the flap is passed through the tunnel and into it. The vascular branches from the thoracodorsal vessels to the serratus muscle are divided should they interfere with flap rotation, but this is not required in every case. If scarring is not extensive and if the thoracodorsal nerve can be freed up without endangering the pedicle, that nerve is divided and a segment of the nerve removed to prevent subsequent unwanted breast movement. The tunnel is partially closed inferiorly, to better define the posterior border of the breast, but is left sufficiently open that the pedicle is not compressed.

Closing the Donor Site

The donor site should be drained (I use a 15-French round Blake drain), and is closed in layers using 2-0 Vicryl (polygalactin 910) sutures for the deep fascia and dermal layers. The skin is closed with running subcuticular sutures of 2-0 Prolene (polypropylene), supplemented with 3-0 or 4-0 chromic sutures at corners or other sites where the closure is less secure. Donor site closure is facilitated by rotating the table past the lateral decubitus position so that the patient is partly prone. Once the skin is closed, the table is rotated again so that the patient is in a more supine position, and the breast skin is closed temporarily over the flap with staples. The wound is then covered with an adherent plastic drape to maintain some degree of sterility during the patient's subsequent repositioning.

Shaping the Breast

After closure of the donor site and temporary closure of the anterior chest, the drapes and beanbag are removed, and the patient is repositioned on the operating table in a supine position. Care is taken to ensure that the positioning is symmetric, and that the back can be safely raised into a nearly upright sitting position. The patient is then washed with antibacterial soap and redraped for the second phase of the operation.

Each ELD flap is different, and there is no one standard all-purpose shaping technique. Certain general principles, however, can be used to achieve a better and more consistent breast shape.

First, the breast pocket dissection should always extend to the limits of the mirror image of the opposite breast, and the flap should be sutured to the medial edges of that pocket so that it cannot drift too far laterally. The inframammary fold should be the mirror image of the opposite side. Gravity will position the flap inferiorly in the pocket, so sutures are not usually required inferiorly, except perhaps toward the midline. The existing native breast skin should be reexpanded to its original position as much as possible by releasing all restricting scar tissue. Any remaining skin deficiency will be made up using skin from the flap.

Care should be taken to re-create a posterior breast border, just as in reconstruction with a TRAM flap. This border should join the inframammary fold in a gentle curve, giving the breast a rounded shape. The most common error is to place the sutures that form this lateral border too far laterally, leading to a breast that is too full under the axilla.

If a star or fleur-de-lis pattern has been used, some of the points of the flap can often be sutured together to give the flap a rounder, more globular shape (Fig 12-13). If a simple horizontal pattern was used, the flap is inset in a fashion similar to that of a TRAM flap. If existing native breast skin covers the lower pole of the breast, the flap can be bunched up beneath that lower pole skin to increase breast projection.

Shaping of the breast is always more difficult with an ELD flap than it is with a TRAM flap because the ELD flap is less soft and more rigid. Often, this rigidity will cause palpable or even visible irregularities in the breast. With time, however, most of this rigidity disappears, and it can therefore be ignored (Fig 12-14). Ultimately, with the passage of time, soft, natural breasts are obtained in most cases.

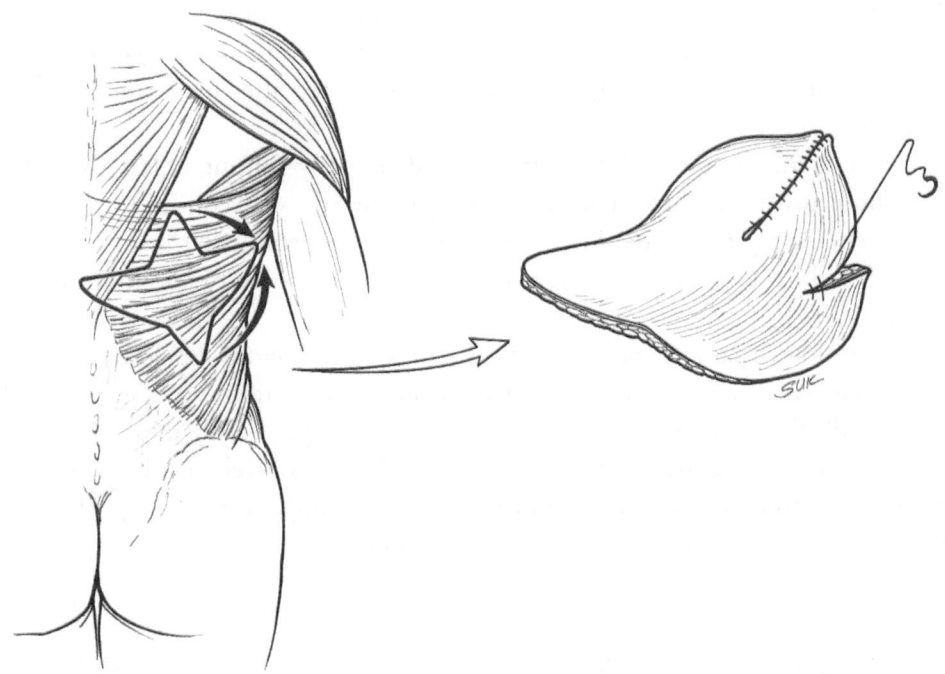

FIG. 12-13   The tips of the star or fleur-de-lis can be sutured together to form a somewhat globular mass of soft tissue.

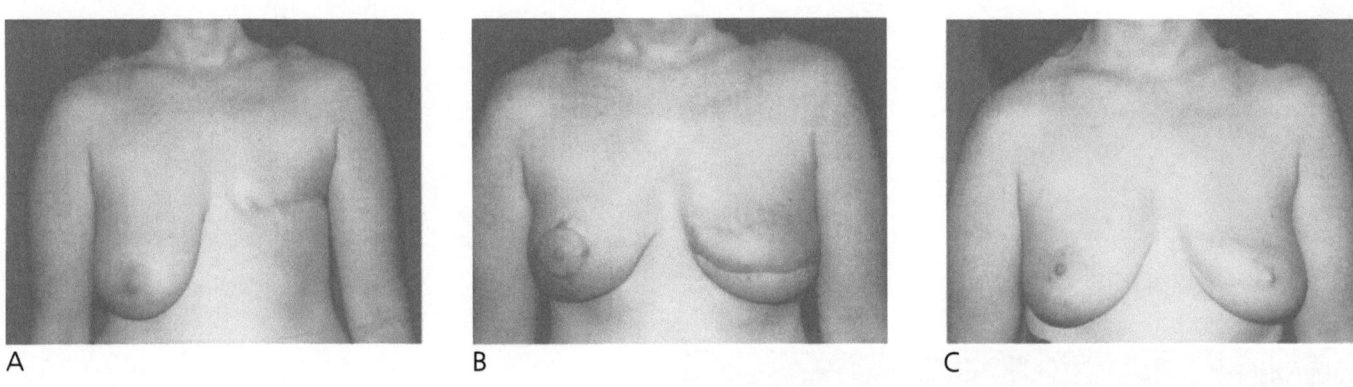

A   B   C

FIG. 12-14   (A) A 31-year-old woman after a left modified radical mastectomy. (B) Immediately after reconstruction with an ELD flap, the reconstructed breast was somewhat irregular and lumpy. (C) With time, the irregularities disappeared and the breast became soft.

Postoperative Care

A 15-French round drain is placed under the flap and led out through a stab wound in the axilla, where it is sutured securely to the skin. Postoperative pain in the donor site can be significant but is usually short-lived. A patient-controlled analgesia pump is helpful for the first few days. Most patients are fully ambulatory the day following surgery and have no dietary restrictions. Most patients can be discharged between the third and fifth postoperative days. Showers are permitted after the second postoperative day.

Each drain should be left in place until its daily output is less than 25 ml for 2 consecutive days. In many cases, the donor site will continue to drain for many weeks. Applying antibiotic or povidone-iodine ointment to the drain site twice daily will reduce local inflammation and make the presence of the drain easier to tolerate.

If a wound separation occurs in the donor site, healing can be delayed for many months (Fig 12-15). For that reason, it is essential not to resect excessive skin when harvesting the flap. This is a complication that is easier to prevent than to treat. If donor wound dehiscence does occur, it must be managed conservatively by obtaining dependent drainage and allowing the wound to heal secondarily. After healing, the wound can subsequently be revised to improve its appearance.

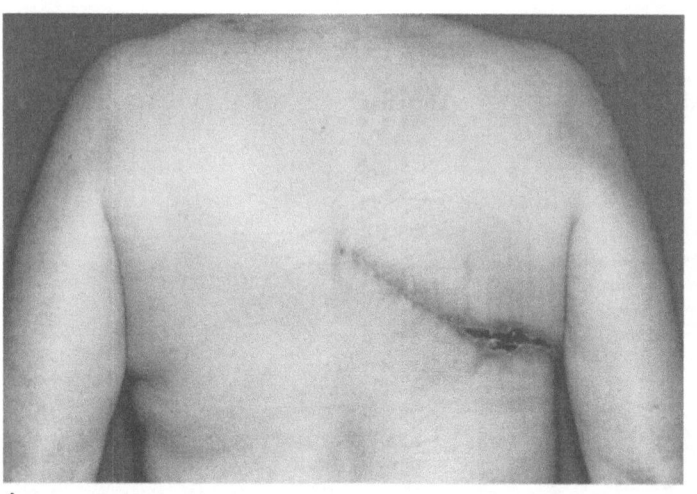

A

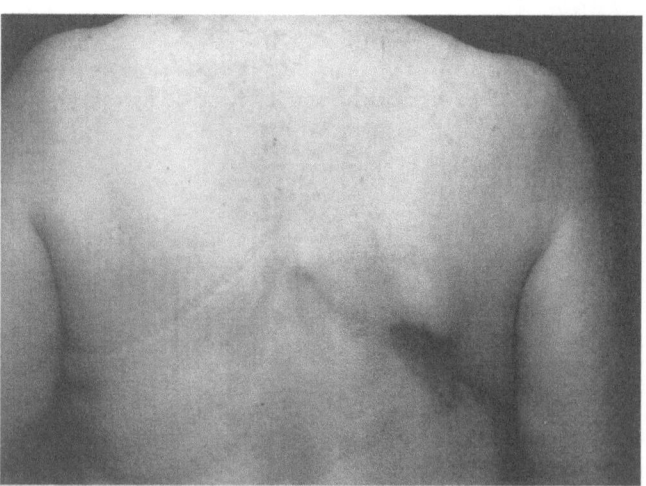

B

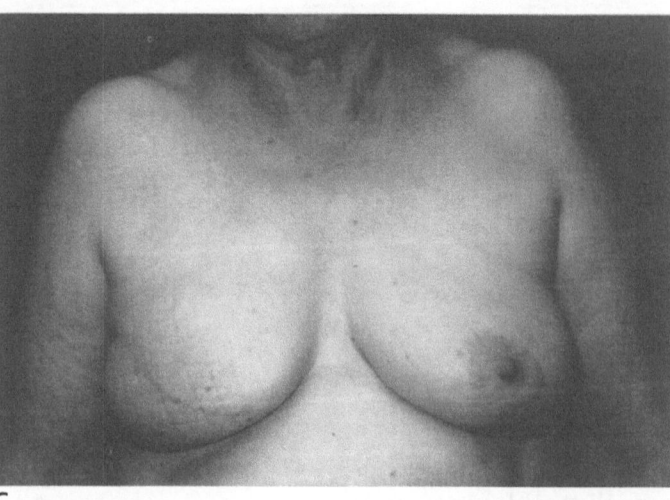

C

FIG. 12-15 (A) Wound separation in the donor site of an ELD flap. This wound remained open for many months. (B) Eventually the wound healed, but the scarring was unattractive. (C) Despite the donor site problems, the result in the breast, augmented with a small saline implant, was reasonably good.

Augmenting the Reconstruction with a Small Implant

Occasionally the ELD flap will not provide sufficient tissue to match the contralateral breast. In most cases, the preferred solution to this problem is a contralateral breast reduction. If the opposite breast is small, however, the patient may prefer to augment the reconstructed breast with a small (150-cc) implant. Although this might seem to defeat one of the principle advantages of extending the standard latissimus dorsi flap, in fact the implant is tolerated better under an ELD flap than under a standard latissimus dorsi flap because there is more autologous tissue overlying the implant to camouflage capsule contracture. This is especially true when the implant is small relative to the size of the breast. Although I prefer not to use an implant if possible, I do not hesitate to use one if the overall result will be improved and the patient is willing to accept the necessary risks. When I do use an implant, I generally prefer a saline-filled one since the risk of capsular contracture is lower than it is when silicone gel–filled implants are used.

Summary

The ELD flap is a useful technique for breast reconstruction in patients who are not good candidates for TRAM flaps. The ELD flap is technically simple yet capable of achieving excellent results. It is most useful for very obese patients and for patients older than 65 years. It can also be used successfully in patients who have very small breasts and therefore do not require transfer of much tissue volume. The ELD technique has the disadvantage of leaving a significant donor site scar, but many patients do not find that objectionable and believe that the donor site scar is more than compensated for by the technique's simplicity and relatively short convalescence.

References

1. McCraw JB, Penix JO, Baker JW. Repair of major defects of the chest wall and spine with the latissimus dorsi myocutaneous flap. *Plast Reconstr Surg*. 1978;62:197.
2. Biggs TM, Cronin ED. Technical aspects of the latissimus dorsi myocutaneous flap in breast reconstruction. *Ann Plast Surg*. 1981;6:381.
3. Bostwick J, Vasconez LO, Jurkiewicz MJ. Breast reconstruction after a radical mastectomy. *Plast Reconstr Surg*. 1978;61:682.
4. DeMay M, Lejour M, Declety A, Meythiaz A. Late results and current indications of latissimus dorsi breast reconstructions. *Br J Plast Surg*. 1991;44:1–4.
5. Maxwell GP. Iginio Tansini and the origin of the latissimus dorsi musculocutaneous flap. *Plast Reconstr Surg*. 1980;65:686–692.

6. McCraw JB, Papp C, Edwards A, McMellin A. The autogenous latissimus breast reconstruction. *Clin Plast Surg.* 1994;21:279–288.

7. Germann G, Steinau HU. Breast reconstruction with the extended latissimus dorsi flap. *Plast Reconstr Surg.* 1996;97:519–526.

8. Wagner DS, Michelow BJ, Hartrampf CR Jr. Double-pedicle TRAM flap for unilateral breast reconstruction. *Plast Reconstr Surg.* 1991;88:987–997.

9. Kroll SS, Netscher DT. Complications of TRAM flap breast reconstruction in obese patients. *Plast Reconstr Surg.* 1989;86:886–892.

10. McCraw JB, Papp C. Latissimus dorsi myocutaneous flap: "fleur-de-lis" reconstruction. In: Hartrampf CR, ed. *Hartrampf's Breast Reconstruction with Living Tissue.* New York: Raven Press; 1991:211–250.

13 The Superior Gluteal Free Flap

Advantages of the Superior Gluteal Free Flap

In the early days of autologous tissue breast reconstruction, the superior gluteal free flap was a popular technique with surgeons who advocated free flaps for breast reconstruction.[1,2] Its advantages are a reasonably inconspicuous donor site, an abundance of available tissue, and the potential to be used for bilateral breast reconstruction (harvesting a second flap from the contralateral side) without requiring that both breasts be reconstructed simultaneously.

In its heyday, the superior gluteal flap was considered an important alternative for patients in whom a transverse rectus abdominus myocutaneous (TRAM) flap was contraindicated. It could be performed in patients who had undergone previous TRAM flaps or abdominoplasties, and it had the advantage (significant for patients with a potbelly habitus) of not weakening the abdominal wall.

Today, the superior gluteal flap is used much less frequently than in years gone by, in large part because of the current availability of new alternatives (such as the inferior gluteal flap,[3–5] the extended latissimus dorsi flap,[6,7] and the Rubens fat pad flap[8]), all of which are technically easier to perform. However, a new and improved version of the superior gluteal free flap, the superior gluteal artery perforator (S-GAP) flap, has recently revived interest in superior gluteal free flaps. Consequently, these flaps may once again become used as a donor site for breast reconstruction.

Disadvantages of the Superior Gluteal Free Flap

The superior gluteal free flap has two main disadvantages. First, and most important, is its technical difficulty. Even for experienced microsurgeons, the very short pedicle of the flap

(2 to 3 cm) makes performance of the anastomoses technically difficult and often mandates the use of vein grafts. Also, the vessels forming the pedicle (especially the vein) are fragile and tedious to dissect. Technically, the free TRAM flap is a much easier operation.

Second, even though the donor site is covered by clothing, harvest of a superior gluteal flap changes the contour of the buttock in a way that can be visible through clothing, especially when the patient is wearing pants (Fig 13-1). Although this contour alteration is not severe and is symmetrical in patients undergoing bilateral breast reconstruction, it can be a significant disadvantage for patients undergoing unilateral reconstruction. Surgical alteration of the opposite buttock can correct this asymmetry, but that approach precludes the possibility of performing a contralateral superior gluteal flap in the future, negating one of the chief advantages of the technique.

Indications

The superior gluteal free flap can be performed in any patient who has excess tissue in the buttock and who desires autologous tissue breast reconstruction. In practice, this technique is rarely a first choice but is considered primarily for patients who cannot be

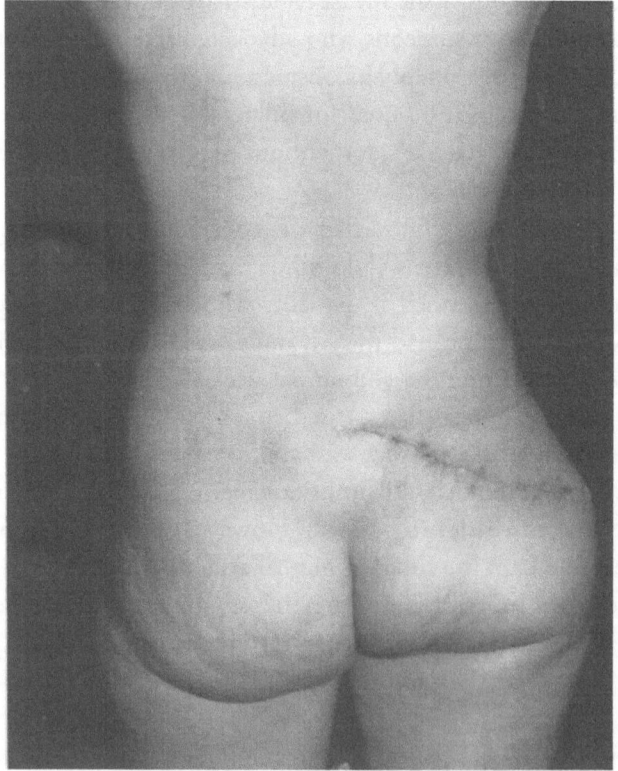

FIG. 13-1 Donor site of a superior gluteal free flap. Although the deformity is not severe, it is not always concealed by clothing, especially if the patient is wearing tight pants. (From Kroll SS: The superior gluteal free flap for breast reconstruction. In: Schusterman MA, ed. *Microsurgical Reconstruction of the Cancer Patient.* Philadelphia: Lippincott-Raven; 1997: Used with permission.)

reconstructed with TRAM flaps. Even in that situation, because of the shortness of the pedicle, the superior gluteal flap is usually not the alternative of choice. In my own practice, I rarely use the superior gluteal flap. Nevertheless, microsurgeons who perform autologous tissue breast reconstruction should be aware of this technique and know how to do it. This is especially true if they wish to progress to the use of S-GAP flaps.

Contraindications

The superior gluteal flap is contraindicated in patients who have insufficient tissue in their buttocks to donate a flap of adequate size. The technique is also best avoided if the patient will not allow harvesting of a vein graft. As with any free flap, absence of adequate recipient vessels and abnormal blood clotting are also contraindications.

Flap Design

The flap is oriented transversely on the upper buttock, with the medial portion of the flap overlying the superior gluteal vessels. Flap design begins by outlining the sacrum and then marking the location of the posterior superior gluteal spine (Fig 13-2). A line is then drawn connecting the posterior superior gluteal spine and the greater trochanter of the femur. The superior gluteal artery is usually located on that line, one third of the way between the spine and the greater trochanter.

The flap's skin paddle should be no wider than is necessary to obtain the tissue required to reconstruct the breast. Excessive tissue harvest greatly increases donor site deformity and should be avoided. The exact shape and orientation of the flap will depend on the patient's anatomy and on where laxity exists in her buttock.

Surgical Technique

The superior gluteal flap can be used for either immediate or delayed breast reconstruction. In immediate reconstruction, the reconstructive surgeon begins elevating the flap from the buttock immediately following the mastectomy. In delayed reconstruction, dissection of the recipient site should precede flap elevation, to ensure that adequate recipient vessels exist before committing to the procedure.

Positioning

The patient must be positioned on the operating table in such a way that access to both the breast and the buttock is possible. This is accomplished by placing the patient supine with her arms outstretched and her legs crossed so that the ipsilateral buttock is exposed (Fig 13-3). Leg compression boots are used to reduce the risk of thrombophlebitis.

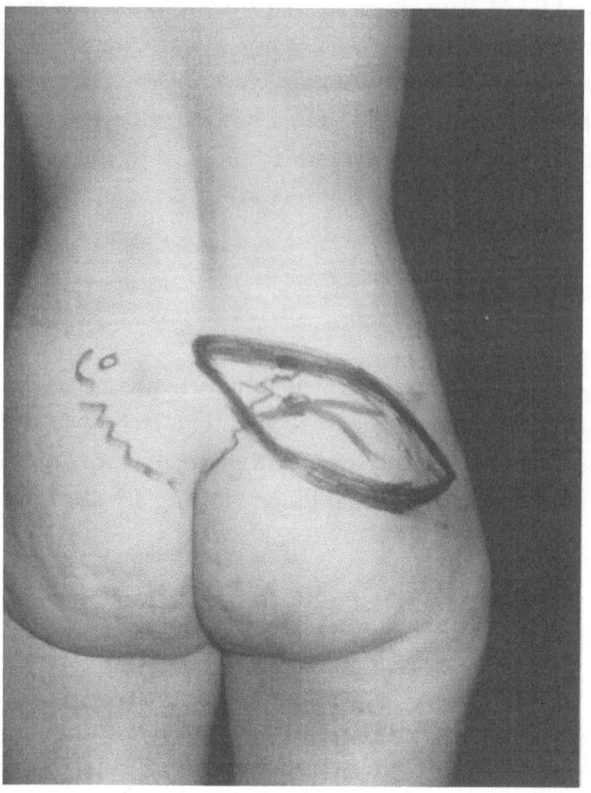

FIG. 13-2 Designing the superior gluteal free flap. The first step is to outline the sacrum and mark the location of the superior gluteal vessels, which the skin paddle is designed to overlie. (From Kroll SS: The superior gluteal free flap for breast reconstruction. In: Schusterman MA, ed. *Microsurgical Reconstruction of the Cancer Patient.* Philadelphia: Lippincott-Raven; 1997: Used with permission.)

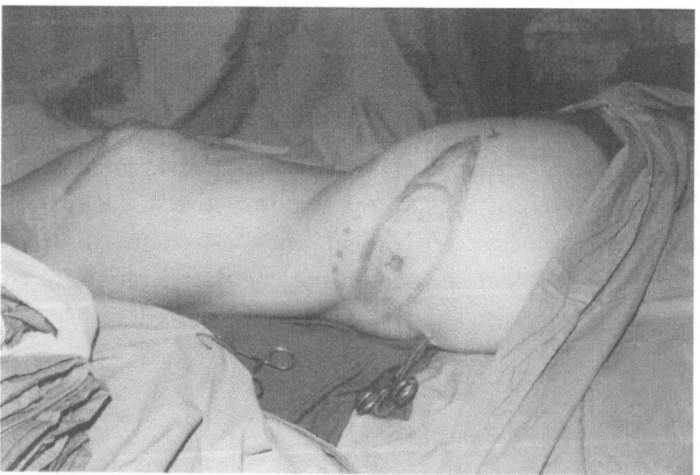

FIG. 13-3 The patient is positioned supine on the table, with her legs crossed so that access to both the breast and the buttock is possible.

Banking the table from side to side will permit access to the buttock for flap harvest and to the chest for transfer of the flap.

Elevating the Flap

The initial incision is made with a scalpel, following the predetermined markings. Most of the subsequent dissection is performed with electrocautery, however, to permit better visualization of the anatomy. The dissection begins superiorly and is deepened to the level of the gluteus maximus muscle. The muscle's superior border is identified, and dissection continues around it, separating the gluteus maximus muscle from the underlying gluteus medius muscle. The superior 5 cm of the gluteus maximus muscle is then partially divided laterally, approximately 5 cm from the greater trochanter, so that the muscle's deep surface is visible. Branches of the superior gluteal vessels can then be found entering the deep surface of the muscle. These blood vessels are followed proximally until they join the superior gluteal artery and vein, just above the piriformis muscle.

Once the pedicle has been identified, the gluteus maximus muscle surrounding the pedicle is divided, removing only that part of the muscle required to preserve integrity of the blood supply. The flap is then attached only by its pedicle, composed of the superior gluteal artery and vein (Fig 13-4).

In most cases, the pedicle will be very short. Sometimes it is possible to extend the length of the pedicle slightly by dissecting the superior gluteal vessels proximally for a short distance, to where they emerge from the pelvis. This must be done with great care, however, because if the vessels are disrupted, bleeding may be impossible to control because access is limited. Often the vein will have several branches. Although these branches are fragile and tedious to ligate, the surgeon can make use of their presence by identifying one that matches the size of the recipient vein on the chest wall and using it for the venous anastomosis.

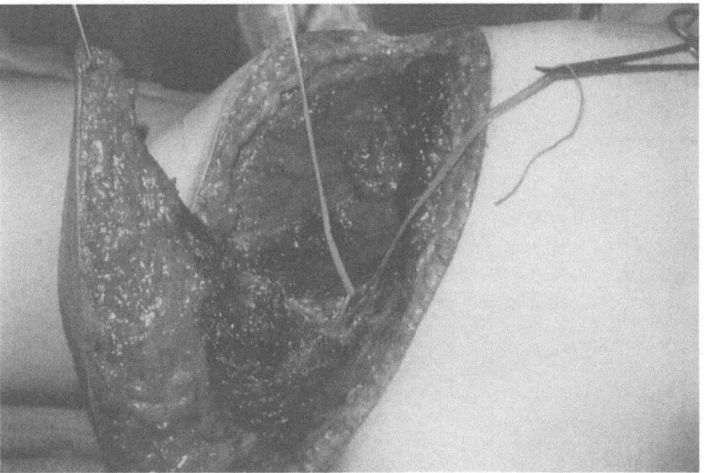

FIG. 13-4   The flap attached to the buttock by the superior gluteal vessels, with vessel loops around them.

Harvesting a Vein Graft

The most common recipient vessels in breast reconstruction with the superior gluteal free flap are the internal mammary vessels. Because these vessels are located close to the reconstructed breast, it is sometimes possible to transfer the superior gluteal flap without using a vein graft. In my experience, however, this transfer can be difficult because the pedicle is so short. In many cases (and always if the thoracodorsal vessels are used as recipients), harvesting of a vein graft will be necessary.

The most common donor site for this vein graft is the saphenous vein of the lower leg. This is a large vein with thick walls, which perhaps makes it a reasonably good substitute for an artery. The walls may be too thick for matching veins, however, especially thin-walled veins like the superior gluteal vein. Moreover, saphenous vein grafts sometimes go into spasm. If this occurs and is not relieved by the application of 2% papaverine solution, substitution of a cephalic vein segment for the saphenous vein graft may be necessary. My own preference is to avoid the use of vein grafts whenever possible, and to use the cephalic vein when a vein graft is necessary.

Transferring the Flap

The flap can be anastomosed to the thoracodorsal vessels (Fig 13-5) or the internal mammary vessels, depending on their availability and the surgeon's preferences. Preparation of these donor sites is described in chapter 9 and will not be repeated here. Most surgeons prefer the internal mammary vessels as recipients for this flap because of the short length of the superior gluteal vessels.[9–12]

If vein grafts are required, and if the flap pedicle is very short, it may be advantageous to anastomose the vein grafts to the flap on a back table, away from the patient. This makes these anastomoses much easier, since they can be performed on a

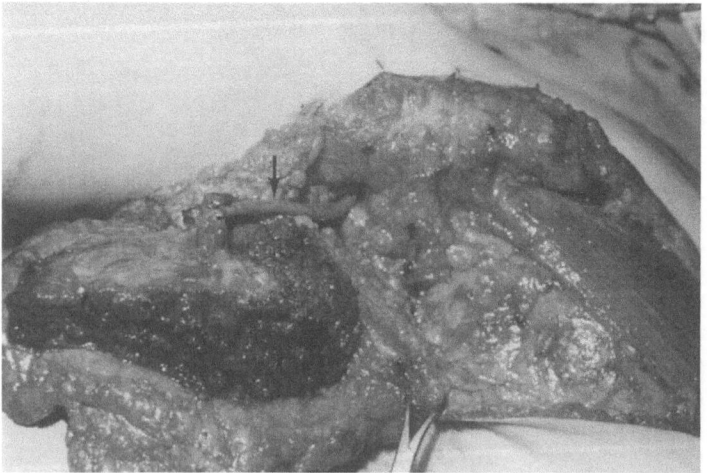

FIG. 13-5   The flap transferred to the axilla, using vein grafts (arrow) to connect the superior gluteal vessels to the thoracodorsal vessels.

level surface with the flap beneath the vessels out of the surgeon's way. When the vein grafts are subsequently anastomosed to the recipient vessels, the longer pedicle length achieved by the vein grafts can make those anastomoses technically easier and more comfortable.

Shaping the Breast

Shaping of the breast is similar to that of a TRAM flap (see chapters 16 and 17) except that the superior gluteal flap is firmer and more difficult to mold. With time, however, the flap will settle and become fuller in the lower pole, improving its shape (Fig 13-6). The deep surface of the medial edges of the flap should be sutured to the medial edges of the defect, using 3-0 Vicryl (polygalactin 910), to prevent lateral flap migration. The inframammary fold and lateral breast border are constructed just as with a TRAM flap. If sufficient tissue is present, the flap is sculpted, around its periphery, into a cone. A drain is placed beneath the flap and led out through a stab wound in the axilla.

Closing the Donor Site

The donor site is closed primarily, in layers. Dead space should be obliterated as much as possible with deep sutures. The wound is drained, using a round suction drain (I prefer a 15-French Blake drain) led out through a separate stab wound and sutured securely to the skin. The skin is closed with buried dermal sutures of 3-0 Vicryl and

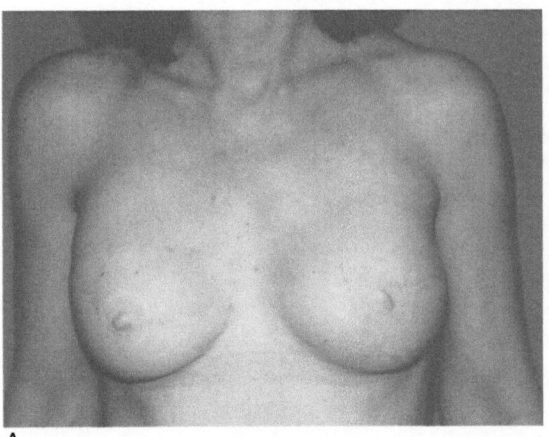
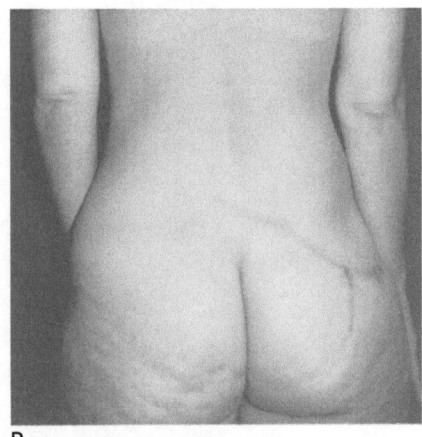

A   B

FIG. 13-6   (A) Result of right breast reconstruction with a superior gluteal free flap. The left breast was augmented for symmetry. Subsequently, the patient had a left mastectomy and underwent another reconstruction, this time with an implant. See color insert, p. I-14. (B) The donor site. See color insert, p. I-14. (From Singletary SE, Kroll SS: *Adv Surg.* 1996: 30:39–52. Used with permission.)

with running subcuticular sutures of 3-0 PDS (polydioxanone) or Prolene (poly-propylene).

Postoperative Care

Postoperative care is similar to that for a free TRAM flap (see chapter 11) except that a nasogastric tube is not required and respiratory function is not interfered with. Patients get out of bed on the second postoperative day and are able to sit on a chair immediately. Ambulation is not restricted. Each drain is left in place until its daily output is less than 25 ml for 2 consecutive days. The running subcuticular sutures are removed in 3 weeks. There are no limitations on lifting, and patients usually can be discharged on the fifth or sixth postoperative day. As with TRAM flaps, revisions are

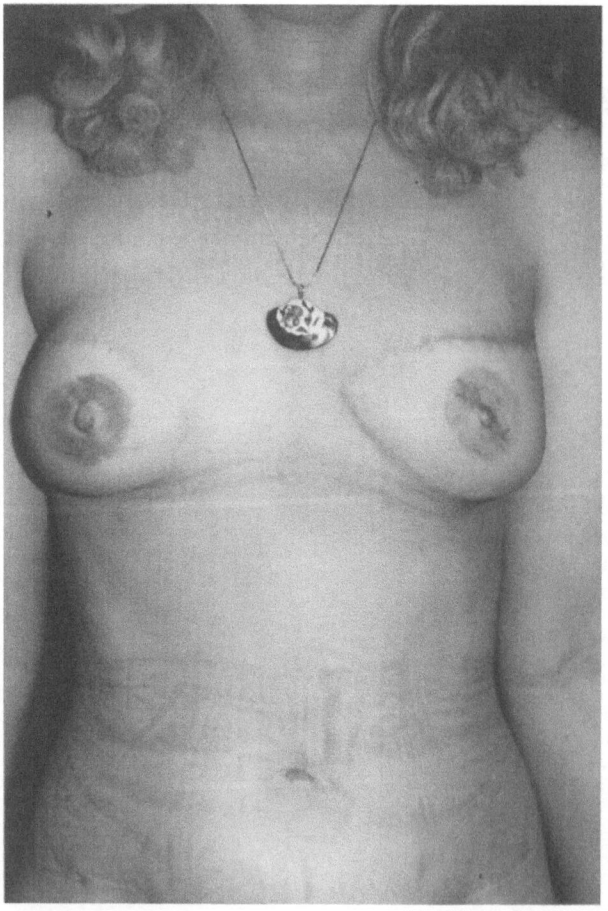

FIG. 13-7 Result of right breast reconstruction with a superior gluteal free flap. The left breast had previously been reconstructed with a TRAM flap. The donor site is shown in Fig 13-1. (From Kroll SS: The superior gluteal free flap for breast reconstruction. In: Schusterman MA, ed. *Microsurgical Reconstruction of the Cancer Patient.* Philadelphia: Lippincott-Raven; 1997: 179–189. Used with permission.)

often necessary and should be expected by the patient. Ultimately, the results can be quite good (Fig 13-7).

Superior Gluteal Artery Perforator Flap

Recently, a new version of the superior gluteal free flap has been described, the S-GAP flap.[13] This flap is based on the same underlying vascular anatomy as the superior gluteal free flap, but leaves the gluteal muscle intact in the buttock. Perforating vessels from the superior gluteal artery and vein are identified where they leave the gluteus maximum muscle and enter the fatty tissues. One or two of these perforators are dissected out of the muscle using loupe magnification. The vessels are followed proximally to the origin of the superior gluteal network. When elevated, the flap consists only of the skin, fatty tissues, and the vascular pedicle. The blood supply is usually excellent, and the results can be quite good (Fig 13-8).

The S-GAP flap has a longer pedicle than the standard superior gluteal free flap and therefore can usually be anastomosed to the internal mammary vessels without using a vein graft. It is still technically much more difficult than a free TRAM flap, however, and the tissues are less pliable and therefore more difficult to shape into a breast. Nevertheless, this is a useful option that will undoubtedly become more commonly used in the future. It is particularly useful for patients with excess buttock tissue who are good surgical candidates but not suitable for a TRAM flap. For this group of patients, it may well become the procedure of choice.

Complications

Although loss of the gluteus maximus muscle can affect ambulation, it is not necessary to sacrifice function of the entire muscle to transfer this flap. Postoperative morbidity is therefore usually limited to alterations in the patient's contour.

Because of the technical complexity and the frequent need for vein grafts, total flap loss is more likely with superior gluteal free flaps (although perhaps not with the S-GAP flap since there is ordinarily no vein graft) than it is with free TRAM flaps. Partial flap loss can occur but is not common.

Summary

The superior gluteal free flap is used for breast reconstruction less often today than in the past. It is technically more difficult than the TRAM flap and has been replaced to some extent by techniques like the inferior gluteal and Rubens fat pad free flaps. Nevertheless, the superior gluteal free flap is capable of excellent results and should be known to surgeons who perform breast reconstruction with autologous tissue. A recent modification of the superior gluteal free flap, the S-GAP flap, is a significant improvement and will probably be used more commonly in the future.

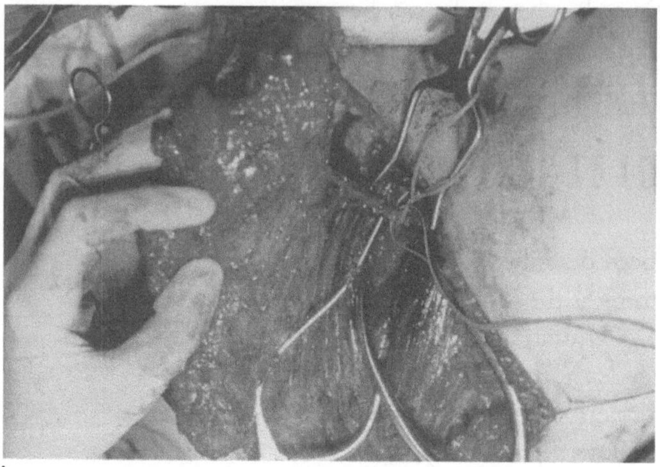

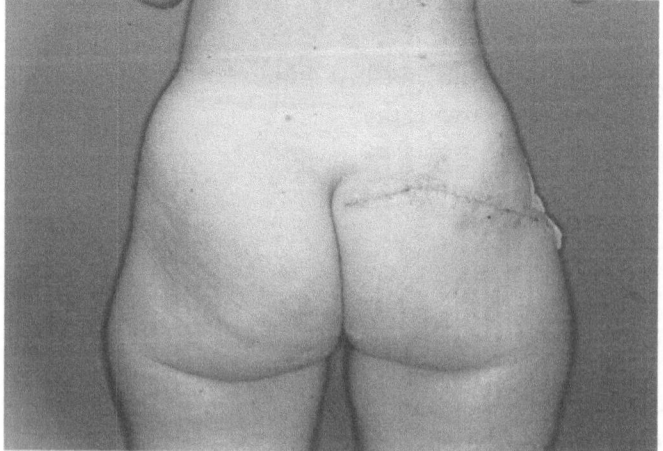

FIG. 13-8   (A) The S-GAP flap being elevated. Only the perforating branches of the superior gluteal vessels are harvested. (B) The elevated flap contains no muscle. (C) The flap was transferred to the chest wall using the internal mammary vessels as recipients. (D) Two weeks later, the result appeared to be excellent. The patient was not allowed to stand up without a brassiere for support for 30 days to avoid tension on the short pedicle. (E) The donor site deformity was not objectionable.

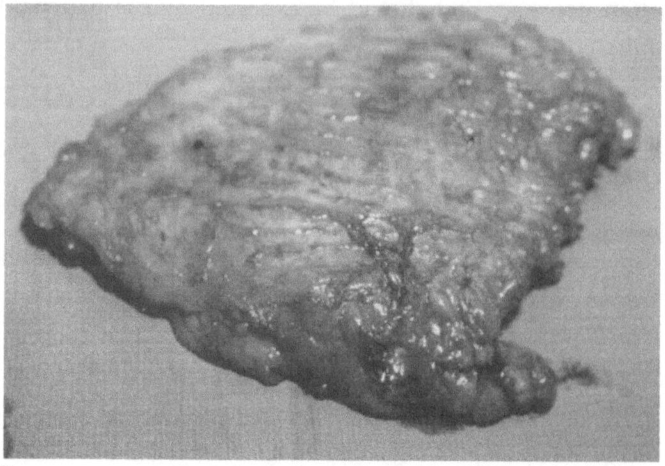

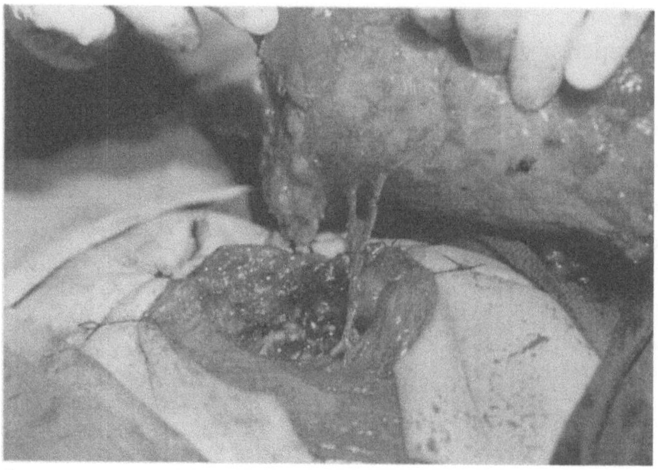

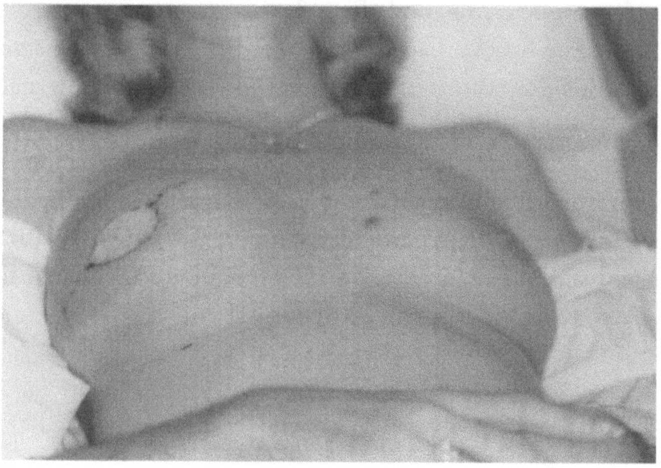

References

1. Shaw WW. Breast reconstruction by superior gluteal microvascular free flaps without silicone implants. *Plast Reconstr Surg.* 1983;72:490.
2. Shaw WW. Microvascular free flap breast reconstruction. *Clin Plast Surg.* 1984;11:333–341.
3. Nahai F. Inferior gluteus maximus musculocutaneous flap for breast reconstruction. *Perspect Plast Surg.* 1992;6:65.
4. Codner MA, Nahai F. The gluteal free flap breast reconstruction: making it work. *Clin Plast Surg.* 1994;21:289–296.
5. Randle PM, Nahai F. Gluteal and other free flaps for breast reconstruction. In: Kroll SS, ed. *Reconstructive Plastic Surgery for Cancer.* Philadelphia: Mosby-Year Book; 1996:295–304.
6. McCraw JB, Papp C, Edwards A, McMellin A. The autogenous latissimus breast reconstruction. *Clin Plast Surg.* 1994;21:279–288.
7. German G, Steinau HU. Breast reconstruction with the extended latissimus dorsi flap. *Plast Reconstr Surg.* 1996;97:519–526.
8. Hartrampf CR Jr, Noel RT, Drazan L, Elliott LF, Bennett GK, Beegle PH. Rubens fat pad for breast reconstruction: a peri-iliac soft-tissue free flap. *Plast Reconstr Surg.* 1994;93:402–407.
9. Dupin CL, Allen RJ, Glass CA, Bunch R. The internal mammary artery and vein as a recipient site for free-flap breast reconstruction: a report of 110 consecutive cases. *Plast Reconstr Surg.* 1996;98:685–689.
10. Feng LW. Recipient vessels in free-flap breast reconstruction: a study of the internal mammary and thoracodorsal vessels. *Plast Reconstr Surg.* 1997;99:405–416.
11. Ninkovic M, Anderl H, Hefel A, Schwabegger A, Wechselberger G. Internal mammary vessels: a reliable recipient system for free flaps in breast reconstruction. *Br J Plast Surg.* 1995;48:533–539.
12. Hefel A, Schwabegger A, Ninkovic M, Moriggl B, Waldenberger P. Internal mammary vessels: anatomical and clinical considerations. *Br J Plast Surg.* 1995;48:527–532.
13. Allen RJ, Tucker C. Jr. Superior gluteal artery perforator free flap for breast reconstruction. *Plast Reconstr Surg.* 1995;95:1207–1212.

14 The Inferior Gluteal Free Flap

Advantages of the Inferior Gluteal Free Flap

The inferior gluteal free flap[1-3] is a useful alternative to the free transverse rectus abdominus myocutaneous (TRAM) flap that allows successful autologous tissue breast reconstruction in patients who cannot have a free TRAM flap but who are otherwise good surgical candidates. The transferred tissue is similar to that of a superior gluteal free flap,[4,5] but the flap pedicle is much longer (8 to 10 cm) and in most cases there is no need for a vein graft (Fig 14-1). The donor site is relatively inconspicuous and is easily concealed by clothing. Bilateral reconstruction is possible without requiring that both breasts be reconstructed simultaneously.

I consider this flap to be one of the best choices for patients who cannot have a TRAM flap and are unwilling to accept the scar on the back that an extended latissimus dorsi flap would create. Although not technically simple, the inferior gluteal free flap is capable of achieving truly outstanding results.

Disadvantages of the Inferior Gluteal Free Flap

The inferior gluteal free flap is easier to perform than a superior gluteal free flap, but remains more technically challenging than a free TRAM flap. The patient must be positioned awkwardly, and the flap takes more time than a TRAM flap to perform. The tissues in the flap are less pliable than those of the TRAM flap, so breast shaping is more difficult. The inferior gluteal flap cannot be harvested at the same time that the mastectomy is being performed, so in immediate reconstruction the reconstructive team cannot begin raising the flap until the mastectomy has been completed.

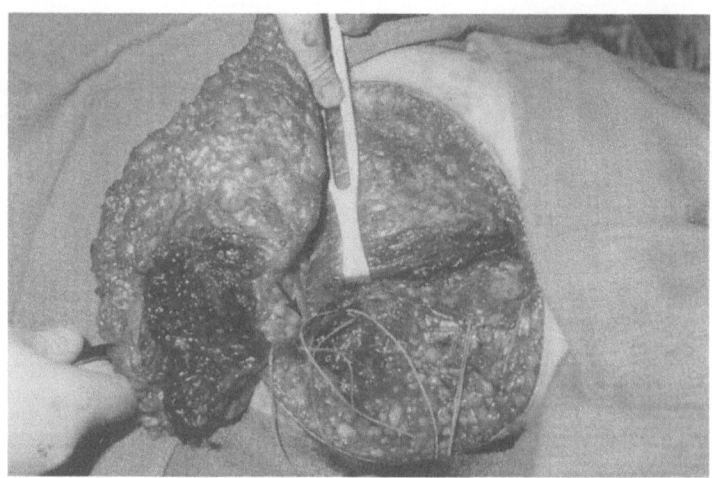

FIG. 14-1   Pedicle of an inferior gluteal free flap (arrow), demonstrating its length.

Indications

An inferior gluteal free flap is indicated when patients cannot have a TRAM flap (because of a previous TRAM flap, a prior abdominoplasty, or a potbelly habitus) but desire autologous tissue breast reconstruction. In rare cases, an inferior gluteal flap may be indicated in patients with excess buttock tissue who could have a TRAM flap but are not ideal candidates. In most cases, patients who require a TRAM flap alternative can choose among an extended latissimus dorsi flap,[6] a Rubens fat pad flap,[7] or an inferior gluteal free flap; the choice depends on the individual patient's anatomy and her personal preferences regarding donor site scars.

Contraindications

The inferior gluteal free flap is contraindicated in patients without sufficient buttock tissue to allow flap harvest without unacceptable donor site deformity. It is also contraindicated in patients who are not in sufficiently good condition to undergo a lengthy surgical procedure. As with any free flap, absence of adequate recipient vessels and any tendency for abnormal blood clotting are also contraindications.

Flap Design

The flap is designed to straddle the inferior gluteal crease, harvesting tissue from the superior posterior thigh as well as from the buttock proper (Fig 14-2). The skin paddle is centered on the mid-axis of the thigh, at a point 2 to 3 cm above the inferior gluteal crease. The skin paddle should be no wider than is necessary to obtain the tissue required

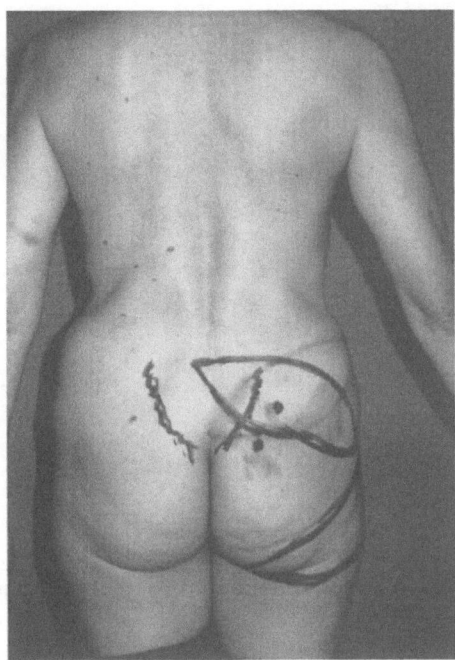

FIG. 14-2 Designs for both superior and inferior gluteal free flaps. In this patient, the inferior gluteal flap was used.

to reconstruct the breast. Although beveling of the incisions can be used to increase the amount of fat harvested, including excessive amounts of soft tissue increases donor site morbidity and can create a deformity that is visible when the patient is wearing pants.

Surgical Technique

Like the superior gluteal flap, the inferior gluteal flap can be used for immediate or delayed breast reconstruction. In immediate reconstruction, the reconstructive surgeon begins elevating the flap from the buttock immediately following the mastectomy. In delayed reconstruction, dissection of the recipient site should precede flap elevation, to ensure that adequate recipient vessels exist before committing to the procedure.

Positioning

The patient must be positioned on the operating table in such a way that access to both the breast and the buttock is possible. This is accomplished by placing the patient supine with her arms outstretched and her legs crossed so that the ipsilateral buttock is exposed (Fig 14-3). Leg compression boots are used to reduce the risk of thrombophlebitis. Banking the table from side to side will permit access to the buttock for flap harvest and to the chest for preparation of the recipient site and transfer of the flap. Because of this table banking, however, it is difficult to work on both sites simultaneously.

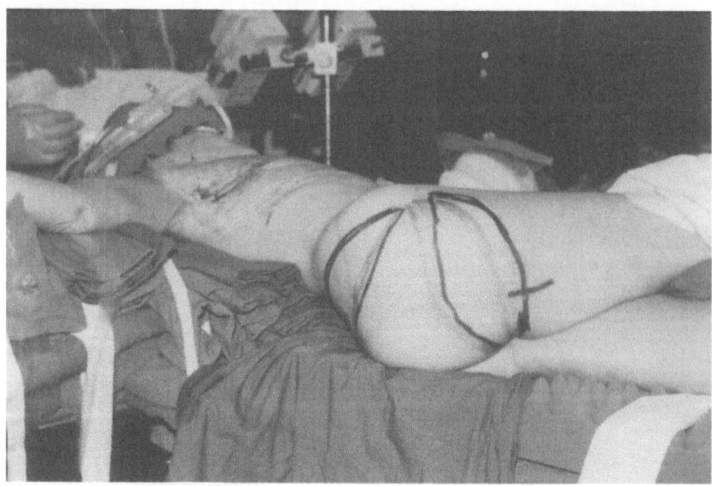

FIG. 14-3 Positioning of the patient for an inferior gluteal free flap. The legs are crossed, and compression boots are placed to reduce the risk of deep venous thrombosis.

Elevating the Flap

The initial incision is made with a scalpel, following the predetermined markings, while most of the subsequent dissection is performed with electrocautery. The dissection begins with the inferior incision, starting approximately 4 cm lateral to the ischial tuberosity. The surgeon then identifies a deep neurovascular bundle consisting of the posterior cutaneous nerve of the thigh and the continuation of the inferior gluteal artery, which

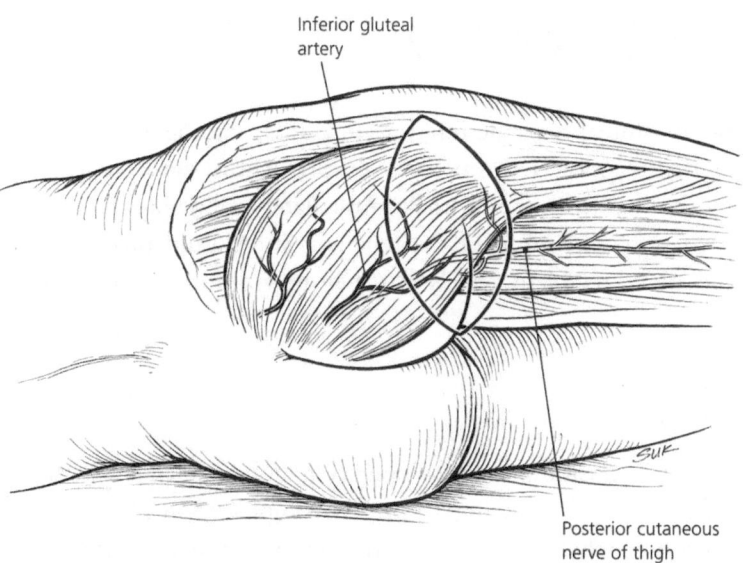

FIG. 14-4 Anatomy of the inferior gluteal free flap, showing the continuation of the inferior gluteal artery (which can often be located with a Doppler probe) running with the posterior cutaneous nerve of the thigh.

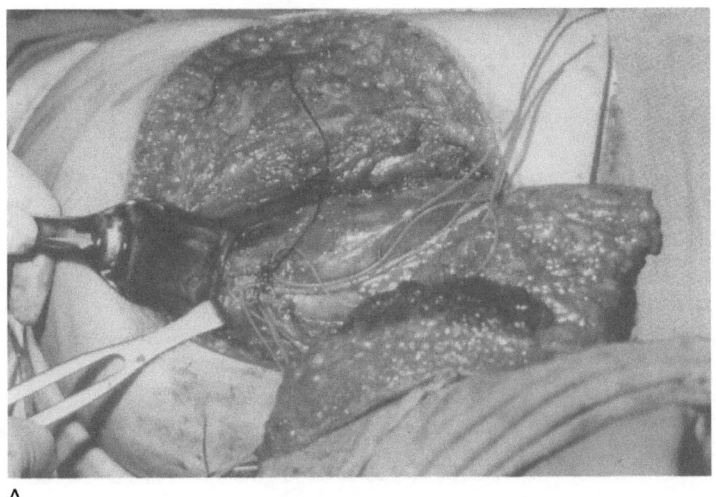

A

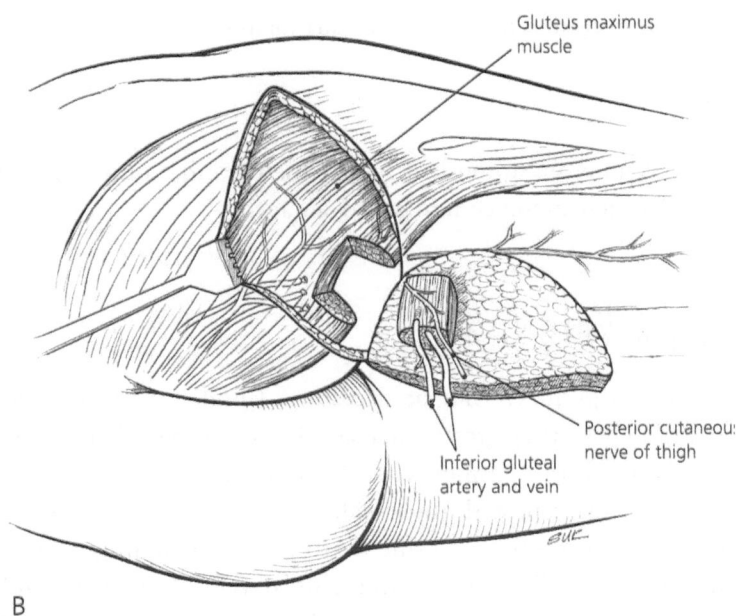

Gluteus maximus
muscle

Posterior cutaneou:
nerve of thigh

Inferior gluteal
artery and vein

B

FIG. 14-5   A small part of the muscle is harvested with the flap.

run together down the posterior thigh (Fig 14-4). This neurovascular bundle is ligated
and divided. The remainder of the cutaneous and subcutaneous portion of the flap is
then circumscribed.

Next, the continuation of the inferior gluteal artery is dissected along the deep
surface of the inferior gluteus maximus muscle. A small part of this muscle is harvested
with the flap (Fig 14-5), taking only what is required to preserve the vascular integrity
of the flap. The sciatic nerve is carefully identified and preserved. Under 4.5 power
loupe magnification the inferior gluteal vessels are traced proximally as far as possible,
ligating and dividing the many branches (Fig 14-6). Although this is tedious because
the venous branches are numerous and fragile, the surgeon can often use one of these

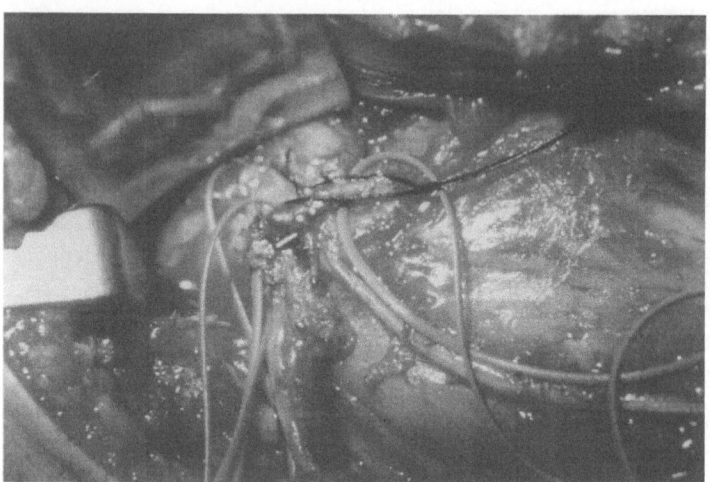

Fig. 14-6   The inferior gluteal vessels have many branches that must be ligated and divided. Often, however, one of them can be used in an anastomosis.

branches for the venous anastomosis if its size matches that of a recipient vein on the chest wall, turning their presence into an advantage.

Harvesting a Vein Graft

In most cases, a vein graft will not be necessary. I prefer to avoid vein grafts whenever possible, as I believe they greatly increase the risk of pedicle thrombosis. If a vein graft is required, the most commonly used donor site is the saphenous vein of the lower leg. This is a large vein with thick walls, which makes it a reasonably good substitute for an artery. The walls are somewhat thick for matching veins, however, especially thin-walled ones like the inferior gluteal vein. Moreover, saphenous veins grafts sometimes can go into severe spasms. If this occurs and is not relieved by the application of 2% papaverine solution, substitution of a different graft may be required. The best alternative, and in fact my preferred vein graft donor site for most patients, is the cephalic vein. This vein is sufficiently strong to be a suitable graft for an artery, but is much less prone to spasm than the saphenous vein is. In patients who are willing to accept a scar on the forearm, I consider the cephalic vein to be the donor site of choice.

Transferring the Flap

The flap can be transferred to the thoracodorsal vessels (Fig 14-7) or the internal mammary vessels, depending on their availability and the surgeon's preferences. Preparation of these donor sites is described in chapter 9 and will not be repeated here. The operating table is banked to render the chest nearly supine. The flap transfer is similar

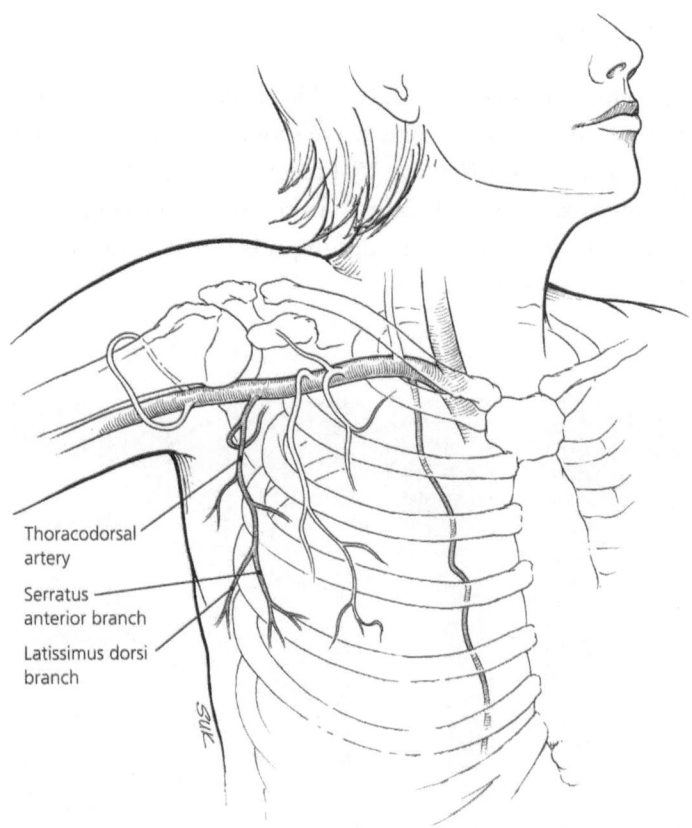

Thoracodorsal
artery

Serratus
anterior branch

Latissimus dorsi
branch

FIG. 14-7   Anatomy of the thoracodorsal and internal mammary vessels, either of which can be used as recipients.

to that of a TRAM flap, except that the caliber of the inferior gluteal vessels is much larger. If the discrepancy in vessel size is too great, using smaller side branches of the inferior gluteal vessels (as noted above) can make the anastomoses easier and less prone to complications.

Shaping the Breast

Shaping of the breast is similar to that of a TRAM flap (see chapters 16 and 17), except that the inferior gluteal flap, like the superior gluteal flap, is firmer and more difficult to mold. With time, however, the flap will settle and become fuller in the lower pole, improving its shape. The deep surface of the medial edges of the flap should be sutured to the medial edges of the defect, using 3-0 Vicryl (polygalactin 910), to prevent lateral flap migration. The inframammary fold and lateral breast border are constructed just as with a TRAM flap. If sufficient tissue is present, the flap is sculpted, around its periphery, into a projecting cone. A 15-French round suction drain is placed beneath the flap and led out through a stab wound in the axilla.

Closing the Donor Site

The donor site is closed primarily, in layers. Dead space should be obliterated as much as possible with deep sutures. The sciatic nerve should be covered by muscle. The wound is drained with closed suction (I use a 15-French round Blake drain) led out through a separate stab wound and sutured securely to the skin. The skin is closed with buried dermal sutures of 3-0 Vicryl and with running subcuticular sutures of 3-0 PDS (polydioxanone) or Prolene (polypropylene).

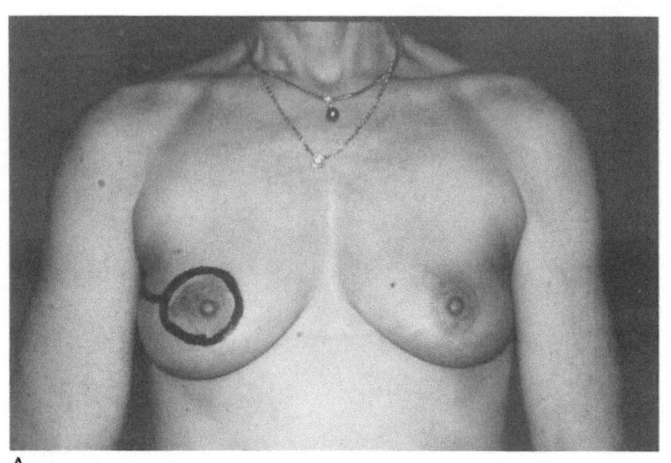

A

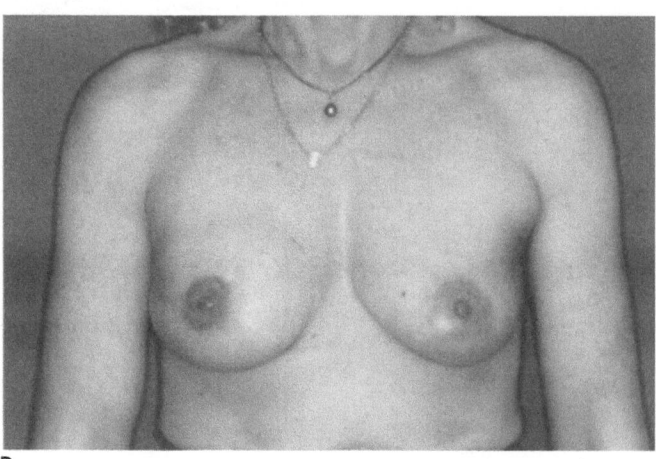

B

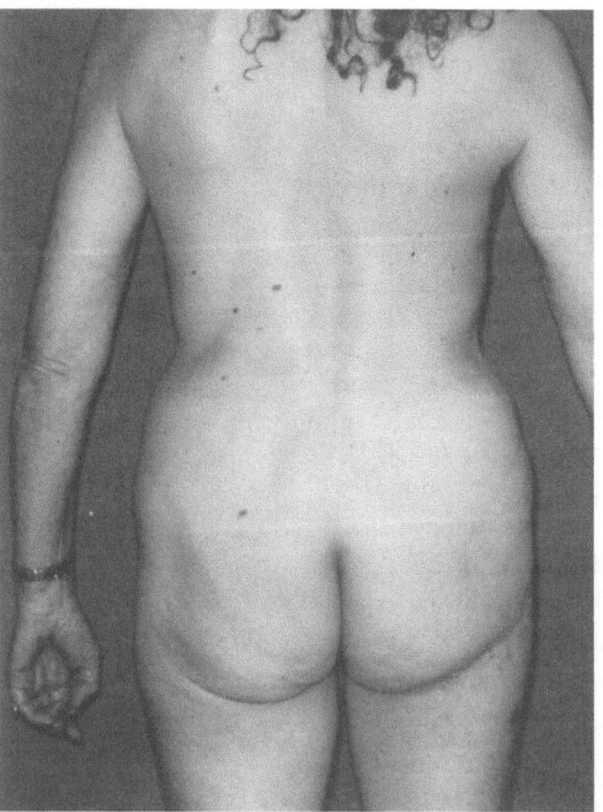

C

FIG. 14-8 (A) A 53-year-old woman scheduled for right mastectomy. She had previously undergone abdominoplasty and therefore was not a candidate for a TRAM flap. See color insert, p. I-16. (B) Result of immediate reconstruction with an inferior gluteal free flap. See color insert, p. I-16. (C) The donor site. See color insert, p. I-17. (From Kroll SS: *Clin Plast Surg.* 1998;25:135–143. Used with permission.)

Postoperative Care

Postoperative care is similar to that for a free TRAM flap (see chapter 11) except that nasogastric tube is not required and respiratory function is not interfered with. Patients get out of bed on the second postoperative day. Ambulation is not restricted. Each drain is left in place until its daily output is less than 25 ml for 2 consecutive days. The running subcuticular sutures are removed in 3 weeks. There are no limitations on lifting, and patients usually can be discharged on the fifth or sixth postoperative day. As with TRAM flaps, revisions are often necessary and should be expected by the patient. Ultimately, the results can be quite good (Fig 14-8).

Complications

The main risk of this procedure is that of total flap loss, which is more likely in a gluteal free flap than in the technically more simple free TRAM flap. Since only a small piece of muscle is sacrificed, ambulation is usually not affected. Postoperative morbidity is usually limited to alterations in the patient's contour, which can be significant if excessive tissue is harvested. Necrosis of part of the flap is possible but not common. Sciatic pain is possible if the sciatic nerve is not protected during the donor site closure, or if it is injured during the dissection.

Summary

The inferior gluteal free flap is only rarely used for breast reconstruction but is capable of achieving outstanding results. It is rarely the flap of choice when a TRAM flap can be performed. It is technically much more difficult than the TRAM flap and cannot be raised simultaneous with performance of the mastectomy. When performed correctly, however, the inferior gluteal free flap leaves an inconspicuous donor site scar and is a good alternative for autologous breast reconstruction when a TRAM flap is not possible.

References

1.   Nahai F. Inferior gluteus maximus musculocutaneous flap for breast reconstruction. *Perspect Plast Surg.* 1992;6:65.
2.   Codner MA, Nahai F. The gluteal free flap breast reconstruction: making it work. *Clin Plast Surg.* 1994;21:289–296.
3.   Randle PM, Nahai F. Gluteal and other free flaps for breast reconstruction. In: Kroll SS, ed. *Reconstructive Plastic Surgery for Cancer.* Philadelphia: Mosby-Year Book; 1996:295–304.
4.   Shaw WW. Breast reconstruction by superior gluteal microvascular free flaps without silicone implants. *Plast Reconstr Surg.* 1983;72:490.

5.   Shaw MM. Microvascular free flap breast reconstruction. *Clin Plast Surg.* 1984;11: 333–341.

6.   McCraw JB, Papp C, Edwards A, McMellin A. The autogenous latissimus breast reconstruction. *Clin Plast Surg.* 1994;21:279–288.

7.   Hartrampf CR Jr, Noel RT, Drazan L, Elliott LF, Bennett GK, Beegle PH. Rubens fat pad for breast reconstruction: a peri-iliac soft-tissue free flap. *Plast Reconstr Surg.* 1994;93:402–407.

The Rubens Fat Pad Free Flap

15

Advantages of the Rubens Flap

The Rubens fat pad free flap (Rubens flap)[1] is a useful alternative to the transverse rectus abdominus myocutaneous (TRAM) flap for patients who have had a previous abdominoplasty or TRAM flap and therefore cannot have another procedure that harvests lower abdominal skin and fat, but who are otherwise good surgical candidates. The Rubens flap supplies tissue with a consistency very similar to that of a TRAM flap, and has an inconspicuous donor site. The pedicle of the flap is sufficiently long that vein grafts are usually unnecessary, and in most cases, the caliber of the vessels is large enough to permit relatively easy microvascular anastomoses (Fig 15-1). There are two potential donor sites (one on each side), so that a second flap is available if required later.

Disadvantages of the Rubens Flap

The Rubens flap has several disadvantages. It is technically more difficult than a TRAM flap, and the blood supply to the flap is less robust. Harvesting a larger section of the abdominal wall musculature improves flap perfusion but can lead to abdominal wall weakness or hernia and increases the intensity and duration of postoperative pain. In approximately 10% of patients, the deep circumflex iliac vein is small, making the venous anastomosis required to transfer the flap more difficult. Finally, depending on how the flap is raised, part of the donor site scar may be visible in a bathing suit.

Indications

A Rubens flap is indicated in patients who are not candidates for a TRAM flap because of a previous abdominoplasty or TRAM flap and who will not accept the donor site scar associated with the technically easier extended latissimus dorsi myocutaneous flap.[2]

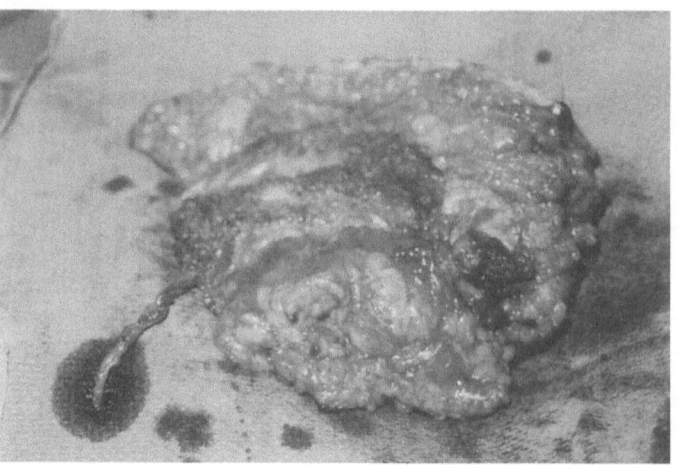

FIG. 15-1   Rubens fat pad free flap, showing the long pedicle that usually allows breast reconstruction without need for a vein graft.

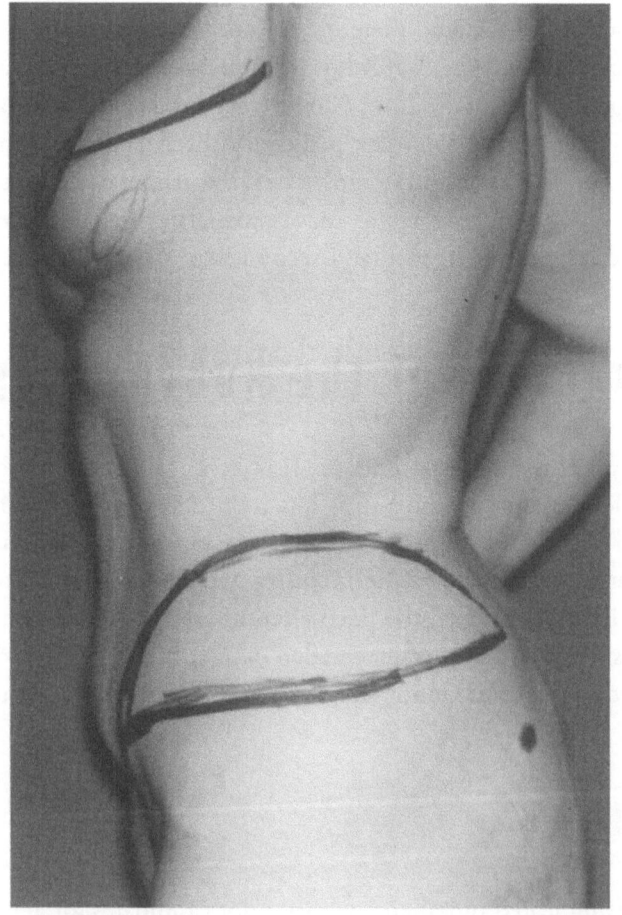

FIG. 15-2   Design of the Rubens flap. The skin paddle is centered over the iliac crest.

The Rubens flap can be ideal for these patients if they have excess tissue in the flank area but not in the buttocks (so that they are not equally good candidates for an inferior gluteal free flap[3,4]).

Contraindications

A Rubens flap is not a good choice for patients with abdominal wall weakness that might make them overly susceptible to hernia formation. Like a TRAM flap, a Rubens flap is therefore contraindicated in patients with a potbelly habitus. It is also contraindicated in patients who have had previous surgery that has interrupted the deep circumflex iliac vessels and in patients with morbid obesity. Like any free flap, the Rubens flap is contraindicated in patients with an abnormal tendency for vascular thrombosis. It is also not a good choice for patients who are very obese.

Flap Design

The flap is designed over the flank, with the skin paddle straddling the iliac crest anteriorly and lying more superior to it posteriorly (Fig 15-2). The skin island is usually approximately 10 cm in width but can be widened in some patients, and can be extended posteriorly to increase the volume of tissue being transferred. The flap can be transferred to either side without any change in technique.

Surgical Technique

The surgical technique is essentially identical to that required to perform a free osteocutaneous iliac crest transfer for mandibular reconstruction,[5,6] except that the bone portion of that flap is left behind and only the soft tissues are elevated.

Positioning

The patient is positioned supine, with pads under one buttock to elevate the hip and improve access to the posterior part of the flap (Fig 15-3). The patient's arms are extended to provide access to the axilla on the side of the reconstruction, and to the opposite arm for anesthesia and monitoring by the anesthetist.

Elevation of the Flap

I prefer to begin the incision directly over the femoral vessels, exposing the origin of the deep circumflex iliac vessels deep to the inguinal ligament (Fig 15-4). This permits the surgeon to evaluate the vascular pedicle of the flap (especially the vein) before com-

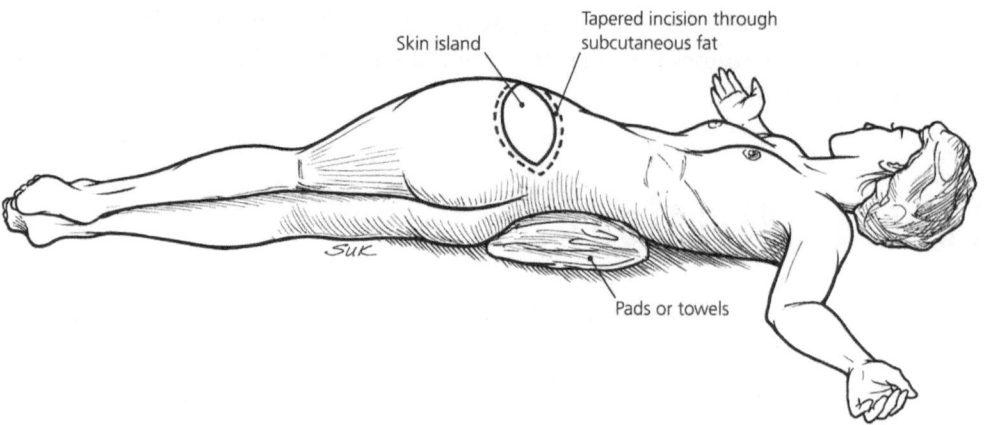

FIG. 15-3 Patient positioning for a Rubens flap. Pads or towels are placed beneath the ipsilateral buttock to elevate the hip.

mitting to making the remaining incisions. If the vein is judged to be inadequate, the opposite side can be explored or an alternative technique selected. Once the decision to proceed is made, the inguinal ligament is tagged with a suture and divided. The deep circumflex iliac vessels are then dissected distally, following them as they curve along the inner surface of the ilium, parallel to and approximately 2 cm from the edge of the crest (Fig 15-5). Loupe magnification is essential to this part of the dissection because many small branches must be clipped and divided. The ascending branch of the deep circumflex iliac artery, which supplies the internal oblique muscle, does not need to be included in the flap.

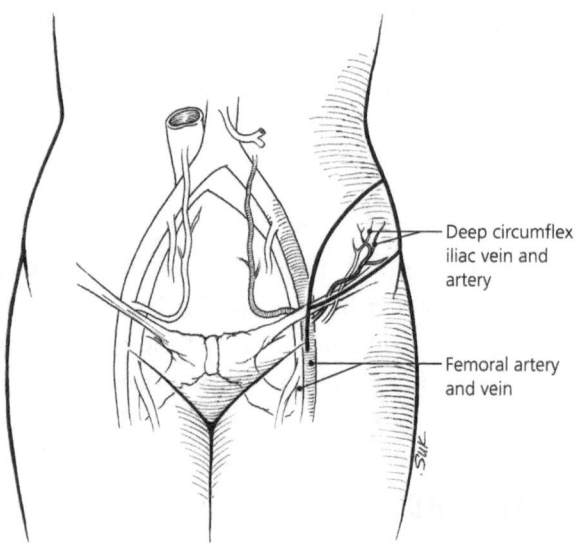

FIG. 15-4 The skin incision begins over the femoral vessels so that the deep circumflex iliac vessels can be exposed and evaluated before the surgeon commits to the remaining incisions.

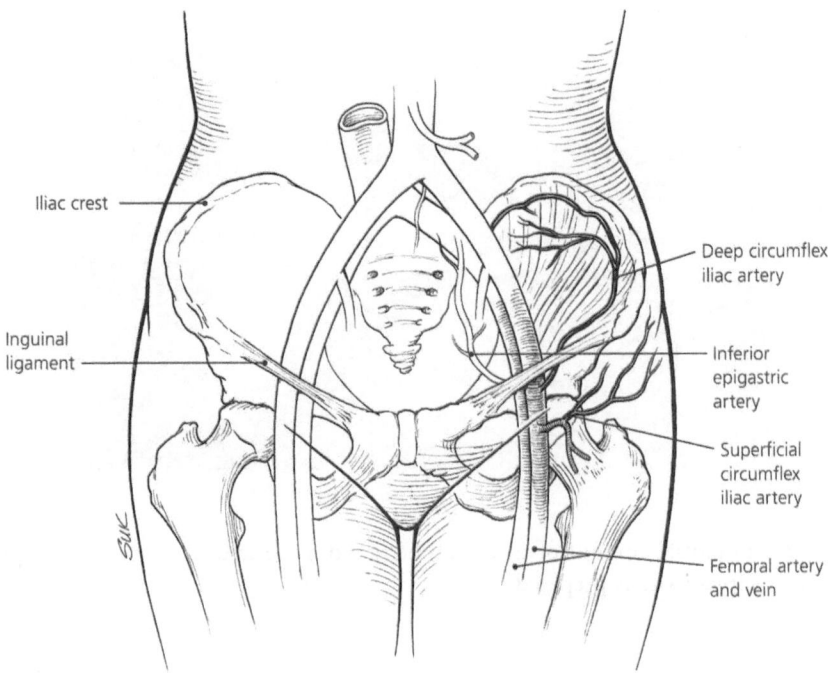

FIG. 15-5 Anatomy of the deep circumflex iliac vessels on the inner surface of the iliac crest.

The lateral cutaneous nerve of the thigh should be identified and if at all possible should be left behind without being injured. If the nerve cannot safely be bypassed, it should be divided cleanly and then microsurgically reapproximated after flap dissection has been completed.

Portions of the internal and external oblique muscles must be harvested with the flap, in continuity with the overlying skin paddle (Fig 15-6). Including more muscle

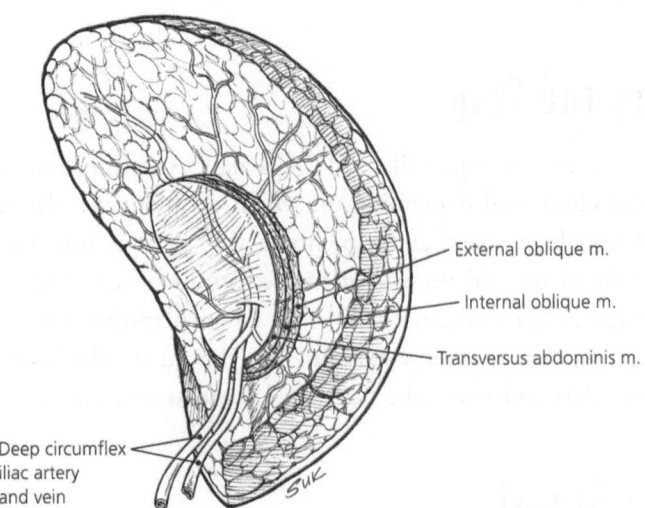

FIG. 15-6 Portions of the internal and external oblique muscles are harvested in continuity with the flap. Increasing the amount of muscle harvested can improve flap blood flow but increases donor site morbidity.

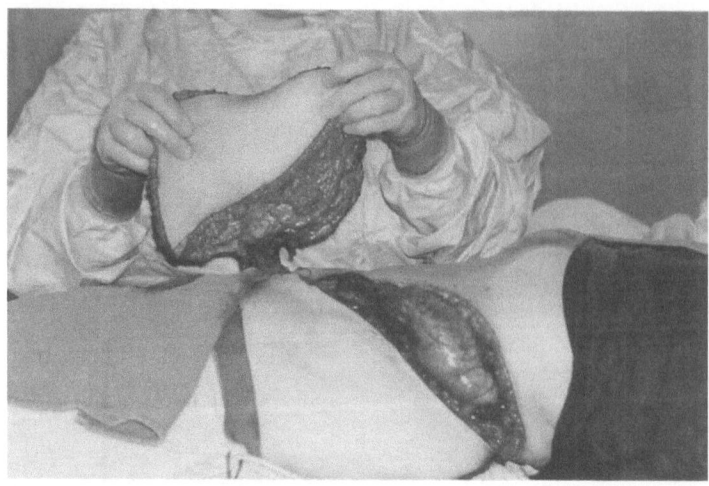

Fig. 15-7   A substantial amount of tissue can be raised, if desired. It is then left to perfuse in situ while the recipient site is prepared.

will improve the flap's blood supply but will make donor site closure more difficult, increase postoperative pain, and increase the risk of postoperative hernia. How much muscle to include is a decision based on surgical judgment, which comes only with experience; but a segment of muscle 4 to 5 cm wide and 10 to 12 cm long would be reasonable. The periosteum overlying the iliac crest should be separated from the bone and included with the flap, to capture any perforators running along the bone.

Once dissection of the flap is completed, it is left attached by the deep circumflex iliac vessels (Fig 15-7) and allowed to perfuse while the recipient site (which can be either internal mammary or thoracodorsal vessels) is prepared. Spasm of the blood vessels, if present, should be treated with local application of 2% papaverine solution and with careful examination of the artery under magnification to ensure that it has no unrepaired open branches.

Transferring the Flap

The Rubens flap is transferred just like a TRAM flap. Anastomoses are performed in the axilla or on the chest wall depending on which recipient vessels are used. Even if the thoracodorsal vessels are used as recipients, a vein graft is not usually required. I usually prefer the thoracodorsal vessels for immediate reconstruction and the internal mammary vessels for delayed reconstruction. As when planning a free TRAM flap, a preoperative color Doppler ultrasonic examination should be obtained to evaluate the internal mammary veins and select the best site for the anastomoses.

Shaping the Breast

Because the Rubens flap tissues are similar in size and consistency to those of a TRAM flap, breast shaping is almost identical to the technique used to shape a TRAM flap.

The flap is sutured to the medial and superomedial edges of the mastectomy defect and sculpted into the form of a breast. Preparation of the breast pocket, the inframammary fold, and the lateral breast border is essential to successful breast shaping and is accomplished as described in subsequent chapters.

Closing the Donor Site

Closure of the abdominal wall portion of the donor site defect must be secure and solid to avoid a postoperative hernia. This is easier if too much muscle has not been removed during flap harvest. The remaining portions of the internal and external oblique muscles are firmly approximated to the iliac crest with heavy (No. 1 Prolene [polypropylene] or Novafil [polyethylene]) running sutures. The lateral attachment can be accomplished either by using drill holes in the iliac crest itself or by suturing the abdominal wall muscles to the proximal tensor fascia lata and gluteal fascia where they attach to the iliac crest. The inguinal ligament is repaired securely with heavy interrupted sutures. The subcutaneous tissues are then closed in layers over a suction drain.

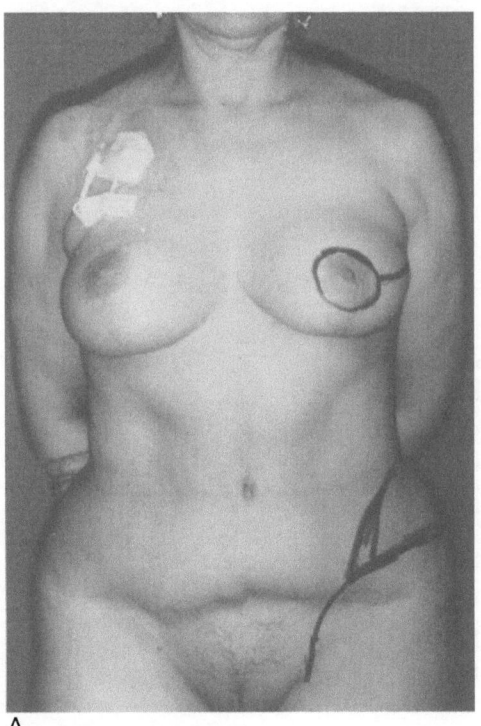
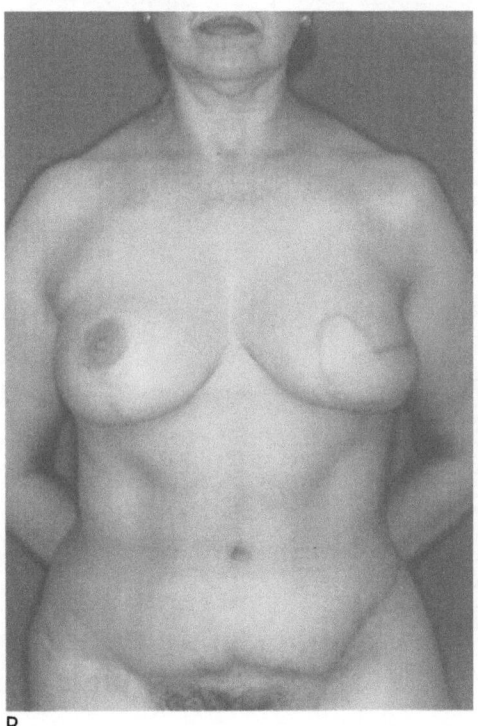

A   B

FIG. 15-8   (A) Patient with a history of previous abdominoplasty and bilateral breast reductions (all performed outside the United States). She required a left mastectomy and desired immediate breast reconstruction. (B) After immediate reconstruction with a Rubens fat pad free flap.

Postoperative Care

Postoperative care is similar to that for a free TRAM flap. The flap should be monitored hourly for 3 full days.[7] The patient is discharged on the fifth or sixth postoperative day when she is fully ambulatory and able to care for herself. Stool softeners should be used to avoid straining. Heavy lifting should be avoided for 3 months, and the patient should not attempt situps for at least 6 months. Postoperative pain may be more intense and last longer than that caused by a TRAM flap, so pain medication should be adjusted accordingly. As in any autologous tissue reconstruction, revision of the flap is often necessary to achieve good breast symmetry. The final results can be excellent and are similar to those achievable with a TRAM flap (Figs 15-8 and 15-9).

Complications

As after any breast reconstruction using free flaps, loss of part or all of the flap is possible and is best avoided by careful technique. Aside from flap loss, the two most seri-

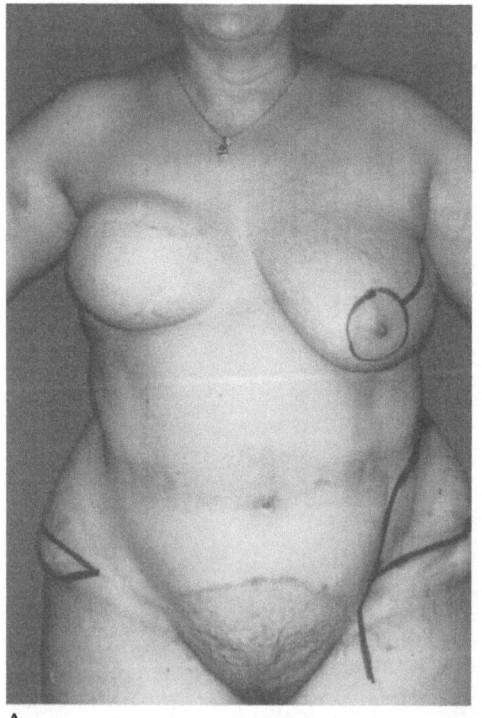
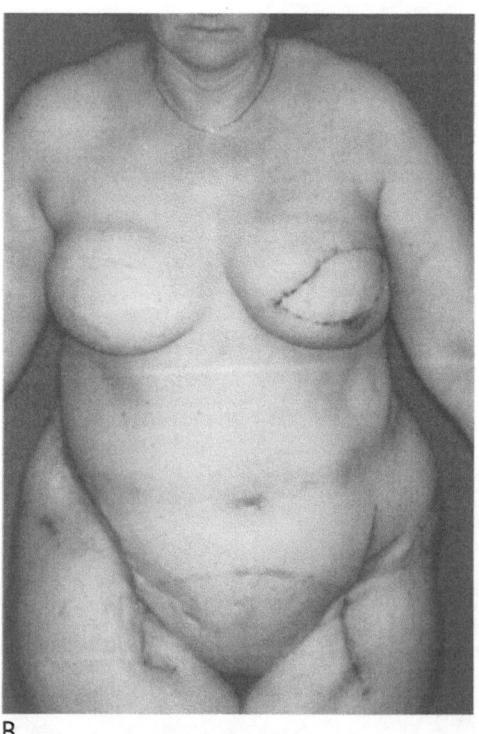

A   B

FIG. 15-9   (A) Patient with previous TRAM flap right breast reconstruction who developed a second primary breast cancer on the left side. (B) The early result of immediate reconstruction of the left breast with a Rubens flap harvested from the patient's right side. The flap was initially planned to come from the left, but after exploration of the donor vessels a change in side was elected. Note the similarity in the shape of the two breasts, suggesting that the tissues have a similar consistency.

ous complications associated with this procedure are abdominal wall weakness and dysesthesia of the anterior thigh. Abdominal wall weakness and hernia can be minimized by harvesting only that muscle required to preserve the integrity of the blood supply to the flap, and by securely closing the donor site. Dysesthesias of the anterior thigh are best circumvented by avoiding any injury to the lateral femoral cutaneous nerve of the thigh when the flap is raised.

Summary

The Rubens fat pad free flap is a relatively new procedure that can provide excellent tissue for breast reconstruction in patients who cannot have TRAM flaps but who are otherwise good surgical candidates. The flap is technically more difficult than a TRAM flap but is capable of achieving equally excellent results. As with a TRAM flap, the donor site scar is relatively inconspicuous, and bilateral reconstruction is possible. Along with the extended latissimus dorsi flap and the inferior gluteal flap, the Rubens flap is a reasonable alternative for patients who desire autologous tissue breast reconstruction but because of previous surgery cannot undergo a TRAM flap procedure. At the time of this writing, experience with this flap is relatively limited. In the future, as surgeons become increasingly familiar with the Rubens flap, it will perhaps grow in popularity.

References

1. Hartrampf CR Jr, Noel RT, Drazan L, Elliott LF, Bennett GK, Beegle PH. Rubens fat pad for breast reconstruction: a peri-iliac soft-tissue free flap. *Plast Reconstr Surg.* 1994;93:402–407.
2. McCraw JB, Papp C, Edwards A, McMellin A. The autogenous latissimus breast reconstruction. *Clin Plast Surg.* 1994;21:279–288.
3. Nahai F. Inferior gluteus maximus musculocutaneous flap for breast reconstruction. *Perspect Plast Surg.* 1992;6:65.
4. Codner MA, Nahai F. The gluteal free flap breast reconstruction: making it work. *Clin Plast Surg.* 1994;21:289–296.
5. Taylor GI. Reconstruction of the mandible with free composite iliac bone grafts. *Ann Plast Surg.* 1982;9:361–376.
6. Shenaq SM. Refinements in mandibular reconstruction. *Clin Plast Surg.* 1992;19:809–817.
7. Kroll SS, Schusterman MA, Reece GP, et al. Timing of pedicle thrombosis and flap loss after free tissue transfer. *Plast Reconstr Surg.* 1996;98:1230–1233.

16 Shaping the Breast Mound in Immediate Reconstruction

I n this chapter I will consider the sequence of steps required to turn a transverse rectus abdominus myocutaneous (TRAM) flap into a breast mound that, after appropriate revision and nipple reconstruction, will become a reconstructed breast that both the surgeon and patient are pleased with. I will use the TRAM flap as the example because it is by far the most commonly used flap for breast reconstruction, but the principles presented here can be applied (with modifications that will be discussed in other chapters) to any autologous tissue flap. In this chapter, I will consider the case of unilateral immediate reconstruction. In chapter 18, I will review the modifications that are required for bilateral immediate reconstruction.

Goal of Shaping in Unilateral Reconstruction

Ideally, the surgeon's goal in shaping the breast mound in unilateral reconstruction is to match the opposite breast so closely that no revision is subsequently required to achieve breast symmetry. Unfortunately, in practice that goal is seldom met. A more realistic goal for most surgeons is to create a breast mound that can be made to match the opposite breast with a reasonable amount of surgical revision (Fig 16-1).[1]

Some defects of shape are easy to correct, while others can be difficult or impossible to rectify. Obviously, the ones that are nearly impossible to correct later must be avoided. The shape abnormalities that are the most difficult to correct are malposition of the inframammary fold and inadequate tissue medially. Correction can also be difficult if the entire breast is positioned too laterally. A simple excess of tissue in the lateral or middle part of the breast mound, on the other hand, is relatively easy to correct and sometimes is best accepted (especially when trying to make a very small breast) during the initial breast mound reconstruction if reducing the mound too much might jeopardize blood supply to the rest of the flap.

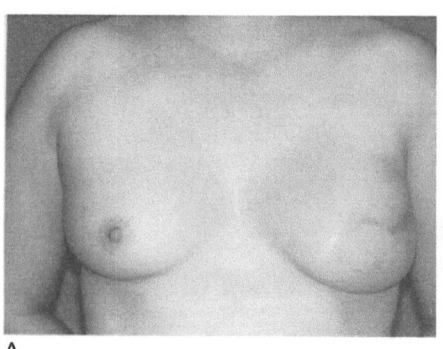
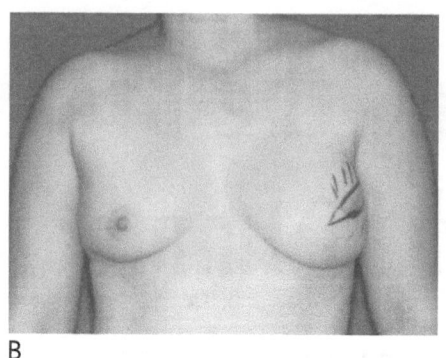
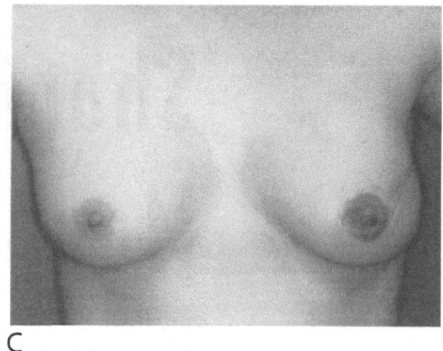

A   B   C

FIG. 16-1 (A) Result of immediate breast mound reconstruction with a free TRAM flap, before revision. (B) Plan for removal of skin and fat from upper outer quadrant. (C) After revision, which was performed using local anesthesia, the symmetry is improved.

Effect of Flap Type and Recipient Site on Shaping

The type of flap that is used can significantly affect the shaping process. Because of the excellent blood supply of the free TRAM flap, aggressive shaping maneuvers like folding or sculpting the flap can generally be performed with relative safety when a free TRAM flap has been performed. Conversely, if a pedicled TRAM flap or a deep inferior epigastric perforator (DIEP) flap has been used, shaping must usually be less aggressive because the blood supply is usually less robust. Naturally, there is considerable variation between flaps, and the blood supply of each flap must be assessed individually. The surgeon should not try to shape a free TRAM flap aggressively if that particular flap has a relatively poor blood supply just because most other free TRAM flaps will tolerate it.

If a free flap is used, the recipient site that is chosen can also affect the shaping process. Shaping is easier if the internal mammary vessels are used as recipients because the vascular pedicle and the muscle around it can be positioned in the center of the breast. Consequently, trimming of the flap around the periphery can be done with relative impunity, without jeopardizing the blood supply of the flap. If the thoracodorsal vessels are used, the flap pedicle may be too short to position the entrance of the blood vessels into the flap in the center of the breast. The surgeon may then be unable to thin the flap laterally as much as he or she desires without risking injury to the vascular pedicle of the flap.

Even so, the thoracodorsal vessels are usually the recipient vessels of choice when performing immediate reconstruction and when an axillary dissection has been performed. In that situation, the thoracodorsal vessels have already been exposed and are readily available for use. This ready availability is a strong argument that carries more weight than the relatively poorer position of the recipient site, a problem that can be overcome in most cases by making the vascular pedicle of the free TRAM flap as long as possible.

In this chapter, I will discuss shaping from the point of view of the surgeon who is using a free TRAM flap with the thoracodorsal vessels as recipients. If the internal mammary vessels are used instead, the shaping process is identical except that (1) reconstitution of the lateral breast border is easier, since the pedicle is not in the way, and (2) trimming the flap peripherally is easier and can be performed more aggressively. If a pedicled TRAM flap is used, folding and sculpting of the flap must be less aggressive, with some of the shaping being deferred until the flap is revised, at which time its blood supply will be more secure.

A Step-By-Step Approach to Breast Shaping

Each patient is unique, with different needs and distinctive challenges. Each breast reconstruction is therefore unique, forcing the reconstructive surgeon to be creative and innovative. Certain patterns repeat themselves, however, so a logical and step-by-step approach to breast shaping can help greatly to achieve a successful result.

The steps required for breast shaping in immediate reconstruction are shown in Table 16-1. If this sequence of steps is followed in a methodical way, breast shaping can proceed fairly rapidly. By having a step-by-step approach, even though originality will sometimes be called for, the surgeon can usually obtain consistent and successful results.

Skin-Sparing Mastectomy

The use of a skin-sparing mastectomy[2,3] simplifies breast shaping by preserving the inframammary fold and much of the breast skin envelope (Fig 16-2). In most cases, the mastectomy incision will be made around the areola and then angle toward the axilla to facilitate an axillary dissection (Fig 16-3). This provides good access for the general surgeon to work in the axilla and allows maximum exposure of the breast mound to facilitate shaping, and is an excellent incision in most cases.

TABLE 16-1   The Step-by-Step Approach to Breast Shaping in Immediate Reconstruction

BEFORE FLAP TRANSFER:
(1) Assess the viability of the mastectomy flaps
(2) Assess and if necessary repair the inframammary fold

AFTER FLAP TRANSFER:
(3) Create the lateral breast border
(4) Trim the flap medially
(5) Inset the flap medially and superiorly
(6) Create projection in the lower pole
(7) Trim the flap excess superolaterally
(8) De-epithelialize the buried skin
(9) Close the wound

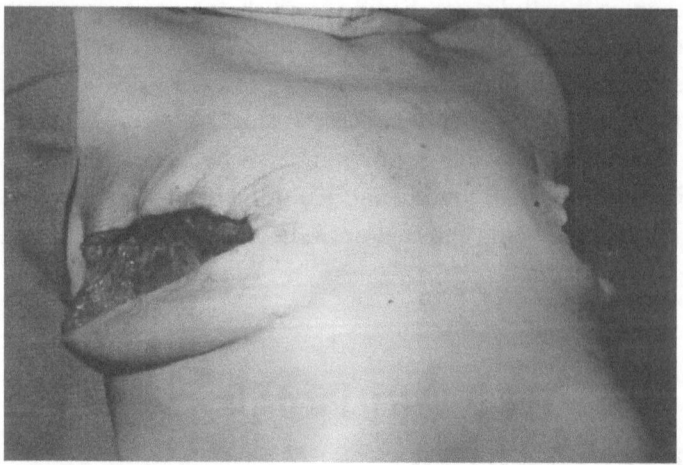

Fig. 16-2   After bilateral skin-sparing mastectomy. The breast skin envelopes and inframammary folds are largely preserved.

It is also possible to perform a mastectomy with free TRAM flap breast reconstruction through a periareolar incision (Fig 16-4). This has the obvious advantage of reducing visible scarring on the breast mound. A separate incision in the axilla is required for nodal dissection and for anastomosis of the flap to the thoracodorsal vessels, but this axillary scar is usually not objectionable to the patient. The main difficulty with this approach is that access to the breast mound is restricted and shaping is therefore more difficult. Because most breast scars fade with time and because the shape of the breast is more important than the scars, in most cases I prefer the standard incision as

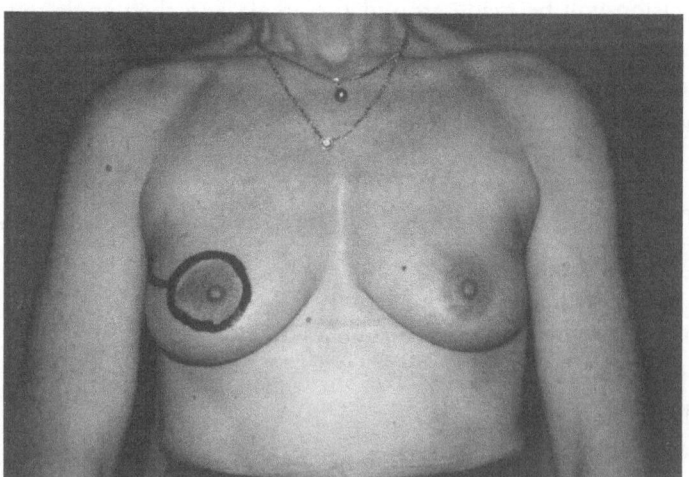

Fig. 16-3   Usual plan for a skin-sparing mastectomy, showing the incision around the areola and the extension toward the axilla. This incision provides good access for both mastectomy and reconstruction and minimizes scarring in the cosmetically important superior and medial parts of the breast.

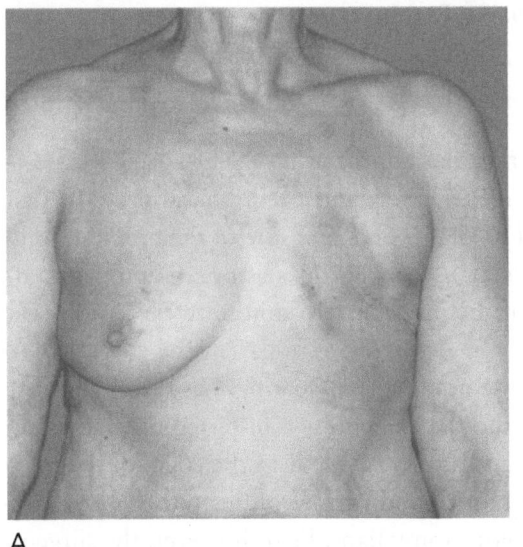

A

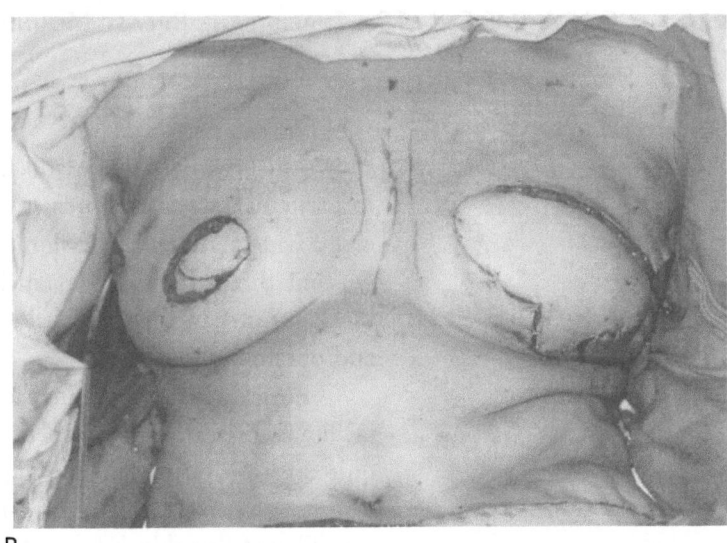

B

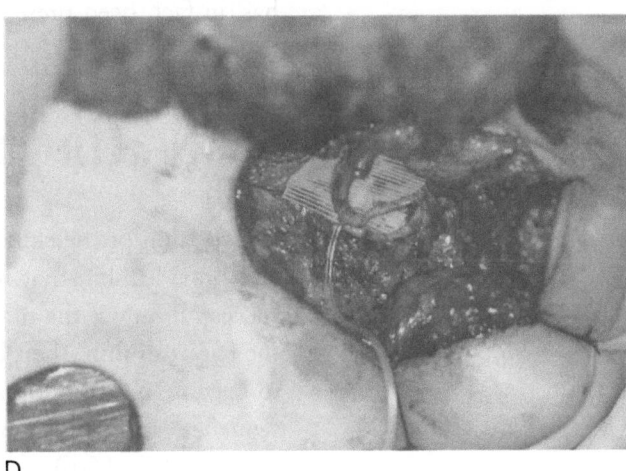

C

D

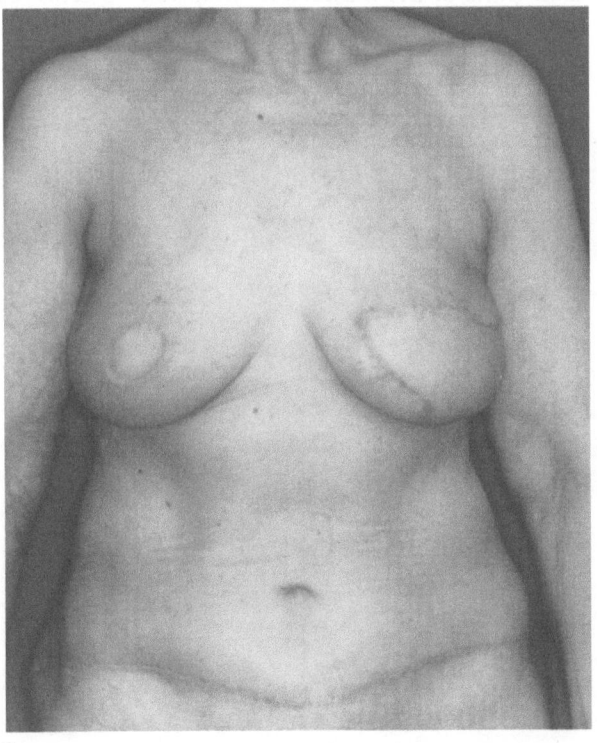

E

FIG. 16-4 (A) Patient with previous left modified radical mastectomy who has a new breast cancer on the right and will need a modified radical mastectomy. (B) Intraoperative view of the bilateral breast reconstruction, showing the periareolar incision used on the right side. A separate incision is visible laterally for access to the axilla. (C) The flap has been transferred to the axilla and anastomosed to the thoracodorsal vessels. (D) Close-up view of the anastomosis, showing that access and exposure are adequate. (E) The result 6 months later shows the cosmetic advantage of the periareolar incision. See color insert, p. I-13.

shown in Figure 16.3, but do find the periareolar approach useful in selected cases—in particular, when the breasts are ptotic preoperatively and need a mastopexy. In that case a wide periareolar incision can be used to allow good exposure of the breast mound without the usual lateral extension of the scar. A concentric mastopexy and a round-block suture can then be used at the end of the procedure to minimize the visible scar and obtain a good result.

Regardless of which incision is used, the use of a skin-sparing mastectomy greatly facilitates breast shaping. In theory, once the flap has been transferred all that is required is to trim the flap to the proper size and shape, suture it to the edges of the mastectomy defect, reestablish the lateral breast border, and remove or de-epithelialize whatever TRAM flap skin is located under the mastectomy flaps. First, however, the surgeon must make sure that the mastectomy flaps are viable and that the inframammary fold has, in fact, been preserved.

Evaluating the Mastectomy Flaps

Preservation of the skin envelope helps to shape the breast, minimizes visible scarring, and provides skin that matches that of the opposite breast perfectly. This is, however, successful only if the mastectomy flaps remain alive. If the oncologic surgeon has made the flaps too thin, their blood supply may be compromised, causing parts of these flaps to become necrotic. Small areas of mastectomy flap edge necrosis are of minimal consequence (Fig 16-5), but large areas can significantly affect the quality of the reconstruction (Fig 16-6).

If inadequate perfusion is discovered before the buried portion of the TRAM flap has been de-epithelialized, the nonviable parts of the mastectomy flap can be debrided

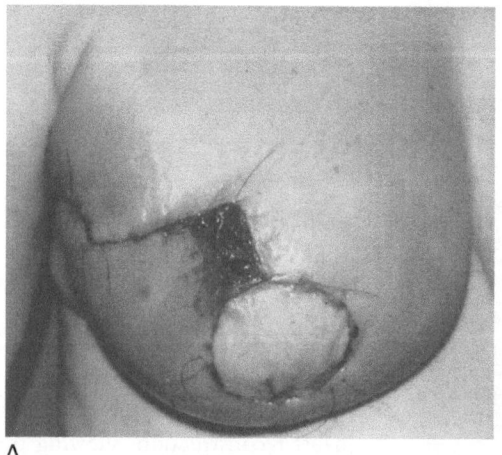

A

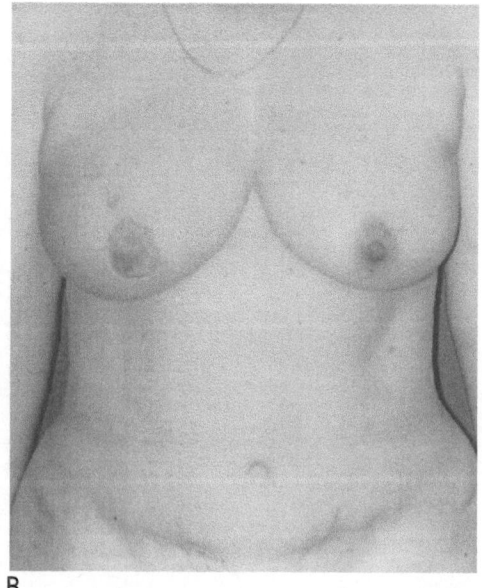

B

FIG. 16-5   (A) Small area of mastectomy flap necrosis overlying a free TRAM flap. (B) Final result shows minimal adverse effects from the mastectomy flap necrosis.

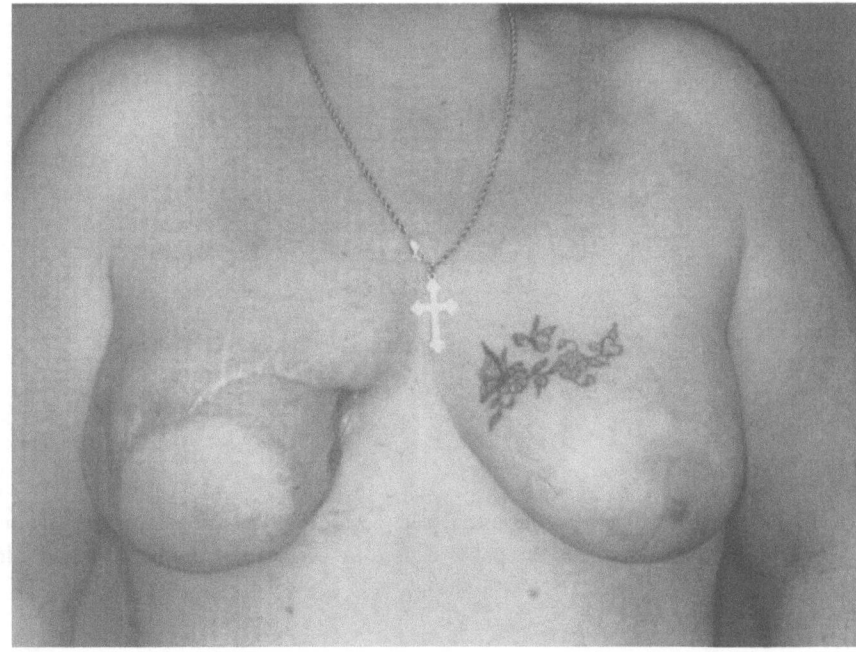

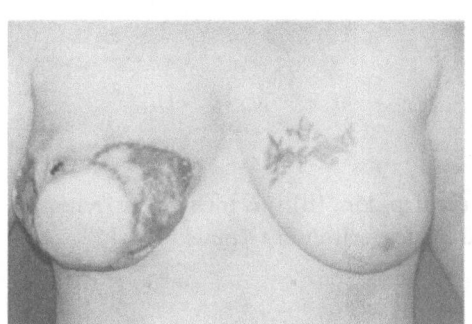

A   B

FIG. 16-6   (A) Large area of mastectomy flap necrosis caused by extension by the general surgeon of the mastectomy dissection below the inframammary fold and across the midline. The patient was also a heavy smoker of cigarettes. (B) After secondary healing, the breast still has residual damage but looks far better than what might have been expected.

and the TRAM flap skin used in their stead. The surgeon should therefore make every effort to determine whether the mastectomy flaps are viable and, if they are not, how much should be debrided, before committing himself or herself by de-epithelializing the unexposed TRAM flap skin.

One simple test of skin viability is the capillary refill time. The surgeon presses the handles of a hemostat against the skin of the flap (Fig 16-7) and then rapidly takes the hemostat away. If the time it takes for the temporary blanching to disappear (the capillary refill time) is 3 seconds or less, the flap is usually viable. If capillary refill takes longer than 3 seconds, the skin in that part of the flap probably will not survive. The test is fairly reliable in nonsmokers; however, in patients who smoke, the perfusion sometimes deteriorates over the first few postoperative days, and more mastectomy flap necrosis occurs than was anticipated.

Another test, but a less reliable one, is evaluation of bleeding at the flap edges. If the mastectomy flap is rubbed or trimmed of 1 or 2 mm of skin along its edge and if the initial bleeding is of bright red blood, viability is likely. If the initial bleeding is dark, even if it subsequently turns a lighter shade of red, the flap edge will probably become necrotic and should be debrided. Again, in patients who smoke, this test may underestimate the eventual extent of skin loss.

The fluorescein test,[4] which involves an intravenous injection of fluorescein followed by evaluation of the skin flaps under a Woods lamp (ultraviolet light), is well known but tends to underestimate the amount of viable skin and is therefore not rec-

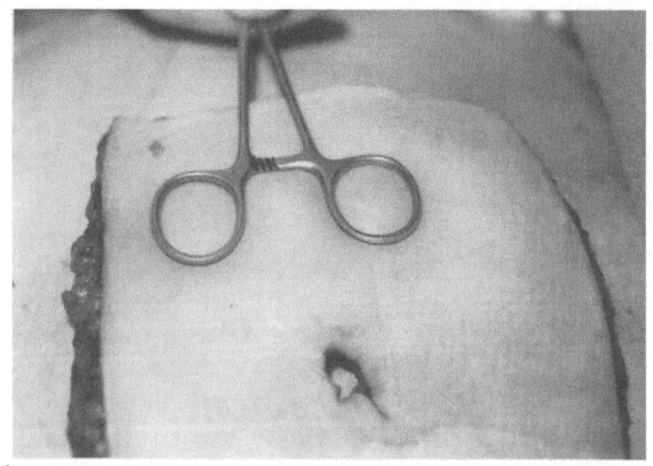
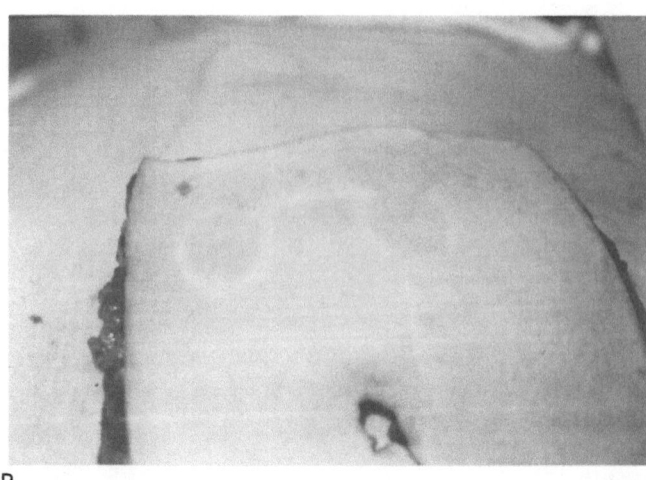

A

B

FIG. 16-7   (A) In the capillary refill test, a hemostat handle is pressed tightly against the flap skin. (B) It is then rapidly removed. If skin circulation is adequate, the pallor caused by pressure of the hemostat should disappear within 3 seconds.

ommended. If the surgeon is very unsure about the extent of mastectomy flap viability, the decision concerning the amount of skin to debride can be deferred by leaving some intact TRAM flap skin under the questionable mastectomy flaps (JW May, personal communication, February 1997). If, after 3 days, the mastectomy flaps are fully viable, the underlying TRAM flap skin can be de-epithelialized with the patient under local anesthesia. Otherwise, the mastectomy flaps are debrided and the preserved TRAM flap skin is used to surface the breast.

Assessing and Repairing the Inframammary Fold

Ensuring that the inframammary fold is correct is one of the most important steps in breast mound reconstruction because an incorrect placement can be difficult or impossible to fix later. Moreover, dissection past the inframammary fold during the mastectomy is a common error, one that can easily go unrecognized and cause the reconstructed breast mound to be positioned too low. It is best to evaluate the inframammary fold prior to transferring the TRAM flap to the chest wall because once the TRAM flap is in place, it is more difficult to repair the inframammary fold, should that be necessary. The fold under the opposite breast should be marked (Fig 16-8), and compared to the position of the fold on the mastectomy side. If the fold on the mastectomy side is too low, it must be reestablished with sutures (usually running 3-0 Vicryl [polygalactin 910] sutures). This can create irregularities and skin dimpling, but these usually disappear with time and in any case are preferable to an inframammary fold that is positioned too low.

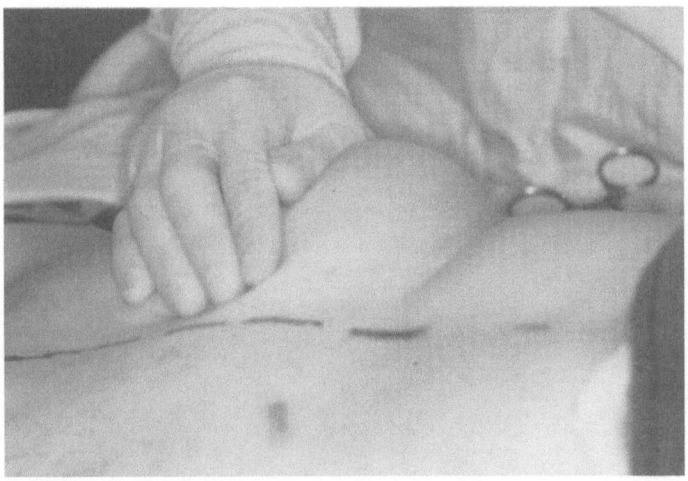

FIG. 16-8 The inframammary fold of the opposite breast is marked after accentuating it by manually displacing it inferiorly.

The inframammary fold should be a smooth arc, which can be difficult to reproduce accurately with sutures. If, after suturing, the new fold is still too low, additional sutures are placed to raise it. If it is much too high, the sutures are removed and replaced. If it is only slightly too high, however, the sutures can be left in place and inferior dissection with electrocautery (just superficial to the sutures) can be used to create a slightly lower fold. This often establishes a smoother fold than could be obtained with sutures alone, but care must be taken not to make the inferior mastectomy flap too thin and thereby jeopardize its blood supply.

Securing the Flap to the Chest Wall

In the case of any free flap, immediately after the anastomoses have been completed, the flap should be secured to the chest wall so that the pedicle cannot inadvertently be subjected to excessive tension. In the case of a free TRAM flap, this is best done by suturing the transferred rectus sheath (which holds sutures better than the muscle does) to the pectoral muscle with 2-0 Vicryl or similar material (Fig 16-9). The surgeon must remember, however, that the pectoral muscle does not hold sutures all that well and will not adequately stabilize a large, heavy flap. If a perforator flap has been used, there will be no rectus sheath and so the flap must be trimmed and then fixed directly to the medial edges of the mastectomy defect, so that the flap cannot slip laterally. With either type of flap, the pedicle should be loose so that arm movements and breast ptosis will not cause tension, but the flap must be advanced medially enough that the breast will not be positioned too laterally. Ideally, pedicle length permitting, the lateral tail of the flap is minimally trimmed to simulate the natural curve of the lateral breast border

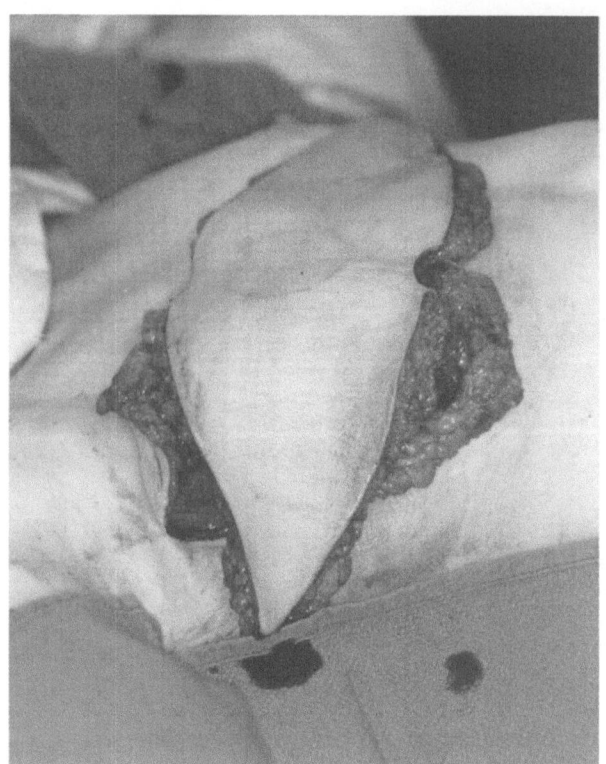

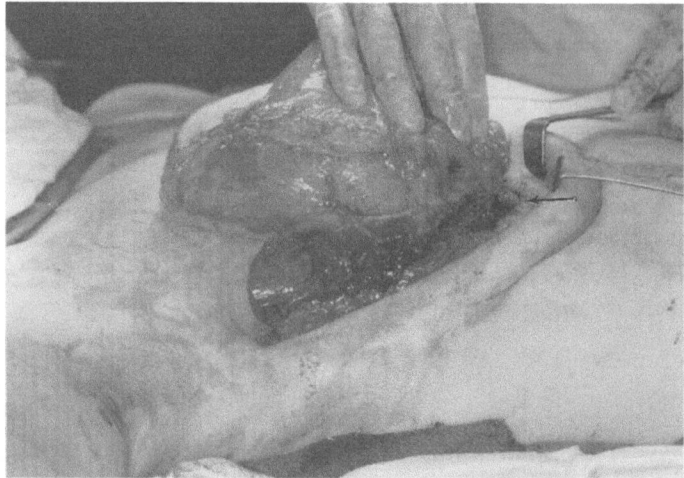

FIG. 16-9 The transferred free TRAM flap is stabilized by suturing it to the chest wall with 2-0 Vicryl. Note the irregularity along the lower edge of the flap at the site of the umbilicus; this will be hidden by the overlying mastectomy flap.

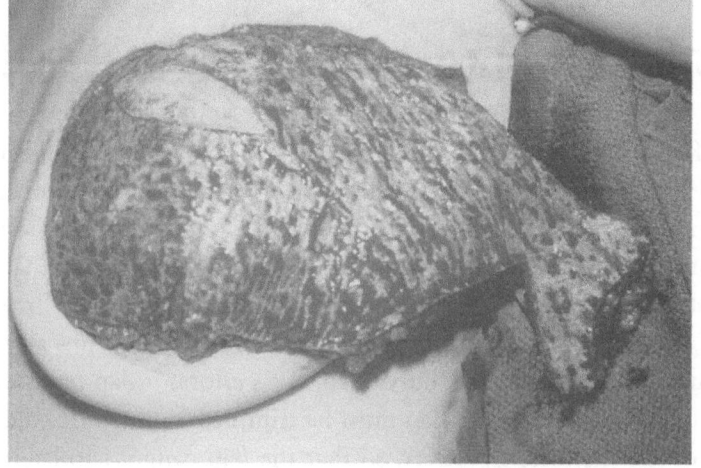

FIG. 16-10 The lateral border of the flap is trimmed to approximate a gentle curve that simulates the normal shape of the breast. In this case a small fish-tail was created at the posterior tip of the flap to replace the axillary contents.

(Fig 16-10) and any remaining trimming is done medially, where the flap's blood supply is weakest.

Establishing the Lateral Border of the Breast

If an axillary dissection has been performed, the latissimus dorsi muscle and adjacent tissues will have been detached from the lateral chest wall, destroying the lateral border of the breast. This lateral border will have to be reestablished with sutures (Fig 16-11). The lateral border is usually located somewhere just anterior to the mid-axillary line but varies slightly among patients; therefore, the opposite breast should be examined to help position the border symmetrically. If the surgeon is lucky, there may be a palpable thickening of the subcutaneous tissues where the oncologic surgeon stopped removing breast tissue. This thicker subcutaneous tissue not only identifies where the lateral border was but can be sutured to the chest wall (usually with 2-0 Vicryl) without dimpling the overlying skin.

If the inframammary fold was correctly preserved, it can also help to position the lateral breast border. The curve of the inframammary fold is followed into the axilla, where it establishes the lower part of the lateral border. Often this maneuver will help identify where the excision of breast tissue ended laterally, at least in the inferolateral quadrant.

By reestablishing the lateral breast border with sutures, the surgeon prevents the breast mound from drifting laterally into the axilla. These sutures also prevent the lat-

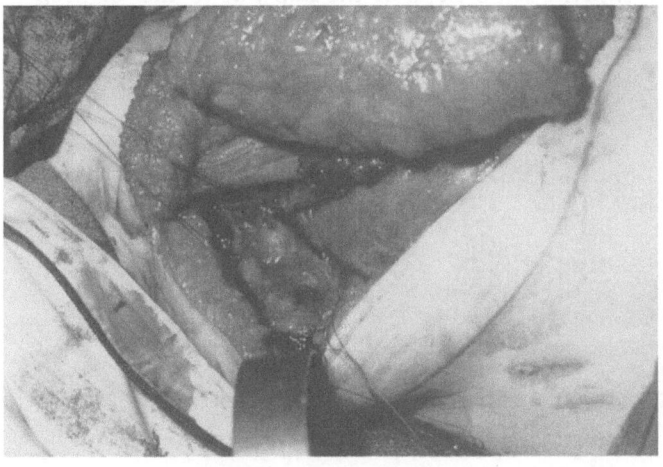
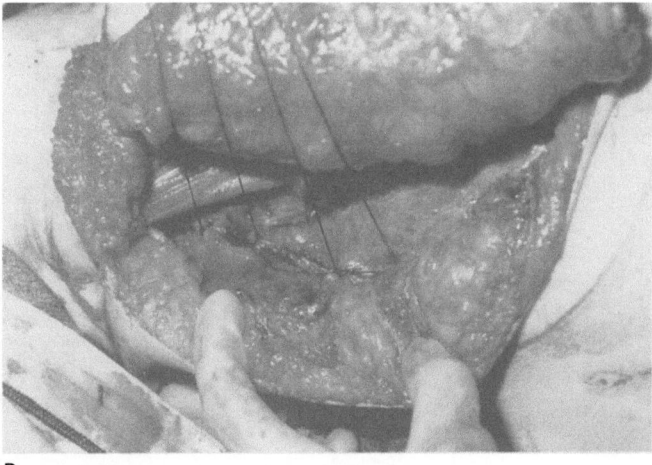

A   B

FIG. 16-11 (A) Sutures are placed to form a lateral breast border by approximating lateral subcutaneous fatty tissue to the chest wall. Here methylene blue was used to mark both the lateral breast border on the chest wall and the subcutaneous tissue that would be sutured to it. (B) The sutures are tied to form a shelf that will support the reconstructed breast.

eral chest wall and axillary subcutaneous tissues from drifting posteriorly and thus reduce the otherwise common tendency toward excess subcutaneous fullness below the axilla.

Trimming the Flap Medially

The easiest way to estimate the size of flap required is to examine the mastectomy specimen (Fig 16-12). Some surgeons weigh the excised breast,[5–7] and this can be helpful. In most cases, the thickness of the TRAM flap will be similar to that of the excised breast, and the dimensions of the mastectomy specimen can therefore be applied to the flap, at least as a rough guide.

A useful approach to medial trimming of the flap is to draw the estimated medial border on the flap skin and then make the actual incision 1 cm medial to the markings (because at this stage it is better to err on the side of having a flap that is too large rather than one that is too small). If vigorous bright red bleeding is found all along the cut edge, hemostasis is obtained and the incised edge becomes the medial border of the flap. If a free TRAM flap has been used, using well-perfused medial tissue in this way effectively lengthens the pedicle of the flap and permits adequate medial fullness even when the thoracodorsal vessels are used as recipient sites. If the flap is too large, it can be trimmed laterally later. If bright red bleeding is not present at the medial incision, a new medial incision is made slightly more laterally, closer to the flap pedicle. The surgeon should not hesitate to move this medial incision more laterally if there is any doubt about the viability of the medial edge of the flap. Otherwise, he or she will sacrifice viable tissue laterally to preserve nonviable tissue medially, and will only end up with medial fat necrosis and an unsatisfactory result.

One of the advantages of the free TRAM flap is its excellent blood supply, which supplies blood not only to the superficial portions of the flap but to the fat deep to

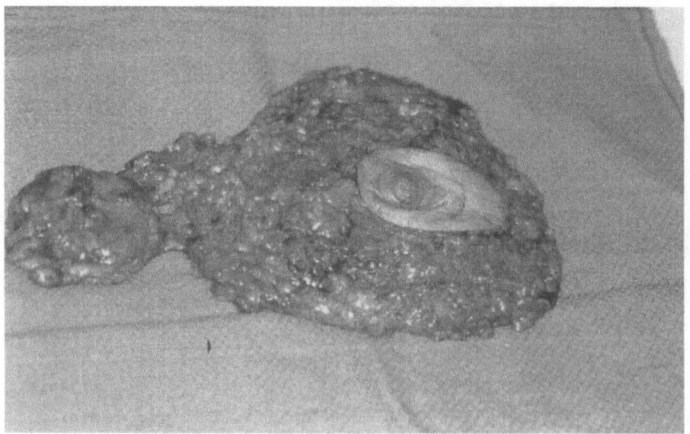

FIG. 16-12 Typical mastectomy flap specimen. The thickness of the breast tissue is usually similar to that of a TRAM flap.

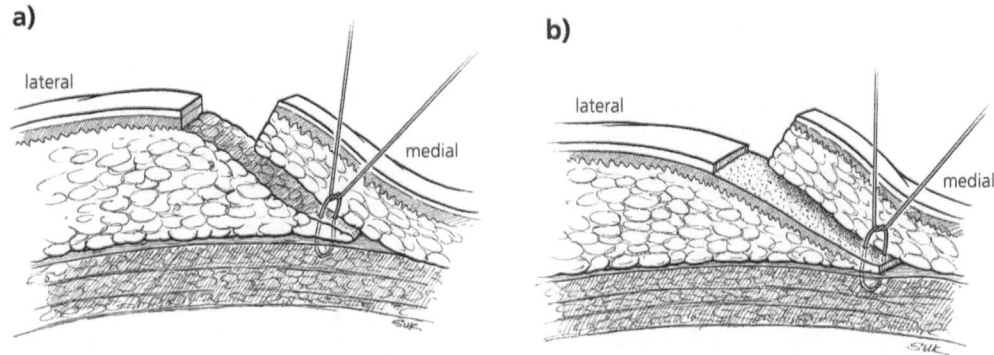

Fig. 16-13   (A) Attaching the medial border of a free TRAM flap. The deep fat is sutured to the medial edge of the mastectomy defect, and the superficial fat is sculpted away to form a cone. (B) After a conventional TRAM flap, the blood supply is less robust so the deeper fat (deep to Scarpa's fascia, which is not shown in this drawing) is usually discarded and the dermis and superficial fat are sutured to the medial edge of the mastectomy defect.

Scarpa's fascia as well. This robust perfusion allows the surgeon to use that deep fat (which is usually discarded at the medial edge of the conventional TRAM flap) and suture it to the medial edge of the mastectomy defect. The surgeon can then sculpt the flap into something approaching a pyramid by removing the more superficial fat (Fig 16-13A). This aspect of breast shaping is not significant when the flap is very thin, but can be important in other patients when the flap is sufficiently thick to be carved and sculpted in this way. If a conventional TRAM flap has been used, or if a free TRAM flap has a blood supply that is less robust than usual, it is usually better to suture the de-epithelialized dermis to the medial edge of the mastectomy defect and to discard any excess fat deep to Scarpa's fascia in order to minimize the risk of fat necrosis (Fig 16-13B).

Suturing the Medial Flap Border to the Medial Defect

Once the flap has been trimmed medially, it is sutured to the edges of the mastectomy defect medially, superomedially, and inferomedially (Fig 16-14). This is done early to help stabilize the flap (supplementing the fixation that has been performed earlier) and make tension caused by pulling on the pedicle less likely. Moreover, this fixation will facilitate subsequent de-epithelialization of buried TRAM flap skin. The sutures should be placed 2 or 3 cm apart, with care taken to secure the flap to deep tissues so the skin is not dimpled.

It is crucial to ensure that there is sufficient tissue in the inferior part of the breast to provide fullness in the lower pole, where projection should be maximized. This should be checked after the first few medial sutures are placed. If the breast is being positioned too high, the sutures should be removed and replaced with the breast positioned more

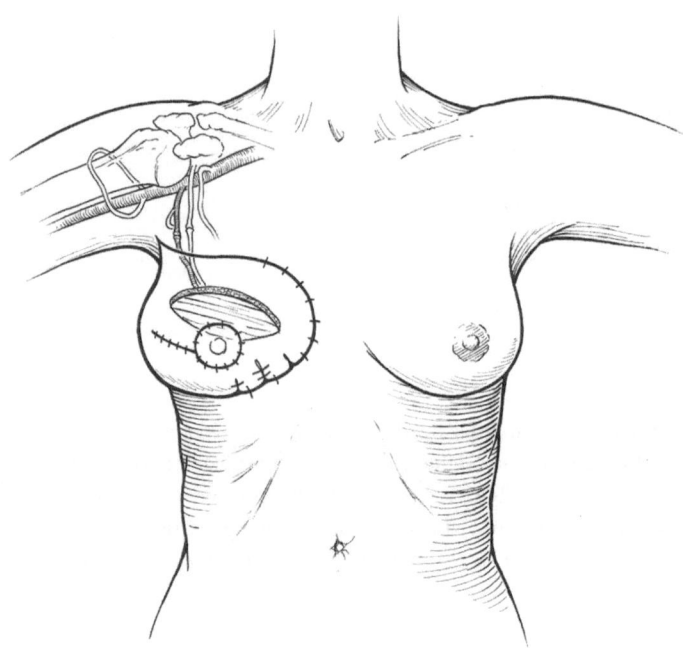

FIG. 16-14   The flap is sutured to the edges of the mastectomy defect medially, superomedially, and inferomedially so that the medial contour of the breast is maintained.

inferiorly. Excess tissue in the medial part of the breast is easily corrected after the medial insetting is complete, simply by removing skin and superficial fat. If the medial flap border causes a noticeable ridge under the skin (Fig 16-15A), removing the dermis along the edge of the flap will usually soften the edge and correct the problem (Fig 16-15B).

Maximizing Projection of the Lower Pole

In the initial breast mound reconstruction, it is difficult if not impossible to reproduce the conical projection under the nipple of a natural breast with a TRAM flap, which by its very nature is flat. Projection can be increased, however, in the lower pole. This is easiest after a skin-sparing mastectomy, because the inferior mastectomy flap can be used to hide bunching or folding of the TRAM flap beneath the breast skin envelope. In thinner patients who have a defect in the TRAM flap caused by removal of the umbilicus, the skin bridge inferior to this hole can be divided and the two parts of the TRAM flap folded over one another (Fig 16-16). If there is no umbilical defect, the TRAM flap in the lower pole is simply bunched together with sutures (Fig 16-17). In either case, any distortion in the TRAM flap itself is disguised by the overlying mastectomy flap.

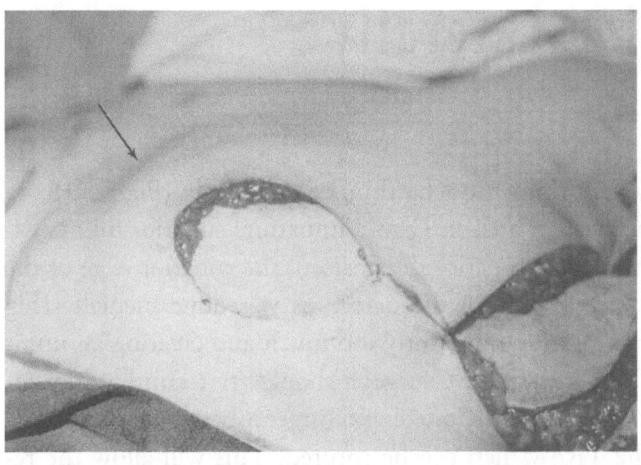

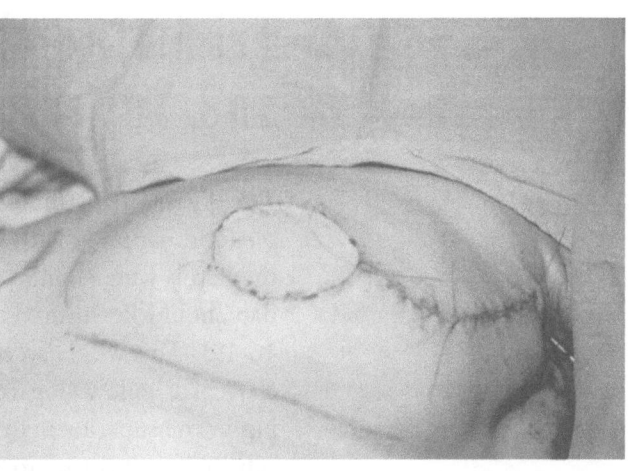

A   B

FIG. 16-15 (A) The medial edge of the flap can sometimes cause a ridge that can be visible through the mastectomy flaps. (B) After the peripheral 1 cm of dermis is removed, the ridge is significantly softened.

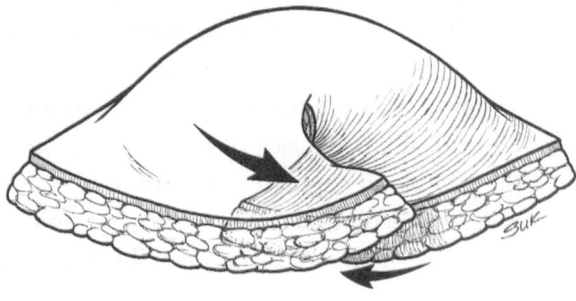

FIG. 16-16 The two parts of the TRAM flap on either side of an umbilical defect can be folded over each other to increase lower pole projection. This is camouflaged by the overlying mastectomy flap.

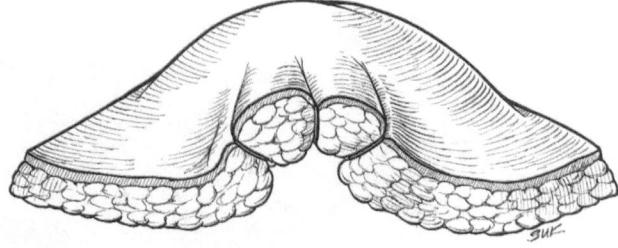

FIG. 16-17 If there is no umbilical defect in the TRAM flap, lower pole projection can be increased by bunching up the lower edge with sutures.

Trimming the Flap Laterally and Superiorly

The TRAM flap (unless already very thin) must be thinned superiorly (Fig 16-18) to blend in naturally with the infraclavicular area and avoid unnatural superior fullness. If the flap is wide enough (in its inferior-to-superior dimension), the superior edge of the flap should be sutured to the superior edge of the defect, as was done medially (Fig 16-19). This will keep the flap from settling inferiorly too much and creating an infraclavicular hollow (Fig 16-20). The reconstructive surgeon should try to find a thickening in the superior mastectomy flap, where the oncologic surgeon began removing less subcutaneous tissue, to which the TRAM flap can be sutured. This will allow the reconstruction to blend into the surrounding tissues as well as provide a place for the sutures to hold without dimpling the skin. The superior sutures can also be designed to include underlying muscle for additional stability.

If the flap is not wide enough and the superior sutures position the flap too high and prevent the flap from being sufficiently full in the inferior pole, the superior sutures can be removed and the risk of an infraclavicular hollow accepted. This is done for the obvious reason that it is more important to achieve lower pole projection than to avoid an infraclavicular hollow. The surgeon should be aware, however, that lower pole projection will usually increase with time because of the effects of gravity. Also, the lack of inferior pole projection can sometimes be corrected later, while an infraclavicular hollow is very difficult to correct. An infraclavicular hollow should therefore not be accepted unless the lack of lower pole projection is significant.

If the flap blood supply is good, thinning can be performed superficially, as was done medially, to sculpt the breast into a pyramid. If the flap blood supply is weaker than usual (especially in a conventional TRAM flap) it is better to discard the deeper

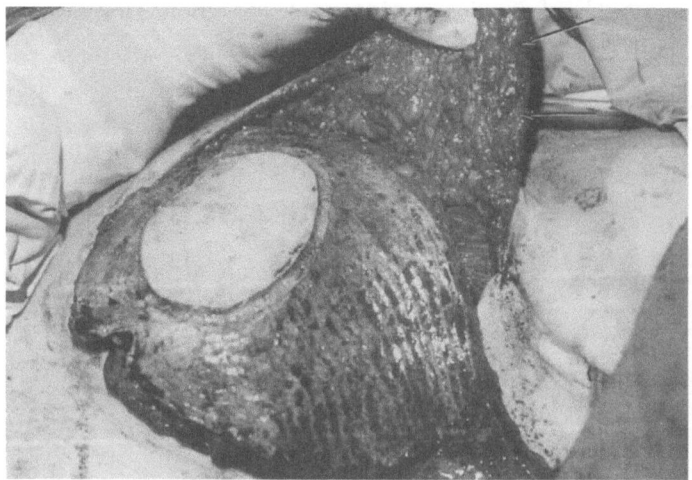

FIG. 16-18   The superior edge of the flap (arrows) is thinned to blend into the infraclavicular chest wall.

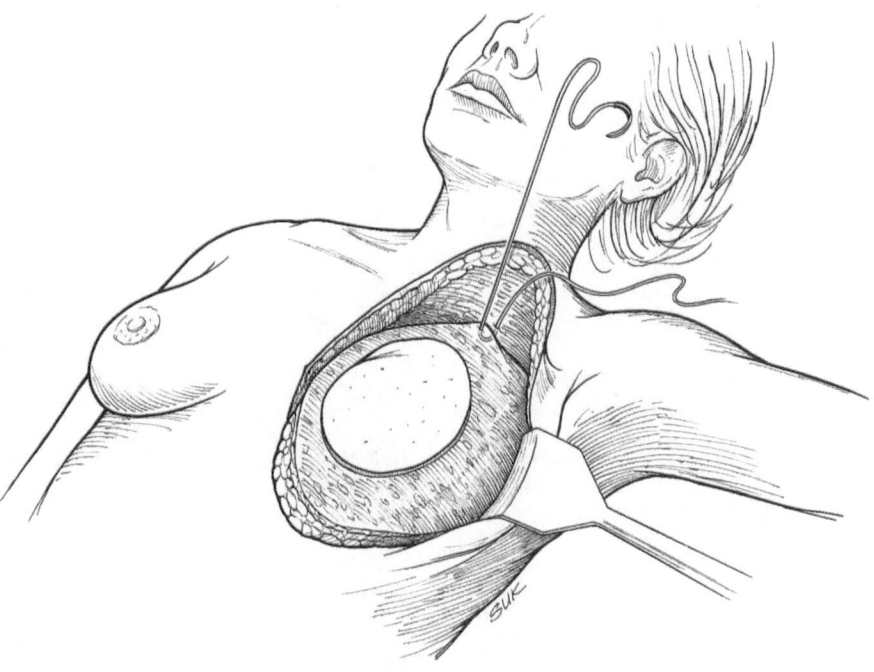

FIG. 16-19   The superior edge of the flap is sutured to the upper edge of the defect to avoid an infraclavicular hollow.

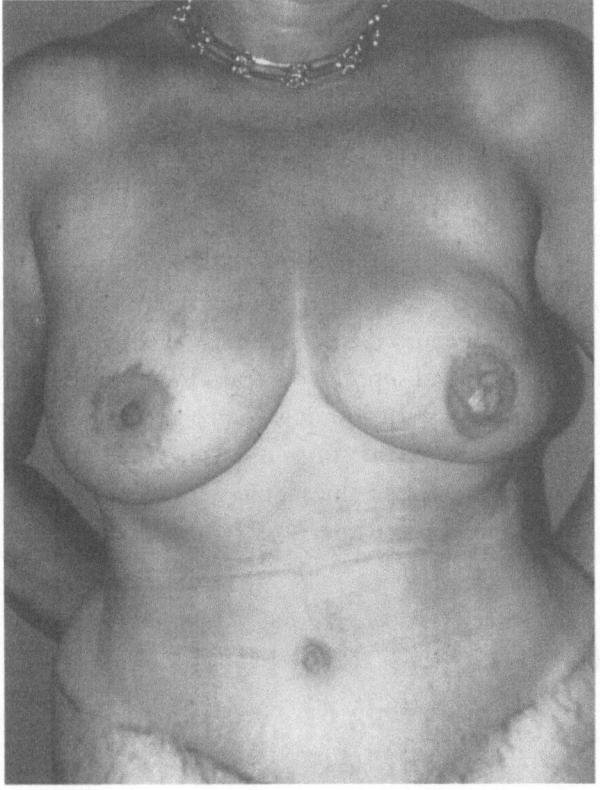

FIG. 16-20   An infraclavicular hollow, which was caused by inadequate fixation of the flap superiorly.

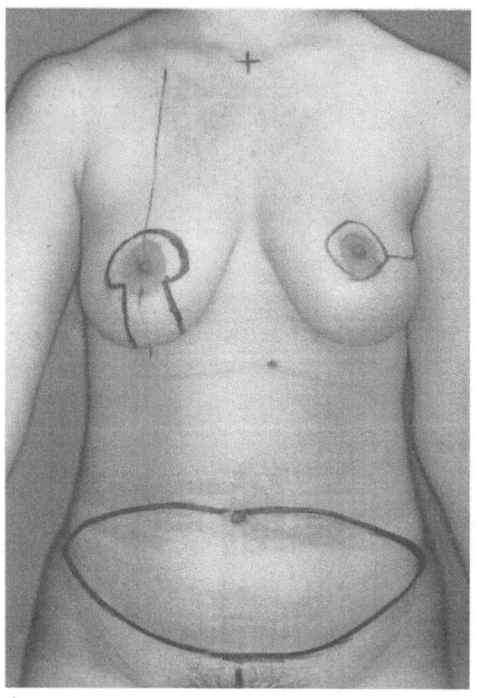
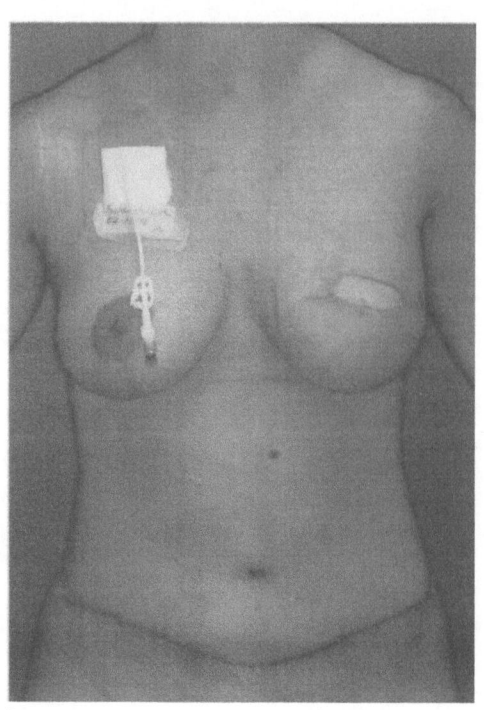

A   B

FIG. 16-21   (A) Preoperative photo. (B) After immediate free TRAM flap reconstruction using the thoracodorsal vessels as recipients, showing the most common postoperative shape abnormality: excess fullness laterally.

fat, which has a greater tendency to develop fat necrosis, and retain the better-vascularized dermis and superficial fat.

The most common abnormality of shape following TRAM flap breast reconstruction is excess tissue laterally, especially superolaterally (Fig 16-21). The surgeon should make special efforts to avoid this by trimming the flap laterally and superolaterally (Fig 16-22), to minimize the need for revision. Often this trimming is accompanied by considerable bleeding because the flap tissue at this point is close to the pedicle and has a particularly good blood supply. It is tempting to put off some of this work until another day because this lateral trimming comes near the end of the operation when the surgeon is fatigued. Unless the surgeon is concerned about jeopardizing the blood supply to the flap, however, he or she should persevere and make every attempt to achieve symmetry in the initial procedure.

Sitting the Patient Upright to Evaluate the Breast

Following any breast reconstruction, the appearance of the patient in the upright position is what determines the quality of the result. After the initial breast mound shaping has been completed, the patient should be placed in a sitting position to

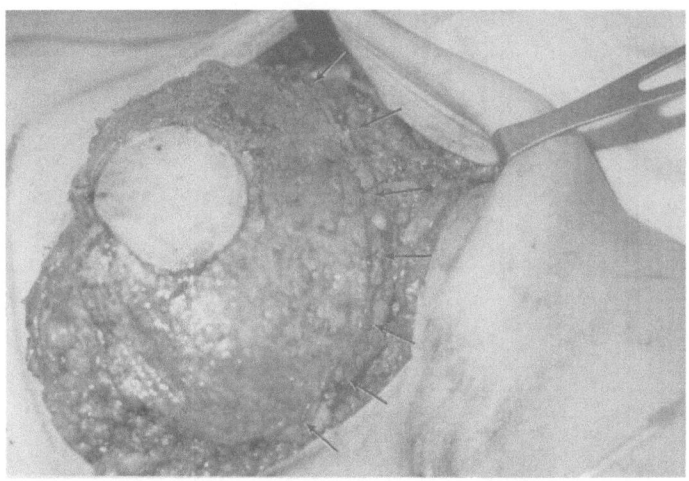

FIG. 16-22   The flap is trimmed laterally and superolaterally.

evaluate the breast and determine the need for adjustments. Although the patient cannot be sat completely upright, the surgeon should try to get her as upright as possible. First, the table should be lowered completely. Next, the back of the table is raised (slowly, and combined with raising the patient's legs as well to avoid a drop in blood pressure). Finally, reverse Trendelenburg position is used to sit the patient up more completely (Fig 16-23). The anesthesiologist will have to ensure that the intravenous lines and airway tubing are long enough to allow this. The surgeon then goes to the foot of the table to evaluate breast shape, size, and position. The operating lights should be turned off or away from the patient, so that they do not illuminate the patient's torso asymmetrically and thereby interfere with the evaluation of symmetry.

The drapes that usually cover the patient's head and shoulders can sometimes make it difficult to tell if she is leaning off to one side. It is helpful to try the sitting position prior to the operation but after anesthesia induction, to make sure that the patient is positioned symmetrically on the operating table. It is also helpful, when possible, to drape the patient so that the tips of the shoulders are exposed (Fig 16-24). That way, if the patient does lean to one side when the anesthesiologist sits her up, the surgeon will be aware of the problem and can compensate for it to some degree by tilting the operating table to one side.

Although the best way to assess breast shape is with the patient in the upright position, the surgeon should also assess the symmetry from below, with the patient supine. If symmetry is good in that view (Fig 16-25), it will more often than not also be excellent when the patient is upright. This view from the foot of the bed can be very helpful in fine-tuning the shaping of the breast both in the initial breast mound creation and in subsequent revisions.

Once the desired volume and shape are achieved, the mastectomy flaps are replaced (Fig 16-26) and once again checked for viability. All that then remains to complete the breast shaping is the TRAM flap de-epithelialization and skin closure.

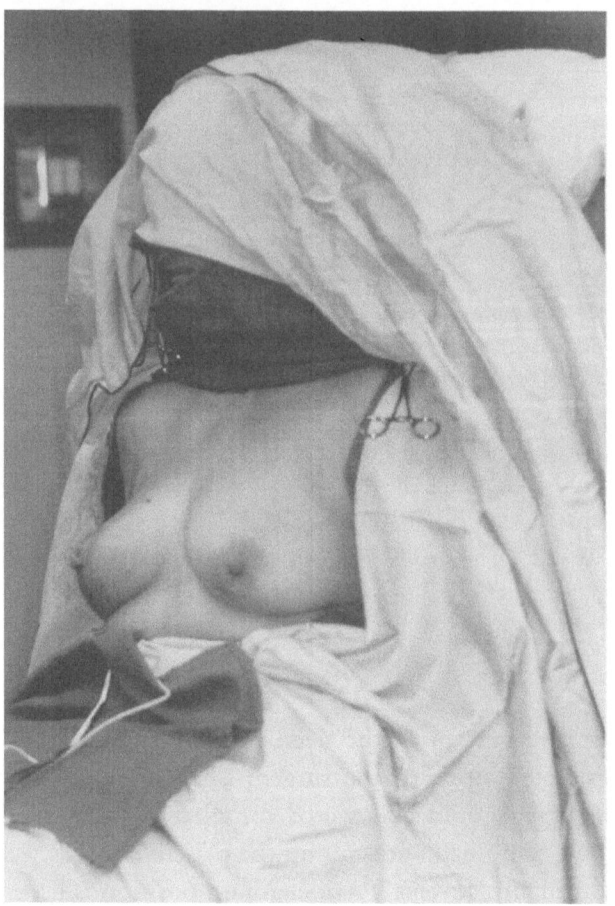

Fig. 16-23   The back of the operating table is elevated to place the patient as close to an upright sitting position as possible. Reverse Trendelenburg position will help to achieve this.

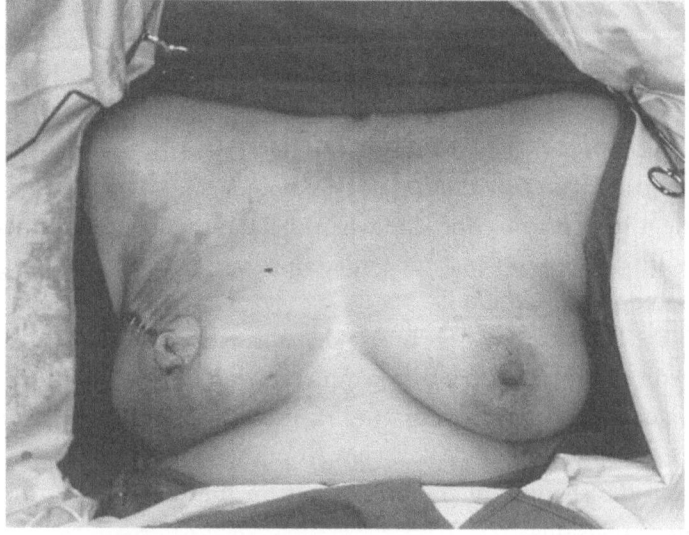

Fig. 16-24   When the patient is draped, the tops of the shoulders should be left exposed so that the surgeon can ensure that the patient is oriented correctly when she is sitting up.

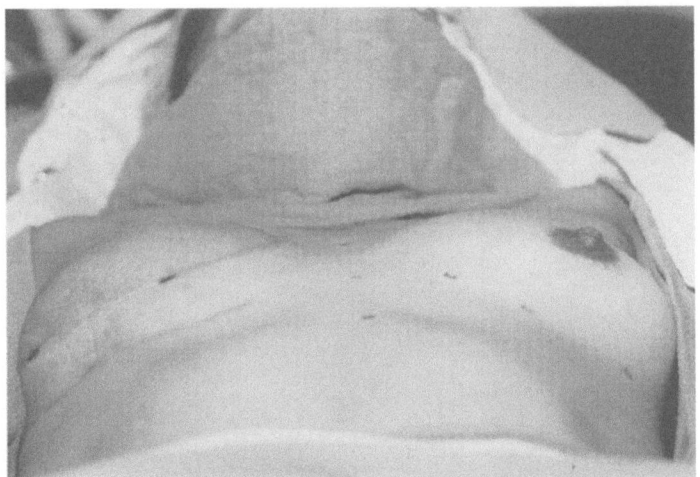

FIG. 16-25   View of the reconstructed breast from the foot of the bed with patient supine. This view is very helpful in evaluating breast symmetry, especially if the patient cannot be sat completely upright.

De-Epithelializing the Buried Skin

Once the viability of the mastectomy flaps has been ascertained, the unexposed skin of the TRAM flap must be de-epithelialized. In doing this, the surgeon should try to keep the de-epithelialization superficial and stay out of the subdermal plexus to minimize bleeding and maintain the circulation to the most distal parts of the flap. At the edges of the flap, however, the dermis is often best removed to soften the contour and avoid

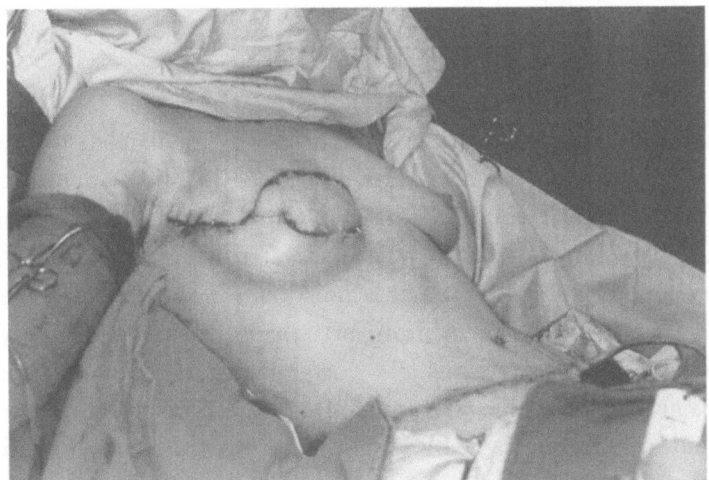

FIG. 16-26   The mastectomy flaps are replaced, and the exposed TRAM flap skin is marked. The remaining skin will be de-epithelialized.

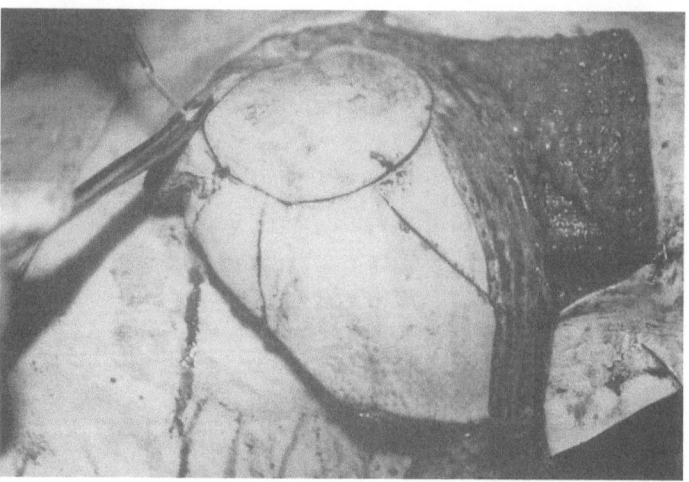

Fig. 16-27   De-epithelializing the skin with large, sharp Mayo or Supercut scissors is effective and allows more than one surgeon to work simultaneously without an assistant.

a visible ridge under the skin. De-epithelialization is tedious. When using electrocautery or a scalpel, it is greatly facilitated by lateral traction on the flap applied by an assistant. The de-epithelialization can be performed with either a scalpel, electrocautery, a laser, or large sharp scissors. Any of these methods can be effective, provided that the subdermal plexus is disturbed as little as possible. The use of large, sharp scissors (Fig 16-27) has the advantage that traction by an assistant is not required so that two surgeons can work on the de-epithelialization simultaneously. Whatever the technique selected (I currently am using Supercut scissors), care should be taken to avoid inadvertent traction on the flap's pedicle.

Incising the Dermis

It is helpful to make an incision through the dermis immediately surrounding the retained TRAM flap skin (Fig 16-28) that will be used to fill the defect created by removal of the nipple/areolar complex (the areolar or "keyhole" area). This allows the exposed TRAM flap skin to be subsequently elevated to the level of the surrounding breast skin envelope (Fig 16-29). If this is not done, the areolar area may be noticeably depressed (Fig 16-30). The incision, best made with electrocautery, ideally extends just barely through the dermis and does not disturb the subdermal plexus. In practice, this is nearly impossible, and some bleeding will be encountered; but the surgeon should endeavor to minimize bleeding by keeping the incision relatively superficial. This maneuver also inevitably causes some disruption of the subdermal plexus and therefore is most appropriate when the flap blood supply is excellent, as it usually is in a free TRAM flap. If the flap blood supply is marginal, the incision of the dermis should be omitted.

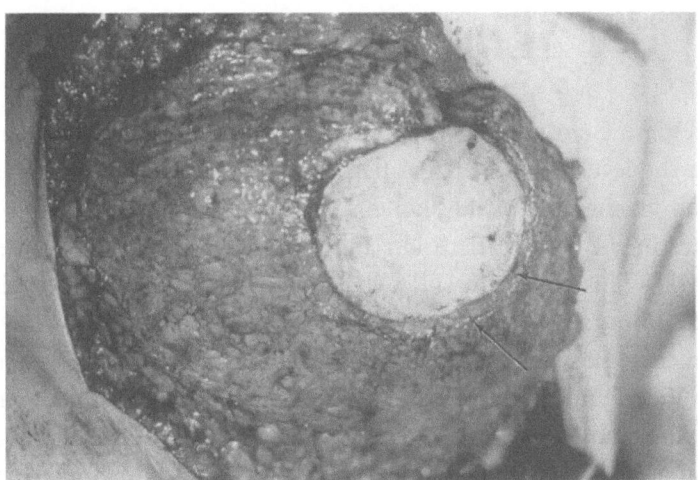

FIG. 16-28   An incision is made through the dermis around the exposed skin paddle so that the TRAM flap skin can be elevated to the level of the surrounding mastectomy flap skin. The arrows point to areas where the incision through the dermis is more obvious.

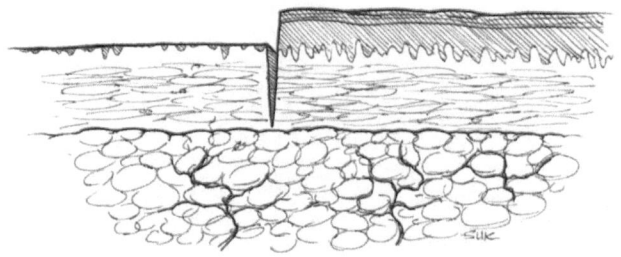

FIG. 16-29   Drawing of the dermal incision. It should extend just through the dermis, but not through the subdermal plexus.

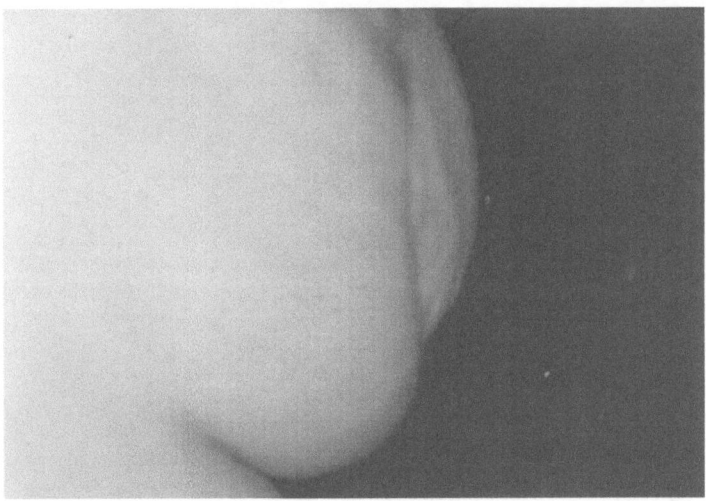

FIG. 16-30   If the TRAM flap skin paddle is not sufficiently elevated with the subdermal sutures, it will be noticeably depressed below the level of the remaining breast skin envelope.

Closing the Skin

Incision of the dermis around the exposed skin paddle, by itself, does not correct the discrepancy in the levels of the TRAM flap and breast envelope skin. Elevation of the TRAM flap skin to the level of the skin envelope is accomplished with sutures, by taking deeper bites in the TRAM flap skin and more superficial ones in the mastectomy flaps (Fig 16-31). This forces the TRAM flap skin to be more superficial, creating a smooth breast contour.

In my practice, I close the dermis of the remaining wounds with interrupted buried sutures of 3-0 Vicryl and then close the skin itself with running subcuticular sutures of 3-0 PDS (polydioxanone) or Prolene (polypropylene) that are removed after 3 weeks. Other suture materials are probably equally effective, however, and most likely make no difference in the final result.

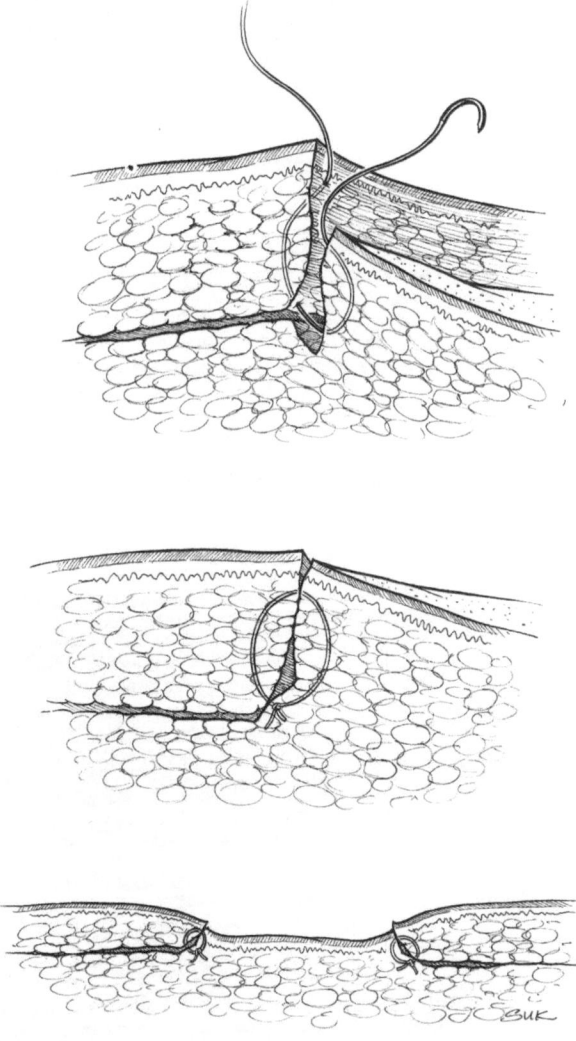

FIG. 16-31 By taking deeper bites in the TRAM flap dermis and more superficial ones in the mastectomy flap skin, the surgeon can bring the TRAM flap skin up to the level of the mastectomy flap. The knot, however, should always be buried rather than placed superficially as in the top drawing.

Draining the Wound

All autologous tissue breast reconstructions require a suction drain, and in most cases the area drained must include the axilla. If the thoracodorsal vessels have been used as recipients, the anastomoses may be adjacent to the drain and care should be taken to keep the drain from impeding blood flow through the pedicle. The surgeon should check this just before completion of the wound closure and, if necessary, reroute the drain so that the pedicle is protected from it. I prefer a 15-French round Blake drain, which rarely clogs and is not painful to remove once it is no longer required.

Summary

Breast mound shaping in large part determines the aesthetic success of autologous tissue breast reconstruction and therefore deserves considerable attention and effort. A logical, step-by-step approach is recommended. The surgeon determines how much tissue is missing and designs the flap accordingly. The mastectomy flaps are evaluated, and any nonviable skin is discarded. The inframammary fold is then evaluated and adjusted if necessary. The flap is transferred and positioned on the chest wall securely so that the pedicle is not under tension. The lateral breast border is formed with sutures. The medial edge of the flap is defined, the excess trimmed off, and the viability of the remaining tissue assessed. The flap is then sutured to the edges of the mastectomy defect medially, superiorly, and inferomedially. The flap is thinned so that it blends into the remaining chest wall, and the lateral excess is trimmed away. The size, position, and shape of the breast are evaluated with the patient in a sitting position; corrections are made if necessary. The wound is then drained and closed.

Optimal breast mound shaping requires artistic judgment, which is not easily taught. Each patient is different, and modifications of the approach presented here are often necessary. My objective, in this chapter, is to present an approach that will facilitate successful breast shaping in the majority of patients and can serve as a framework that the surgeon can build upon as needed to create a breast mound that will satisfy the patient and, after appropriate revision, the fastidious surgeon as well. Unfortunately, breast shaping must be performed toward the end of the procedure, when the surgical team may be tired and eager to finish the operation. The effort required to properly shape the breast at this point, however, will usually pay many dividends in the form of improved results.

References

1. Maxwell GP, Andochick SE. Secondary shaping of the TRAM flap. *Clin Plast Surg.* 1994;21:247–253.
2. Carlson GW, Bostwick J, Styblo TM, et al. Skin-sparing mastectomy: oncologic and reconstructive considerations. *Ann Surg.* 1997;225:570–578.

3.   Carlson GW. Skin sparing mastectomy: anatomic and technical considerations. *Amer Surg.* 1996;62:151–155.

4.   Thorvaldsson SE, Grabb WC. The intravenous fluorescein test as a measure of skin flap viability. *Plast Reconstr Surg.* 1974;53:576.

5.   Hartrampf CR, ed. *Hartrampf's Breast Reconstruction with Living Tissue.* New York: Raven Press; 1991.

6.   Beasley ME. Immediate breast reconstruction with a pedicled TRAM flap. In: Hartrampf CR, ed. *Hartrampf's Breast Reconstruction with Living Tissue.* New York: Raven Press; 1991:161–174.

7.   Salmi A, Tukianinen E, Harma M, Asko-Seljavaara S. A prospective study of changes in muscle dimensions following free-muscle transfer measured by ultrasound and CT scanning. *Plast Reconstr Surg.* 1996;97:1443–1450.

17 Shaping the Breast Mound in Delayed Reconstruction

Differences Between Immediate and Delayed Reconstruction

Delayed breast reconstruction can be far more challenging than immediate reconstruction, with results that are less predictable. Much more tissue is missing, so the flaps must be larger and include more skin (Fig 17-1). Also, because the inframammary fold and skin envelope are missing, the surgeon is forced to re-create them—a step that is usually unnecessary in immediate reconstruction (especially after skin-sparing mastectomy)[1,2] and that can be a potential source of error. Sometimes the patient will have had an aggressive mastectomy and may have large tissue deficits that cannot be corrected (Fig 17-2). Previous radiation therapy may have irreparably damaged the skin surrounding the breast, severely limiting the potential for a successful result (Fig 17-3). Even when the surrounding skin is undamaged, high scar placement and a poor color match can seriously affect the aesthetic quality of the result (Figs 17-4 and 17-5).

Another source of difficulty in delayed reconstruction is the presence of scar tissue. Scar tissue in the axilla may interfere somewhat with the performance of a free transverse rectus abdominis myocutaneous (TRAM) flap by complicating dissection of the thoracodorsal vessels as recipients. Subcutaneous scar tissue, adhering to the skin, also may limit the surgeon's ability to reexpand the native breast skin to its original position.

For these reasons, the average aesthetic outcome of delayed breast reconstruction is generally poorer than that of immediate reconstruction,[3] and outstanding results are not routine. Patients who are undergoing delayed breast reconstruction should understand these limitations and should not expect the same results as with immediate reconstruction and skin-sparing mastectomy. This is especially true if there has been prior irradiation or if a very aggressive mastectomy was performed. Nevertheless, acceptable and even excellent results (Figs 17-6 and 17-7) can be obtained for most patients provided that the surgeon uses a logical, planned approach.

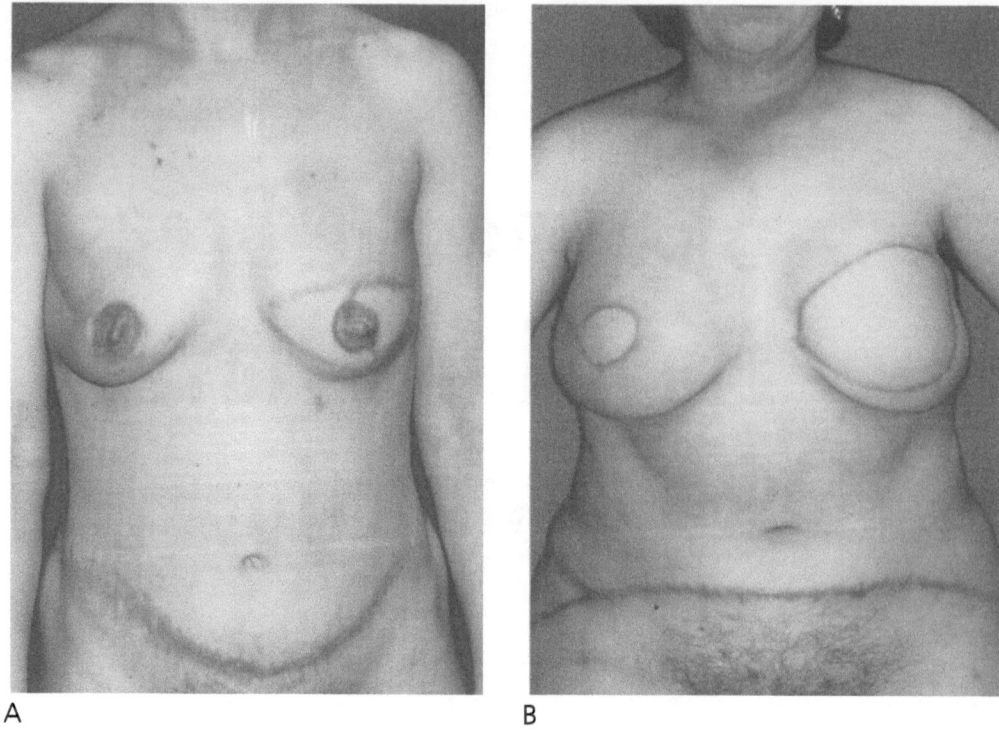

A   B

Fig. 17-1 (A, B) Patients who have had a delayed reconstruction on the left side and an immediate reconstruction on the right. Note the differences in the amount of missing skin that had to be replaced.

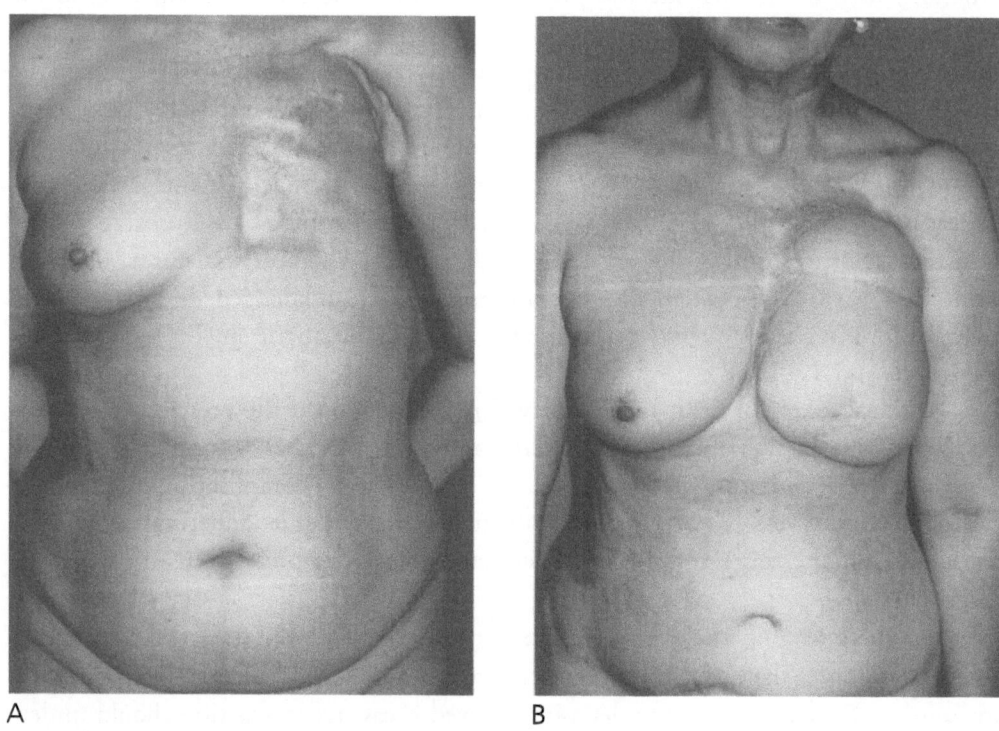

A   B

Fig. 17-2 (A) Patient after a left radical mastectomy and radiation therapy, showing an extensive defect and a large area of radiation-damaged skin. (B) After reconstruction with both a pedicled TRAM flap and a latissimus dorsi myocutaneous flap, the defect is still only partially corrected.

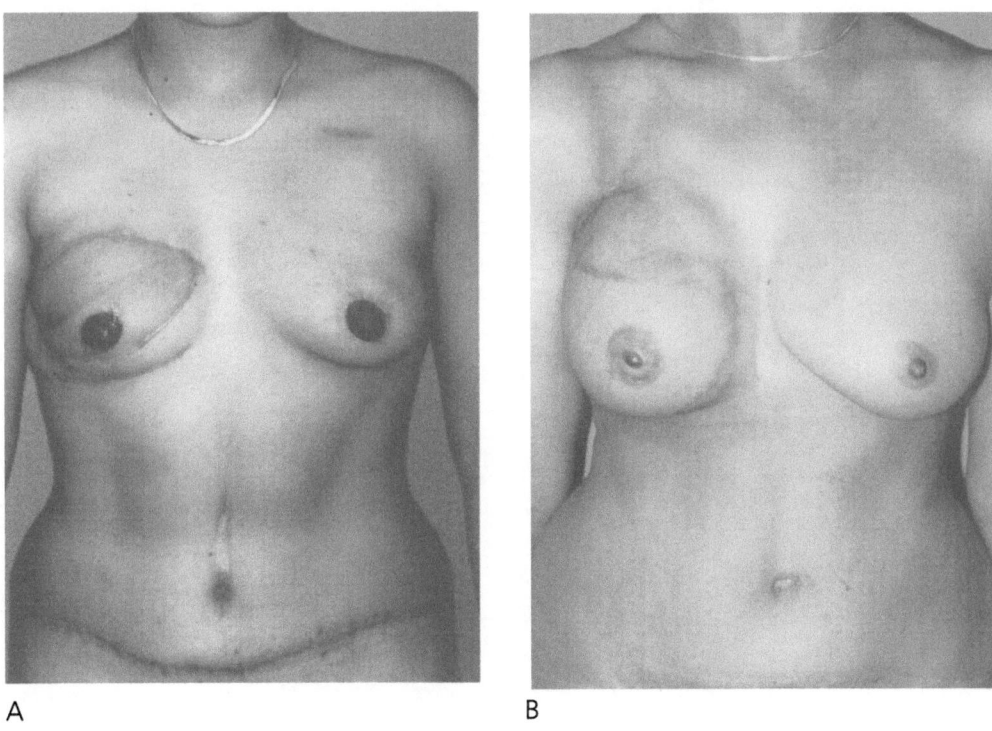

A   B

FIG. 17-3   (A) Patient who had undergone an aggressive right mastectomy and radiation therapy. (B) After delayed breast reconstruction with a pedicled TRAM flap. The result is compromised by the amount of missing tissue and the surrounding radiation-damaged skin.

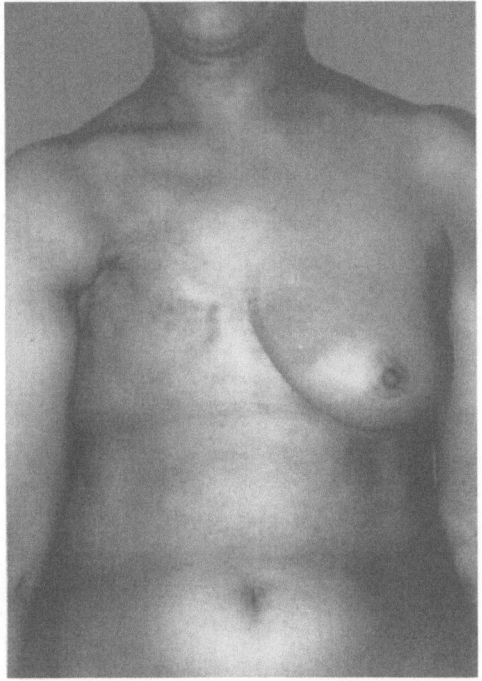

FIG. 17-4   Patient after delayed right breast reconstruction with a free TRAM flap and left concentric mastopexy. Although the form and symmetry are good, the color match is not good and the scar is high.

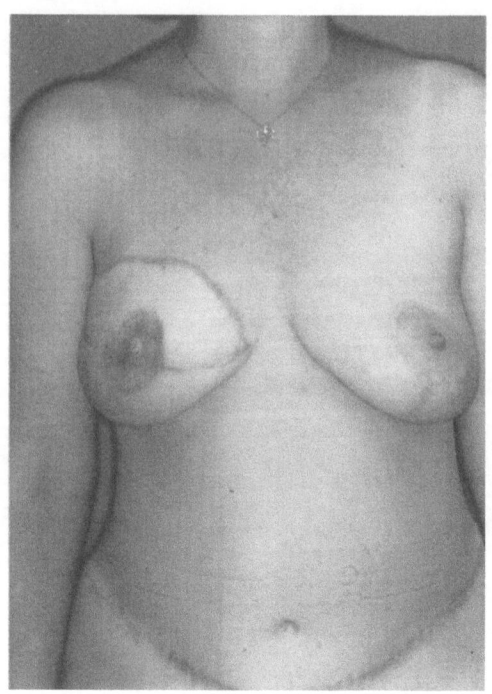

FIG. 17-5 Patient after delayed right breast reconstruction with a free TRAM flap and left mastopexy. Although the form and symmetry are good, the color match is only fair and the scar would be visible in a dress with a low neckline.

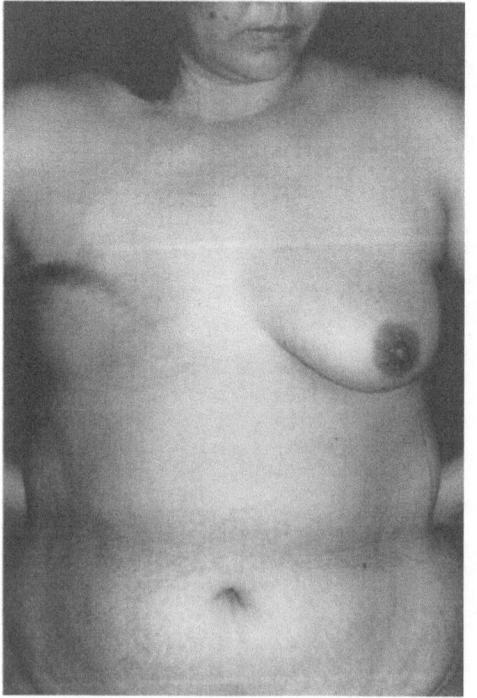 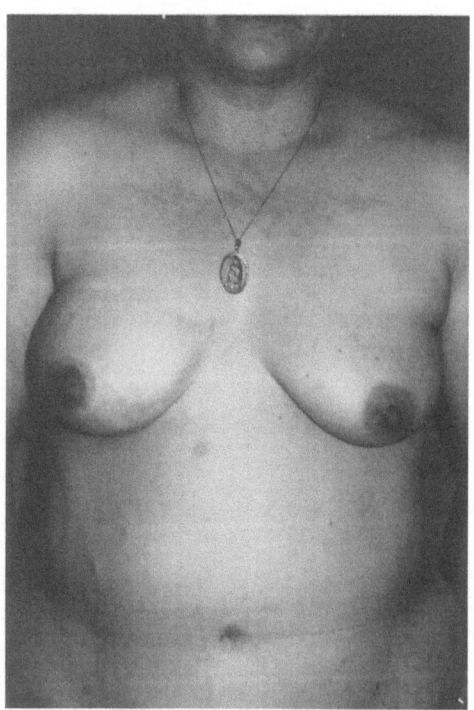

FIG. 17-6 (A) Patient after modified radical mastectomy. See color insert, p. I-15. (B) After delayed breast reconstruction with a pedicled TRAM flap. See color insert, p. I-15.

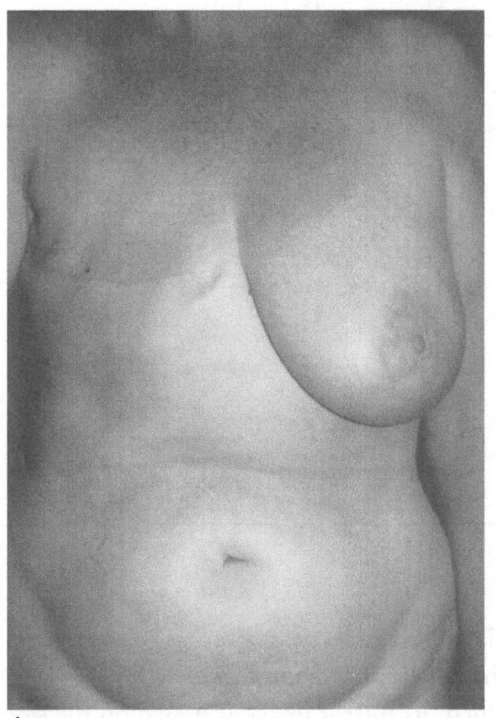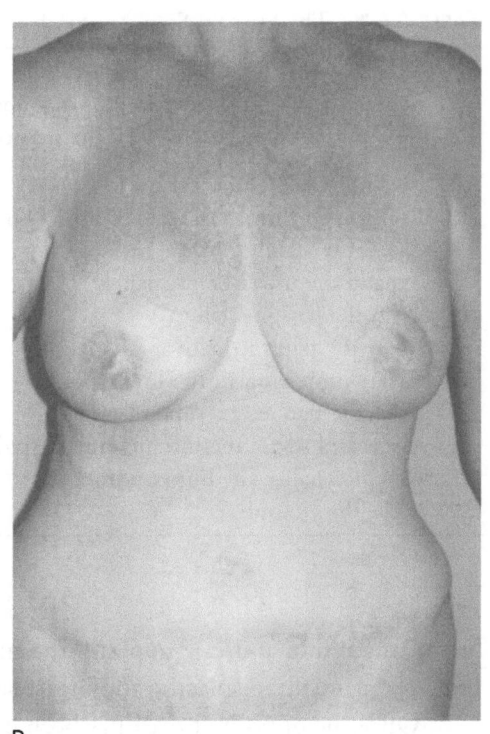

A   B

FIG. 17-7   (A) A 62-year-old woman after modified radical mastectomy. (B) After delayed breast reconstruction with a pedicled TRAM flap and contralateral mastopexy. (From Kroll SS, Miller MJ, Schusterman MA, Reece GP, Singletary SE, Ames F. *Ann Surg Oncol.* 1994;1:457–461. Used with permission.)

A Step-By-Step Approach to Breast Shaping

As in immediate reconstruction, a step-by-step planned approach to breast shaping can help to achieve a successful result. The steps required for breast shaping in delayed reconstruction are shown in Table 17-1. If this sequence of steps is followed in a methodical way, breast shaping can proceed fairly rapidly. By having a plan, even though modifications of it may be required, the surgeon will increase the likelihood of obtaining successful results.

Designing and Creating a Breast Pocket

The first step in shaping the reconstructed breast is designing a pocket into which the autologous tissue flap will be inserted. In planning this pocket, it is helpful to mark the patient's midline and the outline of the opposite, natural breast. The midline can be identified by using the sternal notch and the xiphoid as landmarks. The outline of the

TABLE 17-1   The Step-by-Step Approach to Breast Shaping in Delayed Reconstruction

BEFORE TRANSFER OF THE FLAP:
 (1) Design the breast pocket as a mirror image of the opposite breast
 (2) Re-create the defect: reelevate the mastectomy flaps and dissect a breast pocket

AFTER TRANSFER OF THE FLAP:
 (3) Evaluate and revise the lateral breast border
 (4) Assess the viability of the mastectomy flaps
 (5) Expand the lower breast panel
 (6) Trim the flap medially
 (7) Insert the flap medially and superiorly
 (8) Create projection in the lower pole
 (9) Trim the flap excess superolaterally
 (10) Assess and revise the inframammary fold
 (11) De-epithelialize the buried skin
 (12) Close the wound

breast (the inframammary fold and the medial and lateral breast borders) can be identified by manually displacing the breast so that its limits are emphasized (Fig 17-8).

Once the opposite breast has been outlined, its mirror image is drawn on the side of the reconstruction (Fig 17-9). This mirror image serves as an outline for the pocket

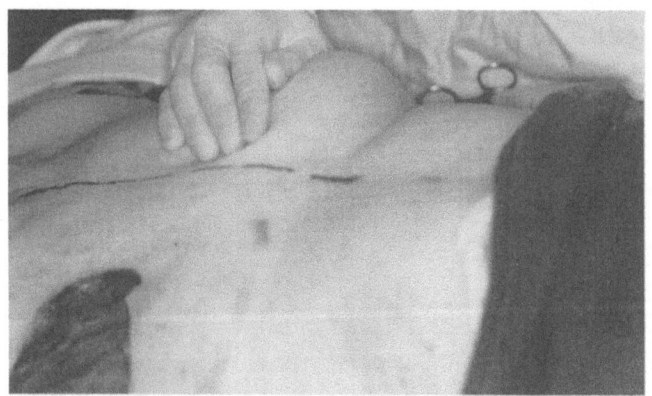

A

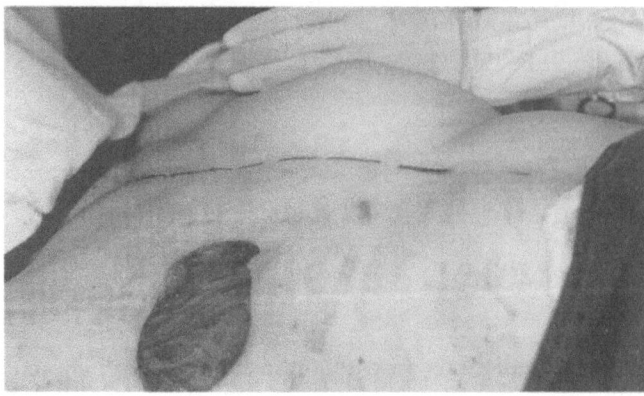

B

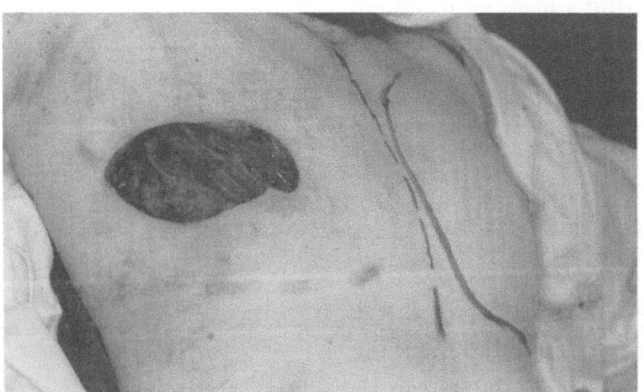

C

FIG. 17-8   Manually displacing the breast inferiorly (A) and medially (B) emphasizes the breast borders so that they are more easily seen. (C) The borders are then outlined with a marking pen to define the position of the breast.

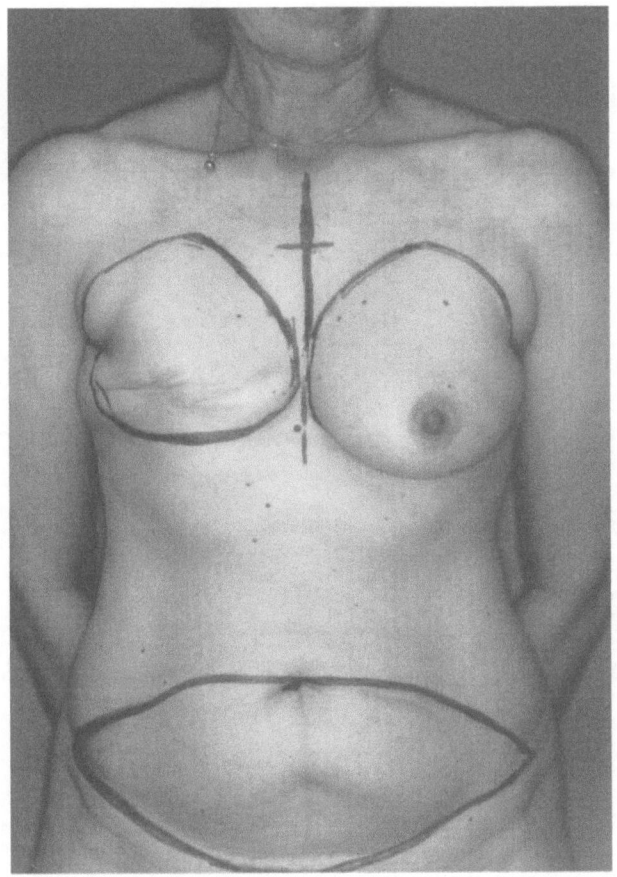

FIG. 17-9 The mirror image of the outlined normal breast is copied onto the side lacking a breast.

that must be created to receive the reconstructed breast. The inframammary fold, however, should initially be dissected to a level approximately 1 cm higher than that of the mirror image, to compensate for any inferior displacement that might occur when the TRAM flap donor site is closed under tension. After the donor site has been closed, the dissection of the pocket can be completed and the inframammary fold lowered to achieve symmetry.

Re-Creating the Defect

Reelevating the Mastectomy Flaps

As in most reconstructions using plastic surgery, the next step is to re-create the defect. For this, the surgeon must reelevate the old mastectomy flaps. There are two possible approaches to the reelevation of the mastectomy flaps. The simplest (and often best) option is to reopen the original mastectomy incision in order to re-create and fill the original defect. In this case, the lower breast panel (analogous to the lower half of a

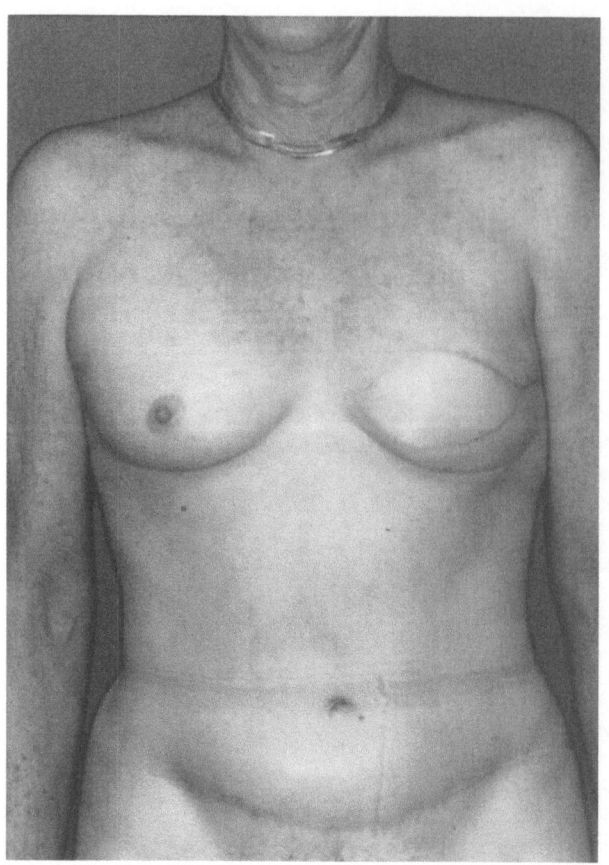

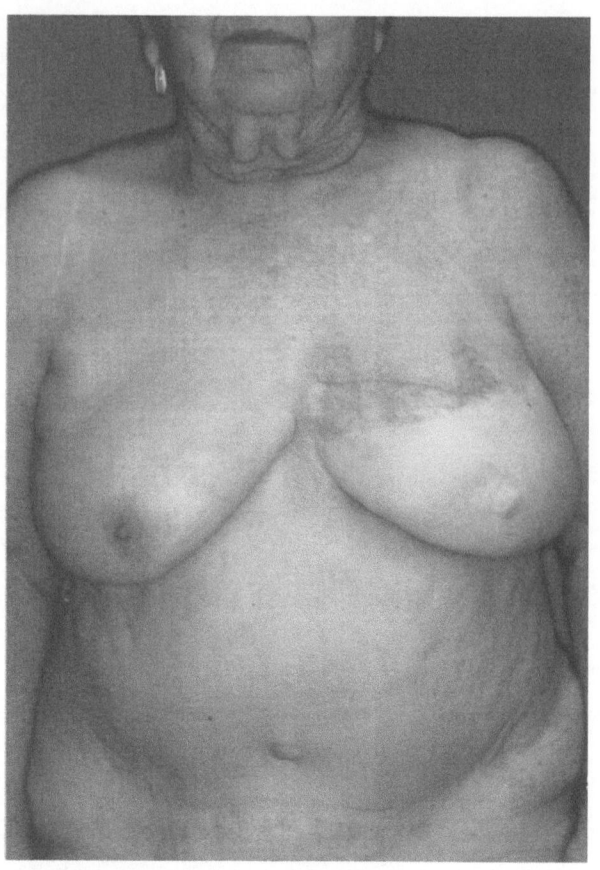

FIG. 17-10 Delayed breast reconstruction using native breast skin to form the lower panel of the breast. This hides the lower edge of the TRAM flap, but leaves a visible scar across the lower pole of the breast.

FIG. 17-11 Delayed breast reconstruction using the TRAM flap itself to form the lower panel of the breast. This hides the lower scar in the inframammary fold, but exposes any irregularities of the lower border of the TRAM flap. Note the surrounding skin changes caused by irradiation. See color insert, p. I-17.

brassiere) will be formed by native breast skin from the old mastectomy flap (Fig 17-10). The second option is to ignore the mastectomy scar and make an entirely new incision along the planned inframammary fold. In this case, the lower breast panel will be formed by skin from the TRAM flap (Fig 17-11).

Each approach has advantages and disadvantages. Reopening the original mastectomy incision minimizes scarring and maximizes blood supply to the mastectomy flaps. It makes delayed reconstruction more like immediate reconstruction and allows the surgeon to hide bunching or folding of the flap (to improve lower pole projection) under the native mastectomy flap skin. On the other hand, it relies on this native breast skin to form part of the new breast skin envelope—native skin that may have been irradiated or be tethered by scar tissue and reluctant to expand. This approach also places the lower edge of the TRAM flap skin paddle in the middle of the breast, where it is more conspicuous than it would be if it were camouflaged in the inframammary fold.

Making a new incision in the inframammary fold allows the surgeon to create the lower breast panel with unscarred TRAM flap skin and places the lower edge of the skin paddle at an aesthetic unit border—the bottom of the breast—where it is relatively inconspicuous. The disadvantages of this approach are that the native breast skin between the old mastectomy scar and the incision can have a precarious blood supply and may have to be discarded, and that any defects or irregularities in the lower part of the TRAM flap will be exposed and visible.

In most cases, I prefer to reopen the original mastectomy incision. If the lower mastectomy flap skin is of poor quality, it can always be discarded, and the lower breast border created with the TRAM flap. If the lower mastectomy flap skin is viable, however, it will hide imperfections in the lower part of the TRAM flap and increase the surgeon's options for breast shaping.

Dissecting the Breast Pocket

As the old mastectomy flaps are reelevated off the muscles of the chest wall, a pocket is created to receive the TRAM flap. This dissection is continued up to the planned medial and lateral borders of the new breast. For the inframammary fold, the limit of the dissection depends on what type of TRAM flap is being performed.

If a free TRAM flap is planned, the level of the new inframammary fold is initially designed approximately 1 cm above the mirror image of the opposite inframammary fold. If a pedicled TRAM flap is planned, however, the inframammary fold is made even higher: 2.5 cm above the mirror image. This higher inframammary fold design is required with the conventional TRAM flap because of the presence of the tunnel, which detaches part of the inframammary fold and allows it to be pulled more inferiorly when the donor site is closed under tension. After either type of flap, the final inframammary fold level is best determined after the abdominal donor site has been closed, with the patient in the sitting position. At that time, the inframammary fold can be lowered until it matches the level of the opposite fold.

If the surgeon chooses to place the lower border of the TRAM flap at the inframammary fold, the incision should be made along the planned fold itself (1 cm above the mirror image of the opposite inframammary fold if a free TRAM flap is planned; 2.5 cm above it if a conventional TRAM flap will be used; Fig 17-12). After the flap has been transferred and the abdominal donor site closed, the inframammary fold can be lowered as necessary by additional dissection or by de-epithelializing or excising additional skin.

Transferring the Flap

After the breast pocket has been created, the flap is transferred, and its viability is assessed. If a free TRAM flap has been performed, the sheath of the rectus abdominis muscle is sutured to the pectoral muscles on the chest wall (Fig 17-13) to stabilize the flap and protect the pedicle from tension. I generally use 2-0 Vicryl (polygalactin 910) sutured deeply into the pectoralis major muscle. It must be remembered, however, that

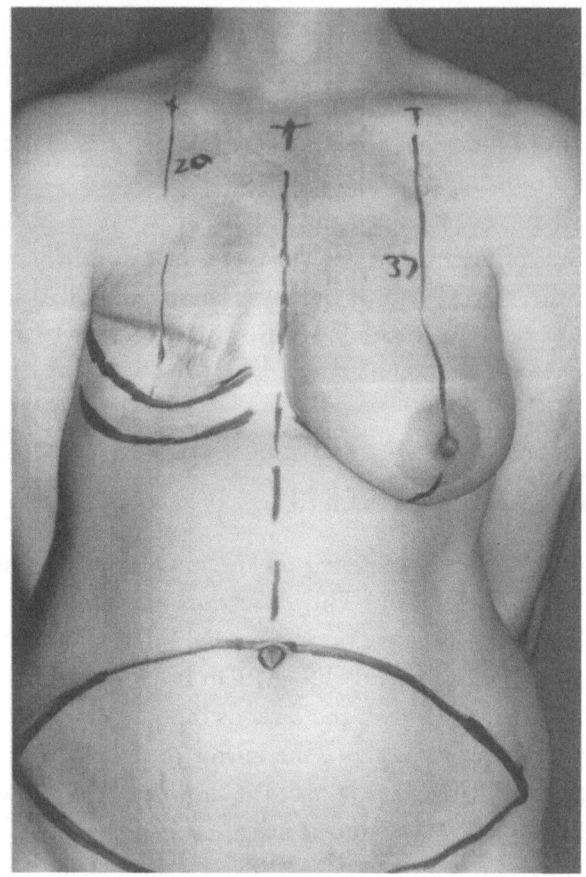

FIG. 17-12   Design of a conventional TRAM flap in a delayed breast reconstruction. The new inframammary fold (upper mark) is initially designed higher than the mirror image of the fold on the opposite side.

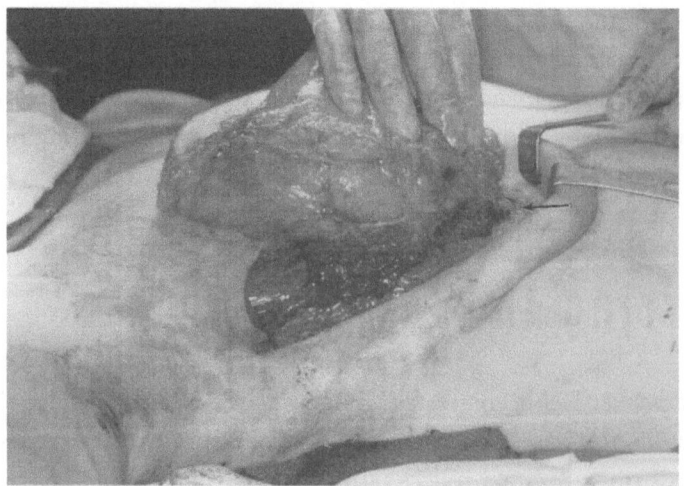

FIG. 17-13   The rectus abdominis fascia of the TRAM flap is sutured to the muscles of the chest wall with 2-0 Vicryl suture.

the muscle does not hold sutures well and these sutures give only partial stability to the flap, especially if it is a heavy one.

If the operating table has been tilted to improve access to the site of an anastomosis, the table is straightened to allow better assessment of breast symmetry. Care should be taken at this point to be sure that the flap has been adequately stabilized and will not fall laterally off the chest wall. Once these steps have been accomplished and the flap is stabilized, the surgeon can proceed with breast shaping.

Forming the Lateral Breast Border

The lateral breast border is normally located just anterior to the mid-axillary line, mimicking the lateral border of the opposite breast. It should join with the lateral portion of the inframammary fold in a gentle curve. If the TRAM flap is pedicled, or is a free flap using the internal mammary vessels as recipients, the lateral breast border will have been established simply by lateral dissection of the breast pocket. If the thoracodorsal vessels are used for recipients, however, the superior part of the lateral breast border will have been transgressed to obtain access to those vessels. In that case, the tissues that form the lateral breast border must be reapproximated with 2-0 Vicryl sutures just as is done in immediate reconstruction (see chapter 16). This is easier if only the superior half of the axilla has been opened to gain access to the thoracodorsal vessels. If that has been the case (Fig 17-14), only one or two sutures will be required to put the tissues back where they belong. If the axilla has been opened widely, more sutures are necessary and the border will be less smooth. The most common error is to make the lateral breast border too posterior, situating the breast too far laterally. Therefore, if the surgeon is unsure of where to place the sutures it is usually better to err on the side of placing them too medial.

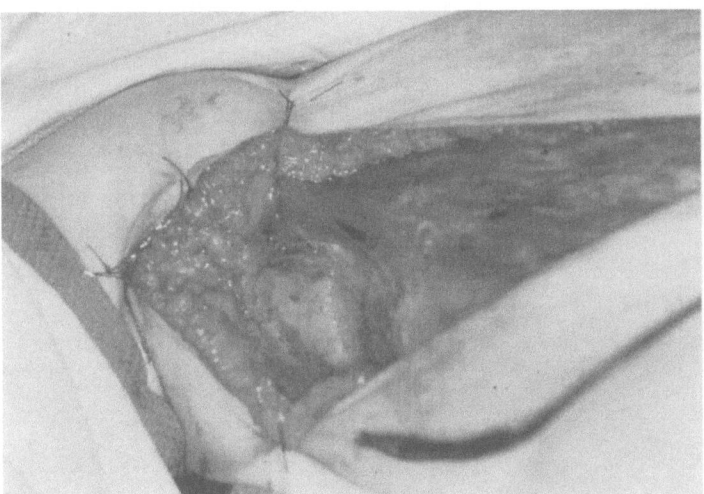

FIG. 17-14 When possible, only the superior half of the axilla is opened for access to the thoracodorsal vessels so that restoration of the lateral breast border requires only one or two sutures.

Assessing the Viability of the Mastectomy Flaps

Once the lateral breast border has been defined, the mastectomy flaps are evaluated for viability. The best way to do this is to press the round handle of a hemostat against the skin and then remove it quickly to assess the capillary refill. If the capillary refill time is 3 seconds or less, the skin is usually viable. If capillary refill takes more than 3 seconds, the skin should be considered ischemic and be discarded. In heavy smokers, mastectomy skin viability is often reduced, and debridement should therefore be more aggressive. Assuming that the lower mastectomy flap is viable, it is then expanded to the position it occupied prior to the mastectomy. In many cases, this skin reexpansion will require extensive release of constricting scar tissue.

If the breast has undergone previous irradiation, all of the chest wall skin will have been damaged. The extent of damage depends on the total radiation dose, its fractionation, and the patient's host response. Each patient will be different and must be managed individually. Chronic radiation injury tends to get worse with time, not better.[4] Any obviously damaged skin (Fig 17-15) is therefore best excised and replaced with nonirradiated skin from the TRAM flap.

In general, irradiated skin that appears grossly undamaged will behave much like normal skin. Some patients who have had previous irradiation can therefore obtain excellent results using normal-appearing irradiated skin as part of the reconstruction (Fig 17-16). Mastectomy flap skin that appears moderately damaged, however, may do very poorly when reelevated, developing ischemia that leads to outright skin loss or to extensive additional scarring. Obviously damaged skin should therefore be replaced, when possible. If there is more obviously damaged skin than the TRAM flap can replace, the outcome will inevitably be compromised and the aesthetic result will be poor.

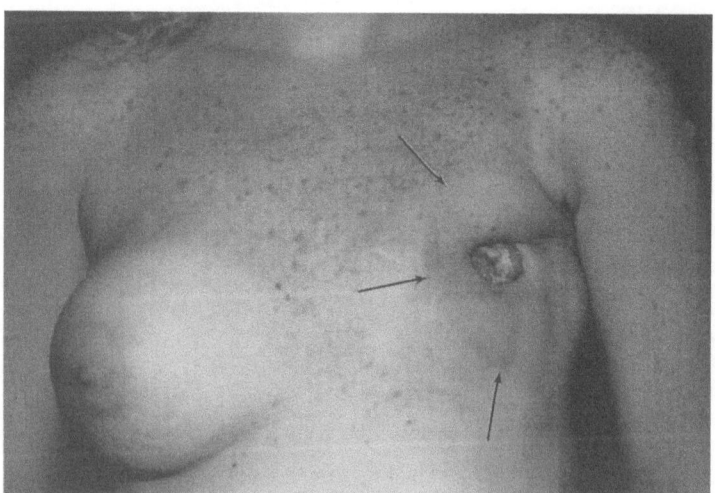

FIG. 17-15 Radiation-damaged skin on the chest wall, which will have to be discarded before beginning the process of breast shaping.

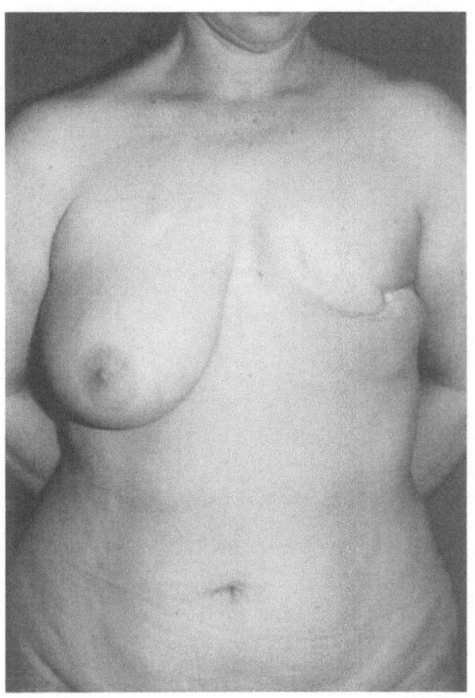
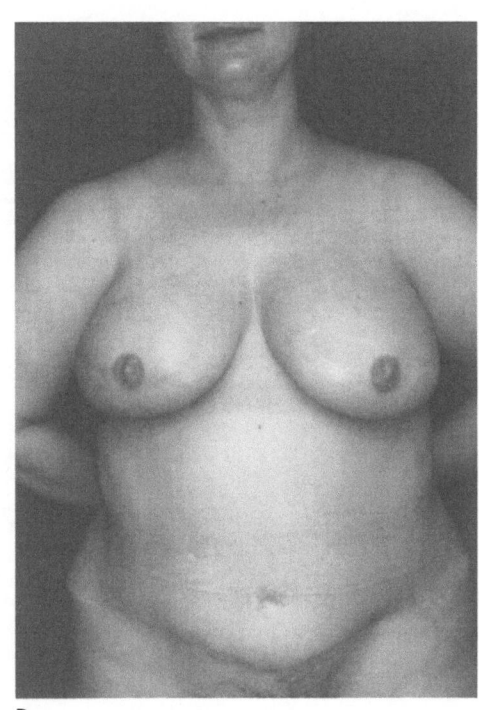

A   B

FIG. 17-16   (A) Patient with a cancer of the right breast and a history of irradiation and mastectomy on the left. (B) After bilateral free TRAM flap breast reconstruction. Despite the irradiation, the reconstruction is only minimally compromised because the radiation injury was not
severe. See color insert, p. I-18.

Expanding the Lower Breast Panel

Releasing Scar Tissue

An important obstacle to achieving good results in delayed breast reconstruction is
the presence of constricting scar tissue. This usually takes the form of a sheet of ci-
catrix deep to the skin at the level of the old mastectomy flap dissection; the scar tissue tethers the skin and prevents it from expanding to its original dimensions. Consequently, it can be difficult to achieve adequate fullness, especially in the lower pole
of the breast, with the original breast skin alone. The scar tissue can also create puckering and other visible deformities if not fully released with scalpel or electrocautery
dissection.

Unfortunately, full release of all subcutaneous scar tissue under the mastectomy
flaps can cause bleeding and decreased mastectomy flap perfusion. This is especially
problematic when the mastectomy flaps were thin and the scar tissue is close to the subdermal plexus. For this reason, scar release may have to be incomplete even when it is
obviously necessary for expansion of the native breast skin and the lower panel of the
breast skin is too tight. One solution to this common problem is to make a vertical releasing incision in the lower breast panel.

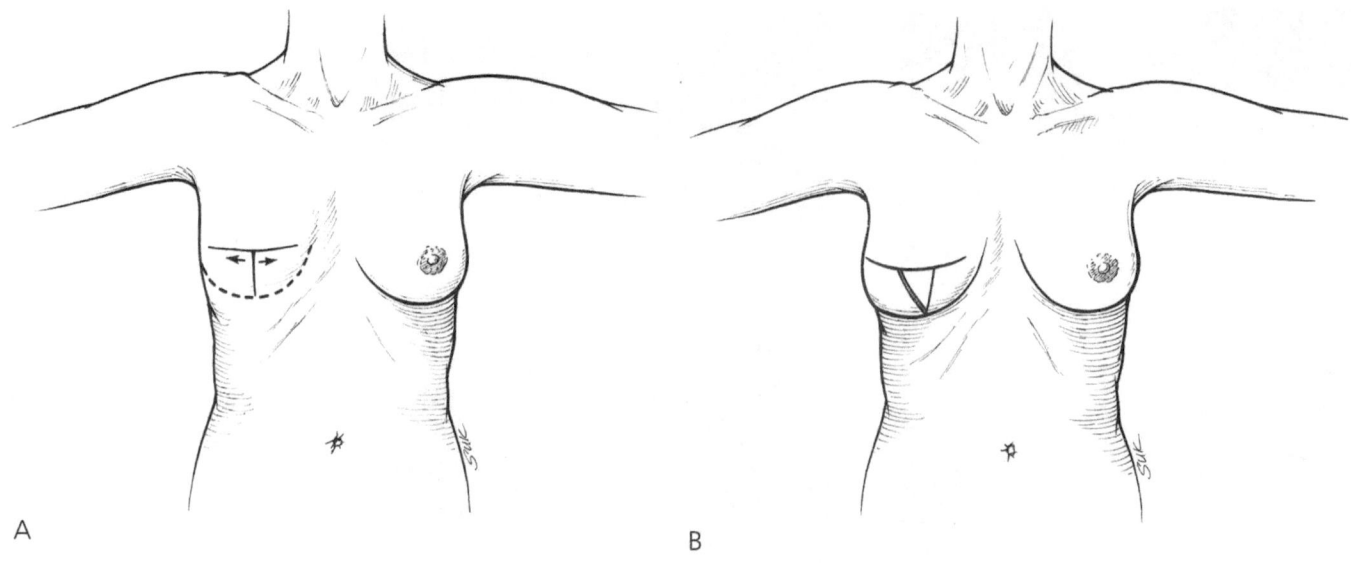

A   B

FIG. 17-17   Vertical incision of the lower mastectomy flap.

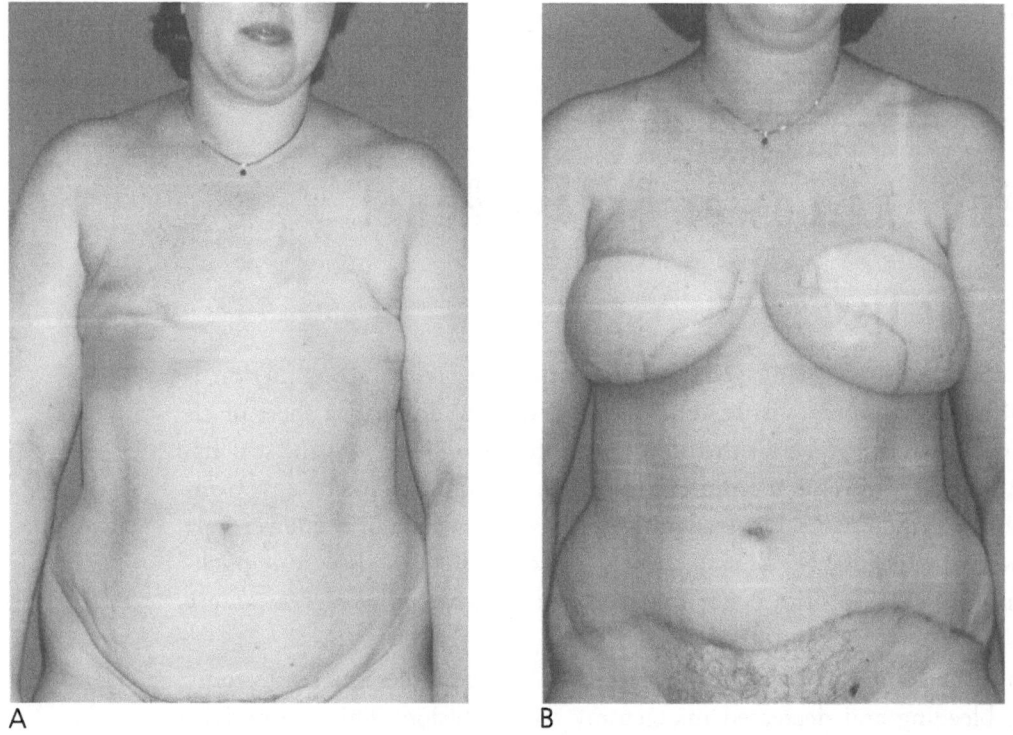

A   B

FIG. 17-18   (A) Patient after bilateral mastectomies, with tight chest wall skin. She also has had radiotherapy on the right side. (B) Result of bilateral breast reconstruction with free TRAM flaps. Vertical incisions were used to expand the lower breast skin panels.

Vertical Releasing Incision in the Lower Breast Panel

If the lower breast panel (formed by the skin of a reelevated mastectomy flap) is too tight, the mastectomy flap skin should be incised vertically down to the inframammary fold (Fig 17-17), to allow the skin to expand and create a V-shaped defect. This V-shaped defect is then filled with skin from the TRAM (or alternative) flap. The surgeon must make the vertical incision where he or she knows that there will be viable TRAM flap skin underneath it. The vertical incision should therefore not be made until the flap has been transferred to the chest and the position of any skin deficiencies (such as a defect in the TRAM flap caused by removal of the umbilicus) is known. If this is done correctly, the results can be quite gratifying (Fig 17-18).

Trimming the Flap Medially

As in immediate reconstruction, the TRAM flap should initially be incised 1 cm medial to where the surgeon judges the medial border of the flap should be (Fig 17-19). Should an error in judgment be made, it is easier to trim off excess than to add tissue to the flap. If the blood supply is judged inadequate, the medial border of the flap is trimmed back until bright red bleeding is observed. Usually, some TRAM flap skin will be exposed nearly all the way to the medial border of the flap. The flap can therefore be fixed temporarily with staples to the medial corner of the mastectomy skin defect (Fig 17-20).

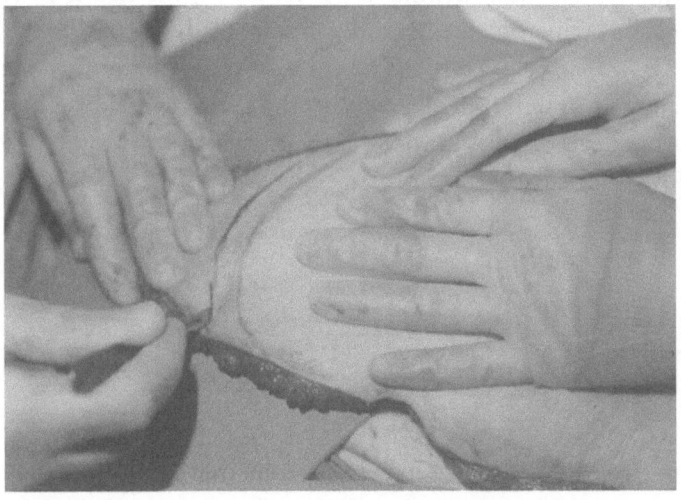

FIG. 17-19 The surgeon makes an initial incision 1 cm medial to the markings made where he or she believes the medial edge of the breast should be on the TRAM flap, to allow for possible error. Additional trimming will be made as necessary.

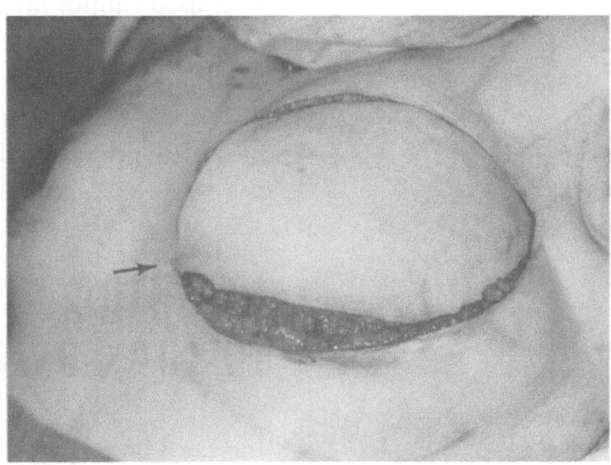

FIG. 17-20 The TRAM flap inset is begun by stapling its skin paddle to the medial corner of the mastectomy skin defect (arrow points to staple).

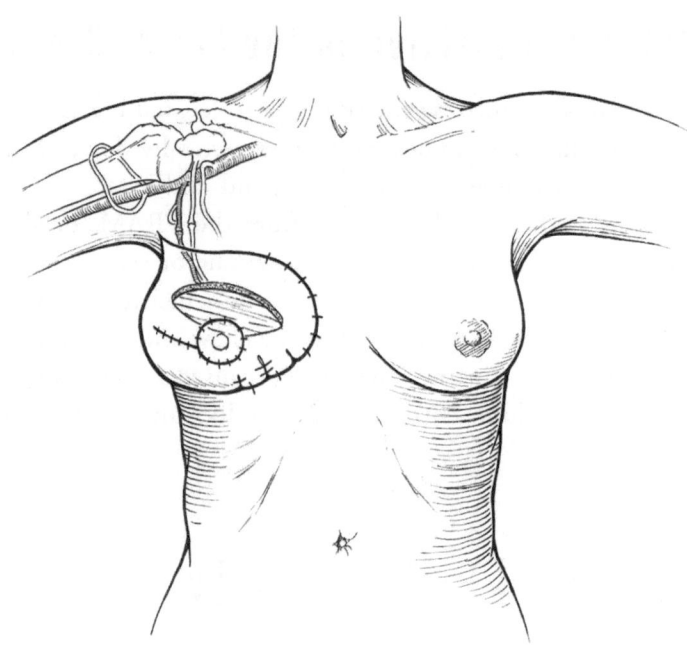

FIG. 17-21   The flap is sutured to the edges of the reconstituted mastectomy defect medially, superomedially, and inferomedially.

Insetting the Flap Medially and Superiorly

Once the medial border of the flap has been definitively determined, the flap is inset with deep sutures placed medially, superomedially, and inferomedially just as in immediate reconstruction (Fig 17-21; see chapter 16). The surgeon must ensure that the flap is not fixed too high to allow it to settle adequately into the lower pole. If the medial part of the breast pocket has been dissected properly, the medial aspect of the two breasts (the cleavage) should by symmetric.

Creating Breast Projection in the Lower Pole

Increased breast projection in the inferior pole can be achieved by folding the flap (Fig 17-22), bunching it inferiorly (Fig 17-23), or increasing the amount of muscle harvested. The most common approach is some combination of folding and bunching the flap. If the lower pole of the TRAM flap is covered by a mastectomy flap, this folding and/or bunching is hidden and can be done with impunity. If the lower breast panel is created only by the TRAM flap, a certain amount of bunching is still permissible, but the increased skin length of the TRAM flap has to be worked into the shorter chest

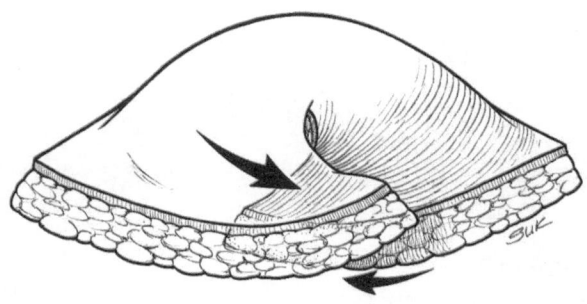

FIG. 17-22   The TRAM flap can be folded inferiorly to increase projection in the lower breast pole. The folding is covered by the inferior mastectomy flap.

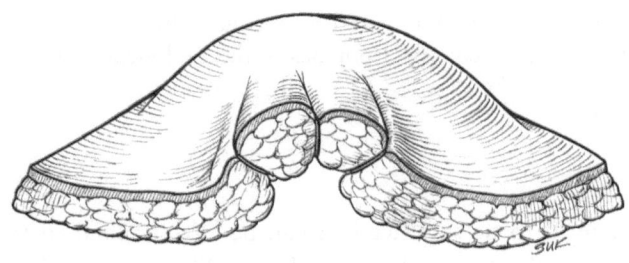

FIG. 17-23   Another way of increasing lower pole fullness is to bunch up the TRAM flap with sutures. This is also hidden by the overlying mastectomy flap.

wall incision with sutures, a little at a time. Obviously, more projection is possible when the TRAM flap is covered inferiorly by an overlying mastectomy flap.

Another method of increasing breast projection is harvesting extra rectus abdominis muscle. This is rarely indicated in any but very thin patients, but can be a reason to select a free TRAM flap over a deep inferior epigastric perforator flap in a patient who has minimal subcutaneous abdominal tissue, provided that the patient agrees that the increased breast volume is worth the loss of muscle function. Although it is widely believed that the transferred muscle atrophies, there is some evidence that this is not true.[5] In any case, the muscle clearly contributes to some degree to breast volume and can be used to increase projection if necessary.

Using the TRAM Flap Itself to Make the Lower Breast Panel

As noted above, using the TRAM flap to provide both volume and skin cover for the lower pole of the breast has the advantage of camouflaging the lower scar in the inframammary fold (Fig 17-7). If the inferior mastectomy flap will not be used for skin

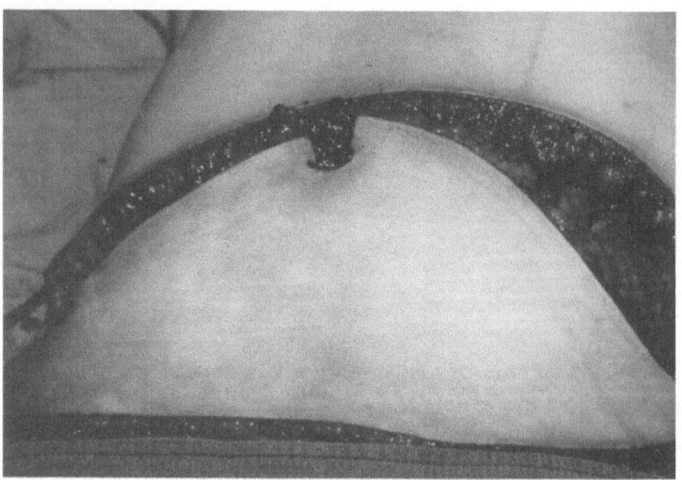

FIG. 17-24 TRAM flap showing the typical defect caused by leaving the umbilicus in situ. If the flap were to be harvested entirely from below the umbilicus, this defect would not be present.

cover, it does not need to be sacrificed; it can be left attached to the chest wall and de-epithelialized, contributing to breast volume. The one problem with using the TRAM flap to make the lower breast panel is that if the TRAM flap has a defect caused by dissection around the umbilicus (as is usually the case; Fig 17-24) and if this defect is positioned inferiorly (as it often is in a free TRAM flap), the defect will cause irregularity and scarring along the lower border of the reconstructed breast (Fig 17-25). Although the defect can be converted into a triangle and closed as a straight line, that approach increases visible scarring and creates scars that may interfere with nipple reconstruction. It also creates a small dog-ear in the upper pole of the breast. In most cases, I prefer to hide the umbilical defect beneath overlying mastectomy flaps, if this is possible.

Trimming the Flap Excess Superolaterally

In most cases, the reconstructed breast mound is too large initially. The surgeon can assess this by cupping both breasts simultaneously with his or her hands, like a push-up brassiere, and comparing the volume and upper pole fullness of the two breasts. In most cases, any excess tissue on the reconstructed side will be primarily lateral and in the upper outer quadrant. The flap should therefore be trimmed laterally and superolaterally until the volume of the two breasts is symmetric. If a free TRAM flap has been performed, the blood supply is usually very robust in this quadrant, so careful hemostasis must be obtained once the trimming has been completed.

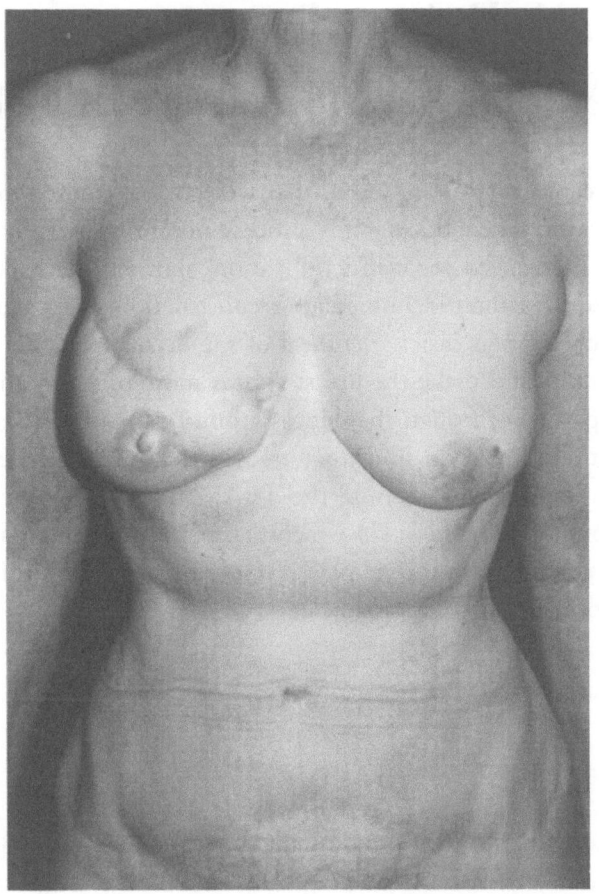

Fig. 17-25   In this patient, the defect in the TRAM flap caused by removal of the umbilicus caused a noticeable deformity just above the inframammary fold.

Assessing and Revising the Inframammary Fold

At this point, it is necessary to sit the patient up (as described in chapter 16) and evaluate the symmetry of the two breasts. The volume is compared, and additional trimming is performed as necessary. The inframammary folds are compared, and the fold on the reconstructed side is revised if necessary. If the reconstructed inframammary fold is too low, it must be elevated with the use of sutures (see chapter 16). The inframammary fold will look less natural than it would had it been created only with dissection, but any puckering of the skin that occurs will usually disappear with time. Taping of the skin below the inframammary fold[6] and use of an underwire brassiere will help to hold the breast mound in position while healing occurs. If the inframammary fold is too high, additional dissection is performed with electrocautery to lower the fold to a more symmetric position.

De-Epithelializing the Buried Skin and Closing the Wound

As in immediate reconstruction, any skin that will not be exposed must be de-epithelialized. Care must be taken during this process not to apply excessive traction on the flap's pedicle. In delayed reconstruction, more skin will be exposed and less de-epithelialization required than in immediate reconstruction. Consequently, postoperative flap monitoring is often easier. Removal of the dermis near the edges of the flap will soften the contour and make the breast appear more rounded and more natural.

An incision partially through the dermis around the exposed skin paddle, as was recommended in the chapter on immediate reconstruction, facilitates suturing of the wound and makes it possible to elevate the TRAM flap skin to the level of the surrounding mastectomy flaps. In cases in which flap perfusion is marginal, however, this step is omitted. A suction drain is then placed under the flap prior to final closure, with care taken not to obstruct the flap's pedicle.

Summary

Delayed breast reconstruction is more difficult than immediate reconstruction and requires more tissue, effort, and artistic judgment to achieve aesthetically good results. Because the inframammary fold and skin envelope have not been preserved, they must be reconstructed. The inferior breast panel can be created using the TRAM flap itself or the original mastectomy flap of native breast skin. Each approach has advantages and disadvantages. The choice of approach depends on the defect, the type of flap being used, and the surgeon's judgment. If the inferior mastectomy flap is used to cover the lower pole of the breast, release of all scar tissue is essential to allow the remaining breast skin to reexpand to its original dimensions. If this is not possible, a releasing incision in the inferior mastectomy flap will often allow adequate expansion of the inferior pole.

Having a logical, step-by-step plan makes shaping the breast easier and faster, and leads to more consistent results. Nevertheless, each patient is unique, so the surgeon must be ready to modify the plan when necessary to attain the best possible results.

References

1.　Carlson GW, Bostwick J, Styblo TM, et al. Skin-sparing mastectomy: oncologic and reconstructive considerations. *Ann Surg.* 1997;225:570–578.

2.　Carlson GW. Skin sparing mastectomy: anatomic and technical considerations. *Amer Surg.* 1996;62:151–155.

3.　Kroll SS, Coffey JA Jr, Winn RJ, Schusterman MA. A comparison of factors affecting aesthetic outcomes of TRAM flap breast reconstruction. *Plast Reconstr Surg.* 1995;96:860–864.

4. Larson DL, Lindberg R, Lane E. Major complications of radiotherapy in cancer of the oral cavity and oropharynx: a 10-year study. *Am J Surg.* 1983;146:531–536.

5. Salmi A, Tukianinen E, Harma M, Asko-Seljavaara S. A prospective study of changes in muscle dimensions following free-muscle transfer measured by ultrasound and CT scanning. *Plast Reconstr Surg.* 1996;97:1443–1450.

6. Maxwell GP, Andochick SE. Secondary shaping of the TRAM flap. *Clin Plast Surg.* 1994;21:247–253.

18 Shaping the Breast Mounds in Bilateral TRAM Flap Breast Reconstruction

Unique Features of Bilateral Breast Shaping

In many ways, shaping of the breast is easier in bilateral transverse rectus abdominis myocutaneous (TRAM) flap reconstruction than it is when the reconstruction is unilateral. For one thing, there is no contralateral breast to imitate. Consequently, the size and shape of the breast can vary considerably so long as the two sides match. Second, the amount of tissue is limited. The surgeon therefore cannot make each breast any larger than the size of one hemi-TRAM flap. This does not necessarily make it easier to achieve a desirable result, but it does make it easier to achieve symmetry, limits the choices, and eliminates some uncertainty about what to do.

In the case of bilateral delayed reconstruction, the surgeon must choose the level of the inframammary folds. This introduces an extra decision with some potential for error but is not overly difficult. The inframammary folds do not have to be at the same level as they were prior to the mastectomy, but they should be within reasonably normal limits and must be symmetric. Even if the inframammary folds are made too high, as long as they are symmetrical the result will usually be acceptable (Fig 18-1).

Transferring Free TRAM Flaps to the Contralateral Side

Breast shaping is somewhat facilitated, when free TRAM flaps are used,[1] by transferring each flap to the contralateral side. When a TRAM flap is divided into two hemi-TRAM flaps the result is two triangular flaps, each having on short and two long sides (Fig 18-2). The two longer sides of each flap form a "tail" that extends laterally. Especially if the thoracodorsal vessels are being used as recipients, I prefer to transfer each

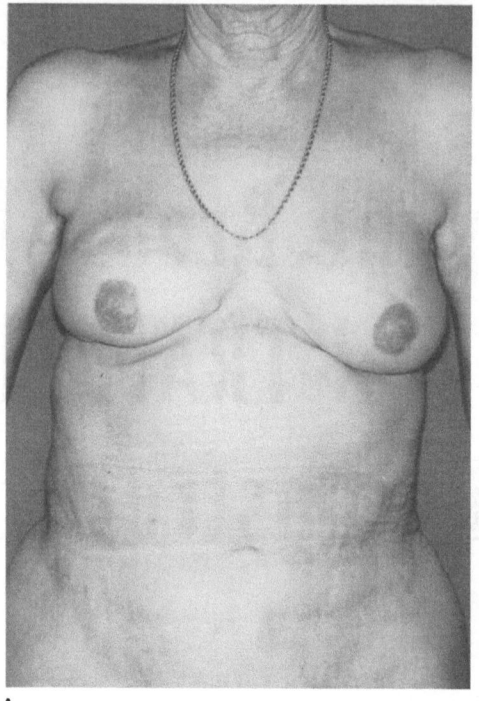
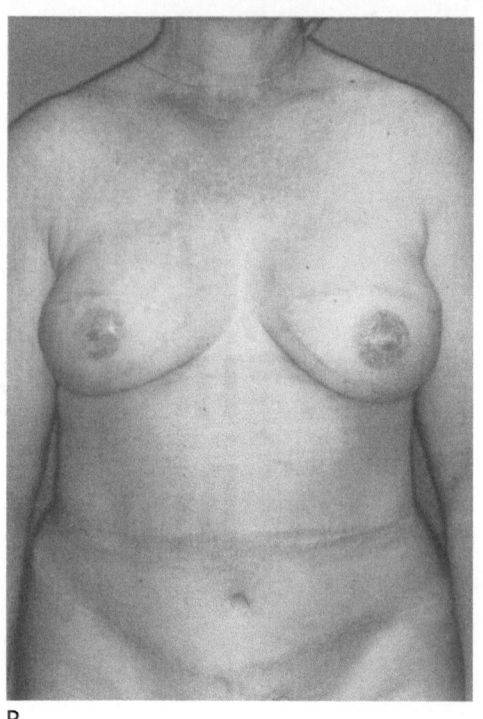

A   B

FIG. 18-1   (A) Result of bilateral delayed breast reconstruction with pedicled TRAM flaps. The inframammary folds are too high, but the result is acceptable because it is reasonably symmetric. (B) Result of bilateral delayed reconstruction with free TRAM flaps. In this case the result is better because the inframammary folds were placed at a more appropriate level. (From Kroll SS: Bilateral TRAM flaps. In: Spear SL, ed. *Surgery of the Breast: Principles and Art.* Philadelphia: Lippincott-Raven; 1998:547–553. Used with permission.)

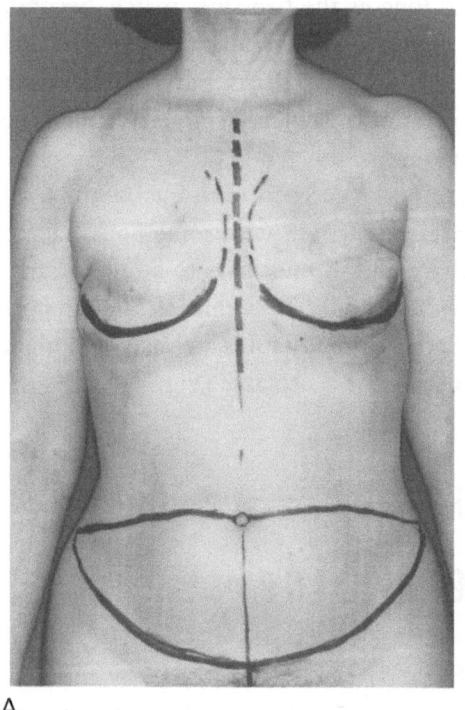
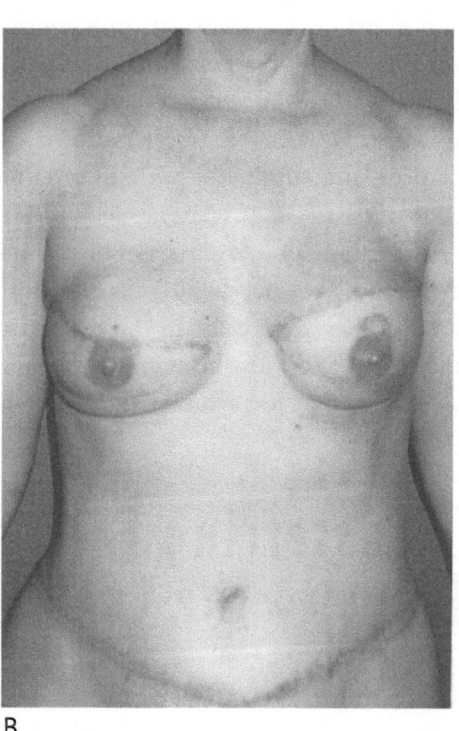

A   B

FIG. 18-2   (A) Plan for a bilateral TRAM flap. Each hemi-flap forms an isosceles triangle, with the two longer sides creating a tail. (B) Result of reconstruction.

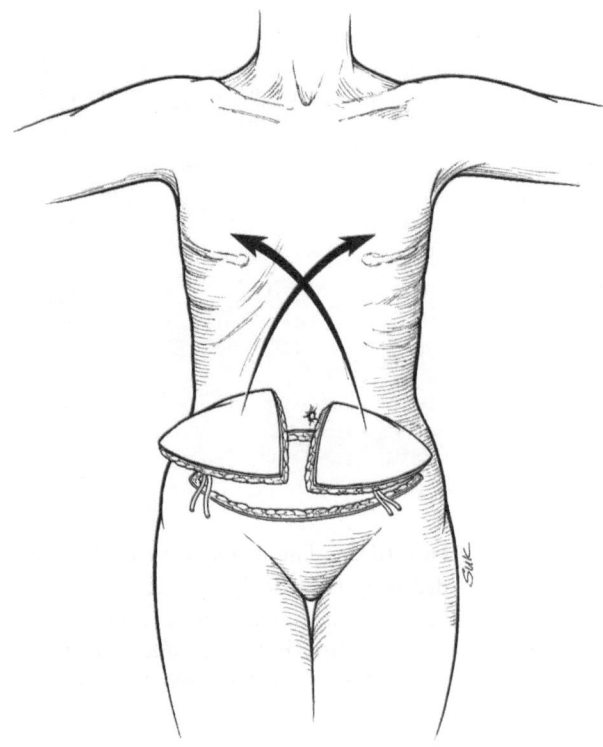

FIG. 18-3 Each hemi-TRAM flap is transferred to the contralateral side.

hemi-TRAM flap to the contralateral side so that the extended tail will be in the lower outer quadrant of the new breast (Fig 18-3). In that location it can be used to increase breast volume, if necessary. Were the flap transferred to the ipsilateral breast, the extended tail would be in the upper inner quadrant, where it could create objectionable fullness and might need to be discarded.

If the internal mammary vessels are being used as recipients[2-4] it is probably not important whether the flap is transferred ipsilaterally or contralaterally, since there is sufficient pedicle length to position the flap however the surgeon wishes, regardless of which side is used. The flap should be oriented, however, so that the tail of the flap lies in the lower outer quadrant of the new breast without the flap's pedicle having to be twisted.

Bilateral Immediate Reconstruction

Shaping of the breast in bilateral immediate reconstruction requires trimming each triangular hemi-TRAM flap into a rounded form. The three points of the triangle are cut off (Fig 18-4) so that they will not show through the overlying skin envelope. If the flap is small and maximum volume must be preserved, the skin and dermis can be trimmed without removal of the underlying fat. As long as the underlying dermis has been rounded, the breast will usually appear globular and not angular.

After the corners have been rounded, the medial edge of the flap is sutured to the deep edge of the mastectomy defect, just as in unilateral reconstruction (Fig 18-5). Su-

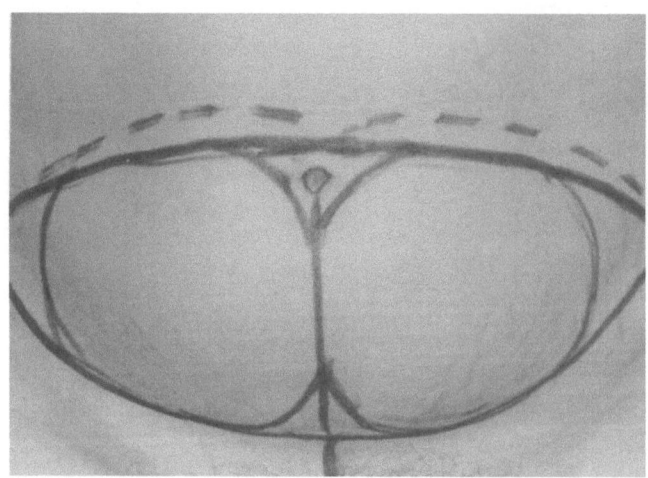

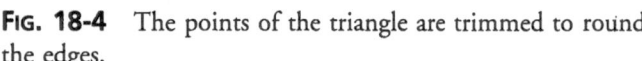

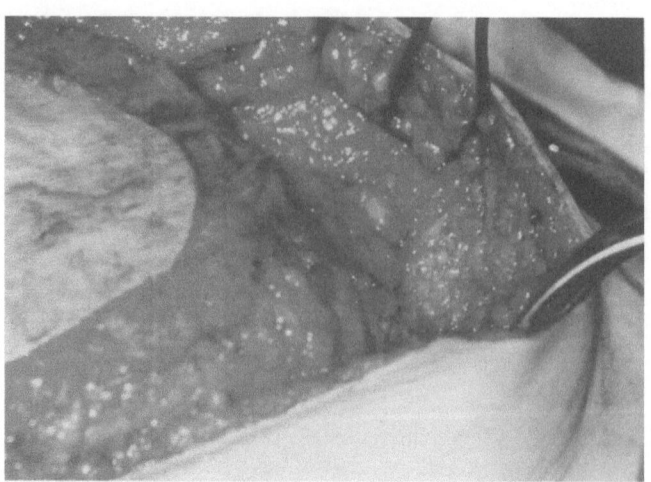

FIG. 18-4   The points of the triangle are trimmed to round the edges.

FIG. 18-5   The medial edge of the flap is sutured to the medial deep edge of the mastectomy defect to create the medial border of the breast. (From Kroll SS: TRAM flap breast reconstruction. In: Kroll SS, ed. *Reconstructive Plastic Surgery for Cancer.* St. Louis: Mosby; 1996:276–285. Used with permission.)

ture fixation should be performed medially, superomedially, and inferomedially, to ensure that the breast cannot migrate laterally. If the flap has sufficient height, it is also sutured to the superior edge of the defect (or alternatively, to the deep surface of the skin flap where it starts to become thicker) so that the flap blends into its surroundings and an infraclavicular hollow is eliminated. This superior suturing should be omitted, however, if it prevents the flap from fully reaching the inframammary fold and filling the lower pole of the breast.

Laterally, the posterior border of the breast is created with dissection or with sutures, just as in unilateral immediate reconstruction (Fig 18-6). In some cases, limiting the lateral border with sutures is relatively unimportant because the flaps may not be wide enough to extend more laterally than desired. In most cases, however, the surgeon should actively create a lateral border (between the mid-axillary and anterior axillary lines) that blends smoothly and naturally into the inframammary fold.

After each flap has been fixed to the medial edges of the defect and the lateral borders have been created, the mastectomy flaps are stapled temporarily in position. The patient is then put into a sitting position, by elevating the back of the operating room table. Reverse Trendelenburg position is then used to increase the elevation until the patient's back is as close to vertical as possible (Fig 18-7). At this point, symmetry is judged and each breast adjusted until the two sides match as closely as possible.

Symmetry is not always easy to achieve, even when both breasts have been reconstructed with the same technique. The mastectomies may have been different, or the inframammary fold may have been violated on one side, or the patient may have been asymmetric prior to the mastectomies. Despite the surgeon's best efforts, the goal of perfect asymmetry may fail to be attained (Fig 18-8). Nevertheless, the surgeon should realize that the best opportunity for achieving symmetry usually occurs during the initial procedure, the breast mound reconstruction.

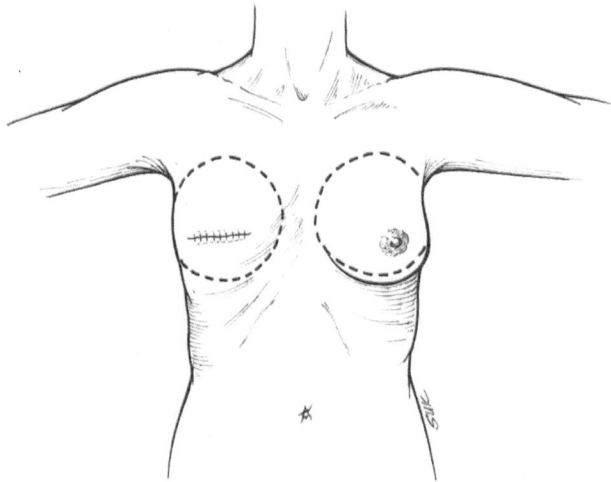

FIG. 18-6 The lateral breast border is created either by the limits of dissection of the breast pocket or with sutures.

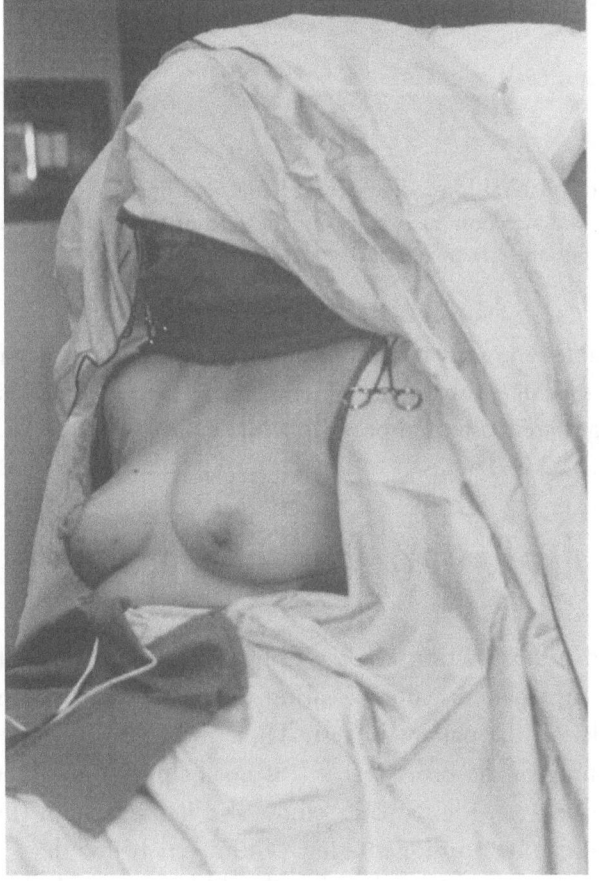

FIG. 18-7 Patient in the near-sitting position. This is accomplished by a combination of elevation of the patient's back and a reverse Trendelenburg position.

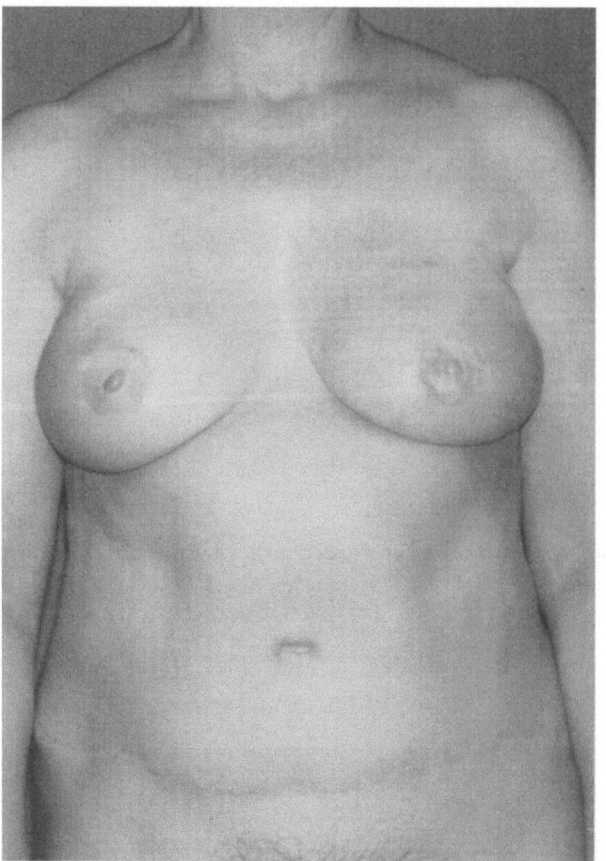

FIG. 18-8   Result of bilateral immediate free TRAM flap breast reconstruction. Even though the same technique was used on each side, and despite my best efforts, the two breasts have slightly different shapes and are not perfectly symmetric.

Once acceptable symmetry has been achieved, the exposed skin paddles are marked, and the covered skin is de-epithelialized. Hemostasis is checked, drains are inserted, and the breast skin edges are closed temporarily with staples.

Bilateral Delayed Reconstruction

In bilateral delayed reconstruction, the level of the inframammary fold must be set by the surgeon. Often, the patient will be wearing a brassiere or an external prosthesis that will have left marks on the patient's chest. These marks can be an excellent guide to the proper positioning of the breasts. If this is not helpful, the nipple level can be set at a point midway between the patient's elbow and her acromion (Fig 18-9), and the inframammary fold can be positioned a few centimeters below that.

In most cases, the mastectomy incision should be reopened, the scar excised, and the mastectomy flaps reelevated to re-create the defect. The hemi-TRAM flaps are then transferred and shaped just as in immediate reconstruction. In delayed reconstruction, however, the mastectomy flaps are often prevented from reexpanding to their original

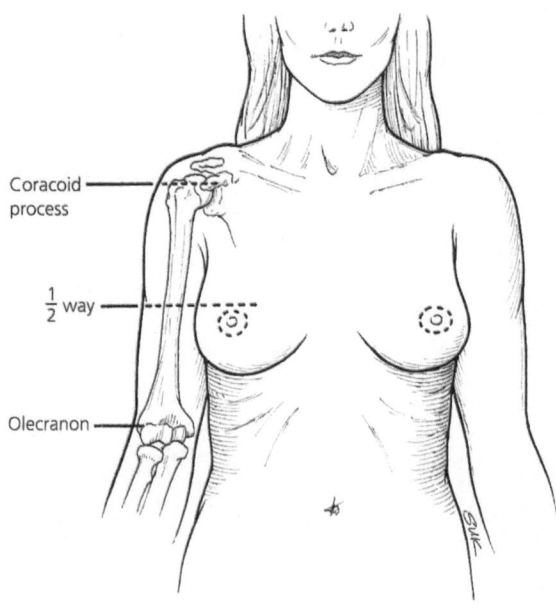

Fig. 18-9 The nipple level should be set 2 to 4 cm below the point halfway between the olecranon and the acromion.

dimensions because of limiting subcutaneous scar tissue. This tissue, which usually forms as a cicatricial sheet deep to the subcutaneous fat, must be aggressively released. If incising this scar tissue does not allow sufficient expansion of the lower mastectomy flap, the skin itself can be released by making a vertical incision down to the inframammary fold (Fig 18-10), as was discussed in chapter 17. This releasing incision will create a V-

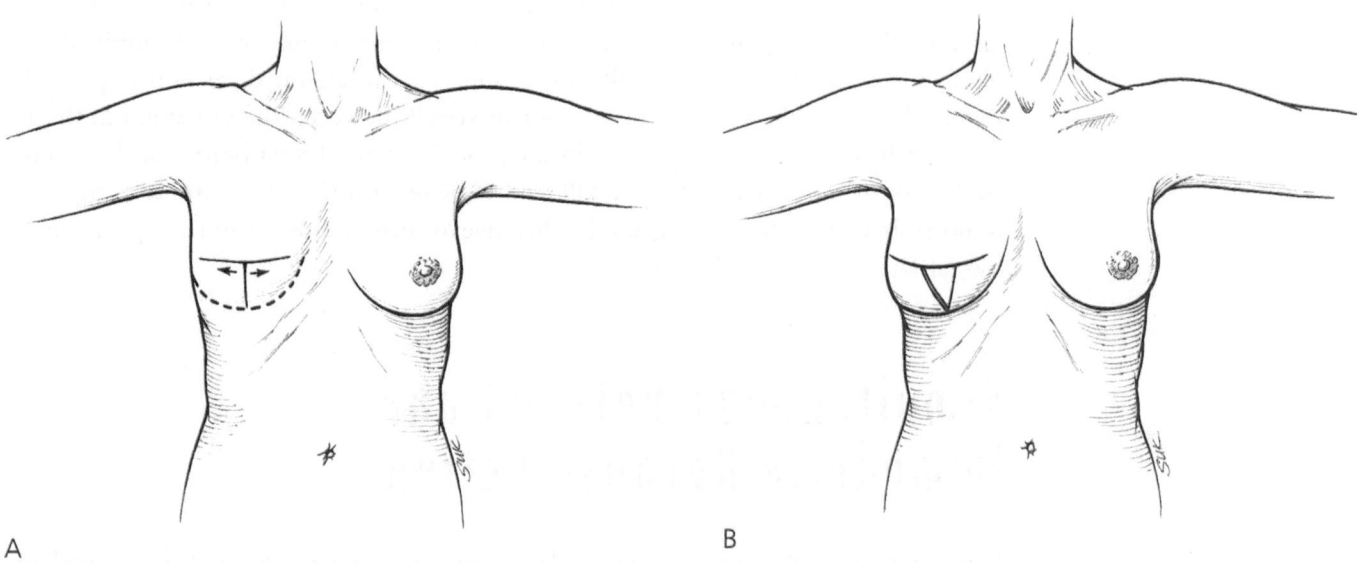

A   B

Fig. 18-10 (A) A vertical incision in a tight lower mastectomy flap allows it to expand to more normal dimensions. (B) This incision, which extends to the inframammary fold, creates a V-shaped skin defect that must be filled by the skin of the underlying TRAM flap.

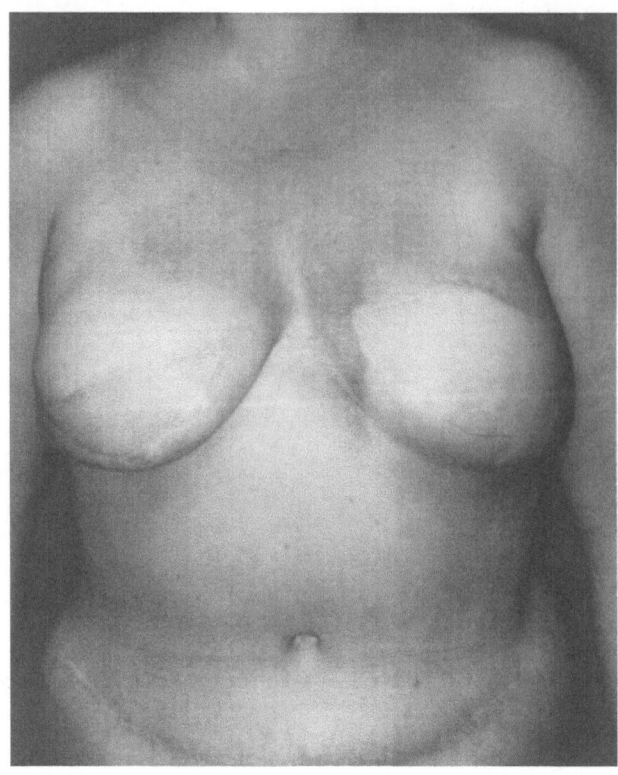

FIG. 18-11 Result of bilateral delayed breast reconstruction in which a vertical incision was used in the lower left mastectomy flap to expand the lower breast envelope.

shaped defect, which in turn is filled by underlying skin from the autologous tissue flap (Fig 18-11).

If the internal mammary vessels are used as recipient vessels in free tissue transfer, both the inframammary folds and the lateral breast borders can be determined simply by the extent of mastectomy flap dissection—i.e., where the dissection stops. If the thoracodorsal vessels are used as the recipient vessels, however, the dissection in the axilla must be carried past the desired location of the lateral breast border (at least superiorly), so part of the lateral border will have to be re-created with sutures after the anastomoses. In either case, the surgeon should strive to keep the breast from being positioned too far laterally.

Simultaneous Delayed and Immediate Reconstruction

It is not unusual that one side of a bilateral breast reconstruction will be immediate, and the other delayed. This situation arises when a patient who had a prior mastectomy without reconstruction subsequently develops a contralateral breast cancer and then requests simultaneous reconstruction of both breasts. The surgeon must therefore perform an immediate reconstruction of one breast, then try to match it with a delayed reconstruction on the contralateral side.

Achieving symmetry is more difficult in this situation because the two mastectomies will usually have been different, leaving different defects. Using the same approach for each side will therefore not automatically ensure symmetry. Ordinarily, the delayed reconstruction side will require more tissue, since the older mastectomy was probably not a skin-sparing one. The surgeon can reduce the breast asymmetry by making the flap for the delayed reconstruction slightly larger than the immediate reconstruction flap. In the case of bilateral TRAM flaps, dividing the flap in two just off the midline will accomplish this; however, the surgeon must be very careful not to compensate excessively because even 5 mm of incision displacement can make a big difference in the volume of the flap.

Reconstruction After Previous Breast Augmentation

If the patient has had a previous breast augmentation, it may be difficult to create breasts of the size the patient desires with autologous tissue alone. In many cases, using extended free TRAM flaps (Fig 18-12) can allow autologous tissue reconstruction of breasts that will satisfy the patient. If the implants were very large, however, and the amount of autologous tissue available is small, the patient must be advised that her reconstructed breasts

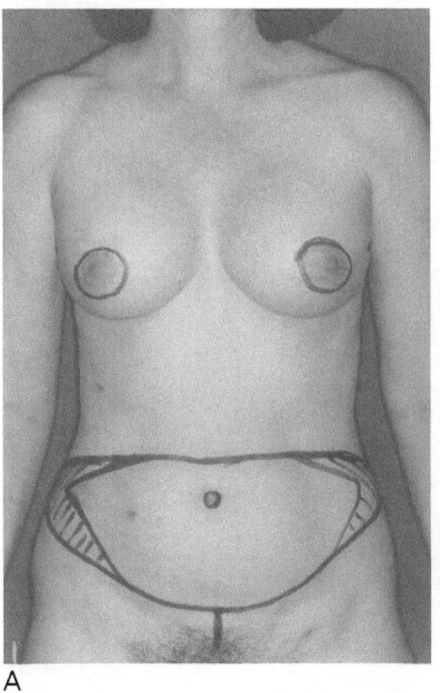
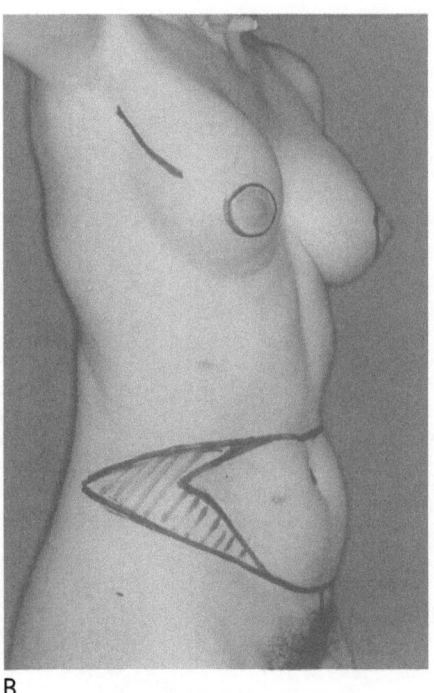
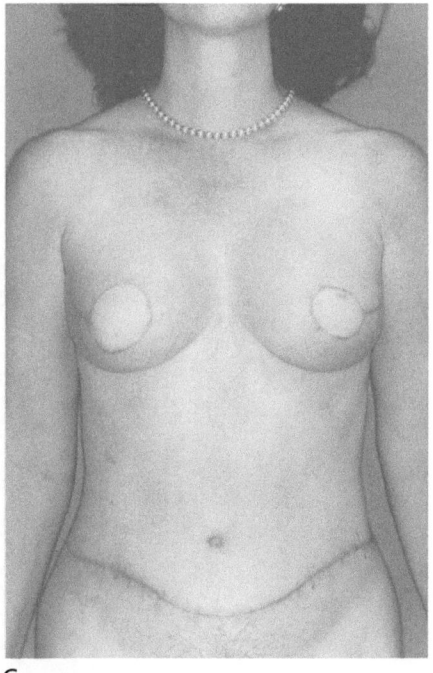

A   B   C

FIG. 18-12   (A, B) Plan for extended bilateral free TRAM flaps in a very thin patient. The flaps extend more laterally than a usual TRAM flap. (B) Because the flaps are longer, they contain more volume and can create larger breasts. (From Kroll SS: *Clin Plast Surg.* 1998;25:251–259. Used with permission.)

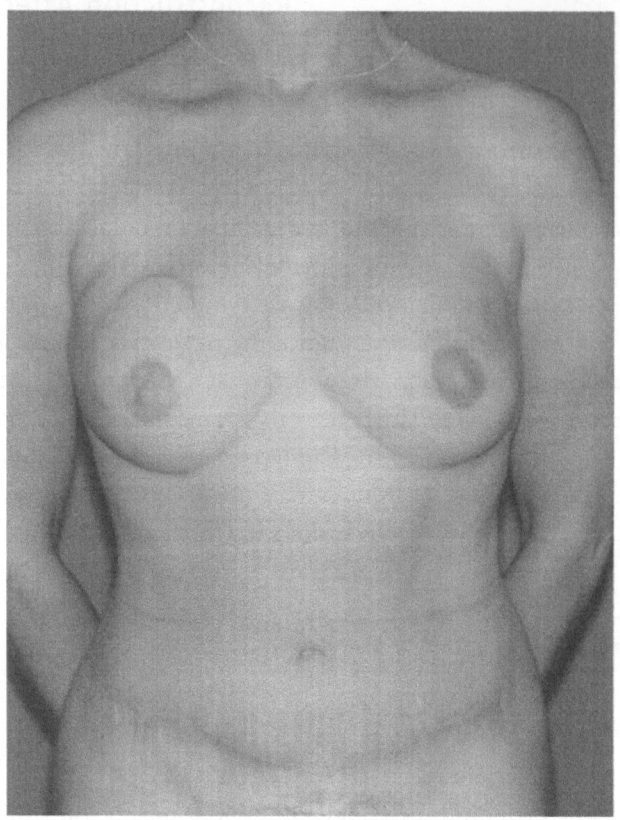

FIG. 18-13 Result of bilateral TRAM flap reconstruction in a patient who had previously had breast implants. Because the inframammary folds were not raised, they are lower than they ideally should be.

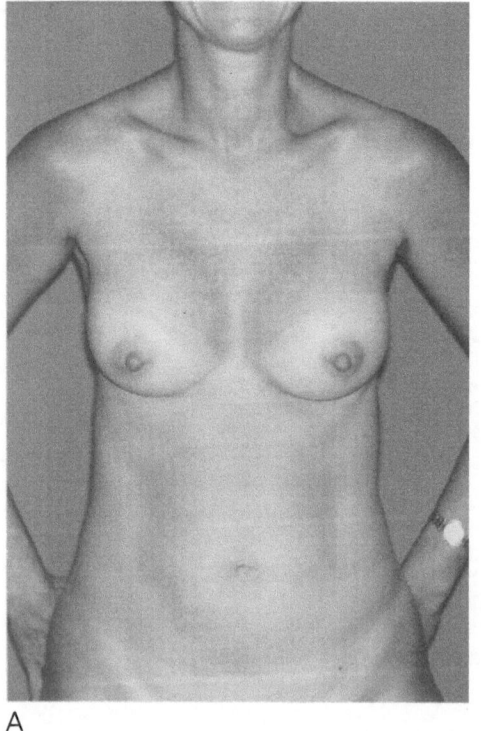

A

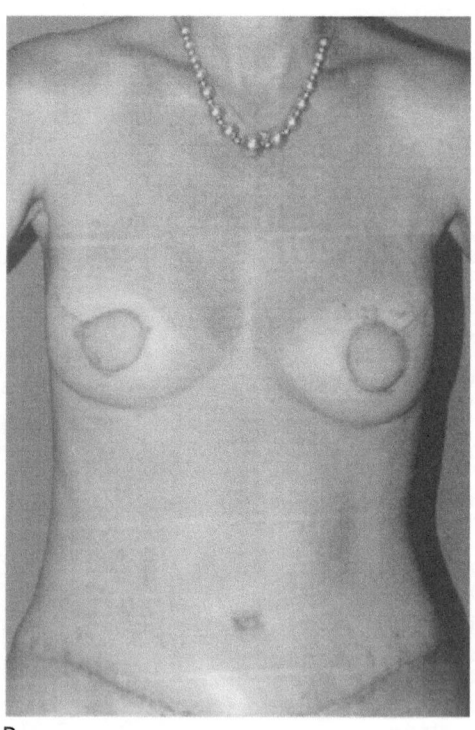

B

FIG. 18-14 In this patient, who had previously had breast implants, (A) the inframammary folds were raised to a higher level during reconstruction so the results (B) look more natural.

will be smaller than her augmented ones were. Although it is possible to augment reconstructed breasts with supplementary implants, I usually discourage this because in most cases the size of the reconstructed breasts without implants is appropriate for the patient's physique. Moreover, the presence of breast implants adds risk and expense to the reconstructive process, and defeats some of the goals of autologous reconstruction.

Another problem associated with previous breast augmentation is the position of the inframammary folds. In most cases, they will have been lowered as part of the augmentation and will no longer be appropriate for smaller breasts reconstructed with autologous tissue (Fig 18-13). It is therefore usually necessary to re-create the inframammary folds at the level where they were prior to the augmentation. This is done by placing running sutures of 3-0 Vicryl (polygalactin 910) 1 cm or so above the existing folds to tack the subcutaneous tissues of the lower mastectomy flap to the chest wall. After the TRAM flaps have been transferred, the new inframammary folds are evaluated with the patient in the sitting position and are lowered by dissection if necessary. If performed correctly, this maneuver can result in very natural breast positioning despite the previous augmentation (Fig 18-14).

Occasionally, an abnormally low inframammary fold can exist without any history of previous breast surgery (Fig 18-15). This is most often due to a marked en-

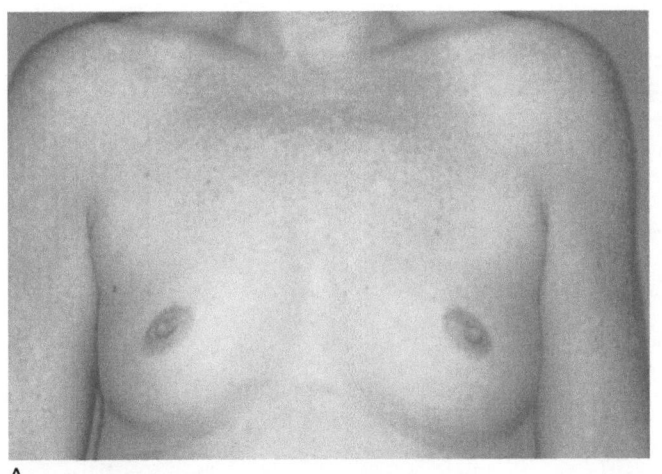

A

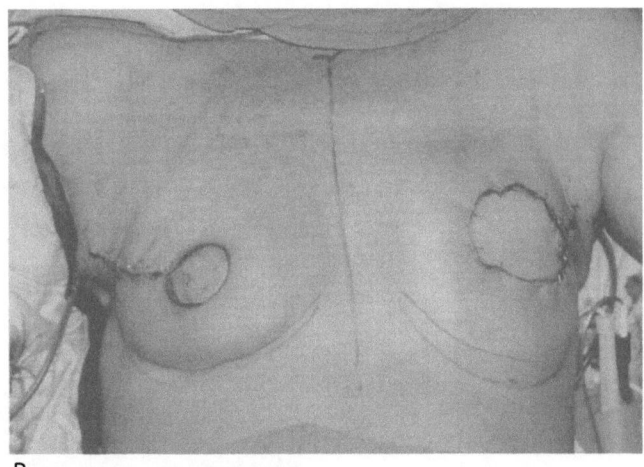

B

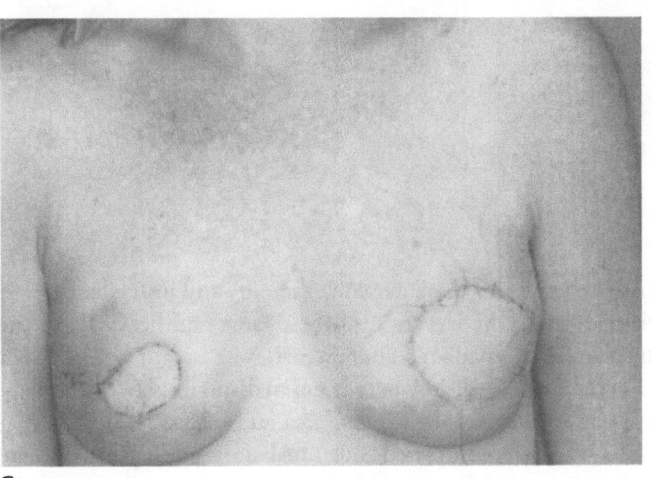

C

FIG. 18-15   (A) Patient prior to bilateral mastectomy, with unusually low inframammary folds and low breast volume. (B) After skin-sparing mastectomy and bilateral free TRAM flap reconstruction, the left breast mound is flat. On the right the breast mound (which was previously like the left) has already had the inframammary fold elevated with sutures so the breast has better position and definition. The left fold was then similarly elevated. (C) Early result, showing a reasonably normal position of both breasts.

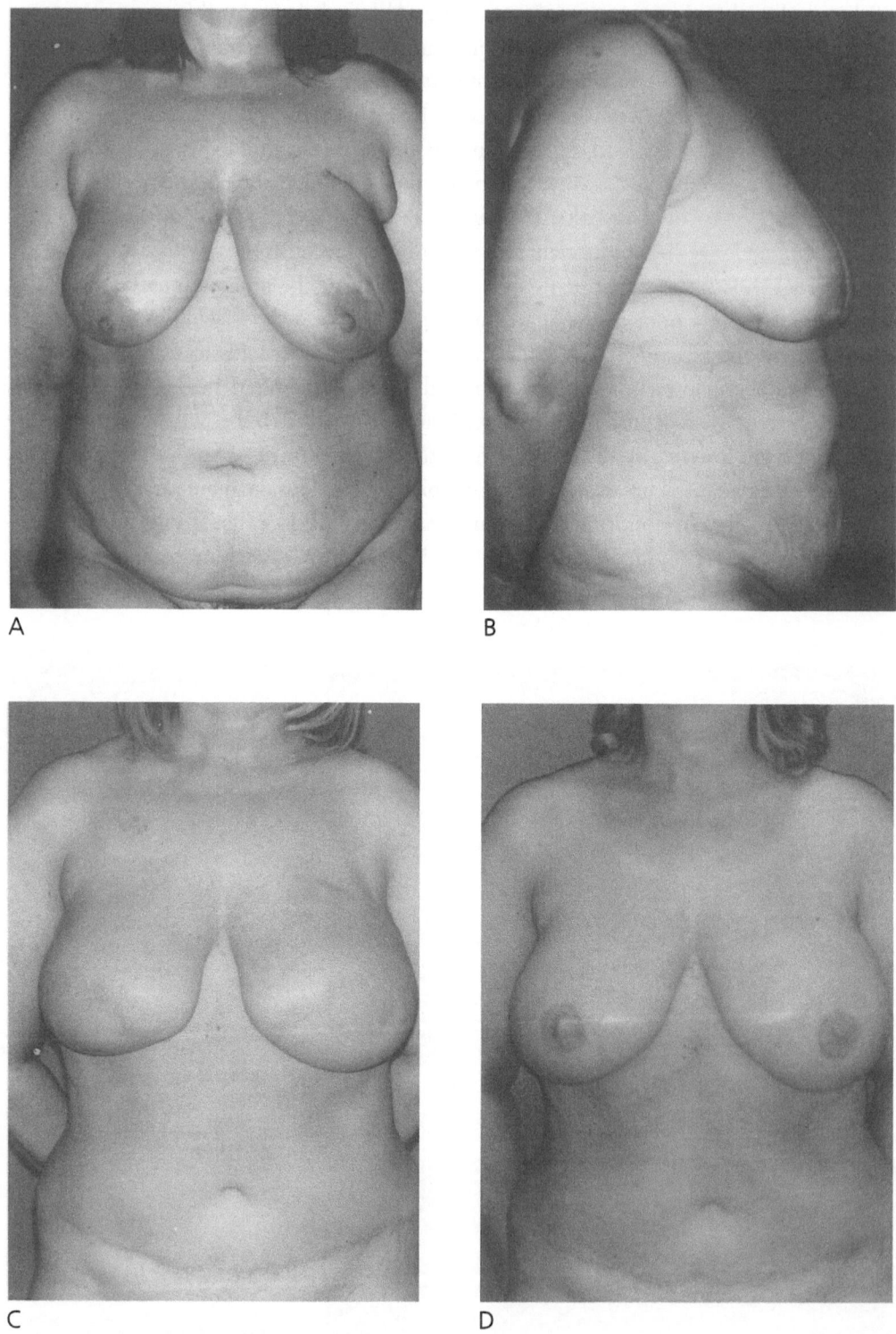

FIG. 18-16 (A, B) Moderately obese patient prior to bilateral mastectomy and immediate breast reconstruction with free TRAM flaps. During the elevation of these large and heavy flaps, the right hemi-TRAM flap slipped and fell off the patient's abdomen. It was caught before it fell on the floor, but not before it had avulsed the pedicle where it entered the muscle of the flap. (C) The early result. Luckily, we were able to excise the avulsed area and repair the pedicle (using 10-0 sutures). The reconstruction was then completed, but not before midnight. (D) The final result was good, despite the unanticipated difficulties. Nevertheless, this case illustrates the problems associated with performing TRAM flaps on obese patients.

largement of the breast during a pregnancy, followed by subsequent involution. This type of low inframammary fold can be managed by making the breast larger if there is sufficient tissue in the abdomen, or by elevating the inframammary folds with sutures. Elevation with sutures can be successful, but must be performed carefully and symmetrically to achieve a normal appearance.

Combatting the Effects of Fatigue

Bilateral TRAM flap breast reconstruction can be a very long operation, and surgeons are often tired and hungry near the end of the procedure when breast shaping must be accomplished. It is tempting to make compromises at that time and accept less than optimal results. The surgeon must remember, however, that his or her goal is aesthetic excellence, and take the time that is necessary to achieve the best possible outcome. Taking short bathroom and food breaks throughout the day will help to combat the effects of fatigue. Having adequate help (two assistants) significantly speeds up the operation[5] and therefore makes shaping easier.

One very significant factor affecting the time required to perform bilateral TRAM flap breast reconstruction is the patient's weight. Obese patients require much more time than patients of normal weight, while thin patients require less time. Obesity also increases the risk of complications and can lead to intraoperative difficulties that can prolong the surgery considerably (Fig 18-16). It is often wise, therefore, to postpone breast reconstruction in obese patients until they lose weight and become more acceptable surgical risks. This not only reduces the risk of complications, but shortens the operative time, which in turn facilitates successful shaping of the breasts. Even so, discipline is still required to spend time shaping the breast at the end of the procedure, but the effort will pay off in the form of better-quality results.[6]

Need for Revisions

Even though symmetry is more easily achieved in bilateral reconstruction and is in fact one of its major advantages, revisions are often necessary. As in any TRAM flap breast reconstruction, excess fullness in the upper outer quadrant of the breast is common and must often be reduced secondarily. Patients should therefore be told to expect at least one revision of their breast reconstruction, even when it is bilateral. The need for revision is particularly likely if one reconstruction is immediate and the other delayed, or if one side has been irradiated. In those cases, symmetry is much more difficult to achieve and more than one revision may be required. In some cases, especially if one mastectomy was very aggressive or if unusually heavy doses of radiation have been used, the goal of adequate symmetry may never be reached.

Summary

Shaping the breast in bilateral reconstruction is similar to shaping the unilaterally reconstructed breast, except that an existing breast need not be matched. In most cases, symmetry is easier to achieve in bilateral reconstruction, and the aesthetic results are better. The actual shaping techniques are the same as those described for unilateral reconstruction (chapters 16 and 17), except that in delayed bilateral reconstruction the level of the inframammary folds is determined by the surgeon. Also, the size of the breasts that can be created may be limited if the patient is thin. Shaping of the breasts occurs near the end of the reconstruction, when surgeons are fatigued and eager to finish the operation. Nevertheless, if a reasonable effort is made, the results can be truly outstanding.

References

1.   Baldwin BJ, Schusterman MA, Miller MJ, Kroll SS, Wang B. Bilateral breast reconstruction: conventional vs. free TRAM. *Plast Reconstr Surg.* 1994;93:1410–1416.
2.   Ninkovic M, Anderl H, Hefel A, Schwabegger A, Wechselberger G. Internal mammary vessels: a reliable recipient system for free flaps in breast reconstruction. *Br J Plast Surg.* 1995;48:533–539.
3.   Hefel A, Schwabegger A, Ninkovic M, Moriggl B, Waldenberger P. Internal mammary vessels: anatomical and clinical considerations. *Br J Plast Surg.* 1995;48:527–532.
4.   Arnez ZM, Valdatta MP, Tyler MP, Planinsek F. Anatomy of internal mammary vessels and their use in free TRAM flap breast reconstruction. *Br J Plast Surg.* 1995;48:540–545.
5.   Khouri RK, Ahn CY, Salzhauer MA, Scherff D, Shaw WW. Simultaneous bilateral breast reconstruction with the transverse rectus abdominis musculocutaneous free flap. *Ann Surg.* 1997;226:25–34.
6.   Kroll SS, Coffey JA Jr, Winn RJ, Schusterman MA. A comparison of factors affecting aesthetic outcomes of TRAM flap breast reconstruction. *Plast Reconstr Surg.* 1995;96:860–864.

19 Correction of Partial Mastectomy Defects

Nature of the Problem

The use of breast conservation therapy as a treatment for early breast cancer has become very popular in recent years.[1-4] In many parts of the United States, it has supplanted mastectomy as the most prevalent form of treatment. Breast conservation therapy consists of partial mastectomy and axillary dissection followed by radiotherapy. When the partial mastectomy is adequate, survival statistics are similar to those obtained with total mastectomy. To avoid an unacceptable recurrence rate, however, the tumor has to be excised with clear, tumor-free margins.

In patients with large breasts and small tumors, partial mastectomy does not significantly deform the breast. In patients with small breasts and larger tumors, however, the deformity caused by partial mastectomy can be significant (Figs 19-1 and 19-2).[5] This is especially true if the surgeon wishes to excise the tumor with a wide margin. The deformity can be reduced by performing a "lumpectomy" with narrower margins,[6] but a price may be paid in the form of a higher local recurrence rate.[7]

At The University of Texas M. D. Anderson Cancer Center, we have found that repairing partial mastectomy defects with local tissue flaps or rearrangement of breast tissue can often greatly reduce the deformity caused by partial mastectomy.[8-10] In some patients, the distortion can be essentially eliminated. In this chapter, I will discuss the indications for this approach and the various techniques that are used.

Indications for Repair of Partial Mastectomy Defects

Repair of partial mastectomy defects is indicated whenever the partial mastectomy would cause significant deformity of the breast. This is most likely whenever the breast is relatively small, or the tumor relatively large. Reconstruction of the defect is usually indi-

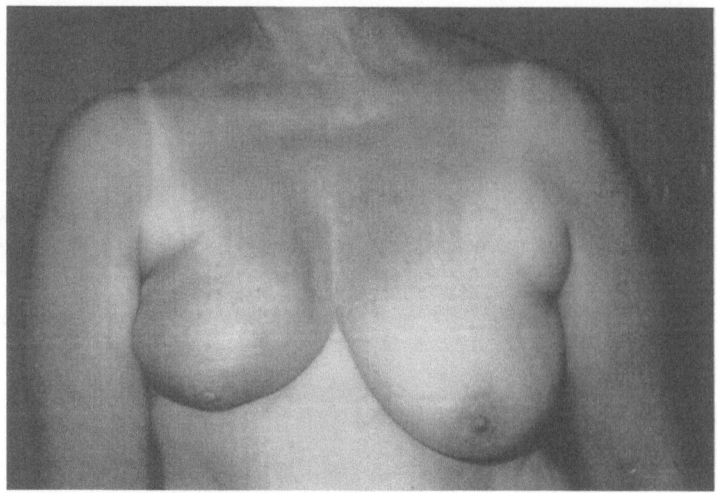

FIG. 19-1 (A) Patient with significant breast asymmetry following partial mastectomy and irradiation for treatment of early right breast cancer. This asymmetry was reduced but not eliminated by a contralateral breast reduction.

cated whenever more than 25% of the breast tissue must be removed. Repair is also indicated whenever the nipple would be significantly displaced by primary closure of the defect. Repair is rarely necessary when the breasts are very large unless the tumor is also correspondingly large.

Repair of a partial mastectomy defect is also usually necessary even for smaller defects if they include any significant amount of skin. If a small defect does not include skin, the cavity caused by the partial mastectomy will sometimes fill in with fluid and scar tissue. This may in some cases leave an acceptable cosmetic result, which is the reason that partial mastectomy defects that do not involve skin should not be drained, and

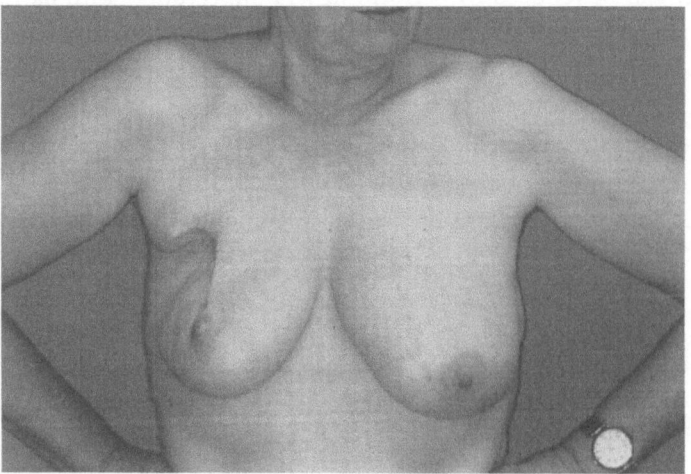

FIG. 19-2 Patient after a partial mastectomy of right breast performed in another country. A significant amount of skin as well as breast tissue had been removed.

the parenchymal tissue is not closed with deep sutures. If skin is missing, however, deformity is usually inevitable unless the breast is so large that the skin defect is relatively insignificant, so reconstruction is indicated.

Contraindication for Repair of Partial Mastectomy Defects

Immediate repair of the partial mastectomy defect with tissue rearrangement should be avoided if there is doubt about the tumor margins. If the margins are not clear or multifocal disease is found on permanent sections, the incisions required to raise and transfer a local flap could interfere with (although would not preclude) a subsequent mastectomy. If the tissue margins are uncertain, the repair can be deferred until the permanent sections have been reviewed by the pathologist and a final opinion rendered.

Repair of a partial mastectomy defect is also contraindicated, in my opinion, if the defect is so large that a transverse rectus abdominus myocutaneous (TRAM) flap would be required for the partial breast reconstruction. In that case, I believe that it is preferable to complete the mastectomy and reconstruct the entire breast with the TRAM flap. This approach reduces the probability that recurrent disease will force sacrifice of the reconstructed breast, making necessary a new breast reconstruction with options limited by the surgeon's earlier partial breast reconstruction.

Use of Distant Tissue

Some very well respected surgeons have recently advocated the use of latissimus dorsi muscle or myocutaneous flaps for repair of small partial mastectomy defects.[11,12] Although this can be effective, it requires the use of a major reconstructive option that could prove useful in the future should mastectomy subsequently be required. Also, the use of a latissimus flap for repair of a small breast defect that includes skin can create a patchwork appearance in the breast that is not attractive (Fig 19-3). My own opinion is that in most cases partial mastectomy defects are best repaired with local flaps if possible, with distant tissue reserved for repair of total mastectomy defects or large defects for which local tissue would not be adequate.

Classification of Defects

I find it helpful to divide partial mastectomy defects into four groups according to how they will need to be reconstructed: Small defects in larger or medium-sized breasts (no reconstruction); medium-sized defects in larger breasts (breast reshaping); medium-sized defects in medium-sized or small breasts (local tissue flaps); and larger defects (distant tissue flaps). The first group, which needs no reconstruction, will not be discussed here.

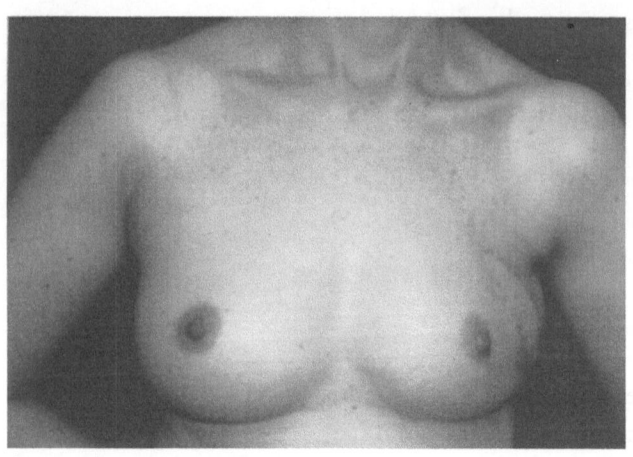
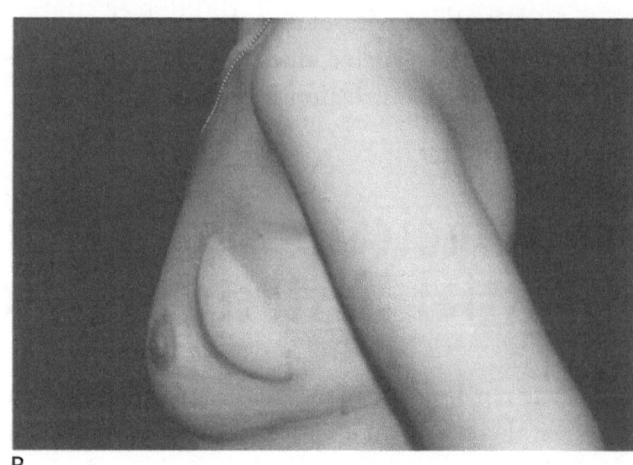

A   B

FIG. 19-3   (A, B) Patient after partial mastectomy and replacement of missing breast tissue with a latissimus dorsi myocutaneous flap. Nipple position has been restored; however, the scars are not located in aesthetic unit borders, so the flap looks like a patch. (From Kroll SS, Singletary SE: *Clin Plast Surg*. 1998;25:303–310. Used with permission.)

The other groups will each be addressed separately. Obviously, many cases could fall into more than one classification, depending on the preference of the surgeon. In those situations, surgical judgment and the wishes of the patient must be taken into consideration.

Medium Defects in Larger Breasts (Breast Reshaping)

If the breast is large enough, the defect can often be managed by converting the partial mastectomy into some form of breast reduction, reshaping the breast with remaining tissue and reducing the opposite breast for symmetry.[13] This approach is easiest if the defect is in the lower pole of the breast, but can be adapted to the medial and lateral parts of the breast in many cases. The main requirement is that the breast be large enough that it would benefit from (or at least tolerate) a reduction mammaplasty.

Defects in the Lower Pole

If the partial mastectomy defect is in the lower pole of the breast, management is simple because the partial mastectomy can just be converted into a reduction mammaplasty (Fig 19-4). This approach will yield a breast that is smaller than before surgery, but that has a normal shape and reasonably well accepted scars. In almost all cases, the opposite breast will need to be reduced for symmetry. This approach can also be used for defects in the area of the nipple (Fig 19-5), except that the nipple itself must be sacrificed and reconstructed secondarily.

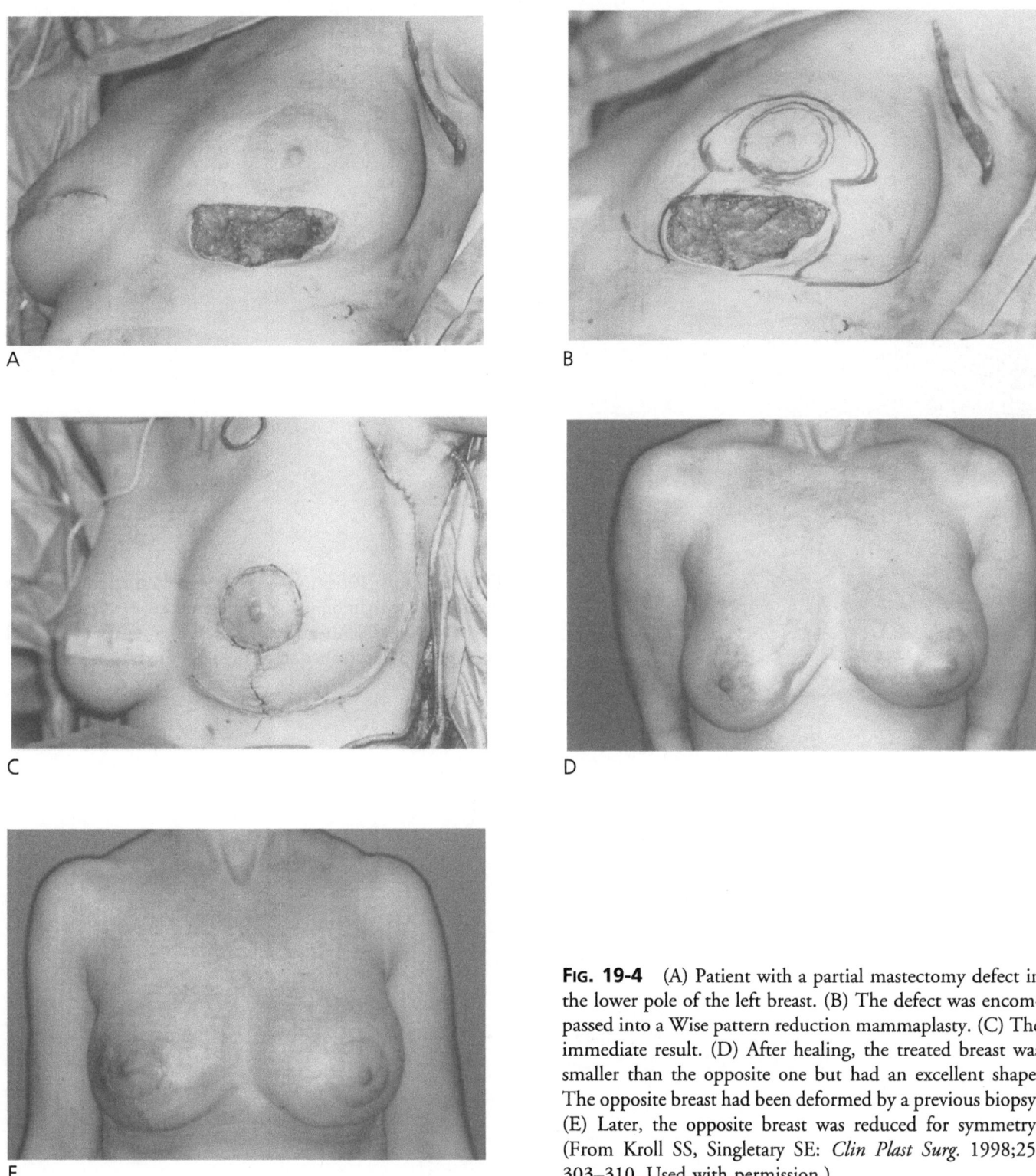

FIG. 19-4 (A) Patient with a partial mastectomy defect in the lower pole of the left breast. (B) The defect was encompassed into a Wise pattern reduction mammaplasty. (C) The immediate result. (D) After healing, the treated breast was smaller than the opposite one but had an excellent shape. The opposite breast had been deformed by a previous biopsy. (E) Later, the opposite breast was reduced for symmetry. (From Kroll SS, Singletary SE: *Clin Plast Surg.* 1998;25: 303–310. Used with permission.)

A variety of breast reduction techniques can be used, all of which are familiar to most plastic surgeons. The only absolute requirement is that the nipple/areolar complex "flap" not be based inferiorly, since any blood supply that would have been relied upon in an inferior pedicle technique will have been resected. Techniques similar to the

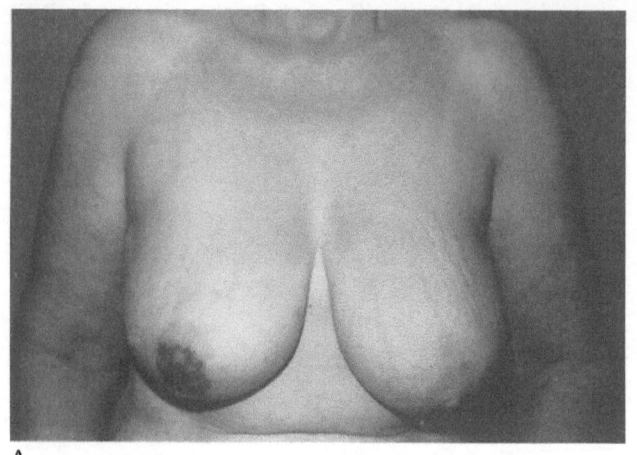

A

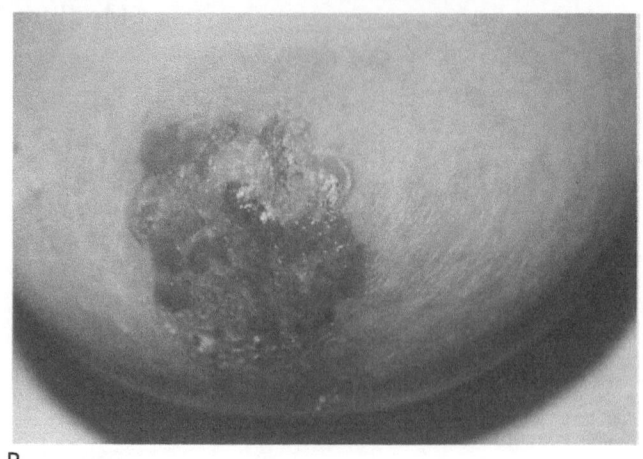

B

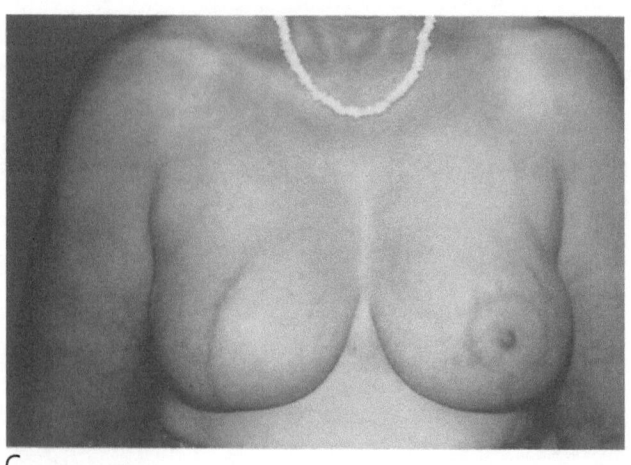

C

FIG. 19-5 (A) Patient with a superficial carcinoma (Paget's disease) in the right nipple/areolar complex. (B) Close-up view of the tumor. (C) After wide local excision using a modified Wise pattern and reduction of the opposite breast.

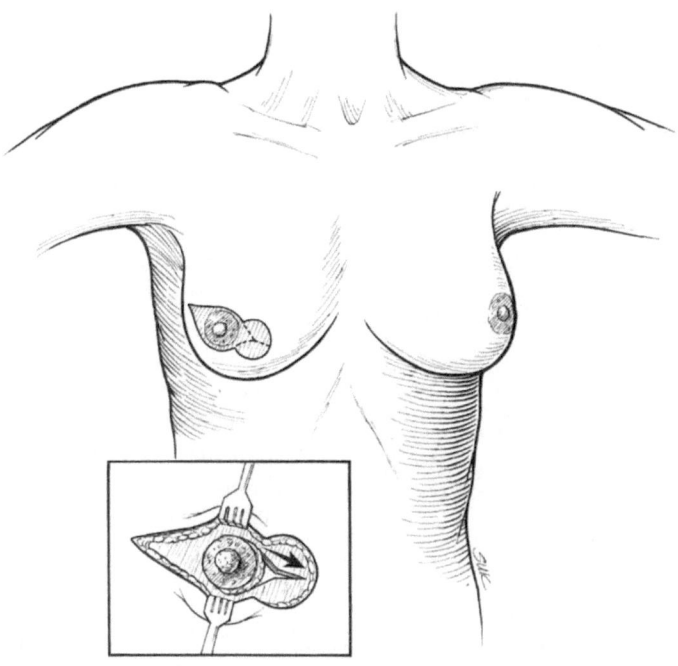

FIG. 19-6 The lateral mastopexy used for nipple centralization. This is like a vertical mastopexy pattern turned on its side.

round-block method of Benelli[14] can also be used provided that no skin outside the usual reduction pattern has had to be removed.

Lateral Defects That Include Skin

If the defect is located laterally, the usual pattern used for reduction mammaplasty can be turned on its side and the equivalent of a breast reduction can be performed by excising a wedge from the lateral breast. The equivalent of a vertical or J-shaped breast reduction pattern works best (Fig 19-6). The nipple/areolar complex must be centralized by relocating it more medially, using the same techniques normally used to elevate the nipple/areolar complex during breast reduction or mastopexy (Fig 19-7).[15] If the

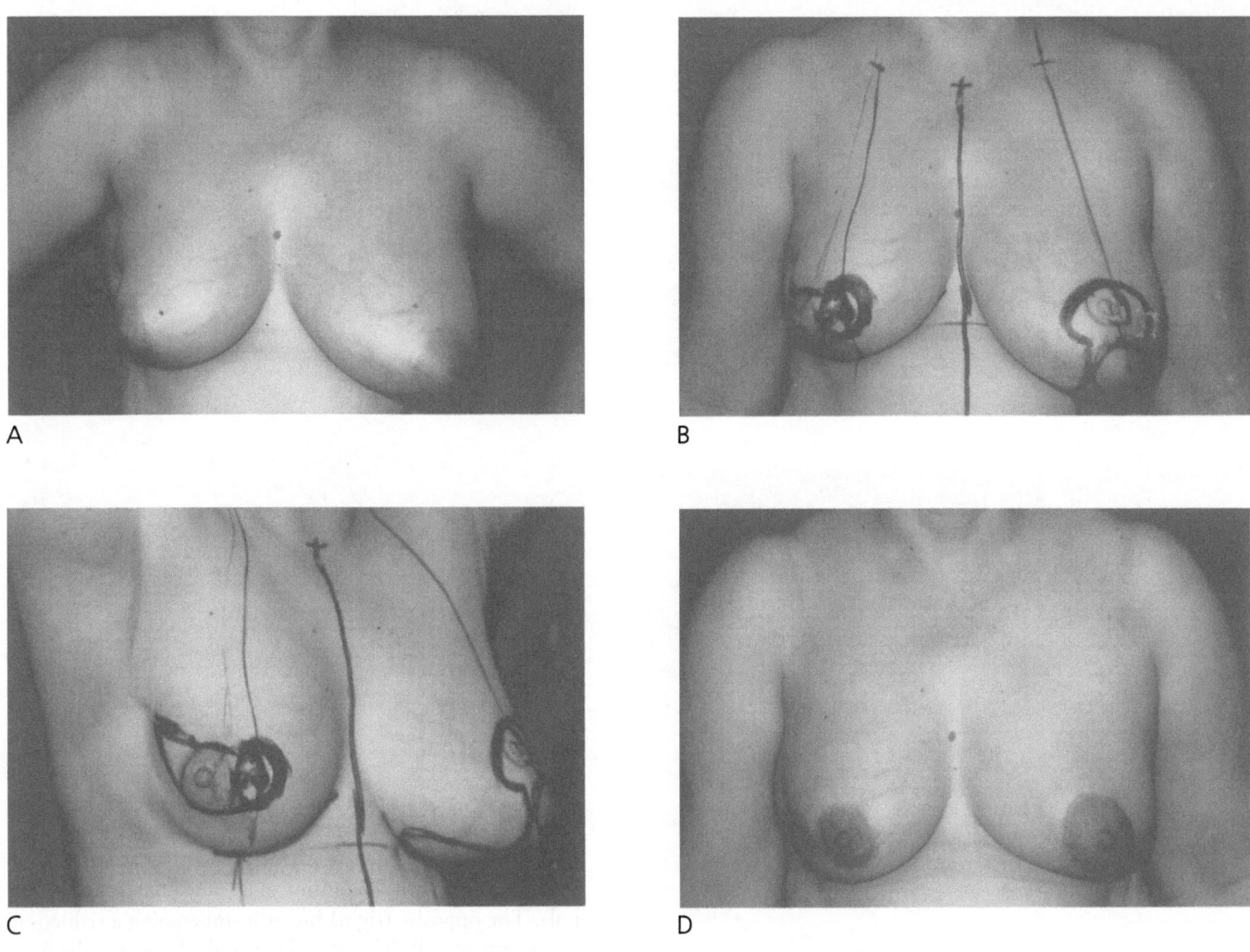

A

B

C

D

FIG. 19-7   (A) A 43-year-old woman 5 years after breast conservation treatment of right breast cancer. The nipple is displaced laterally, and the breast is significantly deformed. (B, C) Treatment plan for nipple centralization and contralateral breast reduction. (D) Result 8 months later, showing better nipple position and improved symmetry. (From Kroll SS: *Ann Plast Surg.* 1990;24:271. Used with permission.)

breast has not been previously irradiated, the glandular tissue can often be rearranged as in the vertical mammaplasty technique of Lassus.[16]

Analogous to the medial and lateral breast flaps in a breast reduction, superior and inferior breast flaps must be developed laterally. The scars will not be hidden in the inframammary fold, but the overall breast shape can be well maintained and a pleasing form achieved. As in treatment of inferior mastectomy defects, if the amount of breast tissue removed was significant a reduction of the opposite breast is indicated.

Another approach to defects in the outer upper quadrant is to use the "plug" flap technique of Daher.[17] In this technique, a centrally based flap is created in the lower pole of the breast, where tissue would ordinarily be resected when performing a reduction mammaplasty. A tunnel is made between the base of this flap and the defect in

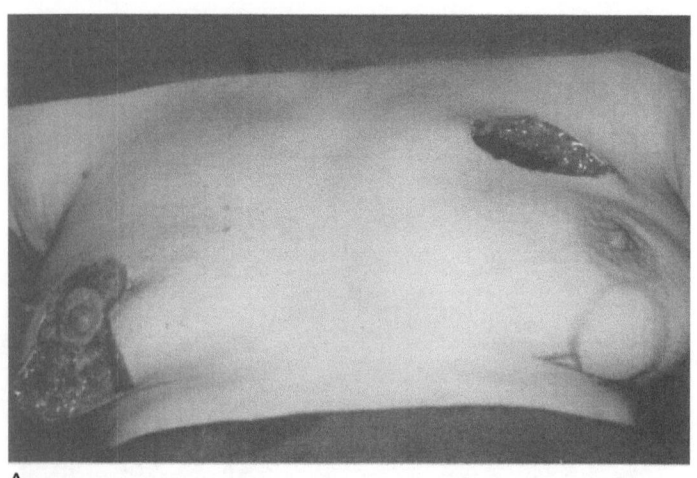

A

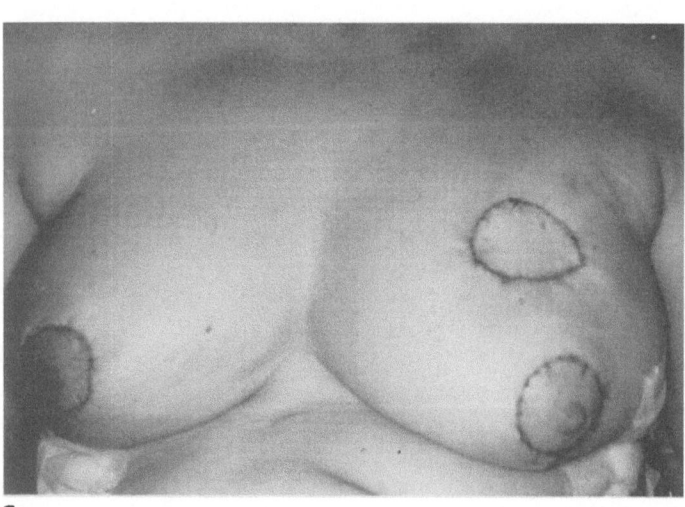

C

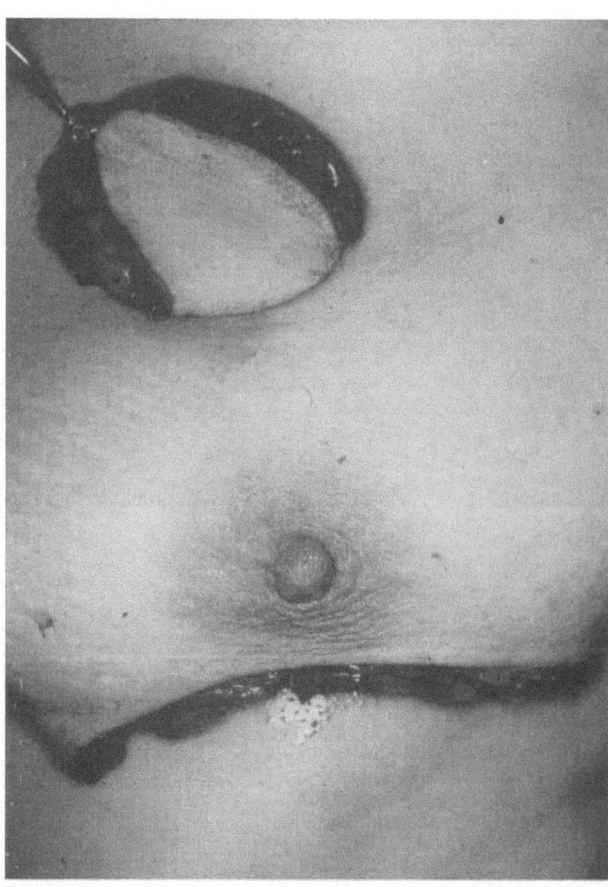

B

FIG. 19-8   (A) Patient with defect in the upper pole of the left breast, with the outline of a "plug" flap in the lower pole. The opposite (right) breast is undergoing a reduction mammaplasty. (B) The plug flap is pulled through the tunnel into the defect in the upper pole of the breast. (C) The immediate result shows good symmetry and breast shape. (Photos courtesy of Fabio Carramaschi, MD, São Paulo, Brazil.)

the upper outer quadrant or upper pole of the breast. The plug flap is passed through the tunnel, then used to repair the defect in the superior portion of the breast (Fig 19-8). The donor defect created by harvest of the plug flap is then repaired as in an ordinary breast reduction. Simultaneously, the opposite breast is reduced to restore symmetry to the two breasts.

Medium Defects in Medium or Smaller Breasts (Local Flaps)

Defects in the Lateral Breast or Lower Pole

If the defect is located laterally or in the lower pole, a local flap can be used to at least partially replace the excised breast with adjacent tissue. For defects in the 12 o'clock position of the lower pole, or for defects situated medial to that, a small thoracoabdominal flap can be very useful. This flap is taken from the skin and subcutaneous tissue just lateral to and below the inframammary fold (Fig 19-9). The donor scar will be partially camouflaged in the inframammary crease, and the defect will be replaced by like tissue.

If the defect is situated more laterally, a rotation flap that transfers redundant skin and subcutaneous tissue from the area just inferior to the axilla can be designed (Fig 19-10). This effectively shifts the defect into the subaxillary region, where it is less conspicuous, and adds tissue to the deficient breast, where it is needed. The rotation flap can work well if there is sufficient subaxillary tissue present to transfer into the breast. If the patient has undergone a very aggressive axillary dissection that included a large amount of subcutaneous fat as well as nodal tissue, however, there may not be sufficient subaxillary fatty tissue remaining to permit this approach to be successful. Here, as in immediate reconstruction with skin-sparing mastectomy, the quality of the result depends to a great extent on cooperation from an oncologic surgeon who is committed to a good aesthetic outcome and is willing to take extra care not to unnecessarily sacrifice tissues that might be required for obtaining a successful reconstruction. Unfortunately, the amount of local tissue available for transfer is never known until the partial mastectomy and axillary dissection have been completed. For this reason, the reconstructive surgeon must be careful during the preoperative consultation with the patient not to make excessive promises concerning the aesthetic result.

Defects in the Upper Outer Quadrant

Defects in the upper outer quadrant can also be managed by moving tissue from the subaxillary area, as described above (Fig 19-11). It may be necessary to use a rhomboid (Limberg) flap rather than a rotation flap because the tissue must be transposed at a more acute angle. In many cases, this approach will restore the breast to a size similar to its preoperative state so that contralateral reduction is not necessary.

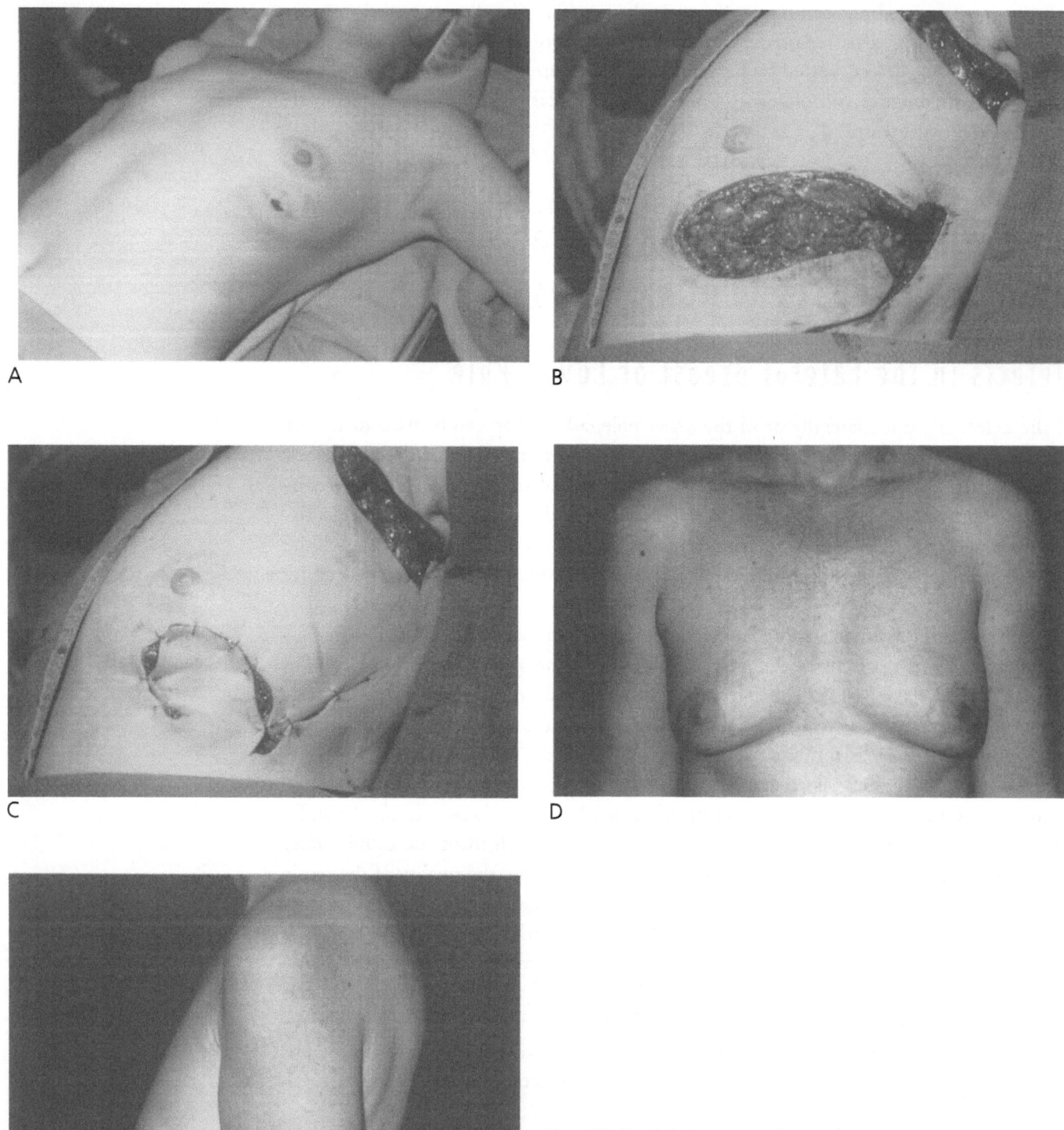

FIG. 19-9 (A) Patient with a melanoma in the lower pole of the left breast. (B) After wide local excision and elevation of a small thoracoabdominal (local) flap. (C) After transfer of the flap into the defect. (D, E) Result at 6 months, showing scarring but good correction of the breast shape.

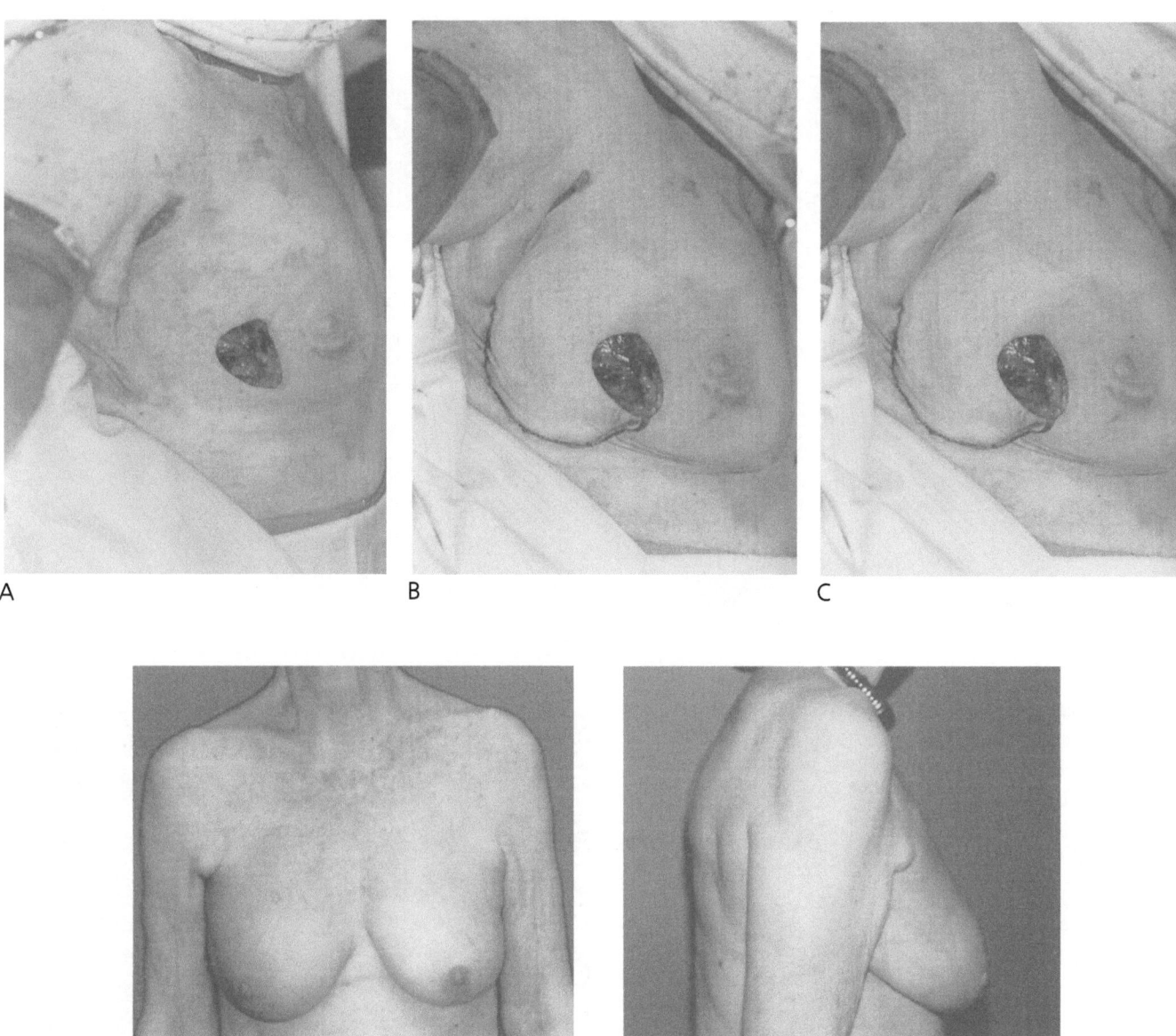

FIG. 19-10   (A) Lateral breast defect following partial mastectomy. (B) Rotation flap designed to transfer subaxillary skin and subcutaneous fat into the breast. (C) Immediate result. (D, E) Patient 4 months later, with a nearly normal breast shape. (From Kroll SS, Singletary SE: *Clin Plast Surg.* 1998;25:303–310. Used with permission.)

Defects in the Upper Pole

Defects in the upper pole can be managed by elevating and transposing a superiorly based composite flap[8] that, like the methods described immediately above, shifts the defect to the subaxillary area (Fig 19-12). The difference between this flap and those described above is that this superiorly based flap contains a significant amount of breast tissue, which gets its blood supply from the overlying skin (Fig 19-13). Because the

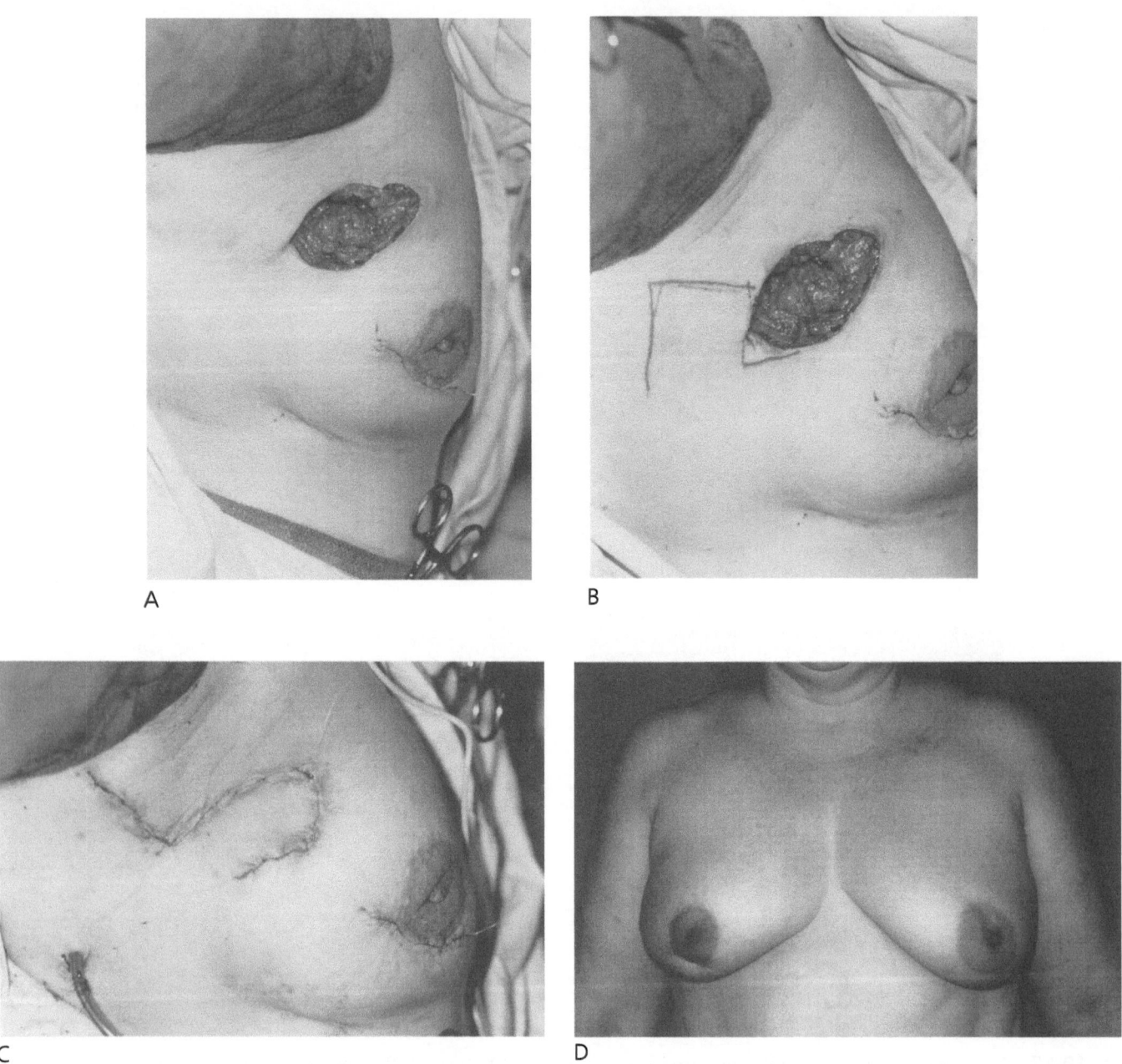

A

B

C

D

FIG. 19-11   (A) A 58-year-old woman with a lumpectomy defect in the upper outer quadrant. She also had a recent biopsy in the subareolar area. (B, C) The defect was repaired with a local flap, shifting the defect to the less conspicuous subaxillary region. (D) Result 9 months later, showing more deformity from the biopsy than from the partial mastectomy.

thickness of the flap matches that of the surrounding breast, the shape of the breast is well maintained and the cosmetic result, aside from the scars, can be excellent (Fig 19-14). Because the scars, like the defect, are in the upper pole of the breast, they tend to be more conspicuous than scars in the lower part of the breast would be. Fortunately, they tend to fade with time, and in any case are less important to the final result than the achievement of correct breast form.

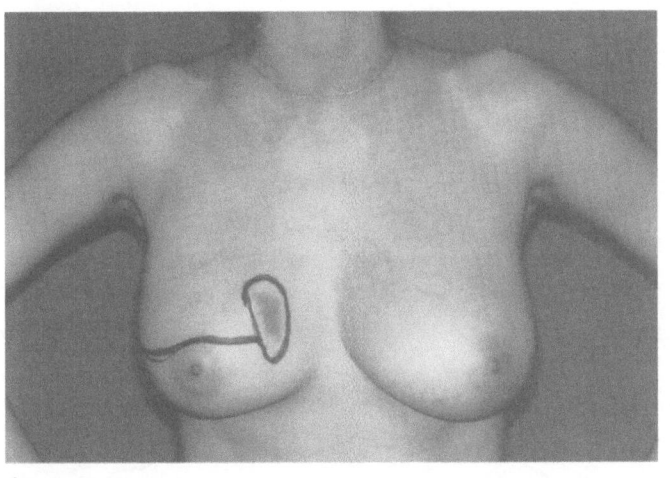
A

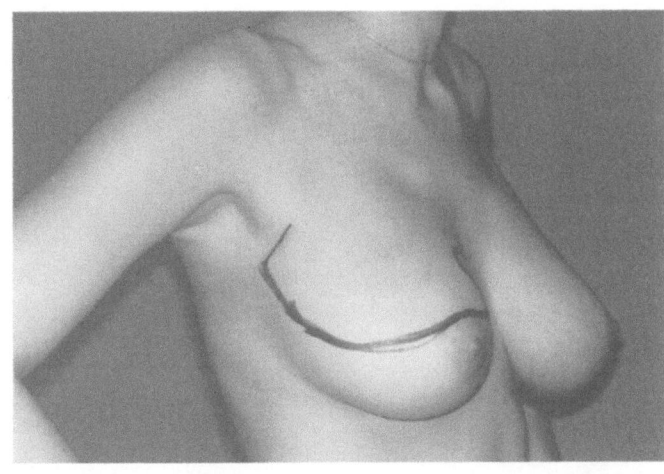
B

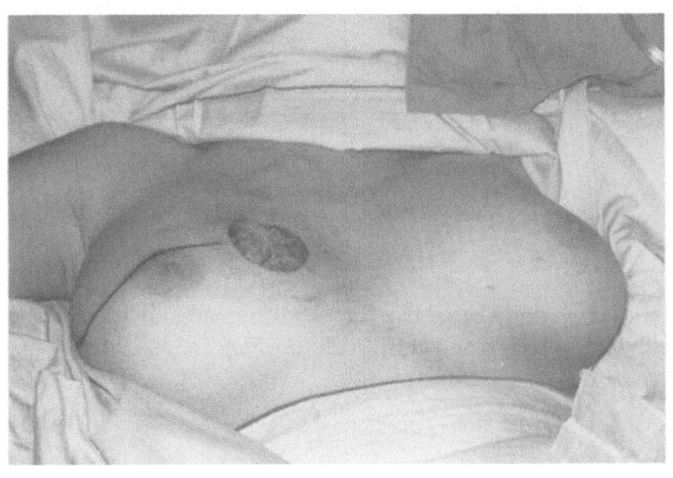
C

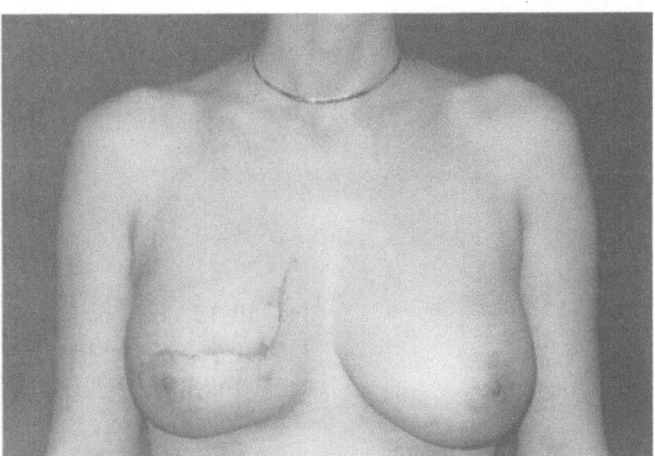
D

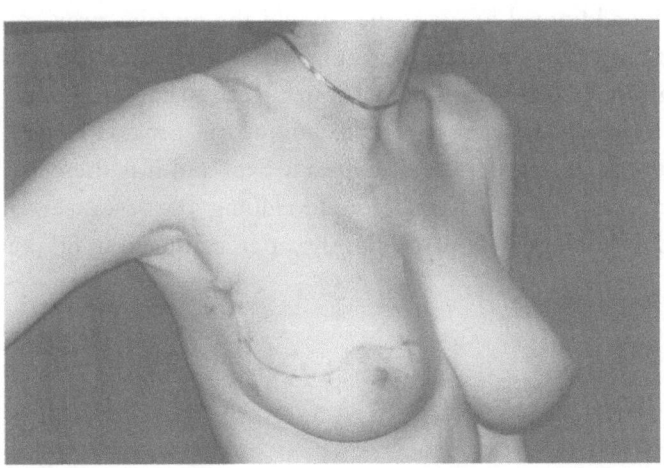
E

FIG. 19-12   (A, B) A 33-year-old woman with early breast cancer, showing the plan for lumpectomy and repair of the defect with a superiorly based local flap. (C) Lumpectomy defect. (D, E) Patient 2 months later, with a breast shape that is almost normal. (From Kroll SS, Singletary SE: *Clin Plast Surg.* 1988; 25:303–310. Used with permission.)

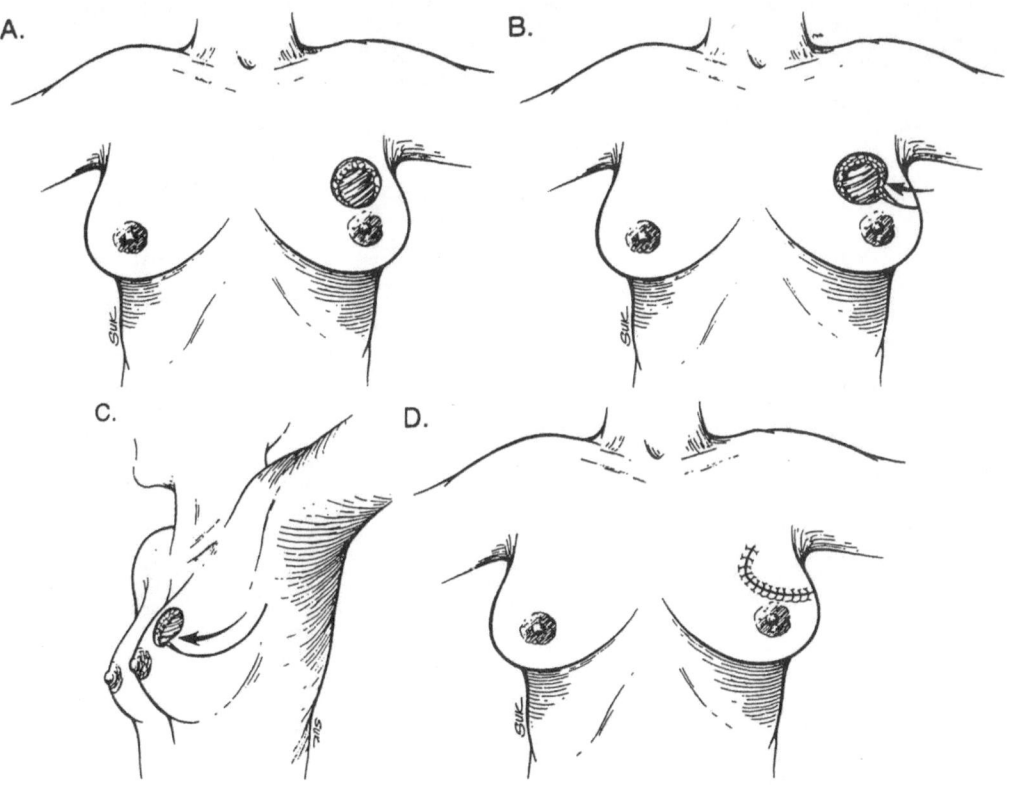

FIG. 19-13   Schematic drawing of the superiorly based flap for reconstruction of defects in the upper pole of the breast. (From Bold RJ, Kroll SS, Baldwin BJ, et al: *Ann Surg Oncol.* 1997;4:540. Used with permission.)

One disadvantage of this approach is that it creates internal breast scarring that could make it difficult to excise additional breast tissue (should the margins prove to contain tumor) without performing a total mastectomy. Subsequent irradiation can significantly increase the scarring (Fig 19-15). This internal scarring can make subsequent mammograms more difficult to interpret. Even so, this technique can provide an aesthetically superior result without requiring the use of a distant flap, and it is therefore very useful. As in any surgery on a breast at risk for developing breast cancer, a baseline mammogram should be obtained 3 to 6 months after completion of the reconstruction.

Large Defects

Unless the breast is very large, large breast defects caused by partial mastectomy usually require distant tissue for correction. I do not like to use TRAM flaps for this purpose because I prefer to keep the TRAM flap in reserve in case a total mastectomy is subse-

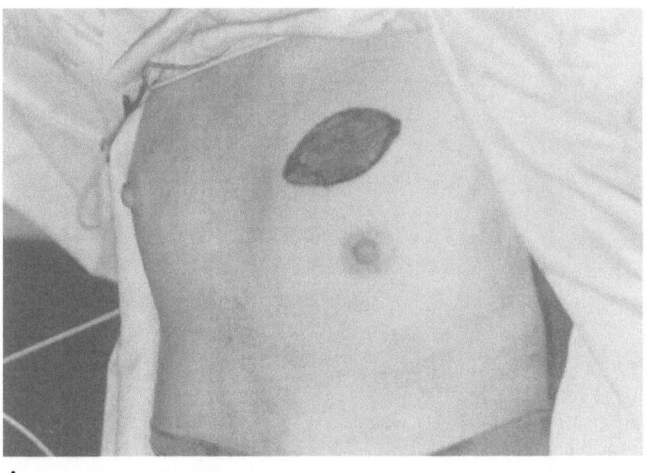

A

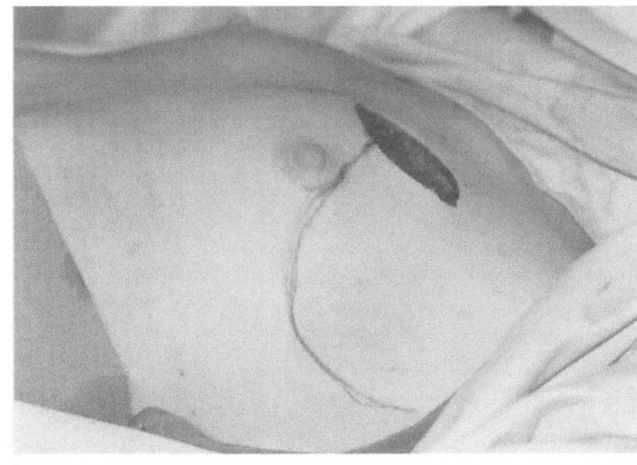

B

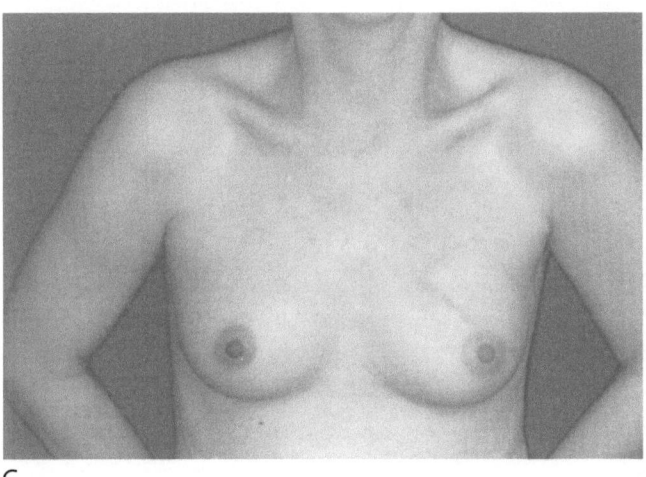

C

FIG. 19-14 (A) A 38-year-old woman with a large lumpectomy defect in the upper pole of the breast. (B) Plan for a superiorly based flap. (C) Result 1 year later. See color insert, p. I-18. (From Bold RJ, Kroll SS, Baldwin BJ, et al: *Ann Surg Oncol.* 1997;4:540. Used with permission.)

quently required. Fortunately, even the largest partial mastectomy defects can usually be managed with a latissimus dorsi flap. The latissimus dorsi flap is technically much simpler than the TRAM flap and has a low incidence of failure. In most cases, a large skin island is not required so the donor site scar is acceptable. The color and texture match of the latissimus flap may not always be ideal, but the patch effect can be reduced by placing at least one of the scars in the inframammary fold or the lateral breast border where it will be less conspicuous.

Late Effects of Radiotherapy

Most of the deleterious effects of breast conservation on breast appearance are due to the partial mastectomy and the distortion of breast shape that it creates. Over the

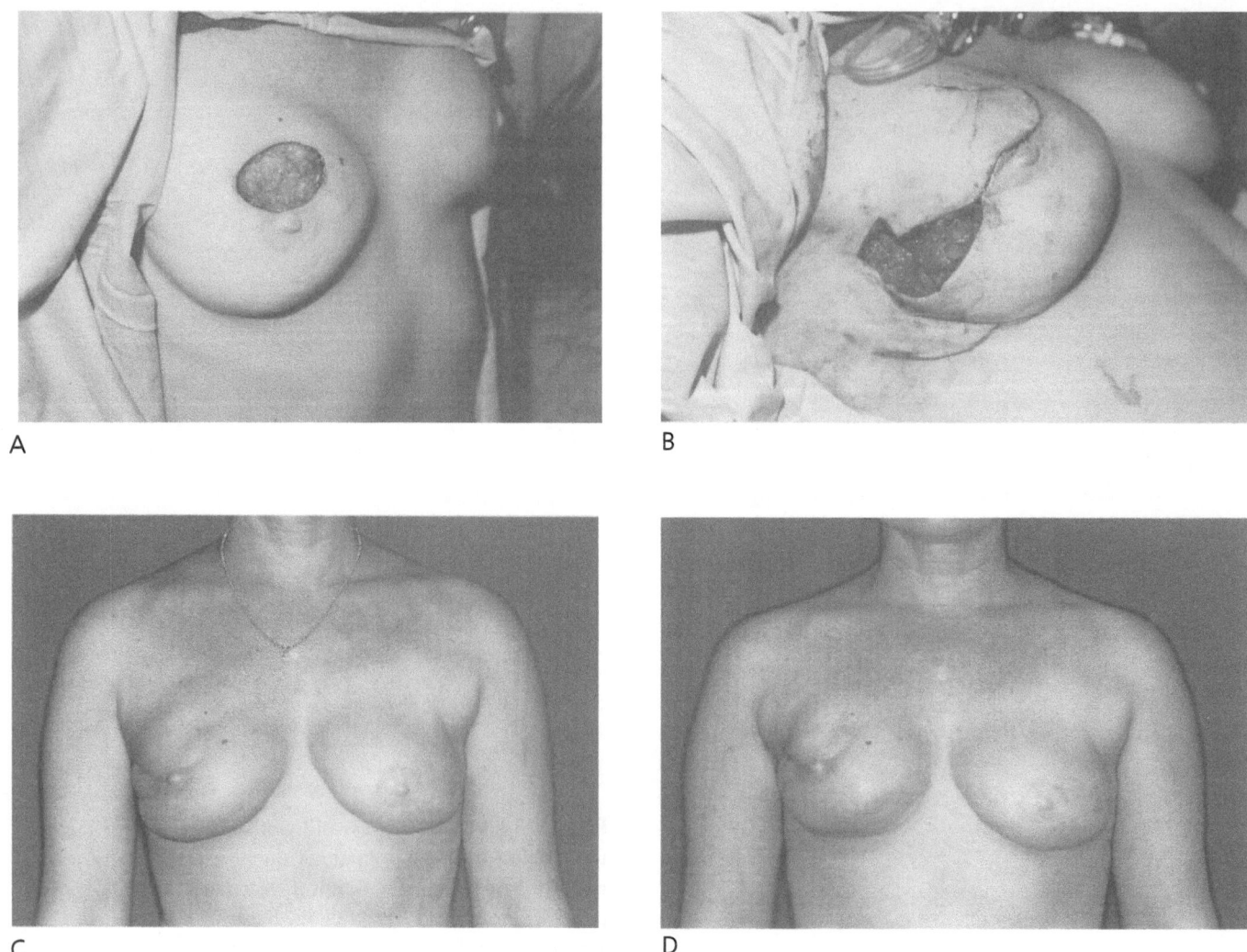

FIG. 19-15 (A) Patient after bilateral free TRAM flap breast reconstruction who underwent excision of a local recurrence in the upper pole of the right reconstructed breast. (B) The defect was repaired with a bilobed superiorly based flap or skin, breast tissue, and subcutaneous fat. (C) Result after 6 months appeared to be good. (D) Unfortunately, the patient then had to be treated with additional radiotherapy, and after 18 months this induced fibrosis, which caused the nipple to become displaced superiorly.

long term, however, irradiation can also induce changes that can harm the appearance of the breast.[8,10] These changes can include skin hyperpigmentation, telangiectasia, and fibrosis. The changes can range from mild to severe, and tend to increase in severity with time. Radiotherapy can even induce sarcomas (Fig 19-16). Although modern radiotherapy treatment methods have reduced the incidence of these problems, deleterious effects from irradiation continue to exist. These effects tend to be more deleterious when the therapy has been aggressive in an attempt to treat an advanced breast cancer with a worse-than-average prognosis, and invariably become more severe with time. Unfortunately, the only treatment for these radiation injuries is to excise the damaged tissue and replace it with a distant flap (Fig 19-17). This

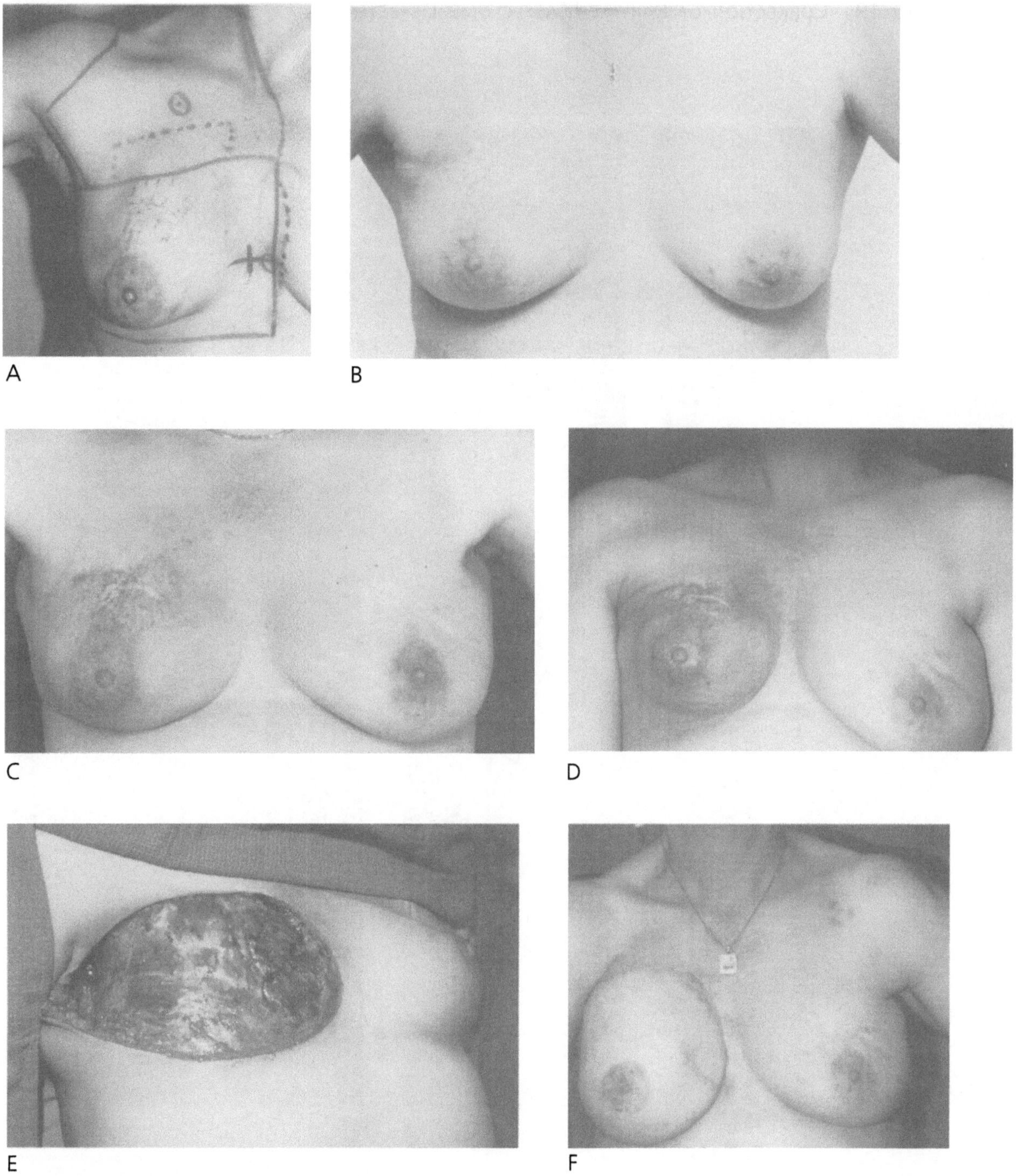

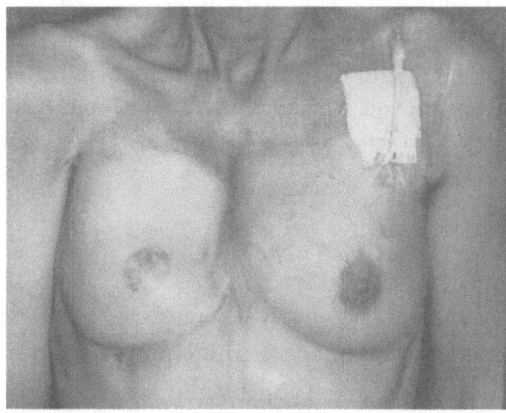

FIG. 19-16 (A) Patient treated for early breast cancer with partial mastectomy and irradiation in 1976. (B) Three years later, the aesthetic result appeared to be excellent. (C) Eleven years after treatment, the breast was showing changes from the radiotherapy. (D) Twelve years after treatment, the breast had changed markedly, and an irradiation-induced sarcoma had appeared. (E) Wide excision of the sarcoma was performed. (F) The chest wall was reconstructed with a TRAM flap, which was shaped into a rough facsimile of a breast. (G) Ultimately (17 years after her radiotherapy), the patient developed systemic metastases. Because of weight loss, the TRAM flap has become much smaller.

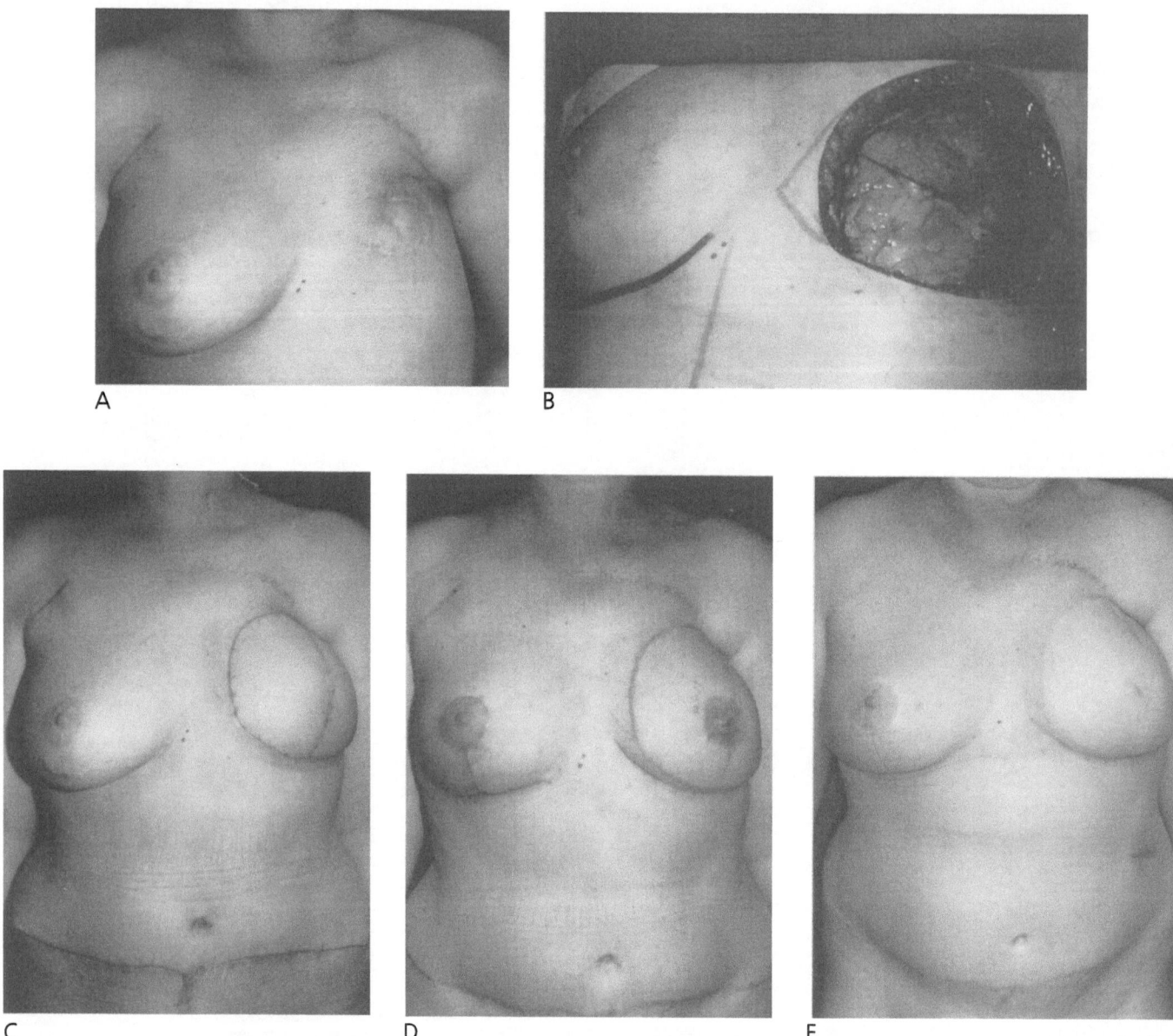

FIG. 19-17   (A) Patient who had been treated for carcinoma of the left breast with mastectomy and irradiation. She subsequently had developed a radiation-induced sarcoma. (B) The sarcoma was treated by wide local excision, leaving a full-thickness defect of the chest wall. (C) The chest wall was reconstructed with a double-pedicled TRAM flap. Fortuitously, there was sufficient tissue to allow creation of a breast mound. (D) The opposite breast underwent reduction, leading to reasonable symmetry considering the circumstances. (E) Nine years later, the patient was free of disease and the reconstruction remained successful. (From Kroll SS, Larson DL: Chest wall reconstruction. In: Kroll SS, ed. *Reconstructive Plastic Surgery for Cancer*. St. Louis: Mosby, 1996; Used with permission.)

treatment is obviously radical and is reserved for only the most severe cases. The best management for radiation-induced collateral tissue damage is therefore avoidance, through careful treatment planning and meticulous execution by the radiation on-cologist.

Summary

Breast deformity caused by partial mastectomy can often be partially or completely corrected by replacing the missing breast tissue with a flap. Local flaps are generally preferred, if sufficient tissue is available. Often, the defect can be shifted to a less conspicuous site, such as the subaxillary region, outside the breast mound. Sometimes the nipple must also be repositioned, using techniques similar to those used in mastopexy. Not every partial mastectomy defect can be satisfactorily repaired with a local flap, however. In some cases, particularly if an aggressive axillary dissection has been performed and the amount of remaining local tissue is limited, distant tissue will be required to successfully restore a normal shape to the breast. In that case, the latissimus dorsi flap is usually the best choice.

References

1. Fisher B, Redmond C, Poisson R, et al. Eight-year results of a randomized clinical trial comparing total mastectomy and lumpectomy with or without irradiation in the treatment of breast cancer. *N Engl J Med.* 1989;320:822–828.

2. Fisher B, Bauer M, Margolese R. Five-year results of a randomized clinical trial comparing total mastectomy and segmental mastectomy with or without radiation in the TX of breast cancer. *N Engl J Med.* 1985;313:665.

3. Fisher ER, Fisher B, Sass R, Wickherham L. Pathologic findings from the National Surgical Adjuvant Breast Project (protocol no. 4) XI. Bilateral breast cancer. *Cancer.* 1984;54:3002–3011.

4. Fisher B, Redmond C, Fisher ER, et al. Ten-year results of a randomized clinical trial comparing radical mastectomy and total mastectomy with or without radiation. *N Engl J Med.* 1985;312:674–681.

5. Matory WE Jr, Wertheimer M, Fitzgerald TJ, Walton RL, Love S, Matory WE. Aesthetic results following partial mastectomy and radiation therapy. *Plast Reconstr Surg.* 1990;85:739–746.

6. Lu LB, Shoaib BO, Patten BM. Atypical chest pain syndrome in patients with breast implants. *South Med J.* 1994;87:978–984. ,

7. Rounet P, Pujol H. Conservative surgery of breast cancer: development of ideas and methods [in French]. *Presse Med.* 1993;22:1005–1009.

8. Bold RJ, Kroll SS, Balwin BJ, Ross MI, Singletary SE. Local rotational flaps for breast conservation therapy as an alternative to mastectomy. *Ann Surg Oncol.* 1997;4:540–544.

9. Berrino P, Campora E, Leone S, Santi P. Correction of type II breast deformities following conservative cancer surgery. *Plast Reconstr Surg.* 1992;90:846–853.

10. Kroll SS, Singletary SE. Repair of partial mastectomy defects. *Clin Plast Surg.* 1998;25:303–310.

11. Monticciolo DL, Ross D, Bostwick J, Eaves F, Styblo T. Autologous breast reconstruction with endoscopic latissimus dorsi musculocutaneous flaps in patients choosing breast-conserving therapy. *AJR Am J Roentgenol.* 1996;167:385–389.

12. Slavin SA, Love SM, Sadowski NL. Reconstruction of the radiated partial mastectomy defect with autogenous tissues. *Plast Reconstr Surg.* 1993;90:854–865.

13. Clough KB, Baruch J. Plastic surgery and conservative treatment of breast cancer. Indications and results [in French]. *Ann Chir Plast Esthet.* 1998;37:682–692.

14. Benelli L. A new periareolar mammaplasty: round block technique. *Aesthetic Plastic Surg.* 1990;14:99.

15. Kroll SS, Doores S. Nipple centralization for the correction of breast deformity from segmental mastectomy. *Ann Plast Surg.* 1990;24:271–275.

16. Lassus C. A 30-year experience with vertical mammaplasty. *Plast Reconstr Surg.* 1996;97:373–380.

17. Daher JC. Breast island flaps. *Ann Plast Surg.* 1993;30:217–223.

20 Breast Mound Revision Surgery

Goals of Revision Surgery

The goal of breast mound revision is to create a mound that matches the opposite breast in size and shape when the patient is standing. Breast mound revisions are frequently required because in the operating room, during the initial breast mound reconstruction, it is impossible to stand the patient up and compare the two breasts in the upright position. Consequently, the surgeon must use artistic judgment and make educated guesses based on the patient's appearance while supine. Some of these guesses will be wrong, and corrections will be needed at a later date. Also, there are limitations to how much shaping can be performed without jeopardizing the viability of the flap while all of its blood supply is coming from one source, the pedicle. Because of these problems, some revision of each autologous tissue breast reconstruction is almost always necessary. Revisions are usually only minor surgery and can often be performed under local anesthesia, but they are extremely important because they can make the difference between results that are only fair and outcomes that are excellent. In revision surgery, the surgeon attempts to correct errors and achieve symmetry.[1] Ideally, this is accomplished without requiring surgical intervention on the opposite breast,[2] but that is not always possible.

During the revision surgery the same difficulty with positioning is present, but the surgeon has the advantage of being able to plan the revision and mark the patient preoperatively in the upright position. Moreover, the breast mound and some degree of symmetry already exist. Because there is less need for radical change, the chance of achieving symmetry is better than was the case in the initial reconstruction. Also, the constraints imposed by the limited blood supply of the flap will have vanished, so more aggressive shaping is possible. Nevertheless, breast mound revision surgery is not always easy. At times, the artistic and technical challenges can be much greater than those presented by the actual transfer of a free transverse rectus abdominus myocutaneous (TRAM) flap.

Surgical Alteration of the Opposite Breast

Sometimes the easiest way to achieve breast symmetry is to alter the opposite, natural breast. This is especially indicated when the natural breast is larger or more ptotic than the reconstructed one. In some cases, alteration of the natural breast is indicated when it is smaller than the reconstructed one but the patient prefers the size of the reconstructed mound and requests contralateral augmentation. This subject will be discussed more thoroughly in chapter 21. When the opposite natural breast is attractive, it is usually preferable to match it by altering the reconstructed breast. In this way, scarring is minimized and the patient's body image is less disturbed. Moreover, any possible interference by scarring with subsequent surveillance of the opposite breast (to detect early signs of a second contralateral primary tumor) is completely avoided.

Common Techniques for Revision of the Reconstructed Breast

The techniques I use most commonly to revise a reconstructed breast mound include suction lipectomy, direct excision of excess tissue, reduction mammaplasty techniques, and internal shifting of tissue within the breast mound using V-to-Y island flaps. Each approach has advantages and disadvantages, and has certain situations for which it would be the method of choice.

Suction Lipectomy

The easiest, and therefore best, approach to reduction of excessive size when overall breast shape is good and the size excess is not substantial would, in theory, be suction lipectomy. Ideally, this would reduce the size of the breast without changing its shape or adding visible scars. In practice, however, suction lipectomy provides variable results. Some reconstructed breasts respond well to suction lipectomy, giving up fat freely and reducing substantially in size, while others seem to respond poorly. Prior injection with saline solution containing very dilute (1:1,000,000) epinephrine will reduce blood loss and make the liposuction more effective.[3–5] In my opinion, liposuction is worth trying whenever a relatively small amount of reduction is desired, but the surgeon should always have a backup plan in case the suction is ineffective. For overall reduction of breast size, suction lipectomy works best when only a moderate reduction is required. For a more radical change, direct excision or a reduction mammaplasty technique is usually necessary.

The most common use of suction lipectomy in my practice is to alter the shape of the breast using localized liposuction within the breast mound. Liposuction is especially useful for reducing areas that are not easily accessible to direct excision, such as the medial or superior part of the breast mound in a patient who has had an immediate reconstruction after a skin-sparing mastectomy (Fig 20-1). Through the use of li-

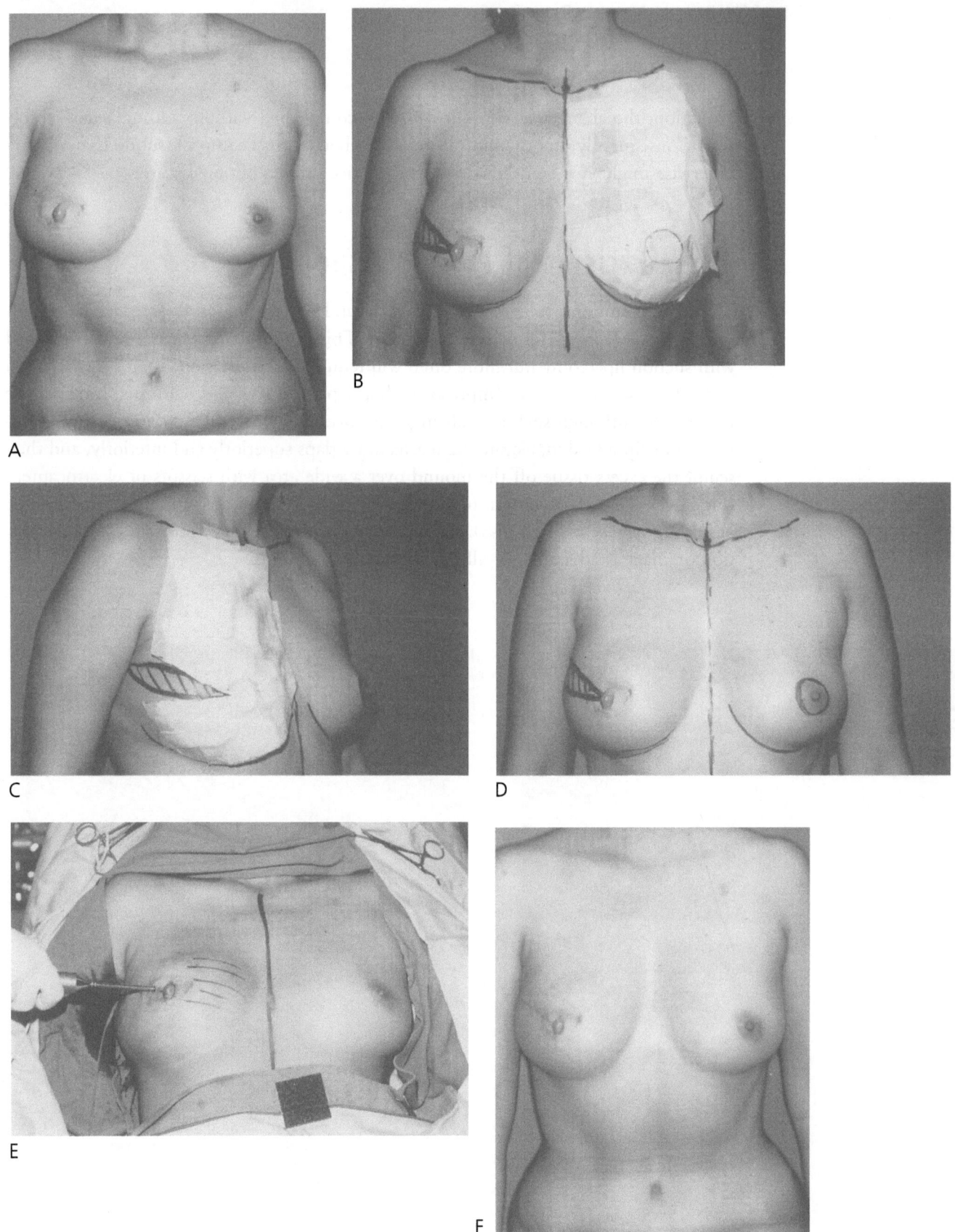

FIG. 20-1 (A) Patient after immediate right breast reconstruction with a free TRAM flap. The reconstructed mound is too large. (B) A paper tape template was made of the opposite breast. (C) The template was inverted and used to design a skin resection from the reconstructed breast. (D) Final pattern for skin and fat resection on the reconstructed breast. (E) Tissue was surgically excised laterally, but liposuction was required medially to reduce the breast without introducing additional scarring. (F) After revision with liposuction, the symmetry is significantly improved.

posuction, the changes in contour can be accomplished without adding a new visible scar. Consequently, liposuction can be used liberally to accomplish subtle changes that otherwise might not be deemed worth the price of an additional scar.

Direct Excision of Excess Tissue

The most common problem after breast mound reconstruction is excessive lateral tissue, particularly in the upper outer quadrant. This can sometimes be adequately reached with suction lipectomy but more often will require direct excision. If an ellipse of skin and subcutaneous tissue is simply excised, a depressed scar and deformed breast shape may result. Although such a result may improve with time, a better approach is to remove an ellipse of skin, elevate the mastectomy flaps superiorly and inferiorly, and then sculpt the excess tissue off the mound over a wide area with scissors or electrocautery (Fig 20-2). This approach can provide a nice result without deforming the breast shape or adding new scars (Fig 20-3). It does not, however, improve breast projection. Suction drainage is advisable for all but the smallest wounds.

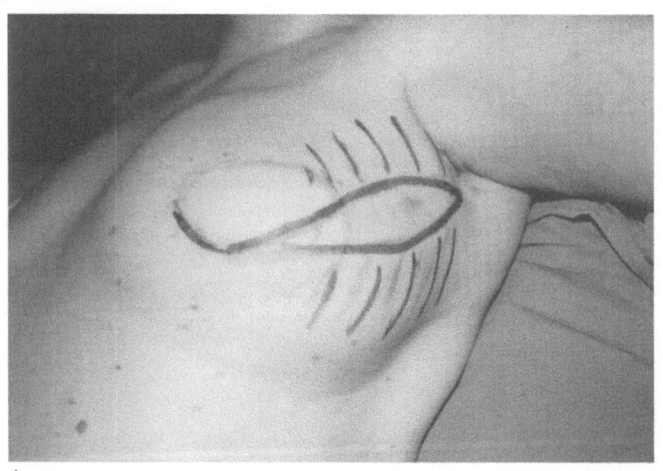

A

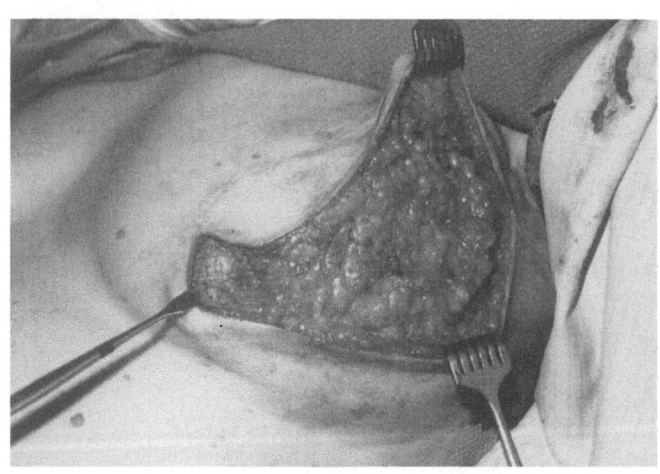

B

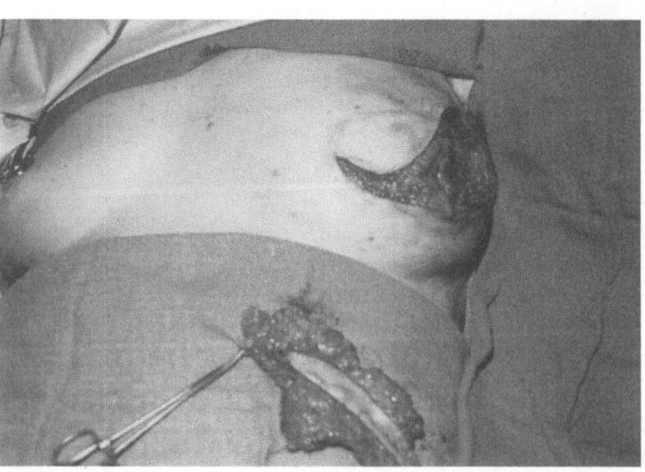

C

FIG. 20-2 (A) Plan for sculpting away excess tissue from the upper outer quadrant. (B) The mastectomy flaps are elevated to expose the TRAM flap. (C) The tissue resected from the reconstructed breast, containing more fat than skin.

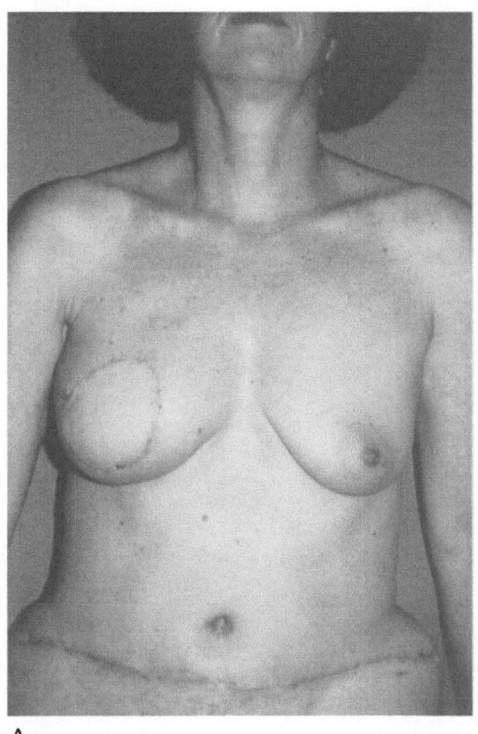
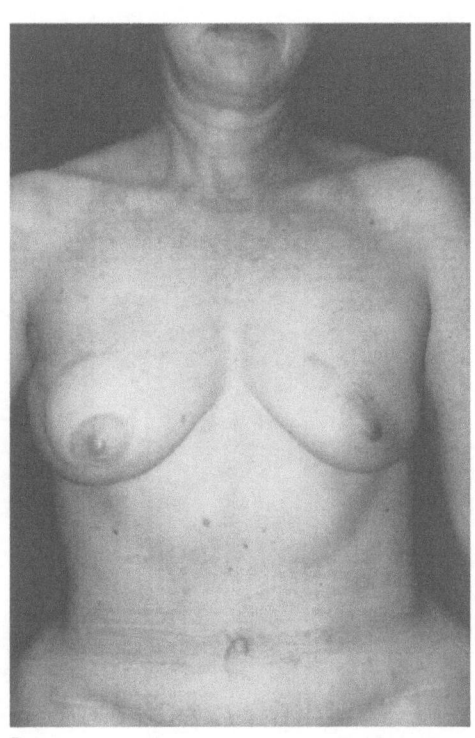

A   B

FIG. 20-3   (A) Patient after breast reconstruction with a free TRAM flap, showing excess lateral fullness. (B) Same patient after revision, showing improved symmetry. See color insert, p. I-19.

Use of Reduction Mammaplasty Techniques

Another very effective way to reduce overall breast size is to resect a triangle of skin and fat from the lower pole, using an approach similar to that used in some reduction mammaplasties. This approach works best when the autologous tissue flap has a superiorly based blood supply (as in a free flap). In fact, the ability to use this revision technique is one of the advantages of using free flaps for breast reconstruction. Medial and lateral breast flaps are developed using an incision along the inframammary fold, and these flaps are mobilized toward the breast meridian where they are sutured together (Fig 20-4). Tissue is sculpted away from the lower border of the breast as necessary. By resection of tissue that includes all of the base of a triangle from the lower pole, but by sparing some of the tissue deep to the superior tip of this triangle, this technique encourages the breast to assume a pyramidal shape that will increase projection under the new areola.

An excellent way to design this revision is to make a paper tape template of the opposite breast, then turn it over and mark the pattern on the reconstructed breast (Fig 20-5). In this way, the skin brassiere of the reconstructed breast becomes a mirror image of the natural one. Moreover, some of the excess skin that would normally be discarded during this maneuver can be used to create a nipple (Fig 20-6), avoiding the flattening of the breast mound usually associated with nipple reconstruction.

A similar approach can be used to resect an ellipse of skin from the lateral breast mound (Fig 20-7). A paper tape template is made of the opposite breast as in the tech-

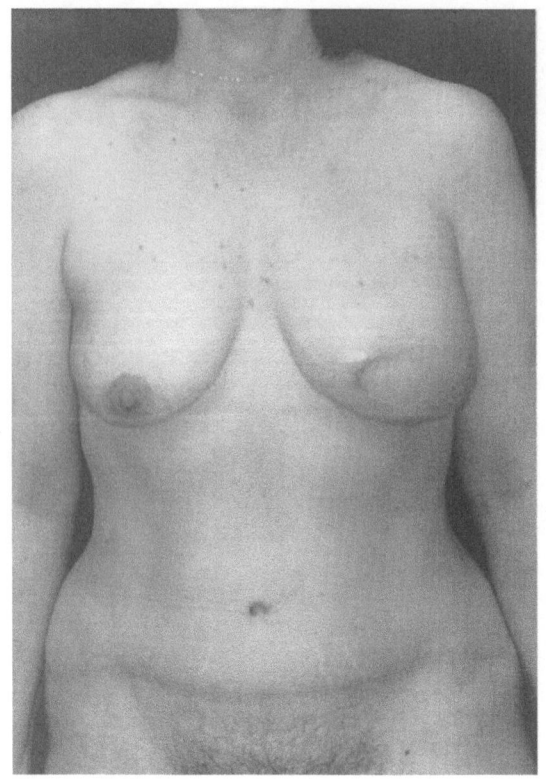

A

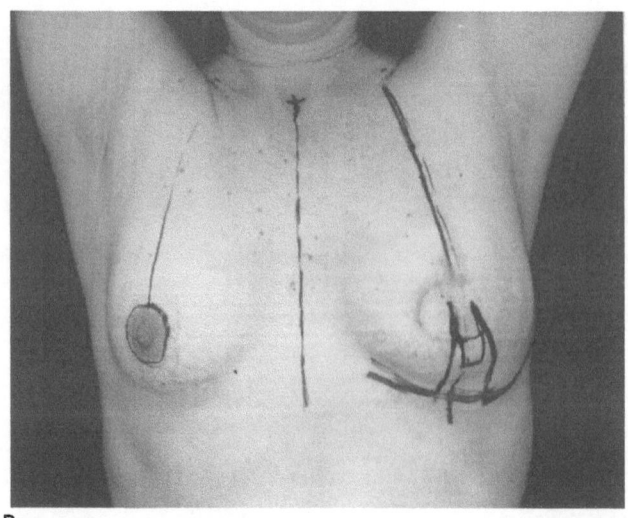

B

FIG. 20-4 (A) Patient with a breast reconstructed with a free TRAM flap that is larger than the opposite, natural breast. (B) Reduction of breast size by resection of a triangle of tissue from the lower pole. A small superiorly based flap is used to provide tissue for nipple reconstruction. Medial and lateral breast flaps are mobilized and sutured together at the breast meridian, as in a reduction mammaplasty. (C) After revision, but before definitive nipple reconstruction. See color insert., p. I-19.

C

nique described above, but the template is opened laterally instead of inferiorly. The template is used to predict how much skin must be resected from the lateral part of reconstructed mound to achieve symmetry with the natural breast. This approach has the advantage of not creating a new scar on the inferior pole of the breast. Redundant skin can still be used to create a nipple, but the projection in the inferior pole is not augmented, and the inframammary fold is not elevated.

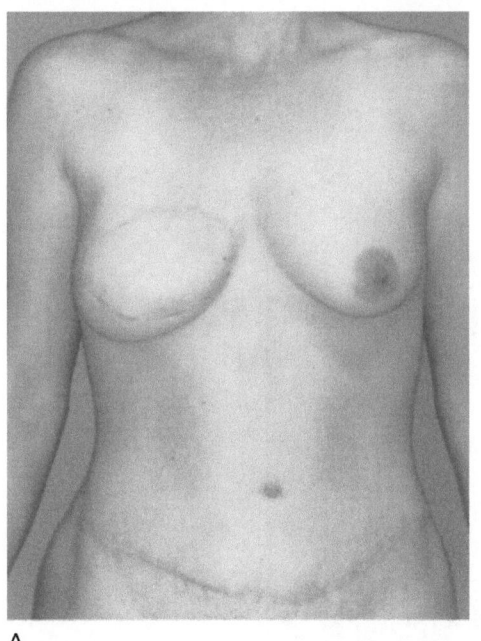

A

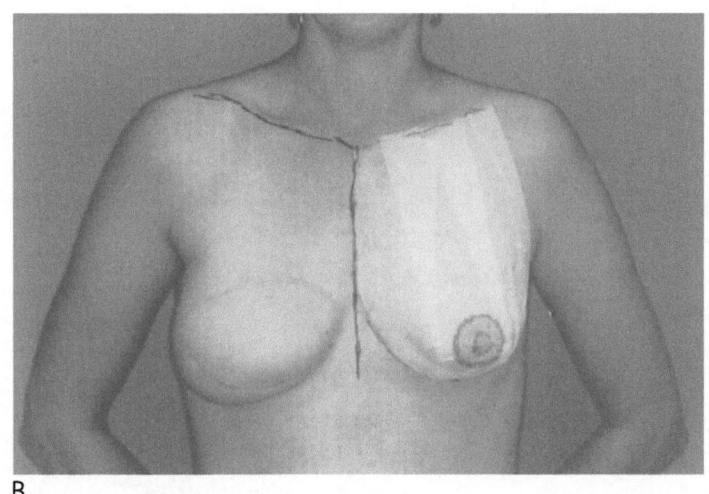

B

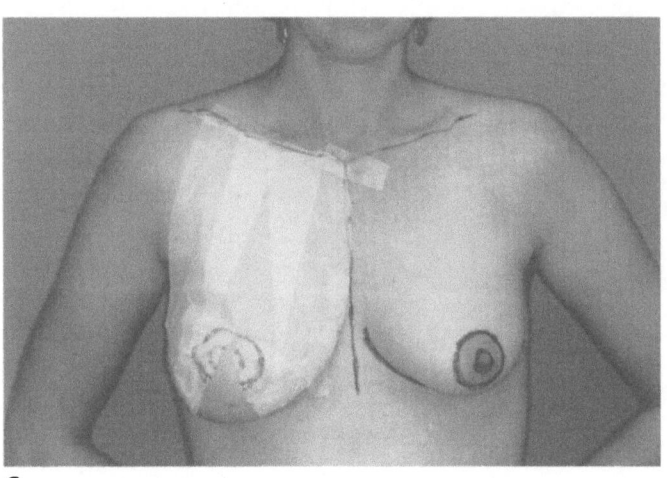

C

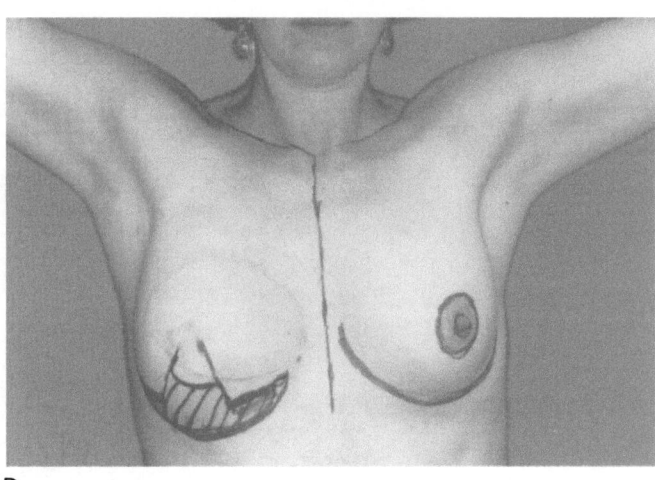

D

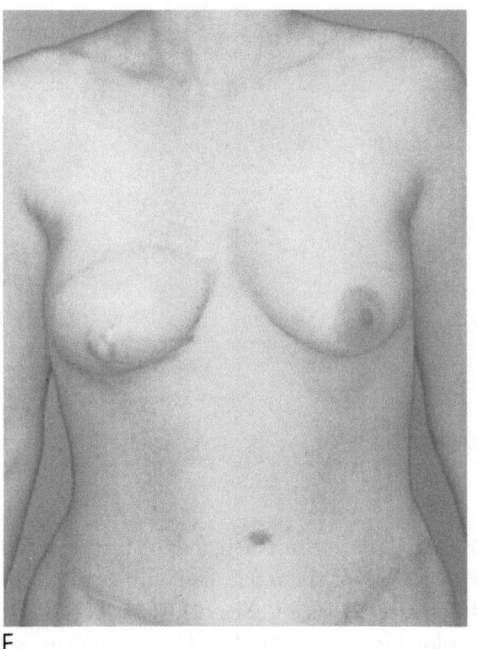

E

FIG. 20-5 (A) Patient with an immediate free TRAM flap breast reconstruction that is larger than her opposite natural breast. (B) The midline, clavicle, and inframammary fold are marked on the natural breast, and a paper tape mask is created to form a template. (C) The tape mask is removed, spit inferiorly, turned over, and placed symmetrically on the reconstructed breast, using the midline and the clavicle as guides. (D) The pattern is used as a plant for reduction of the reconstructed mound. Some of the skin excess becomes a superiorly based flap for nipple reconstruction. (E) After one revision using this approach, symmetry is much improved. Nipple reconstruction is not finished, however.

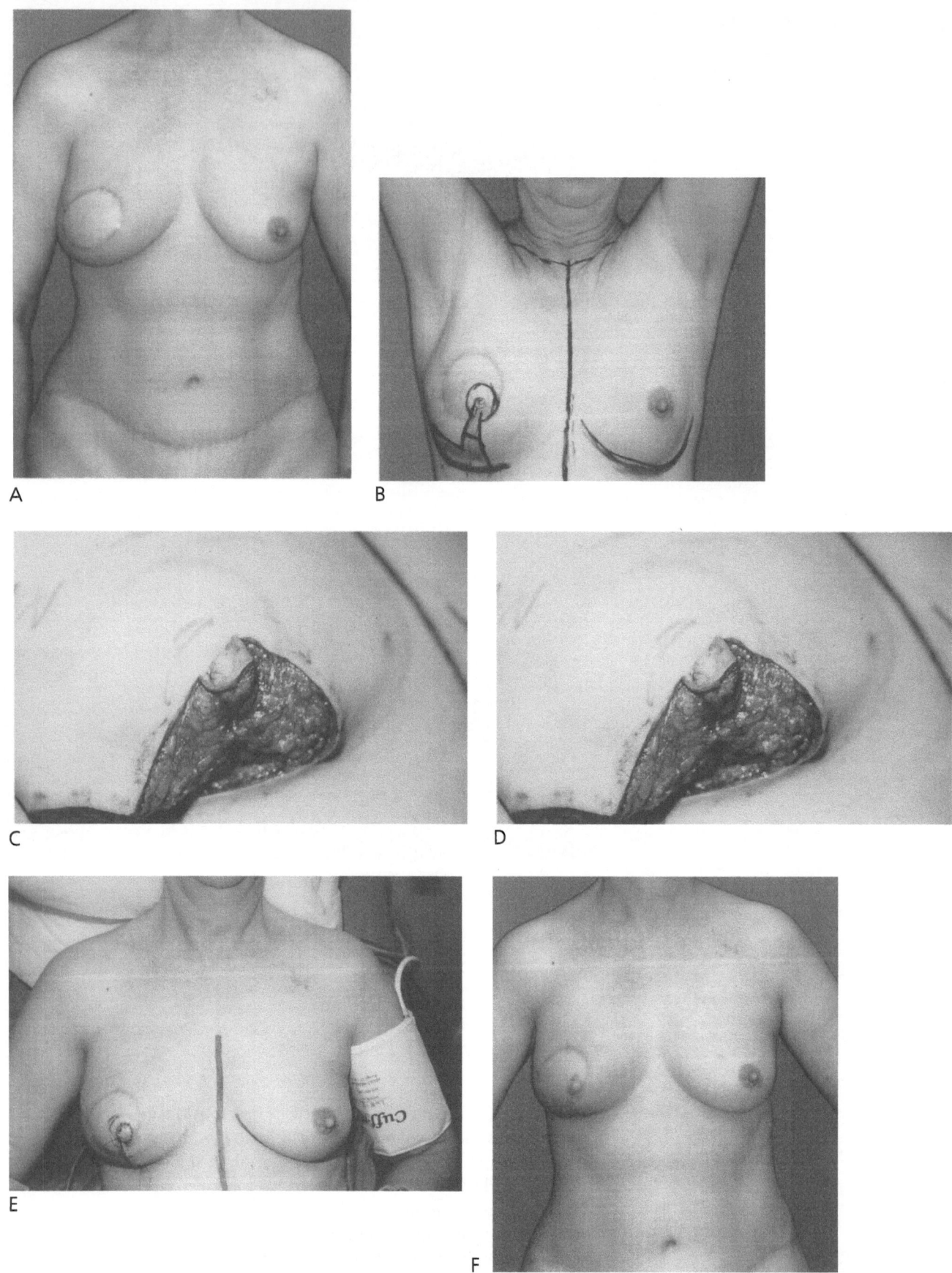

FIG. 20-6   (A) Patient after breast mound reconstruction with a free TRAM flap. The reconstructed right breast is too large. See color insert, p. I-20. (B) Pattern for reduction of reconstructed breast, with use of the redundant skin as a "wrap-around" flap to create a nipple. See color insert, p. I-20. (C) The wrap-around flap after elevation. See color insert, p. I-21. (D) The flap is turned medially upon itself to create a projecting nipple. See color insert, p. I-21. (E) The immediate result in the operating room. See color insert, p. I-22. (F) The same patient 3 weeks later. See color insert, p. I-22.

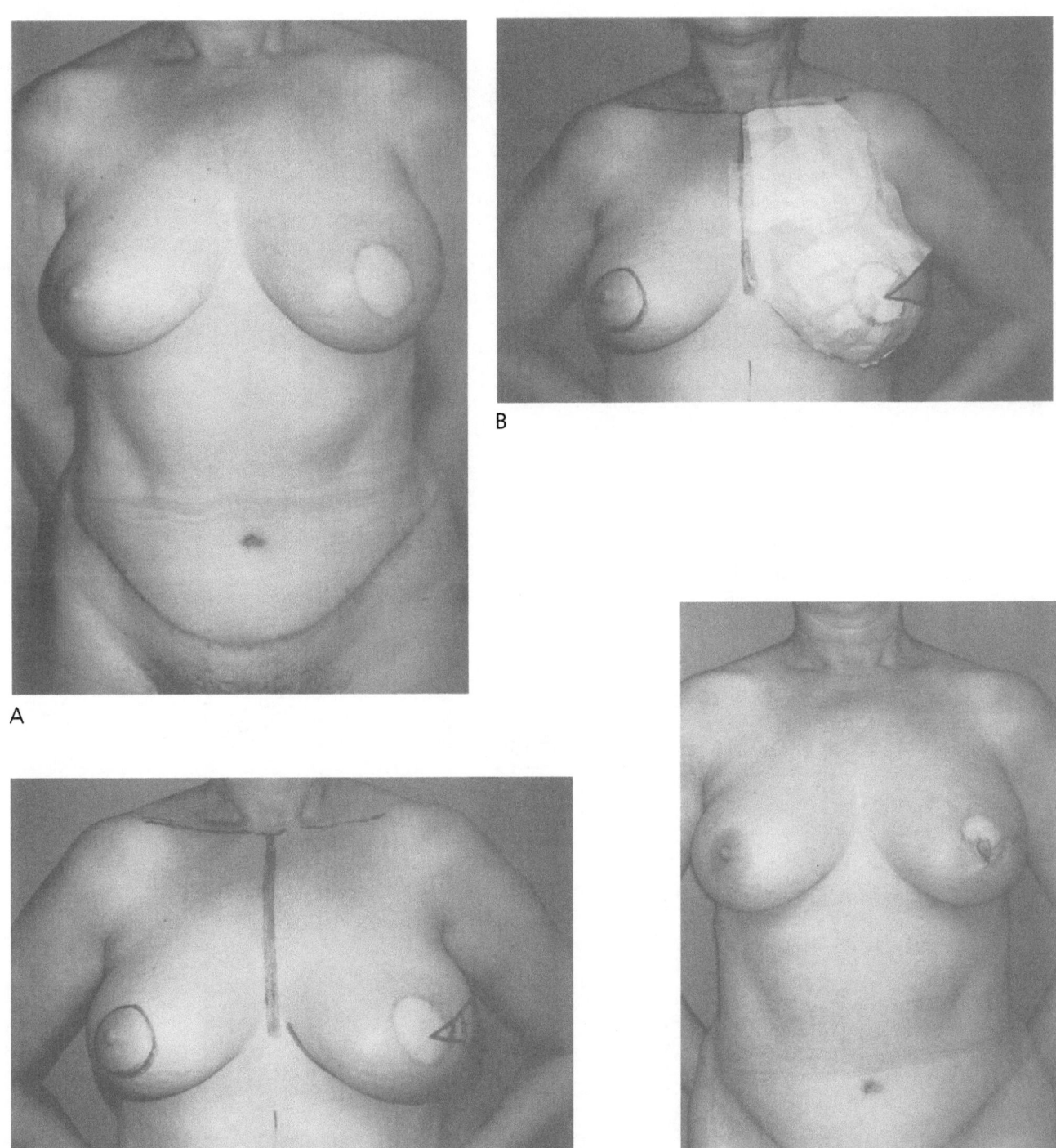

FIG. 20-7   (A) Patient with excess tissue laterally after free TRAM flap breast reconstruction. (B) A paper tape template is made from the opposite breast, then turned inside-out and used to design the reduction of the skin brassiere of the reconstructed breast. (C) Operative plan. (D) Result of revision and of nipple reconstruction using the "wrap-around" flap created from redundant skin.

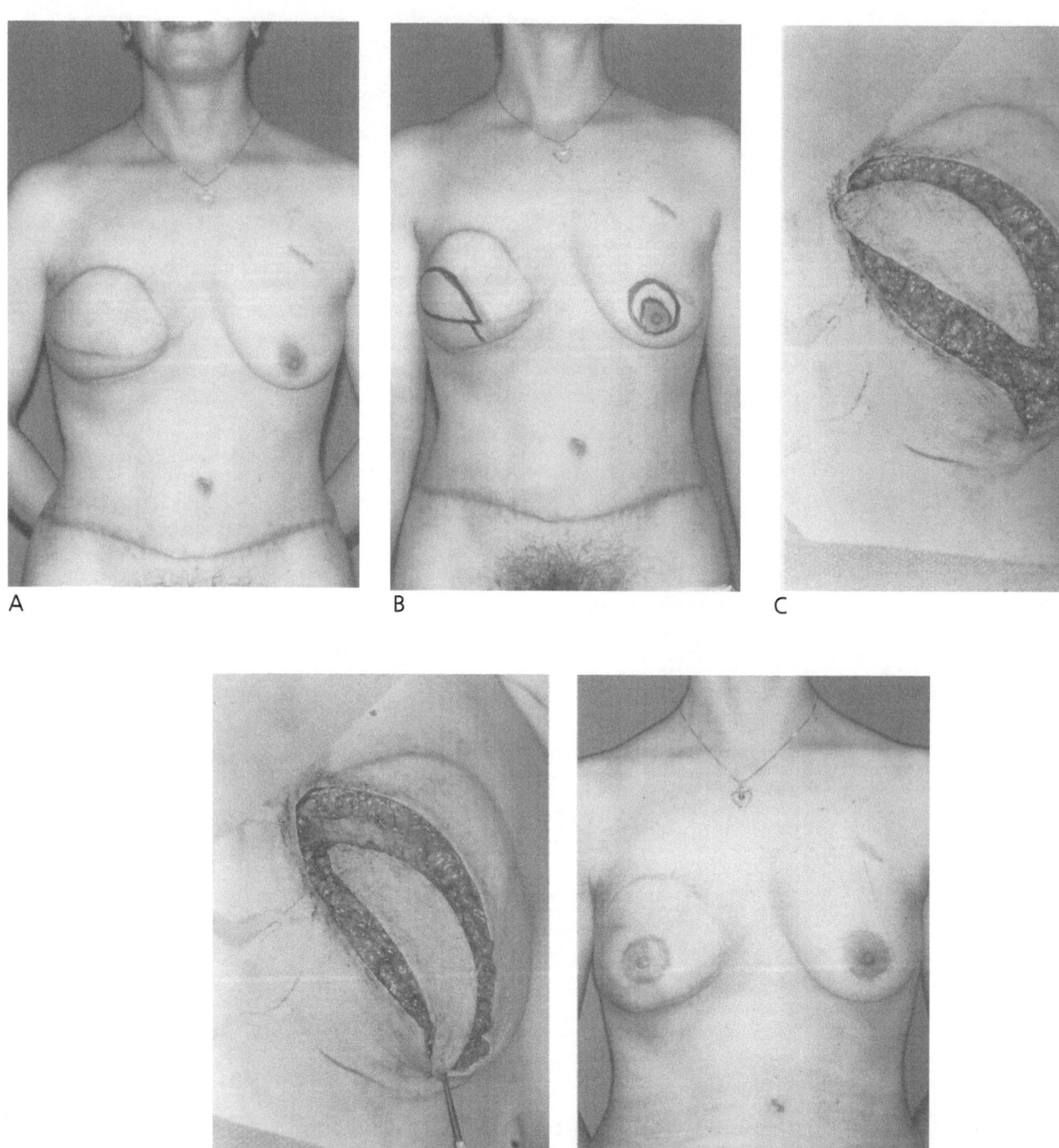

FIG. 20-8 (A) Reconstructed breast mound that is too full in the upper outer quadrant and has insufficient projection inferiorly. (B, C, D) V-to-Y island flap is designed to move tissue toward the lower pole. (E) The result is a better balanced breast with increased projection inferiorly, where it belongs. See color insert, p. I-23.

Internal Shifting of Tissue with V-to-Y Flaps

Not infrequently, a deficiency of tissue in one part of the breast mound will be combined with an excess of tissue elsewhere in the breast. In some cases, this excess can be transferred to the part of the breast that is in need of it by using a large subcutaneously based V-to-Y island flap. The most common indication for this technique is an excess of tissue in the upper outer quadrant of the breast combined with a deficiency of projection and tissue in the lower pole (Fig 20-8). Although the tissue excess may be located far from the deficient area, the flap itself does not move very far. The flap must be large enough to have its tail in the area of excess and the tip within 1 or 2 cm of the area of deficiency. The flap is based on a subcutaneous pedicle, and must be freed up enough that sufficient tissue is transferred to the deficient area (usually the lower pole of the breast) but not so much that viability of the tissue is threatened. The tip of the flap should be expected to move no more than 1 to 2 cm, but the tail and midportion can often advance a greater distance. The skin paddle of the flap should be large enough to include several subcutaneous perforators. Designs with small skin islands, therefore, should be avoided.

This technique is most often used for augmentation of the lower pole of the breast, but can also be used to correct deficiencies medially (Fig 20-9) or even centrally (Fig 20-10). It is especially useful for localized deformities caused by partial flap loss or excision of areas of fat necrosis that have failed to resolve spontaneously.

Less Commonly Used Techniques

Increasing the Reconstructed Breast Mound Size

A reconstructed breast that is smaller than the opposite one is best corrected by reduction of the natural breast unless the reconstructed breast is obviously too small. In some cases, however, the patient will not consent to this and insists on enlarging the reconstructed breast. By far, the easiest way to do this is with an implant (Fig 20-11). If the implant is relatively small, any casular contracture that occurs can be effectively camouflaged by the soft overlying tissue of the autologous tissue reconstruction. I generally prefer saline-filled implants, which have a lower rate of capsular contracture than silicone gel–filled implants but are more likely to leak and require eventual replacement. The smaller the implant, the more likely it will be to look natural and avoid the symptoms of capsular contracture.

Small autologous tissue augmentations of the reconstructed breast mound can sometimes be accomplished with local flaps from the subaxillary or inframammary skin. If much tissue will be needed, however, a large flap like a latissimus dorsi flap may be required. This approach was often necessary in the early days of TRAM flap breast reconstruction, when partial flap losses were more common. Today, with free TRAM flaps, partial losses are much rarer, and supplementary latissimus dorsi or other major flaps are rarely required.

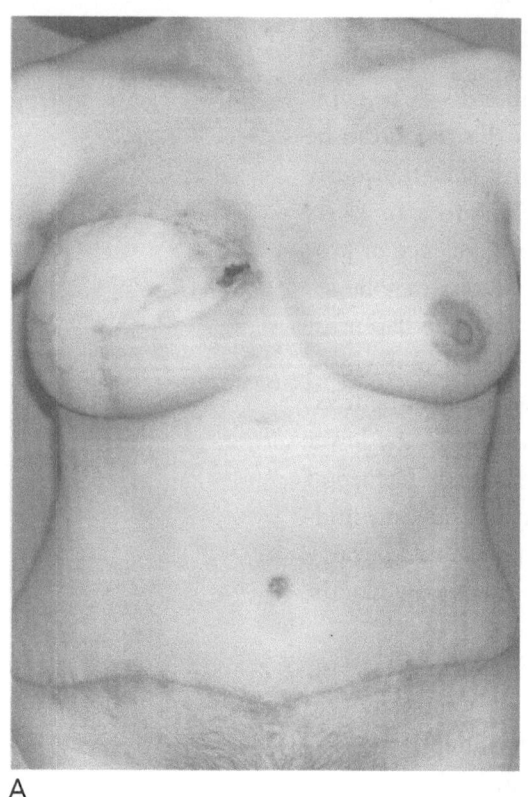

A

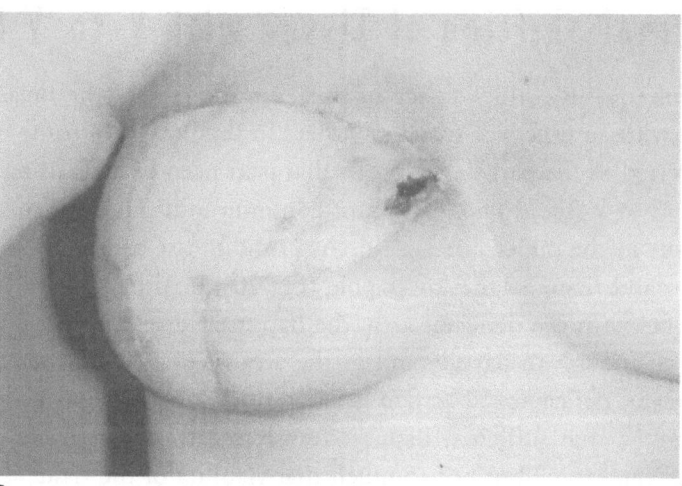

B

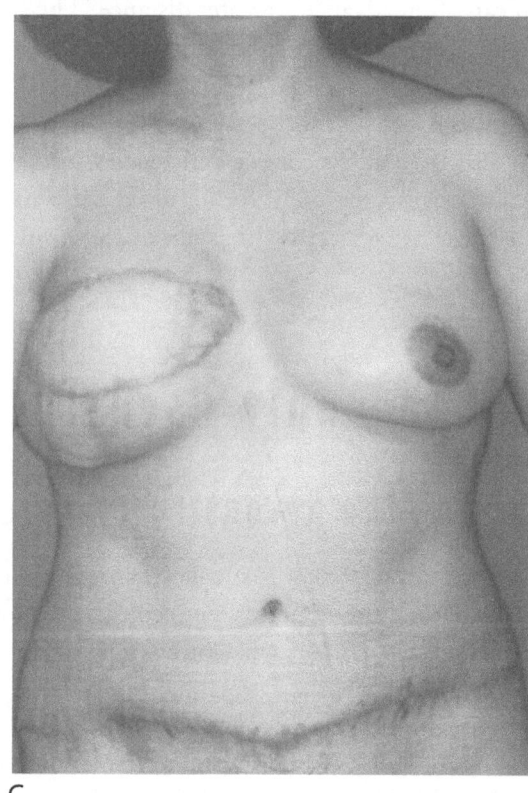

C

FIG. 20-9 (A) Patient after a deep inferior epigastric perforator flap who had medial fat necrosis that was resected in the clinic. (B) Close-up of breast mound after resection of the fat necrosis. (C) After correction of the medial defect with a V-to-Y island flap that consisted of most of the upper portion of the flap. Note the new scar crossing the midportion of the breast.

Moving the Breast More Medially

Occasionally, the surgeon will find that the overall breast size is correct but the mound has been placed too laterally, making clothing and brassieres fit poorly. After a free flap (TRAM or other) reconstruction, this can be corrected effectively by making an inframammary incision, freeing up the lower pole of the breast (taking care not to injure the flap pedicle), and advancing the entire lower breast medially (Fig 20-12).

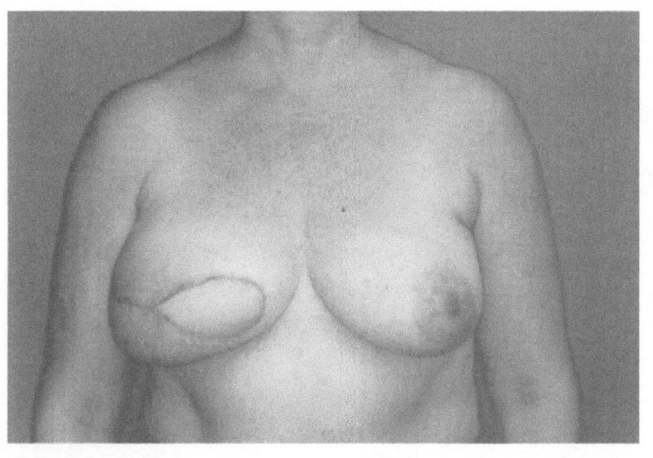
A

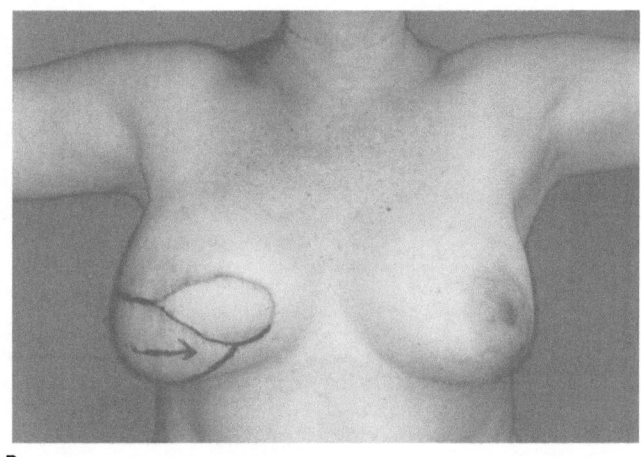
B

C

FIG. 20-10 (A) Patient with a breast mound reconstructed with a free TRAM flap who has a great deal of excess tissue laterally. The breast lacks projection inferiorly, however, and has an inframammary fold that is too flat. (B) A large subcutaneously based V-to-Y island flap is created laterally, then advanced inferomedially to augment the lower pole of the breast. (C) This revision resulted in better inferior pole projection and a more rounded inframammary fold.

Essentially, this approach converts the breast reconstruction into a huge superiorly based flap. It can be successful only when the flap has a superiorly based blood supply. A new inframammary fold is created more medially, with de-epithelialization of the skin between it and the original fold as necessary. The breast is then rotated medially and inset into the new inframammary fold, improving breast symmetry and reducing lateral fullness in one step. A modification of this procedure can also be used to lower the inframammary fold, should that be necessary. The disadvantage of this

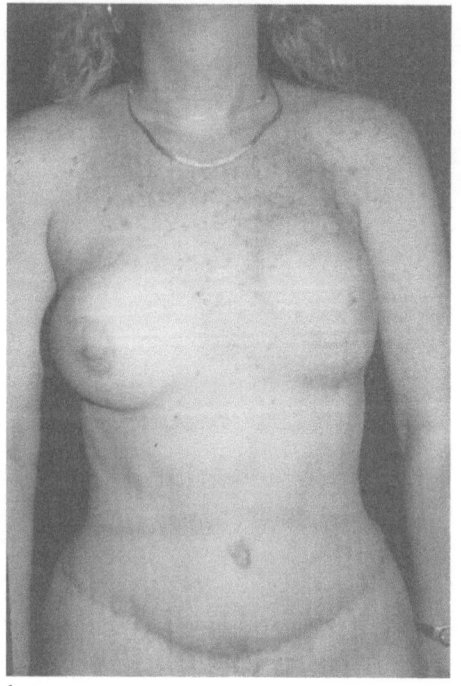
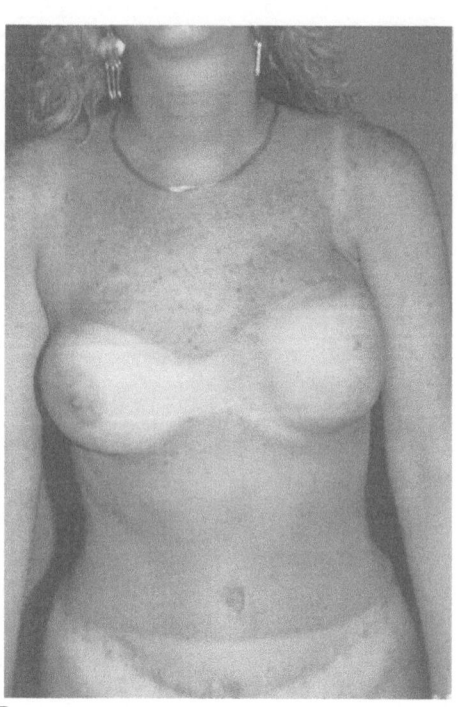

A   B

FIG. 20-11 (A) Patient who underwent previous heavy irradiation and whose reconstructed breast was smaller than the opposite breast. (B) After augmentation of the reconstruction breast with a saline-filled implant, the symmetry is improved, although because of the irradiation it is far from perfect.

approach is a long inframammary scar, but this scar is partially hidden by breast ptosis and in any case is preferable to a malpositioned breast. This method of moving the breast mound might theoretically also be used for mounds reconstructed with pedicled TRAM flaps, but the intervening pedicle would make the process technically more difficult.

Raising the Inframammary Fold

Raising an inframammary fold that is too low can be extremely difficult. Performing a mastopexy by simply excising skin using existing scars is tempting and will achieve a temporary change, but the inframammary fold will usually settle back to its original low position with time. Similarly, freeing up the fold and the surrounding soft tissues and suturing the fold to a higher position on the chest wall will usually achieve only temporary success. This is especially true if the breast mound is large, in which case gravity will work to defeat the surgeon's best efforts.

One approach that I have found effective is to reelevate the inferior mastectomy flap, sculpt fatty tissue away from the lower pole of the breast, and then artificially recreate an inframammary fold with sutures attaching the mastectomy flap to the chest wall at a more superior position (Fig 20-13) or using other suturing techniques similar

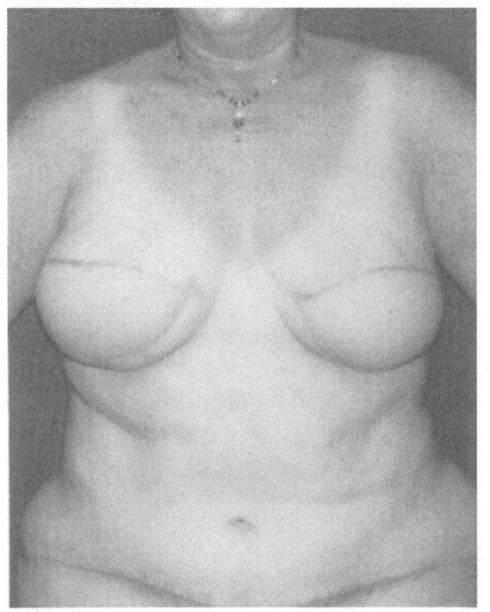

A

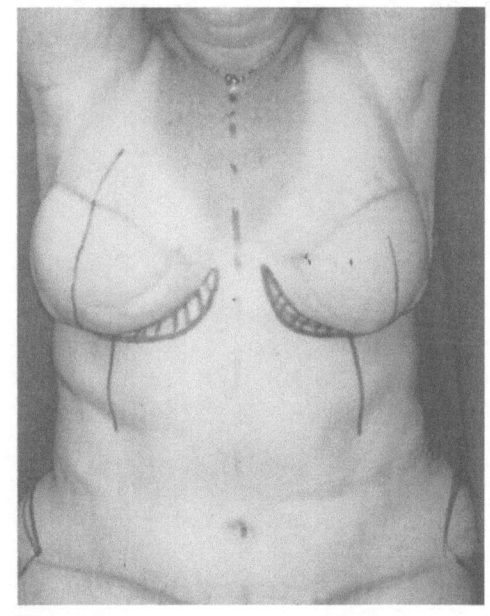

B

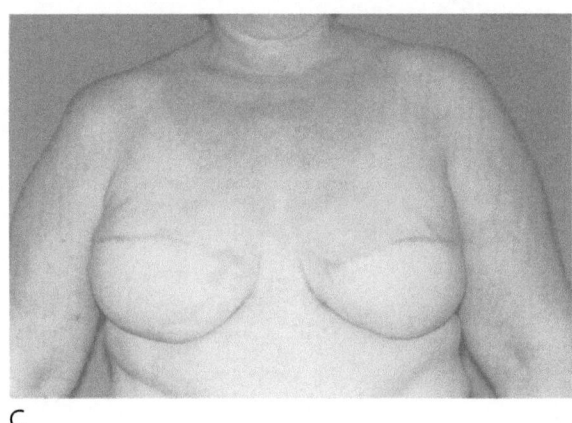

C

FIG. 20-12   (A) After breast mound reconstruction, the breasts are positioned too far laterally. (B) The breasts are made into superiorly based flaps to allow them to move medially. (C) The mounds were moved medially, giving the breasts a slightly more natural appearance although even more medial movement might have been better.

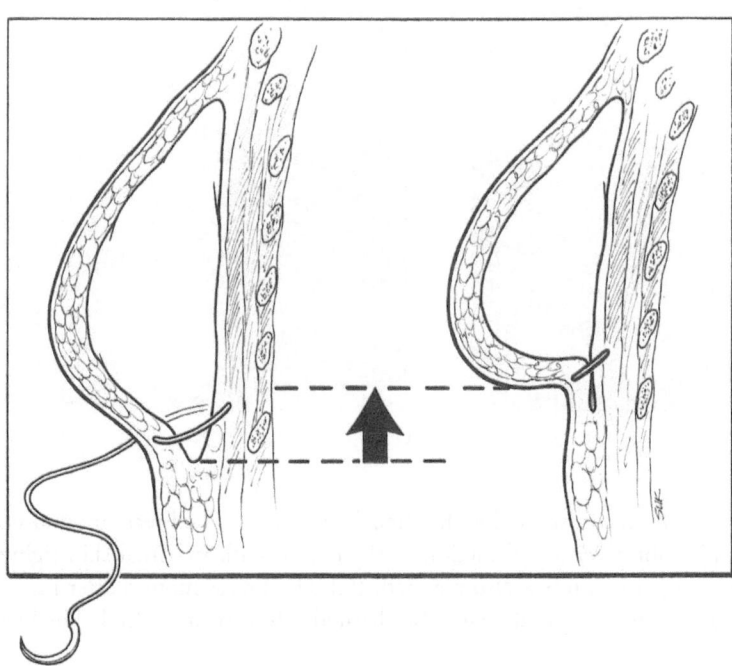

FIG. 20-13   The inframammary fold is positioned more superiorly, creating it with continuous sutures.

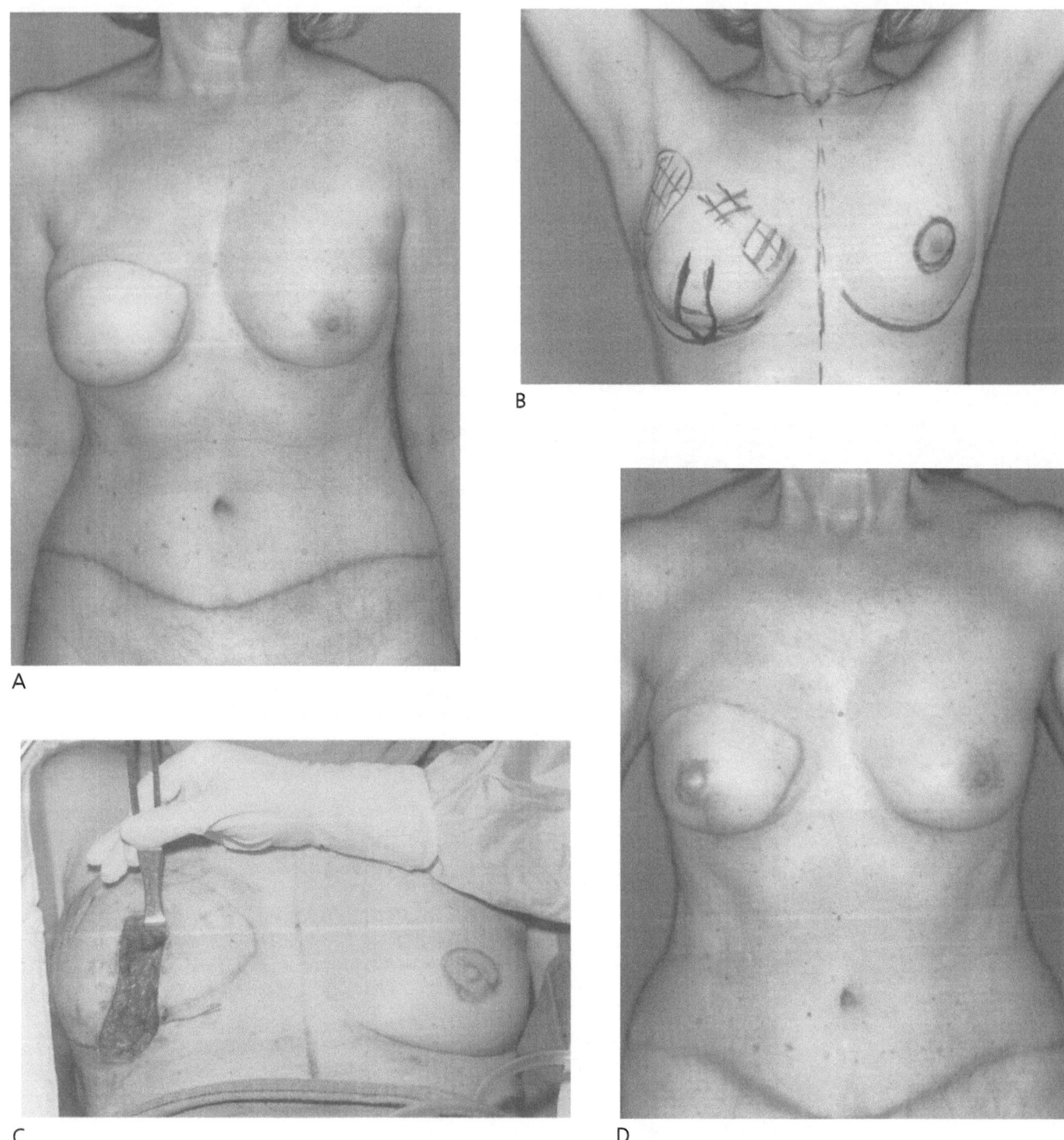

FIG. 20-14 (A) Patient with a right breast mound reconstructed with a free TRAM flap. The breast mound is slightly too large and the inframammary fold is too low. (B) Plan for a vertical reduction of the breast, with maximal skin tightening at the level where the inframammary fold is desired. Some liposuction was also planned. (C) The breast mound after resection of the excess tissue from the lower pole of the breast. (D) The result, clearly showing the elevated inframammary fold. The breast mound, however, was slightly overreduced.

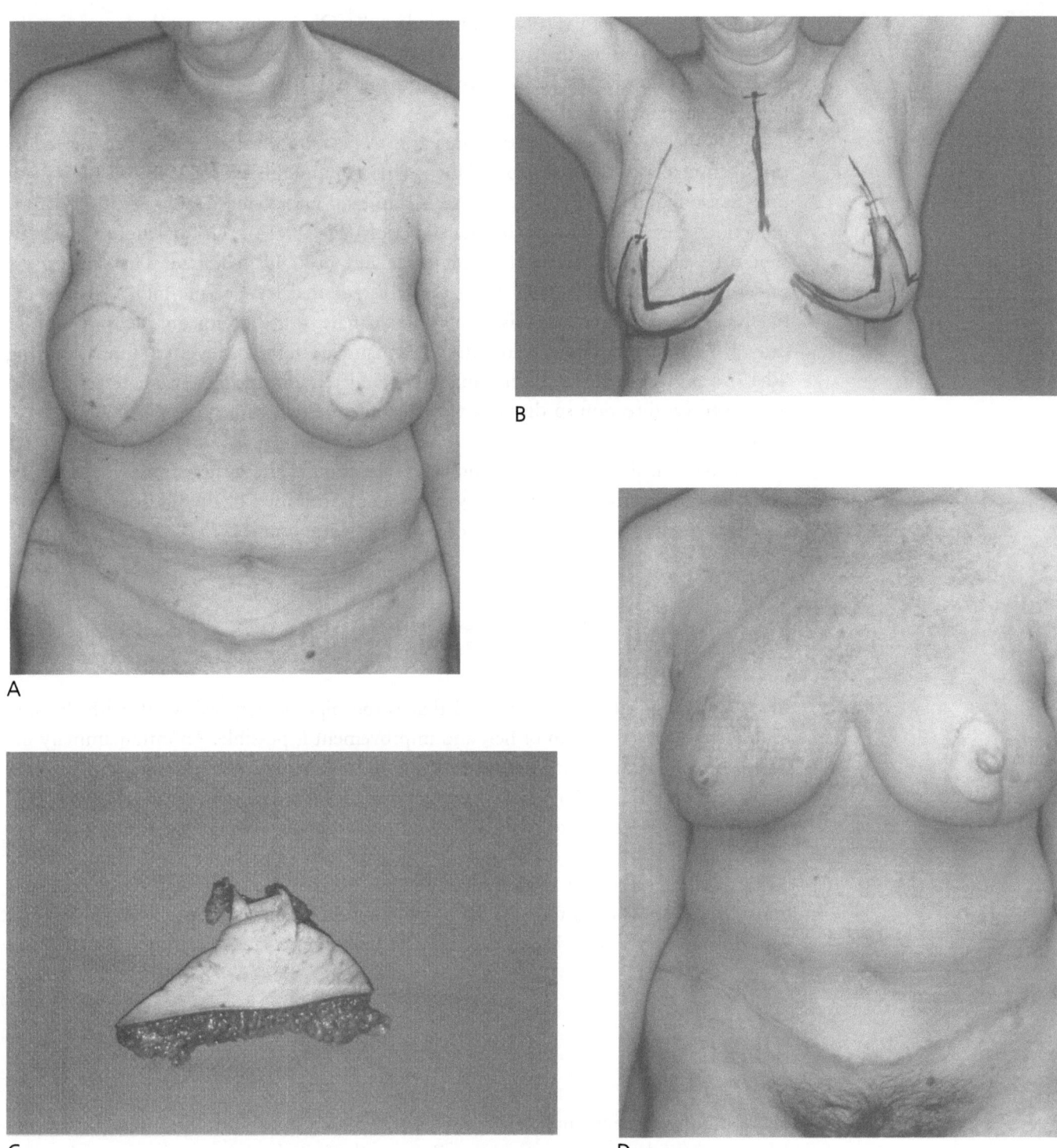

FIG. 20-15   (A) Somewhat obese patient after bilateral breast reconstruction with free TRAM flaps. The breasts are both too large and too pendulous. There also are bilateral dog-ears lateral to the abdominal donor site scar. (B) Plan for reduction of breast size and elevation of the inframammary folds using inverted T-shaped patterns. Nipple reconstruction with wrap-around flaps is also planned. (C) Tissue removed from lower pole of right breast. (D) Early result, before complete settling of the breasts. The breasts are smaller and less ptotic.

to those employed in a vertical mammoplasty.[6,7] Obviously, this works best when the breast mound is larger than the opposite breast and must be reduced. Taping of the chest wall skin under the breast with foam tape and use of an underwire brassiere may help to maintain the fold's position.

Another even more useful approach is to perform a variation of a vertical reduction mammaplasty or mastopexy. This is especially useful if a reduction in breast volume is also required. The surgeon resects skin (and underlying tissue as well, if volume reduction is desired) in a horizontal direction (Fig 20-14). The maximum tightness should be at the level where the new inframammary fold is desired. The skin can be undermined and tissue excised from below the desired level of the fold, to better define its location. If access to this tissue is inadequate or if the surgeon does not want to extend the vertical incision below the inframammary fold, an inverted T incision (Fig 20-15) can be used instead. The surgeon should refrain, however, from resecting skin in the vertical direction so that any tendency for the fold to be pulled back downward is minimized.

Even with these approaches, however, elevation of the inframammary fold can be difficult and uncertain. For that reason, correct positioning of the fold during the initial breast mound reconstruction is of paramount importance.

Lowering the Inframammary Fold

In the case of an inframammary fold that is too high, gravity will work with the surgeon instead of against him or her, and improvement is possible. An inframammary incision, mobilization of the lower part of the reconstructed breast mound, and removal of skin between the old and new inframammary folds will allow the breast to descend. This approach is similar to that used to correct a breast mound that is positioned too laterally, and will be successful provided that there is enough skin and internal tissue laxity to allow the breast to descend. It is not likely to be successful in an irradiated breast, however, where internal scarring may prevent the breast from moving inferiorly. Also the amount of lowering of the fold is usually limited to 1 or 2 cm.

Summary

Breast mound revision surgery is frequently necessary and is an important part of autologous tissue breast reconstruction. Because the initial reconstruction must be performed with the patient supine, achieving symmetry when the patient is upright can be difficult. Correction of the reconstructed breast mound to match the opposite side is ideal, but sometimes it is more practical to achieve symmetry by altering the opposite, natural breast. The most common asymmetry requiring revision is excess tissue in the lateral part of the reconstructed breast; this is usually corrected by removing an ellipse of skin, reelevating the mastectomy flaps, and removing excess fat from the mound over a wide area. Alternatively, reduction mammaplasty techniques can be used to improve breast projection and shape at the same time that the size is reduced. A breast mound that is too lateral can sometimes be moved medially without removing tissue by making an inframammary incision, separating the lower half of the breast mound from the chest wall, and moving it medially as a superiorly based flap. If there is insufficient tissue in the lower pole, a V-to-Y island flap can be used to move excess tissue in the upper breast to a more inferior position. Suction lipectomy can be effective for modestly reducing overall breast size or to make small localized corrections.

Breast mound revision surgery is not always easy, but it is crucial to the goal of attaining the best possible outcome. Mastery of this aspect of breast reconstruction allows the surgeon to significantly improve the quality of the patient's results with relatively little expense, and is well worth the investment of time and effort required.

References

1. Maxwell GP, Andochick SE. Secondary shaping of the TRAM flap. *Clin Plast Surg.* 1994;21:247–253.
2. Godfrey PM, Godfrey NV, Romita MC. Restoring the breast to match the normal side. *Ann Plast Surg.* 1993;31:392–397.
3. Klein JA. Tumescent technique for local anesthesia improves safety in large-volume liposuction. *Plast Reconstr Surg.* 1993;92:1085–1098.
4. Hunstad JP. Body contouring in the obese patient. *Clin Plast Surg.* 1996;23:647–670.
5. Burk RW, Guzman-Stein G, Vasconez LO. Lidocaine and epinephrine levels in tumescent technique liposuction. *Plast Reconstr Surg.* 1996;97:1379–1384.
6. Lejour M. Vertical mammaplasty and liposuction of the breast. *Plast Reconstr Surg.* 1994;94:100–114.
7. Lassus C. A 30-year experience with vertical mammaplasty. *Plast Reconstr Surg.* 1996;97:373–380.

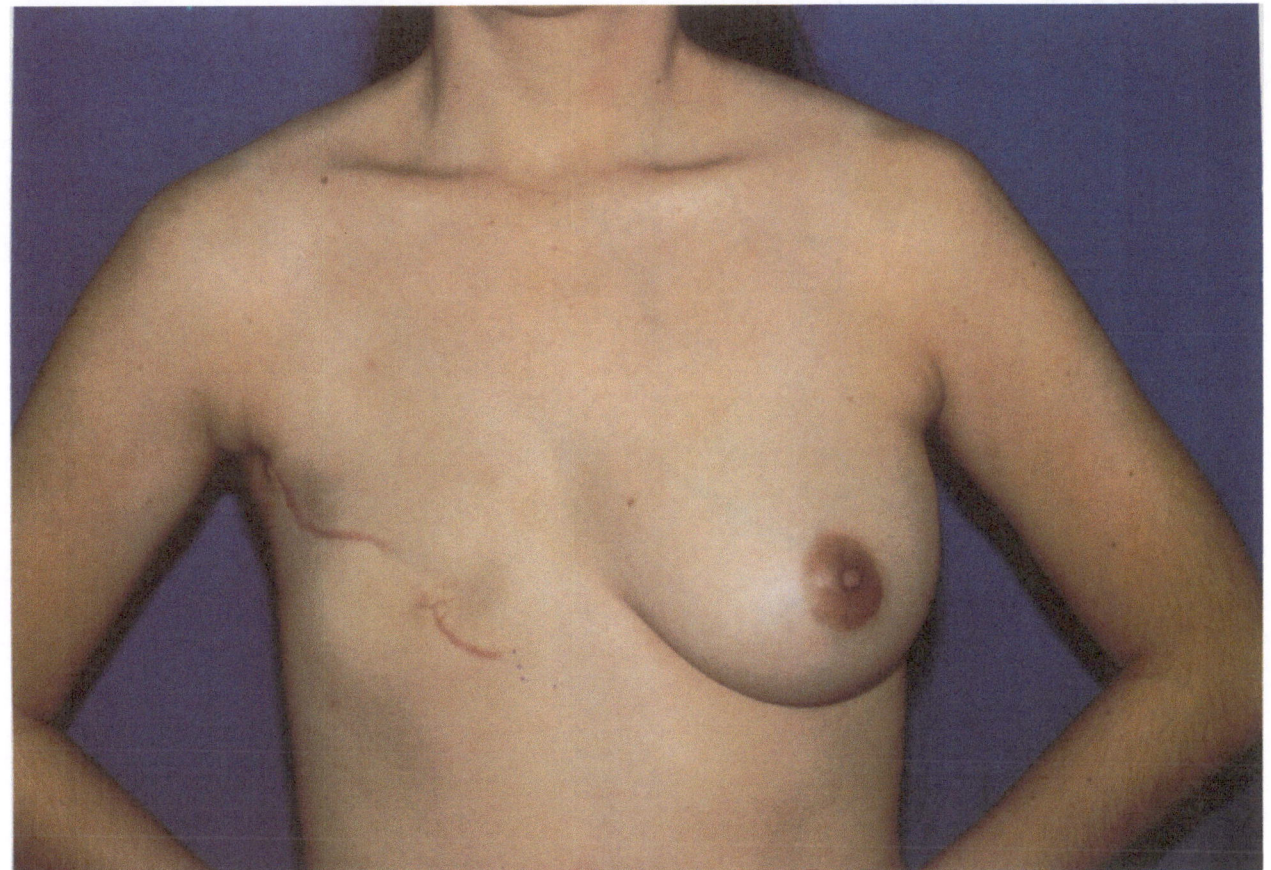

A

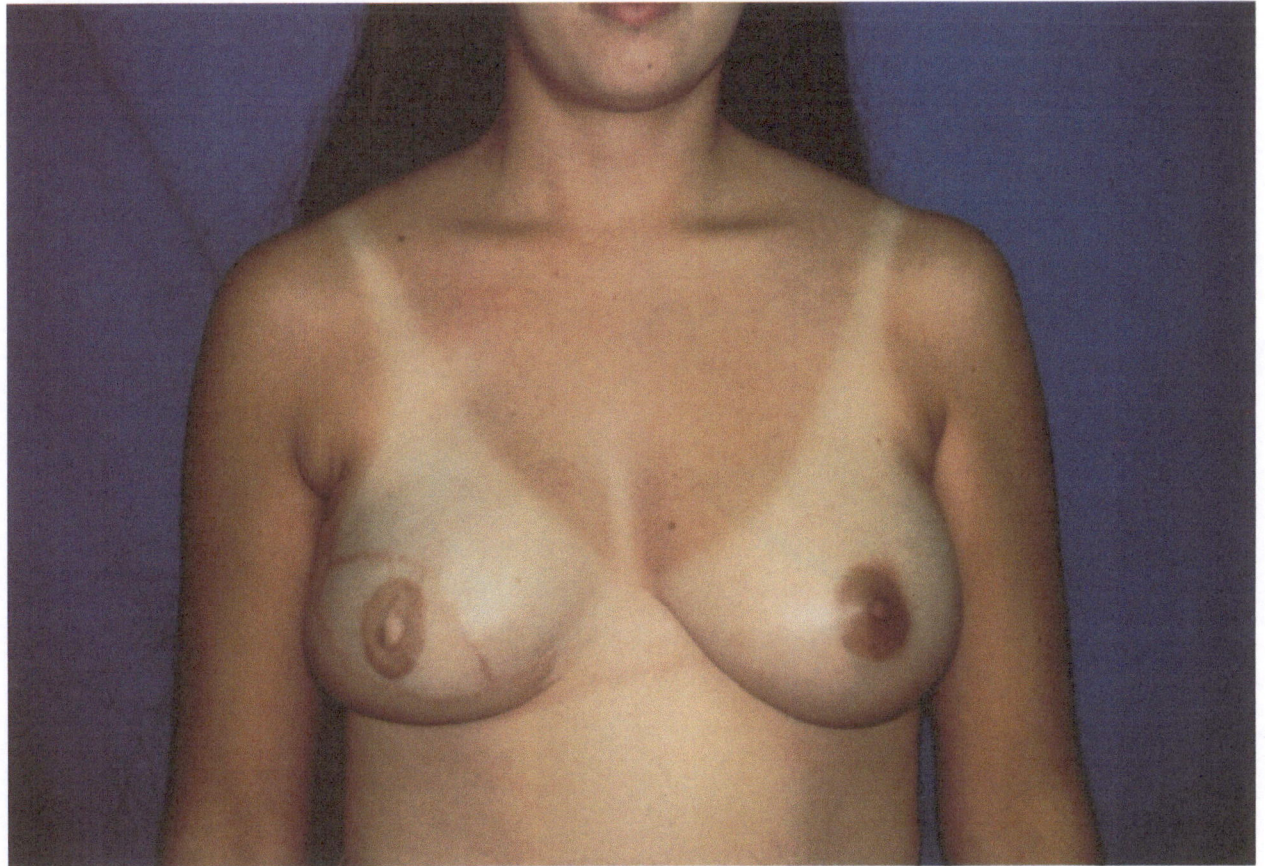

B

FIG. 1-1 (A) A 22-year-old woman following right modified radical mastectomy for breast cancer. (B) After breast reconstruction with a latissimus dorsi flap and a silicone implant. The patient sunbathes and has resumed an active life. (From Kroll SS: *Clin Plast Surg* 25: 135–143, 1998. Used with permission.)

FIG. 1-2   The result of bilateral immediate
breast reconstruction with free transverse rectus abdominis myocutaneous (TRAM) flaps.

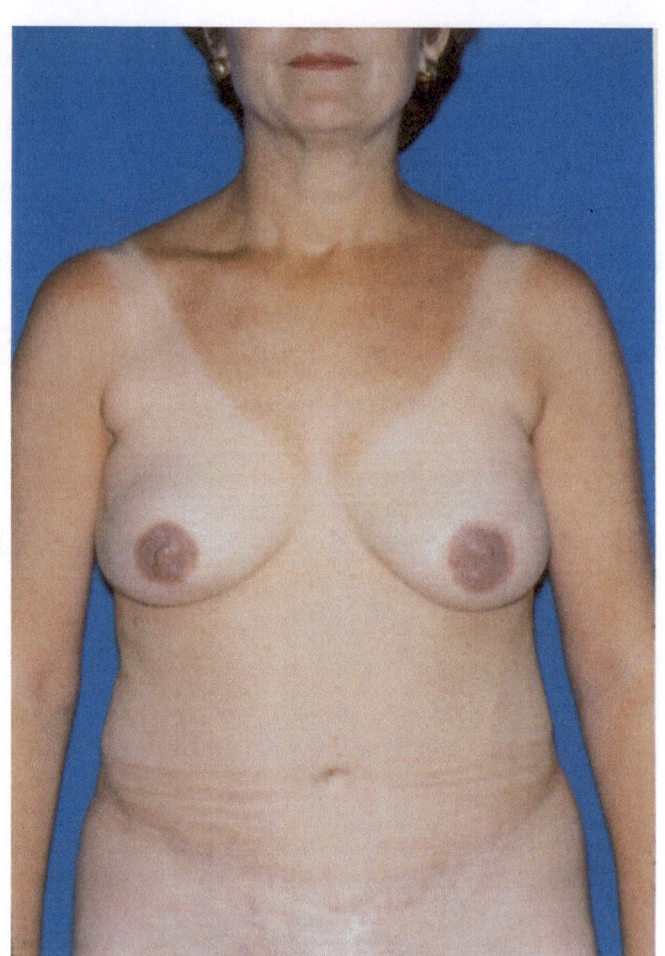

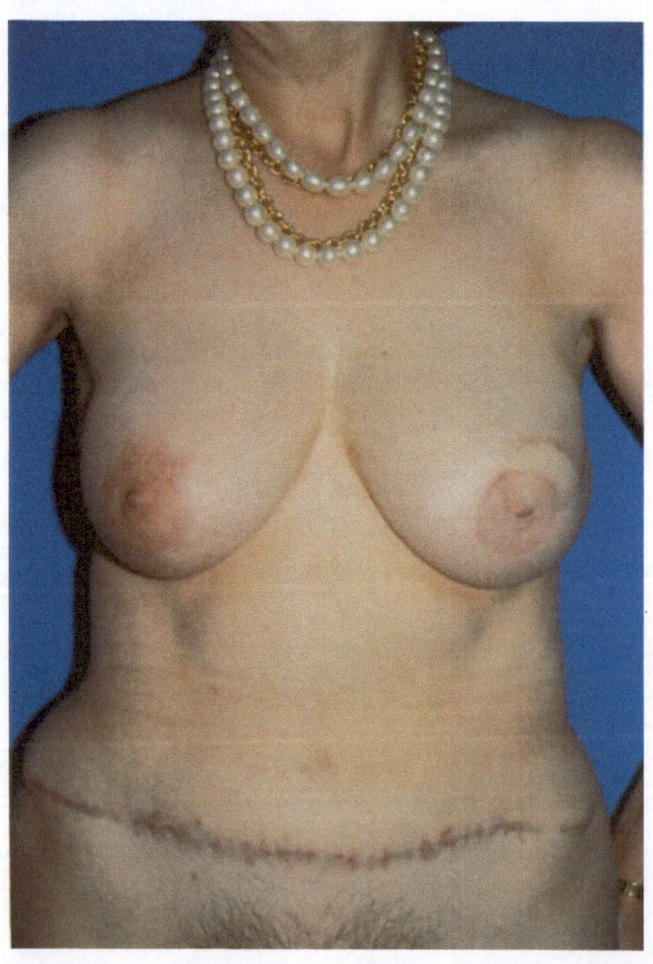

FIG. 3-5   A free TRAM flap breast reconstruction, showing a completely smooth inframammary fold.

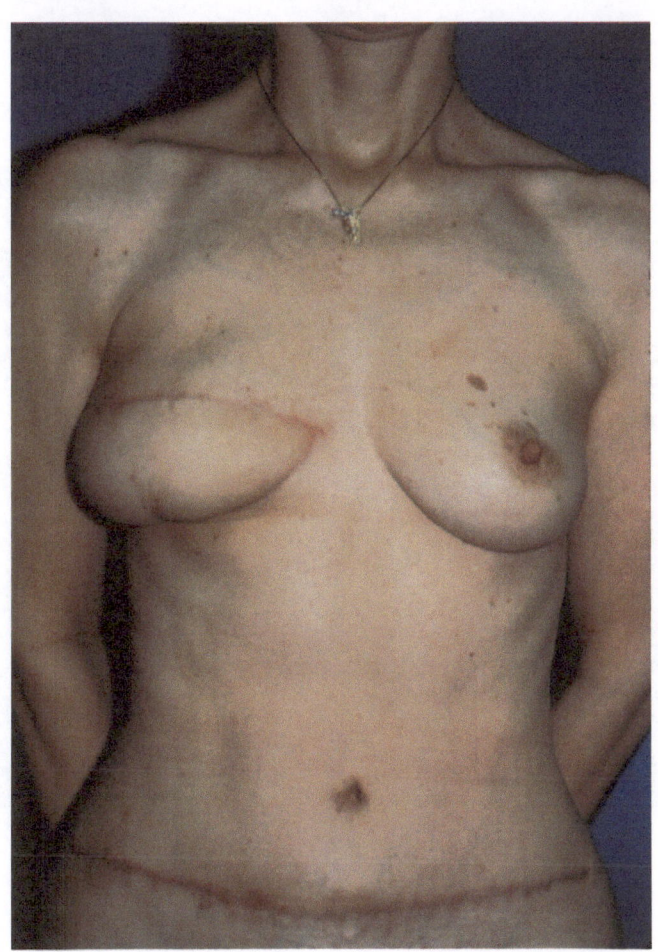

A

FIG. 1-4   (A) A patient after breast mound reconstruction with a free TRAM flap. (B) The same patient after revision of the breast mound and reconstruction of the nipple, showing significant improvement in her appearance. (From Kroll SS: Nipple and Areolar Reconstruction; in Kroll SS, Ed. *Reconstructive Plastic Surgery for Cancer.* Mosby, St. Louis, 1996. Used with permission).

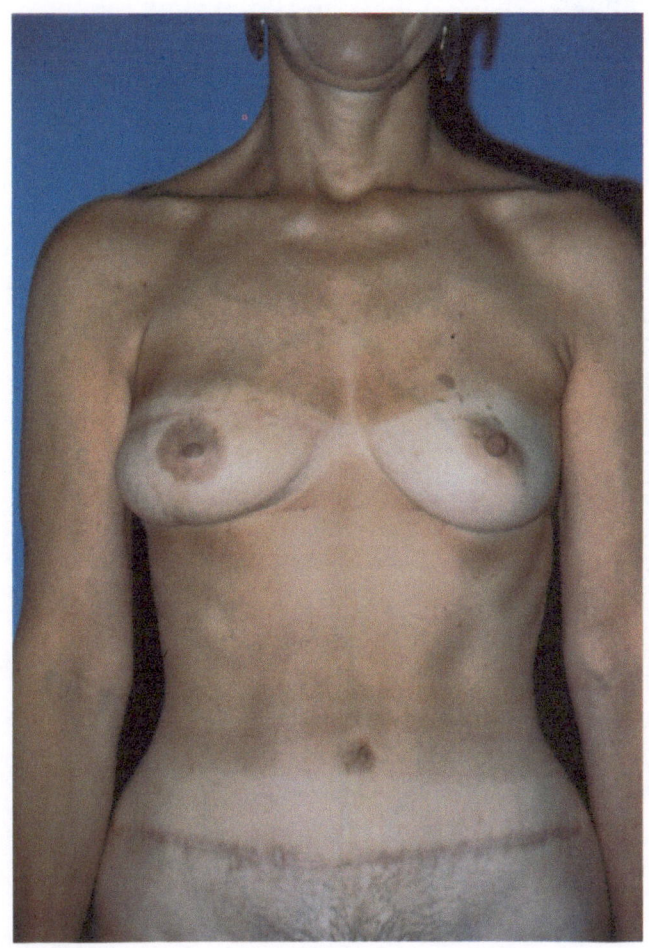

B

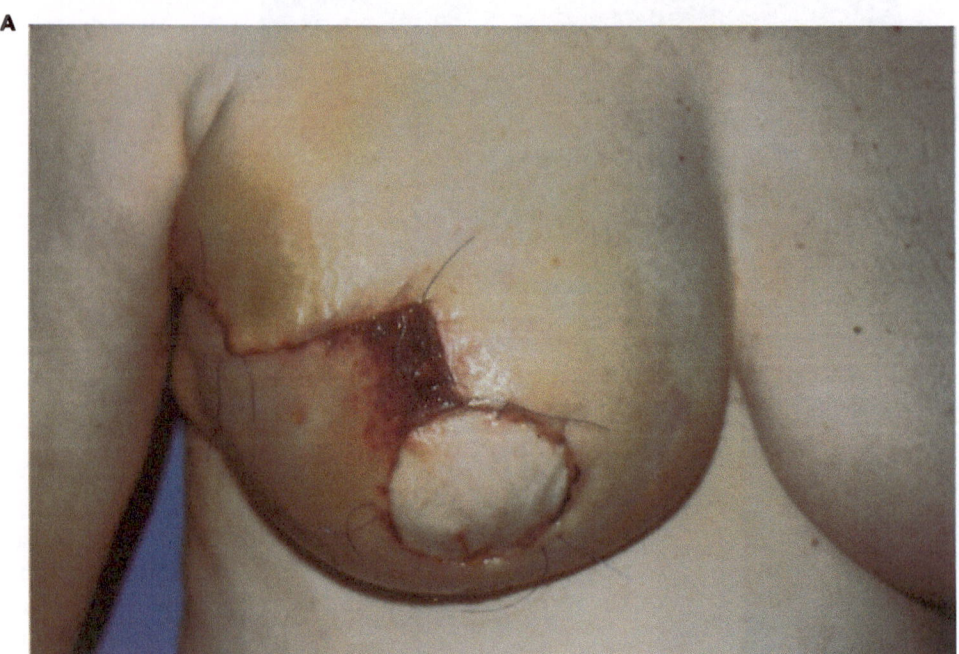

FIG. 2-7 (A) A patient with mastectomy flap edge necrosis after immediate breast reconstruction with a free TRAM flap. (B) The same patient after secondary healing, revision, and nipple reconstruction. The final result was not significantly impacted by the exposure of the underlying TRAM flap.

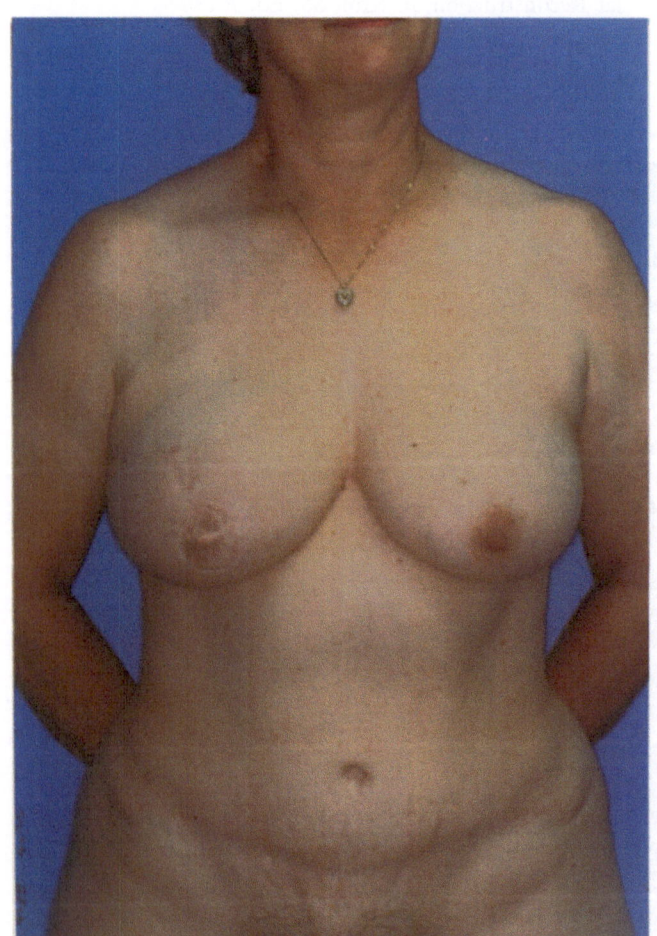

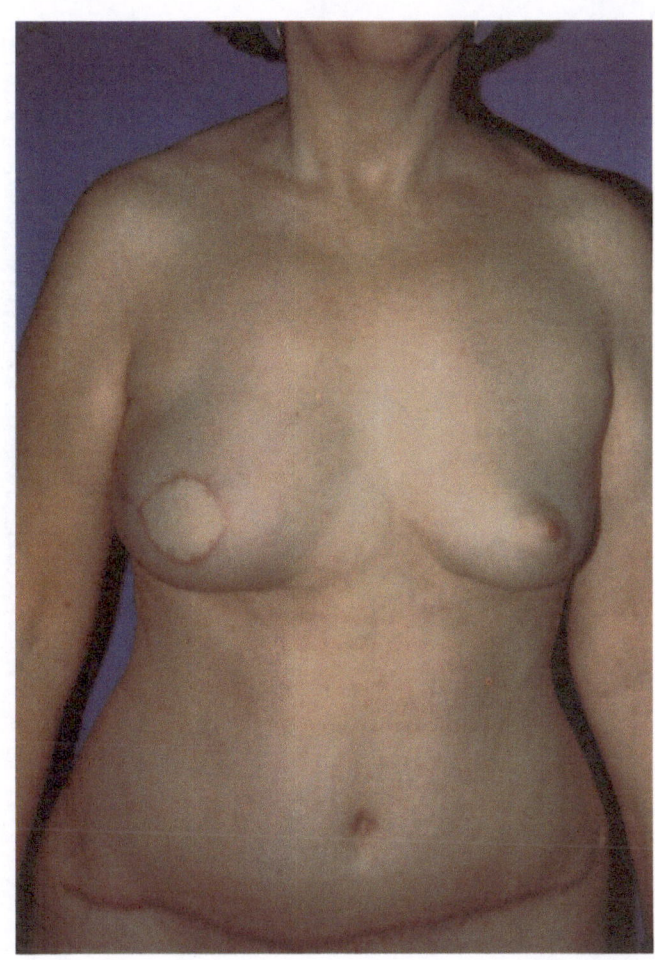

A

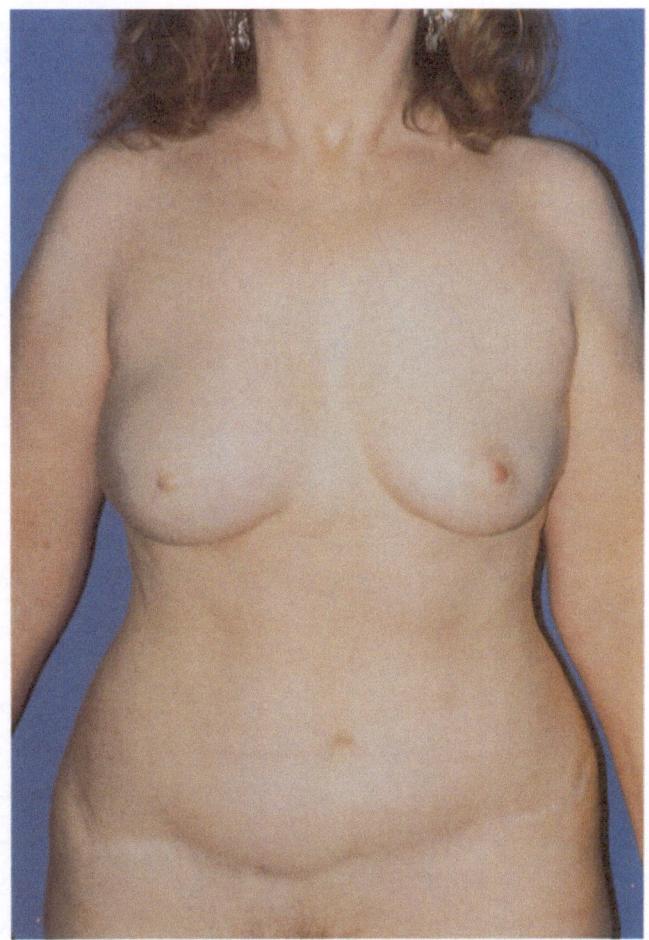

B

FIG. 2-9 (A) Early result of a pedicled TRAM flap breast reconstruction. (B) After 4 years, the scars have faded and the patient looks better than she did immediately after the reconstruction.

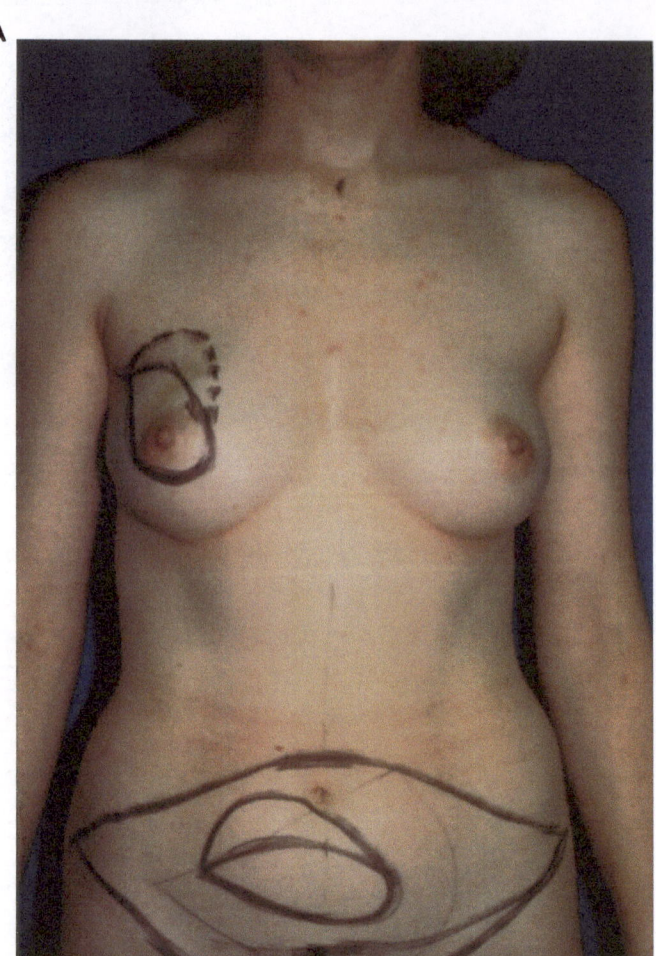

FIG. 4-1 (A) Preoperative plan for a skin-sparing mastectomy. (B) Result of immediate reconstruction with a TRAM flap (From *Plast Reconstr Surg* 90:455, 1992. Used with permission.)

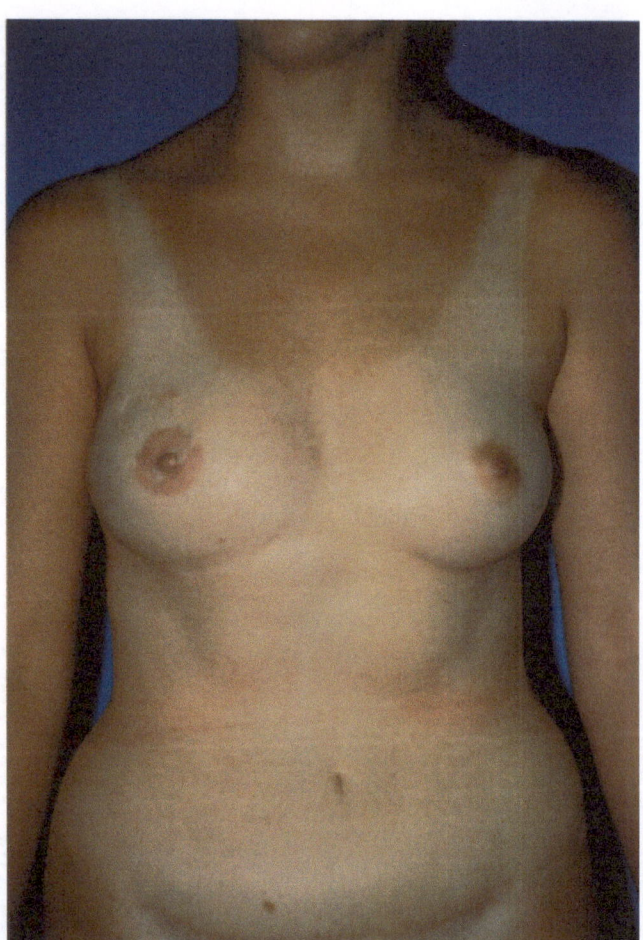

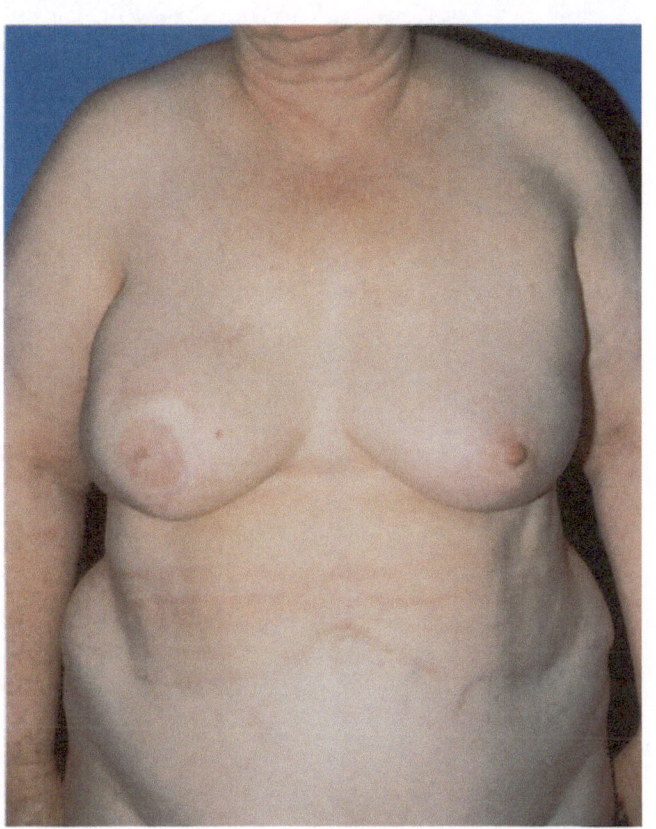

Fig. 4-2 (C) Patient shown in 4-2 A and B after debridement, healing, revision, and nipple reconstruction. Because autologous tissue was used, the mastectomy flap necrosis did not significantly compromise the final result. (From *Plast Reconstr Surg* 94:637, 1994. Used with permission.)

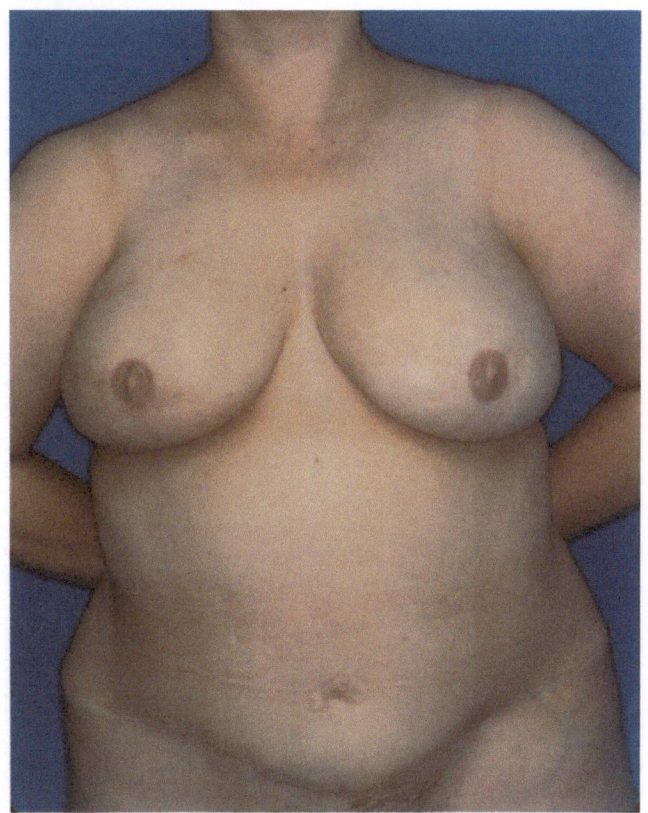

Fig. 5-9 A patient 4 years after bilateral free TRAM flap breast reconstruction. She had been treated previously with mastectomy and radiotherapy on the left side, but there is no apparent difference between the irradiated (left) and non-irradiated (right) sides.

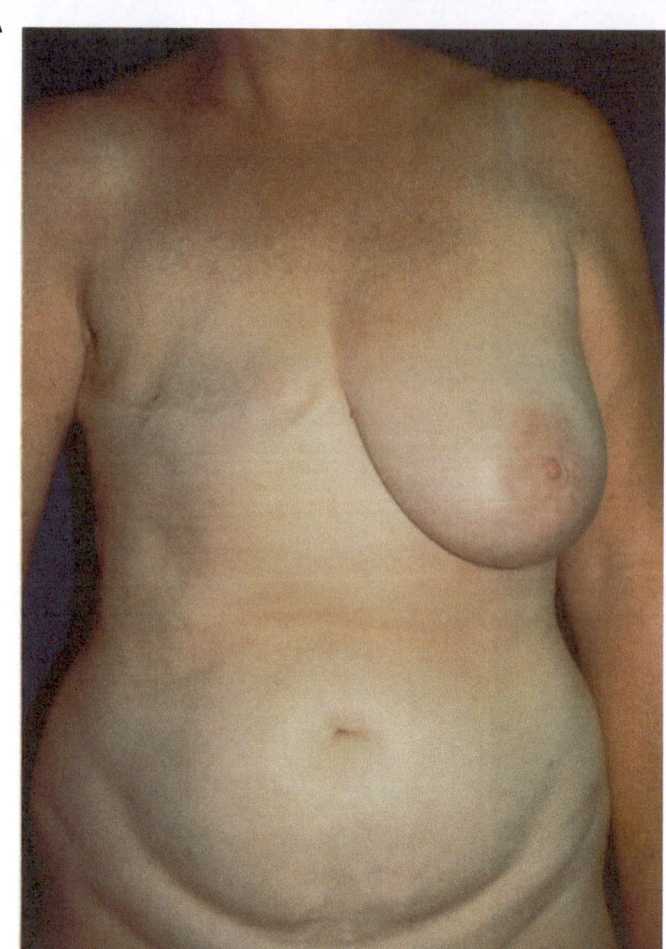

FIG. 5-1 (A) A 49-year-old patient after right mastectomy. (B) The same patient 1 year after delayed breast reconstruction with a pedicled TRAM flap. (From *Ann Surg Oncol* 1:457, 1994. Used with permission.)

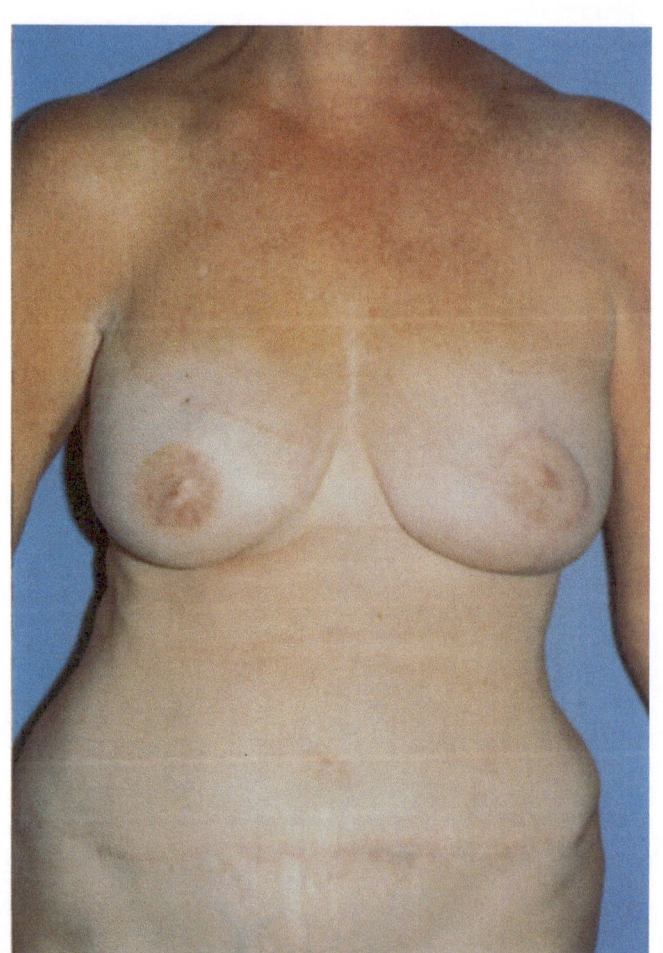

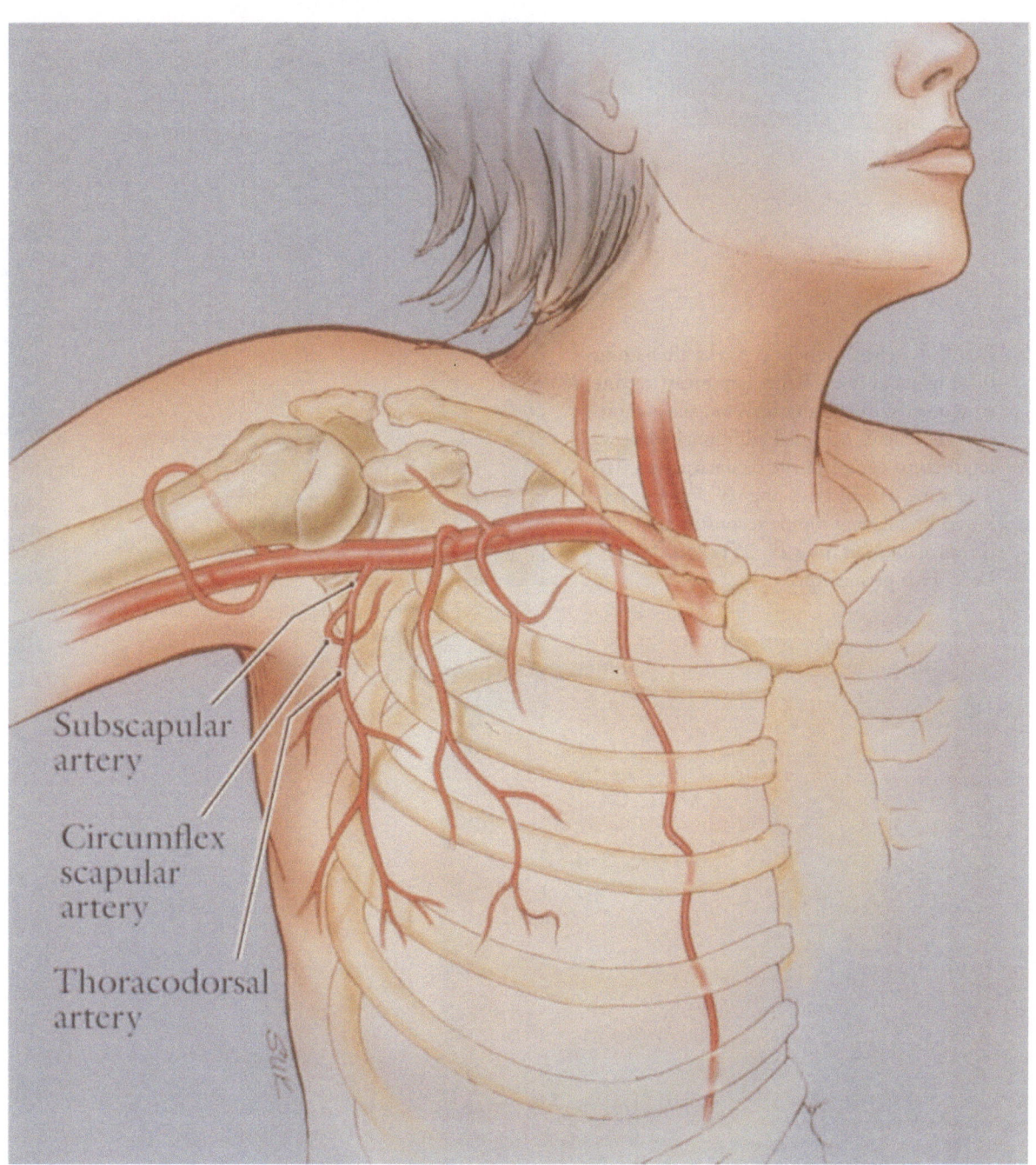

FIG. 5-4 The subscapular vascular system. The most commonly used recipient vessels are the thoracodorsals. If these are too small, the circumflex scapular or subscapular vessels may be suitable.

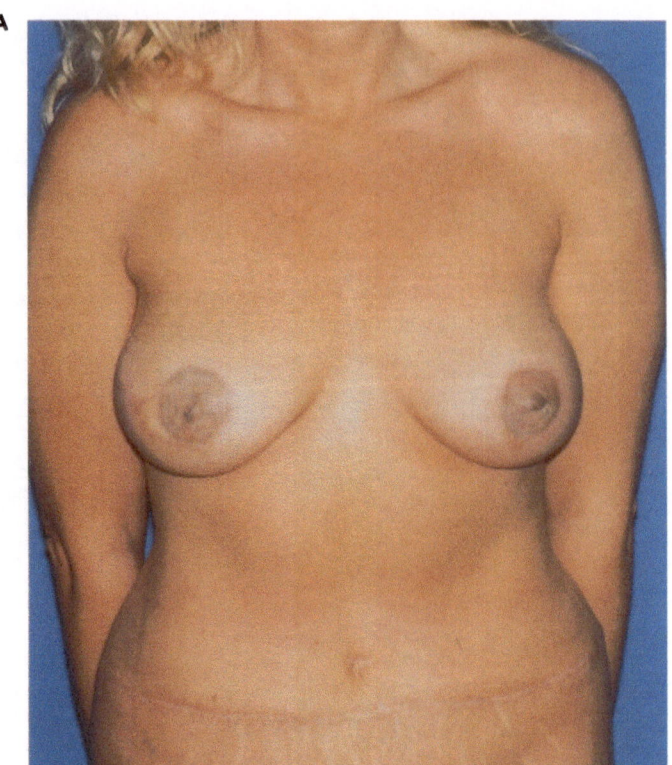

FIG. 6-4 (A) A patient 3 weeks after immediate bilateral free TRAM flap breast reconstruction. Without any revision, the symmetry is excellent. Minimal additional work was required to complete the reconstruction. (B) The same patient after one revision and followed by bilateral nipple reconstruction. (From *Clin Plast Surg* 25: 251–259, 1998. Used with permission.)

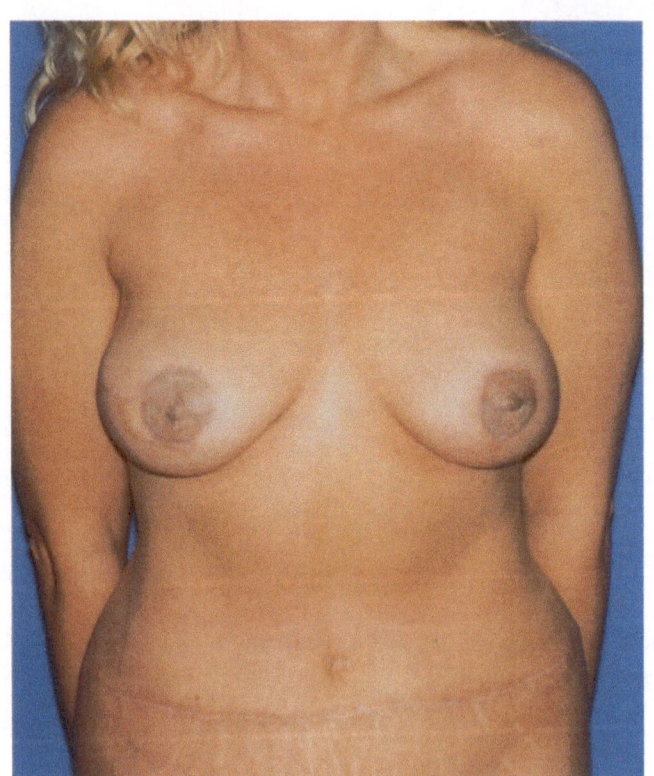

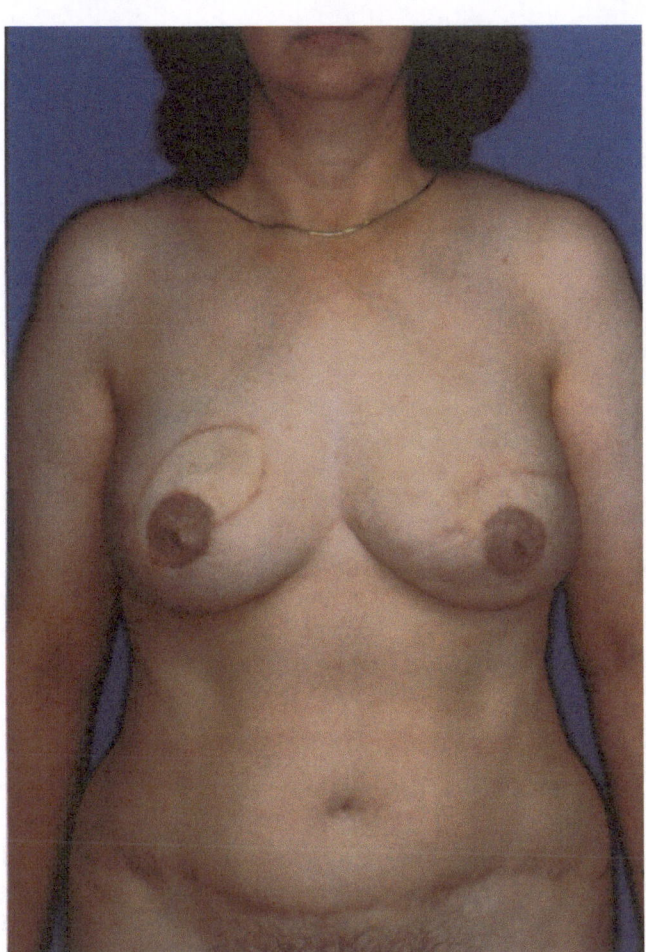

Fig. 6-3 Bilateral simultaneous breast reconstruction with free TRAM flaps. In this patient, who had bilateral breast cancer, the symmetry is good because the same technique was used for both sides (From *Clin Plast Surg* 25: 251–259, 1998. Used with permission.)

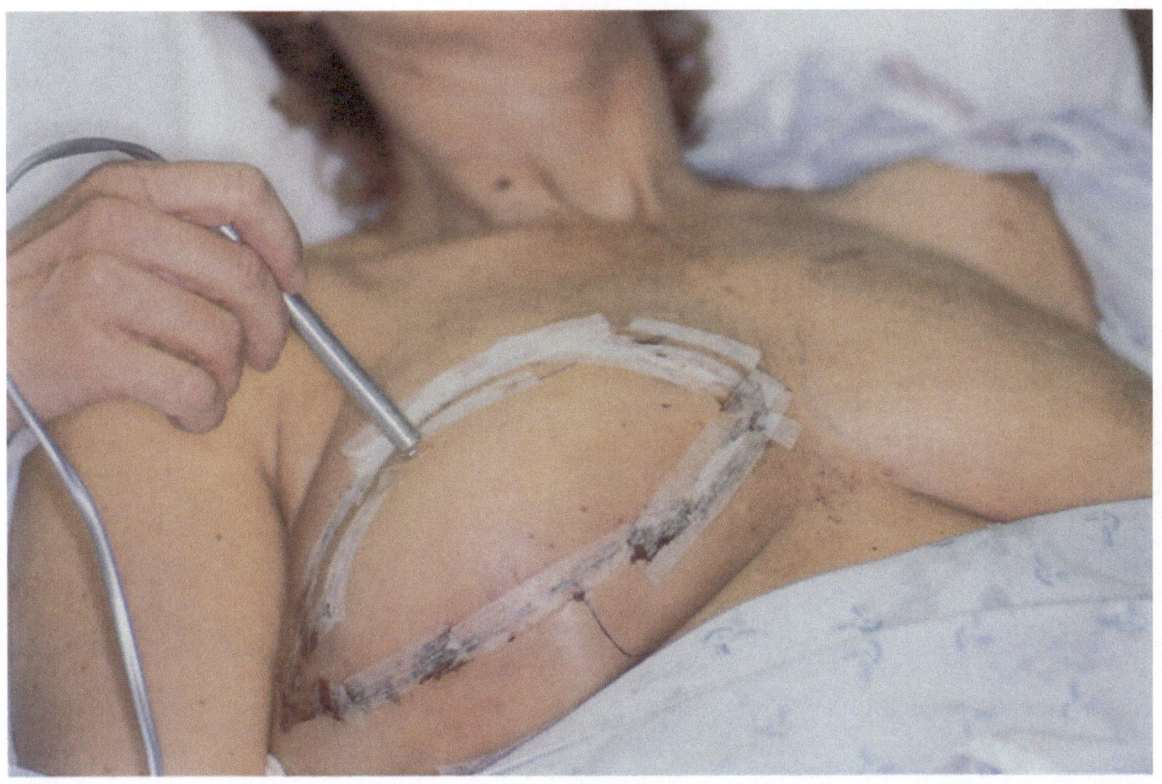

Fig. 11-1 Monitoring the flap with a hand-held pencil Doppler probe. This is the simplest method of flap monitoring and is therefore preferred if a signal can be located.

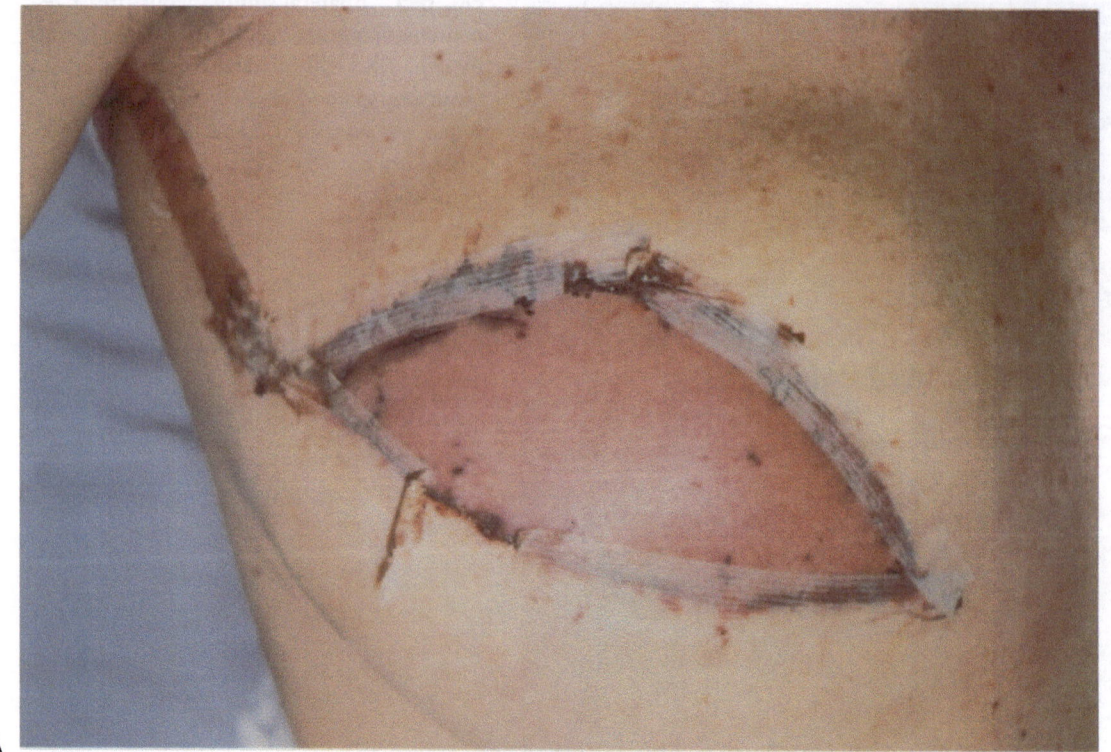

A

Fig. 11-2   (A) Free TRAM flap compromised by venous obstruction. The flap is blue. (C) Six days after revision of the venous anastomosis, the flap is viable.

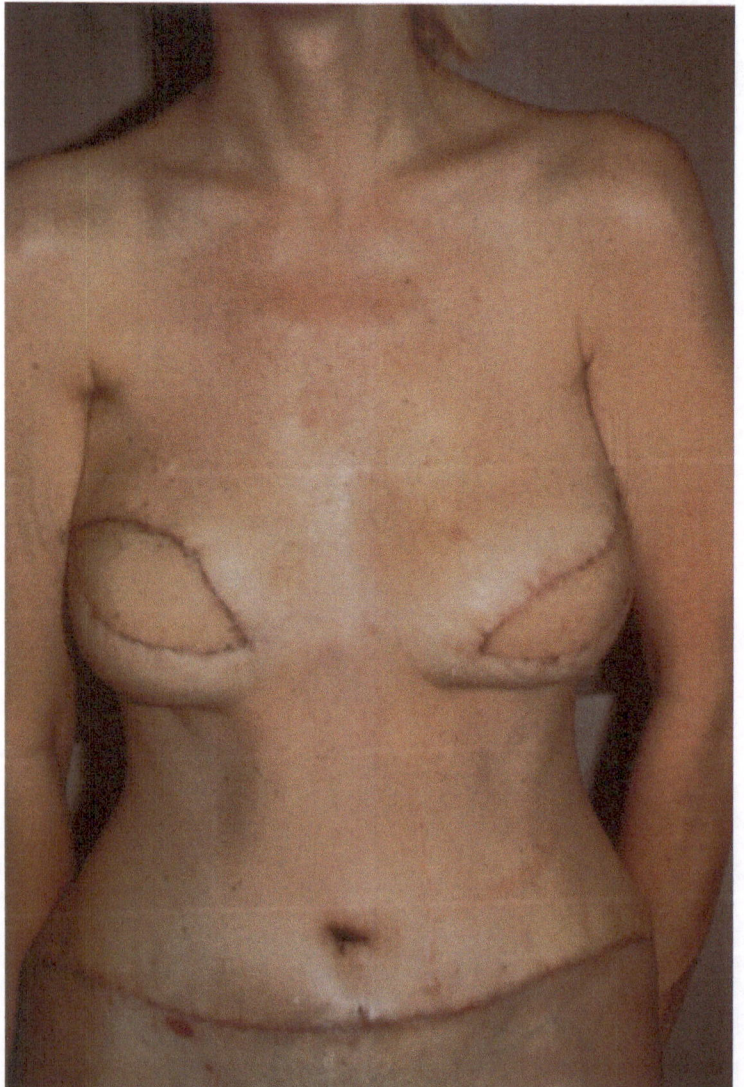

C

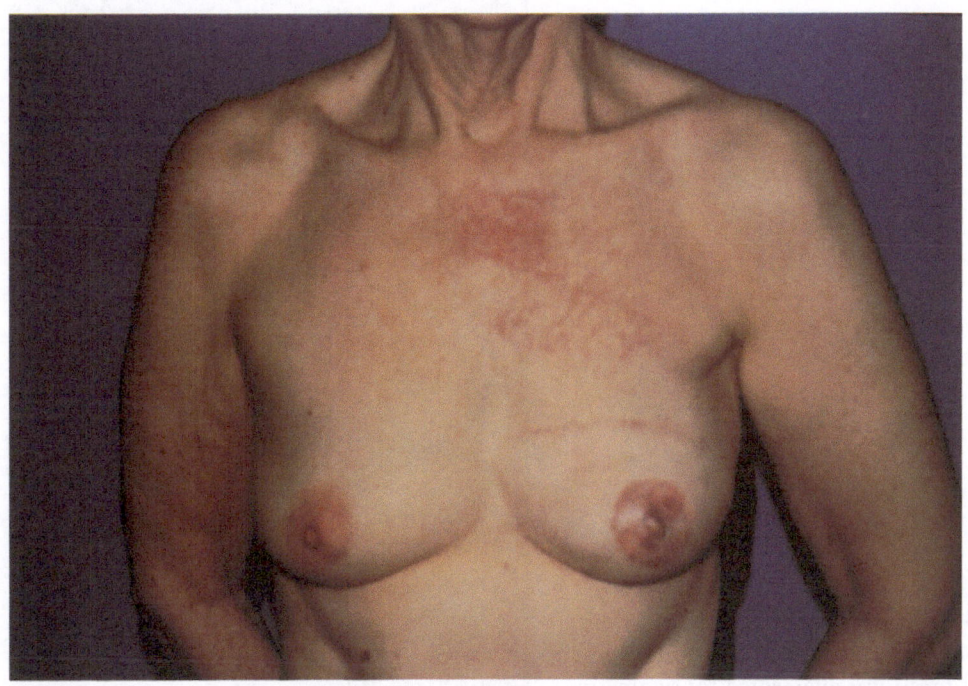

Fig. 12-2 (C) Result 2 years later.

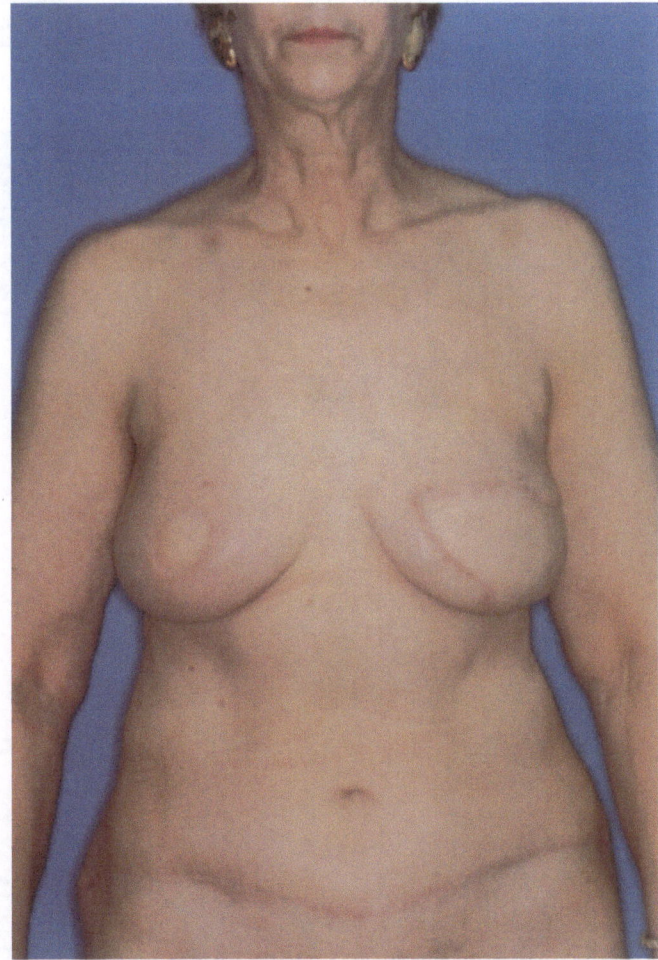

Fig. 16-4 (E) The result 6 months later shows the cosmetic advantage of the periareolar incision on the patient's right side (the left side had a delayed reconstruction).

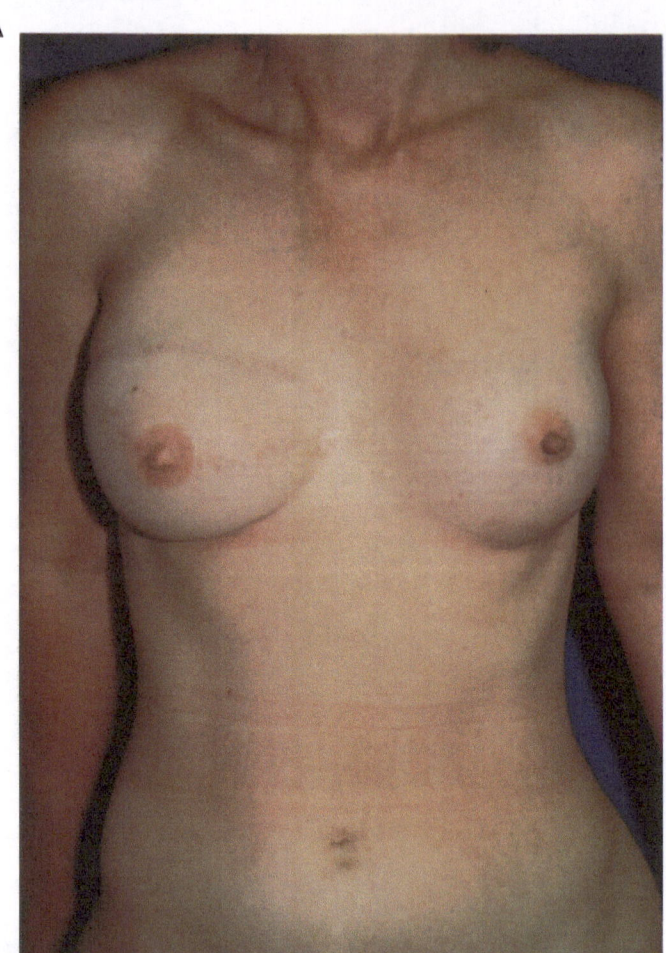

FIG. 13-6 (A) Result of right breast reconstruction with a superior gluteal free flap. The left breast was augmented for symmetry. (B) The donor site. (From Singletary SE and Kroll SS: Skin-sparing mastectomy with immediate breast reconstruction. *Advances in Surgery* 30:39–52, 1996. Used with permission.)

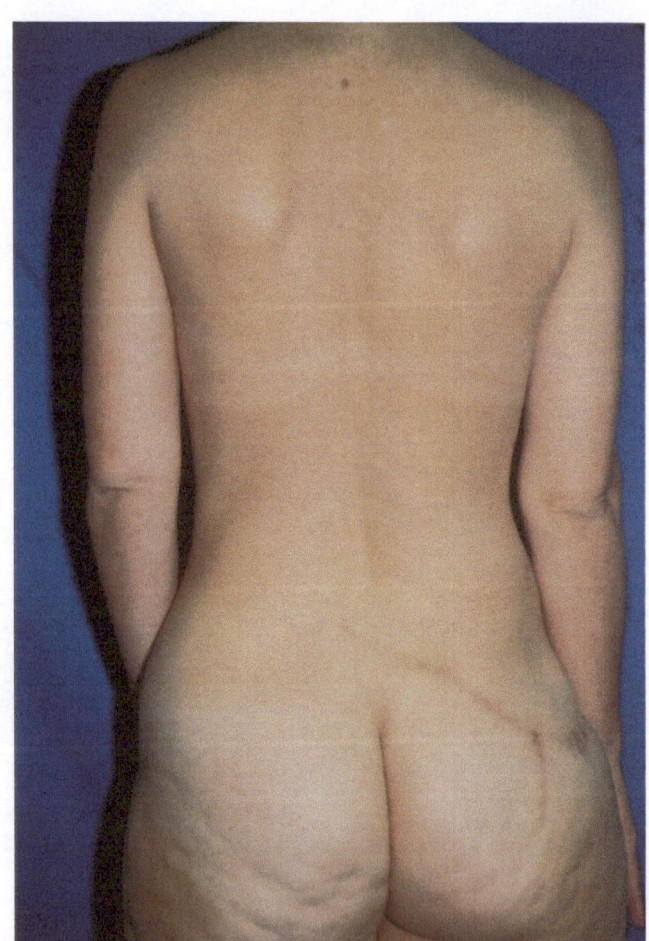

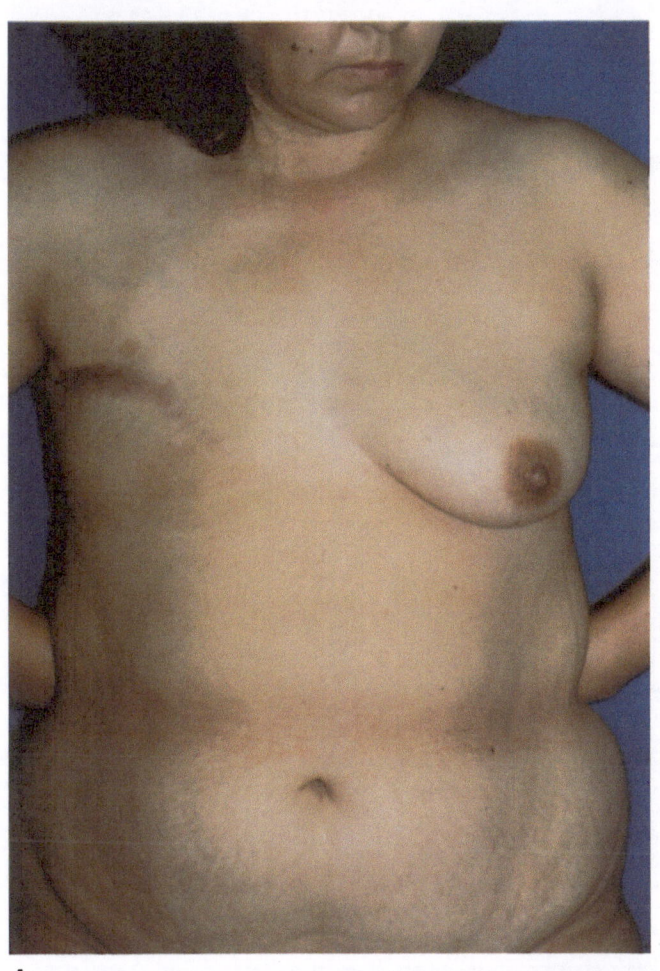

A

FIG. 17-6 (A) Patient after modified radical mastectomy. (B) After delayed breast reconstruction with a pedicled TRAM flap.

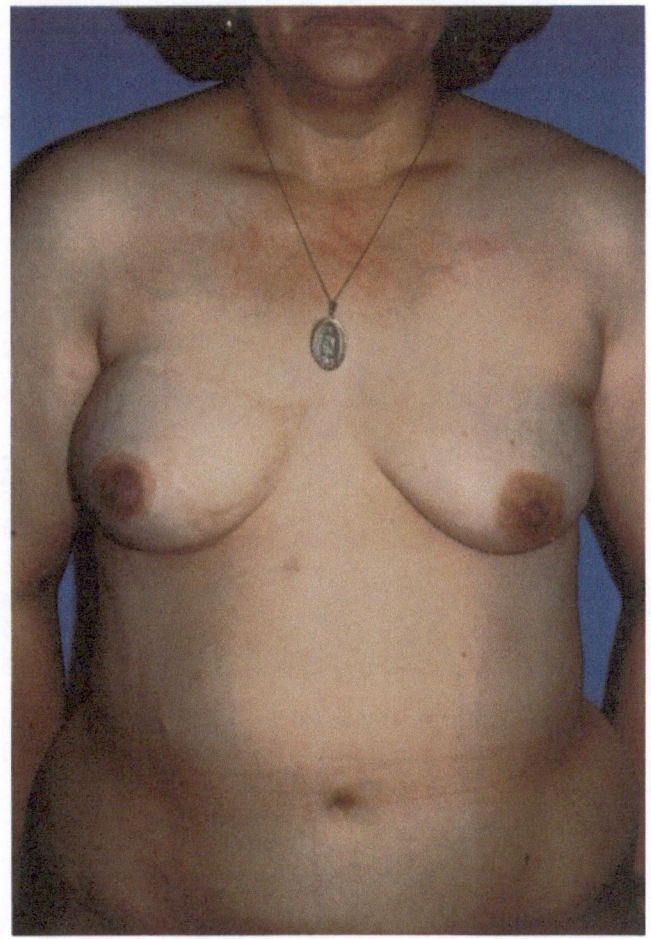

B

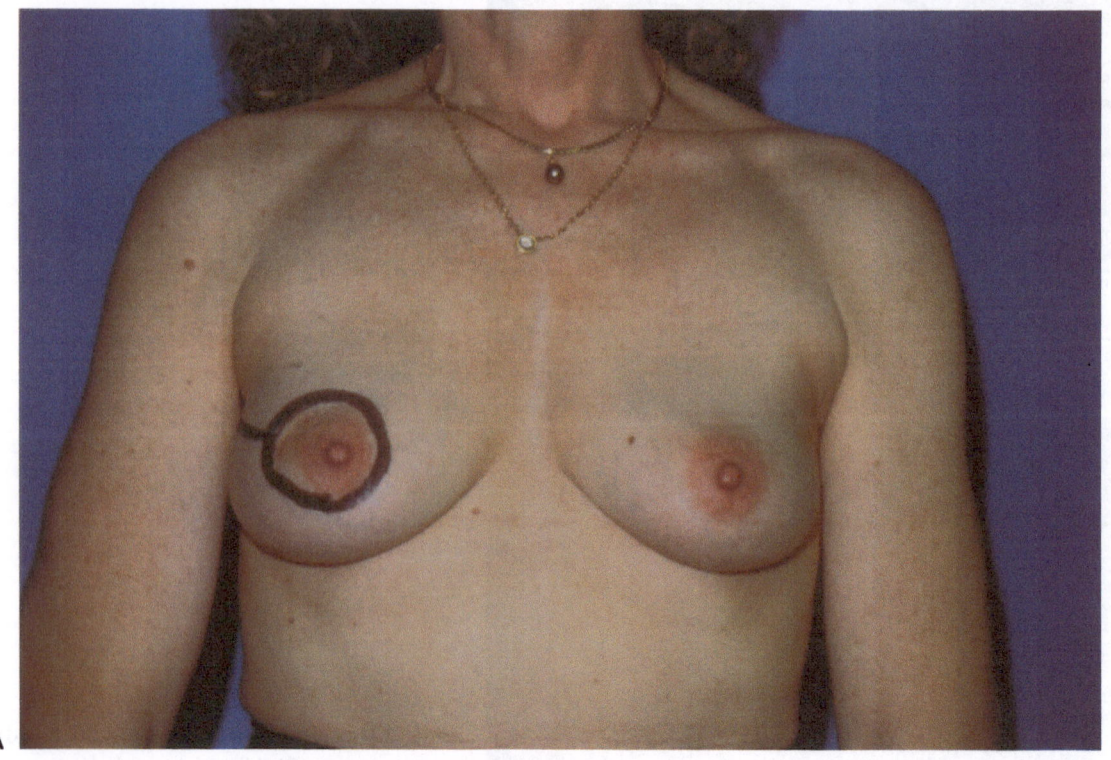

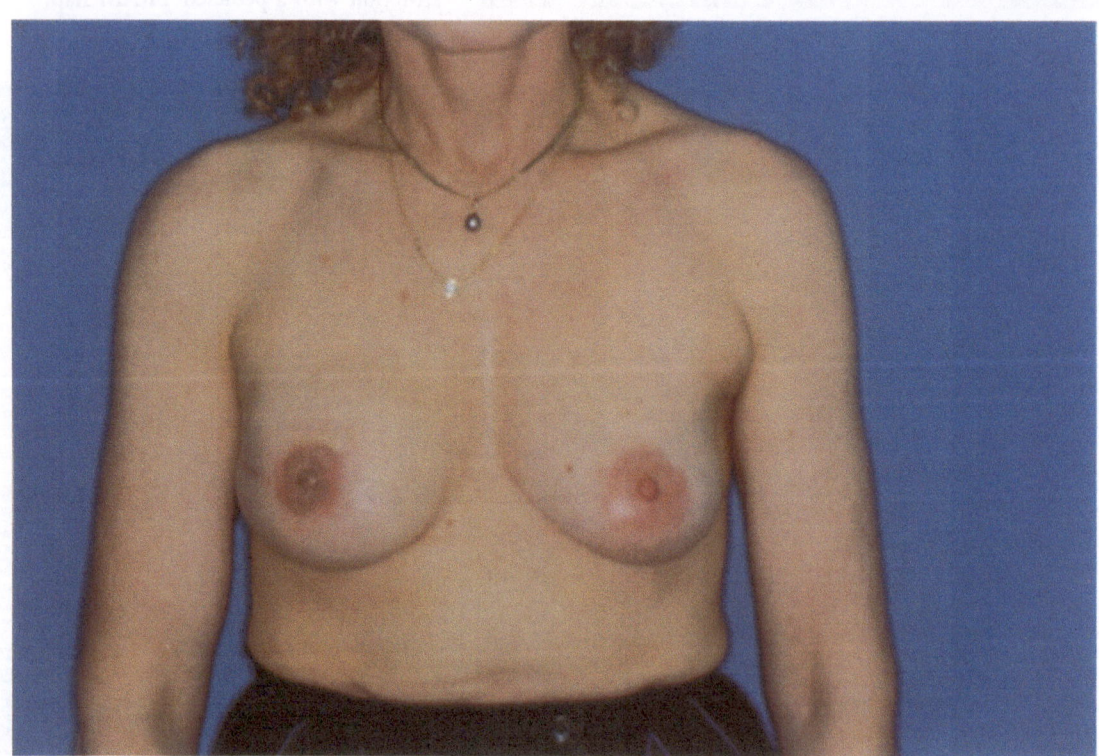

Fig. 14-8 (A) A 53-year-old woman scheduled for right mastectomy. She had previously undergone abdominoplasty and therefore was not a candidate for a TRAM flap. (B) Result of immediate reconstruction with an inferior gluteal free flap.

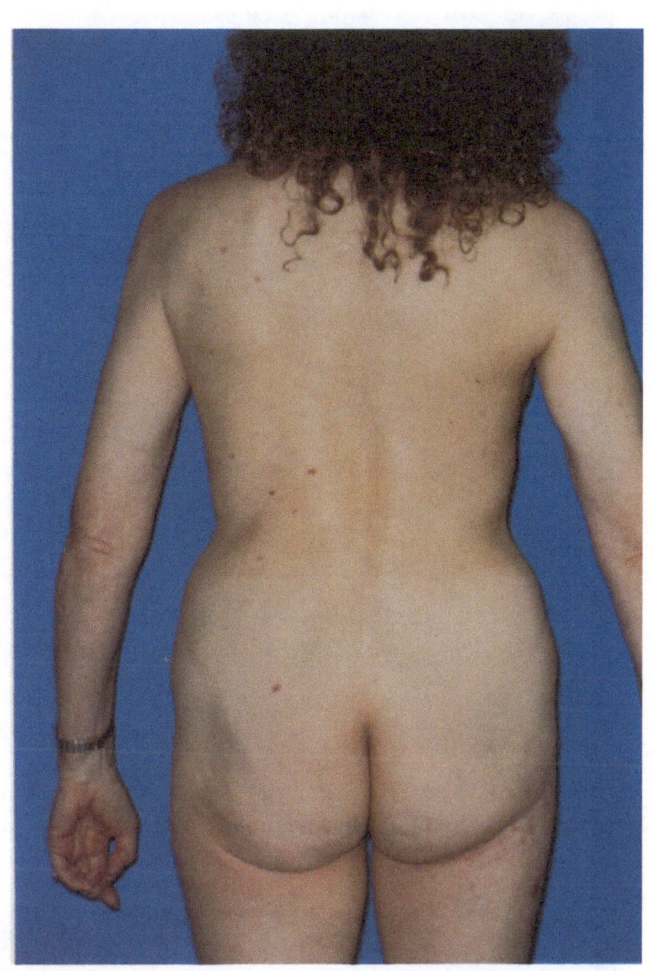

FIG. 14-8 (C) The donor site. (From Kroll SS: *Clin Plast Surg* 25: 135–143, 1998. Used with permission.)

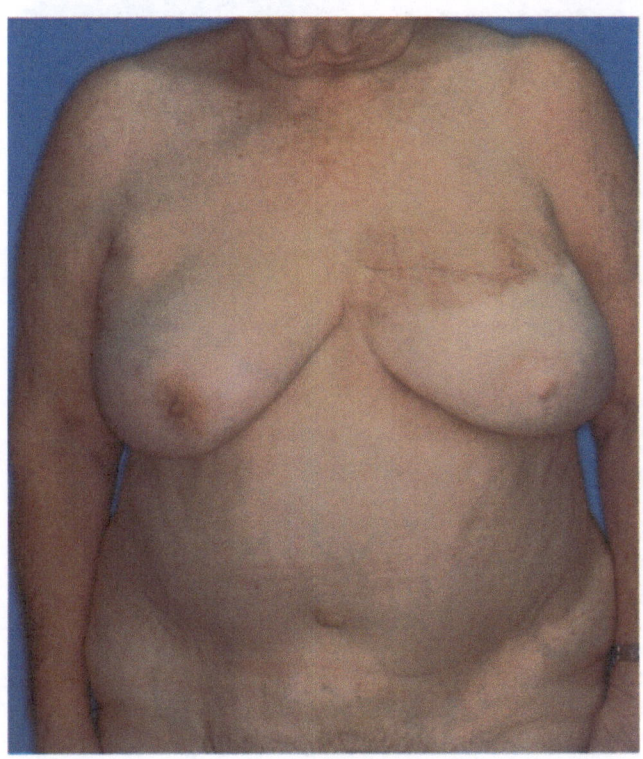

FIG. 17-11 Delayed breast reconstruction using the TRAM flap itself to form the lower panel of the breast. This hides the lower scar in the inframammary fold, but exposes any irregularities of the lower border of the TRAM flap. Note the surrounding skin changes caused by irradiation.

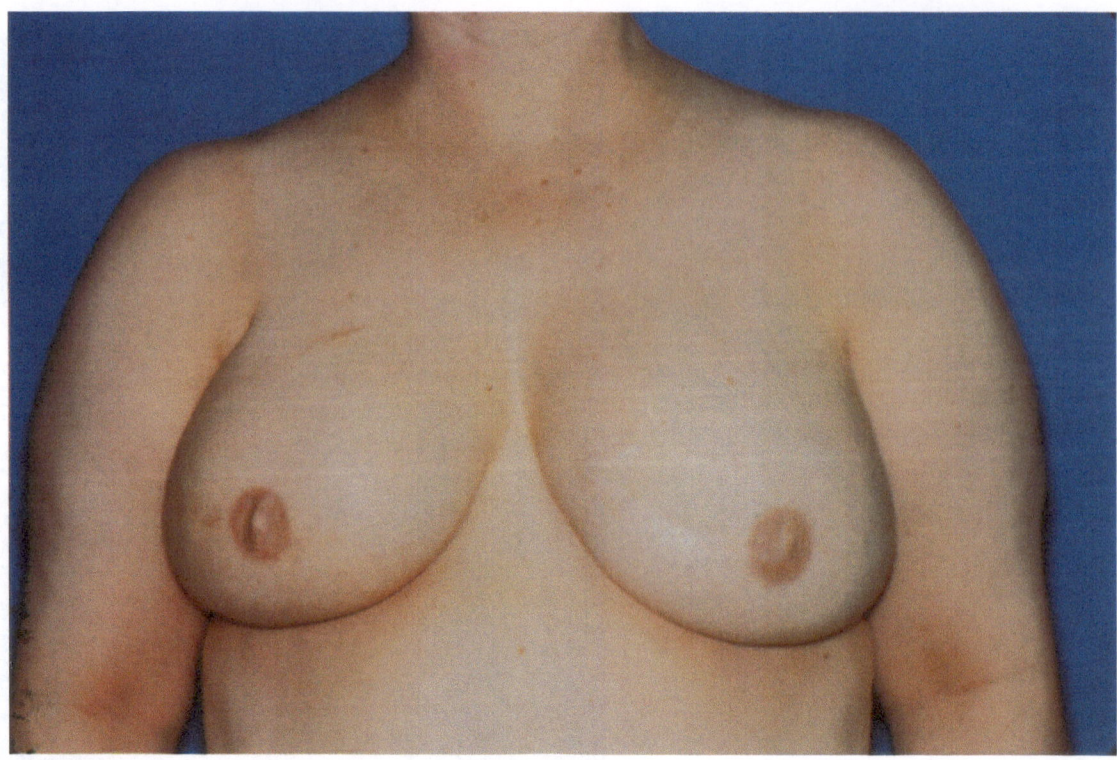

FIG. 17-16 (B) After bilateral free TRAM flap breast reconstruction. Despite the irradiation, the reconstruction is only minimally compromised because the radiation injury was not severe.

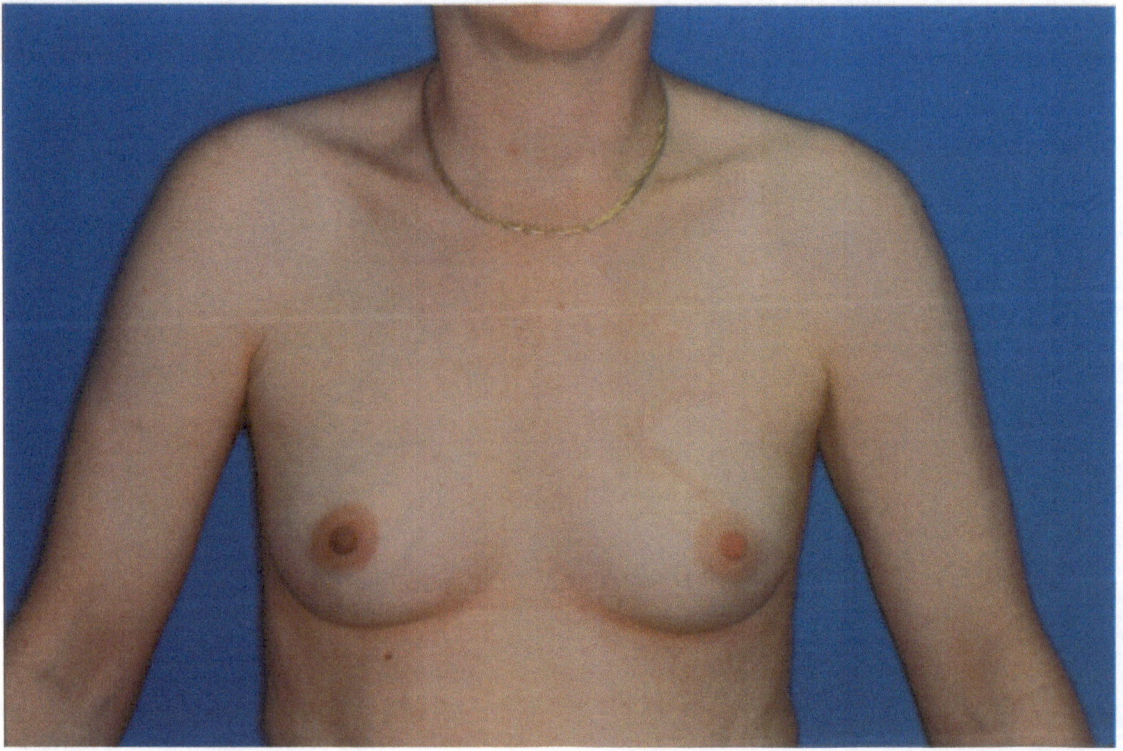

FIG. 19-14 (C) Result 1 year after reconstruction of a partial mastectomy defect in the upper pole of the breast using a superiorly-based composite flap. (From Bold RJ, Kroll SS, Baldwin BJ, et al: Local Rotational Flaps for Breast Conservation Therapy as an Alternative to Mastectomy. *Ann Surg Oncol* 4:540, 1997. With permission.)

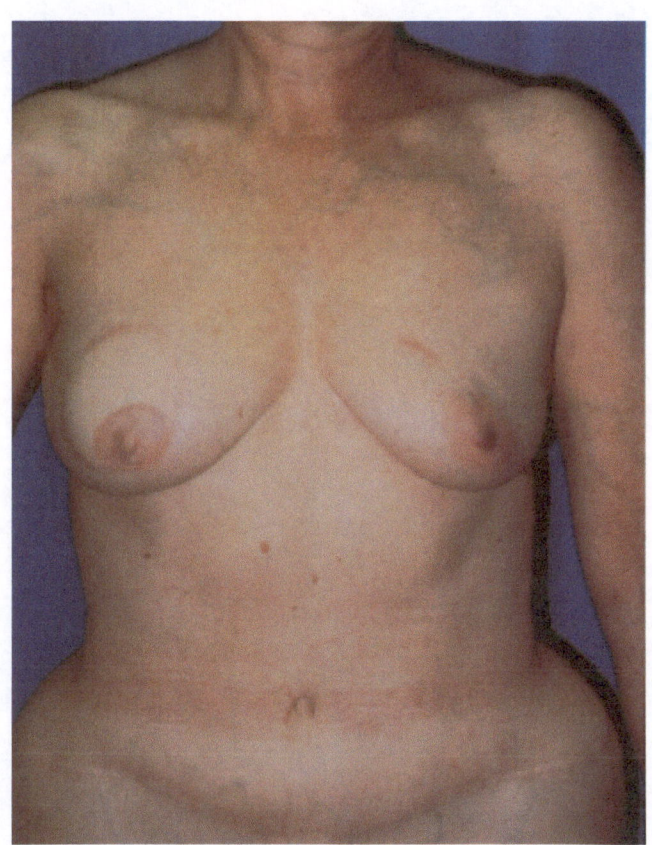

FIG. 20-3 Patient after revision, showing improved symmetry.

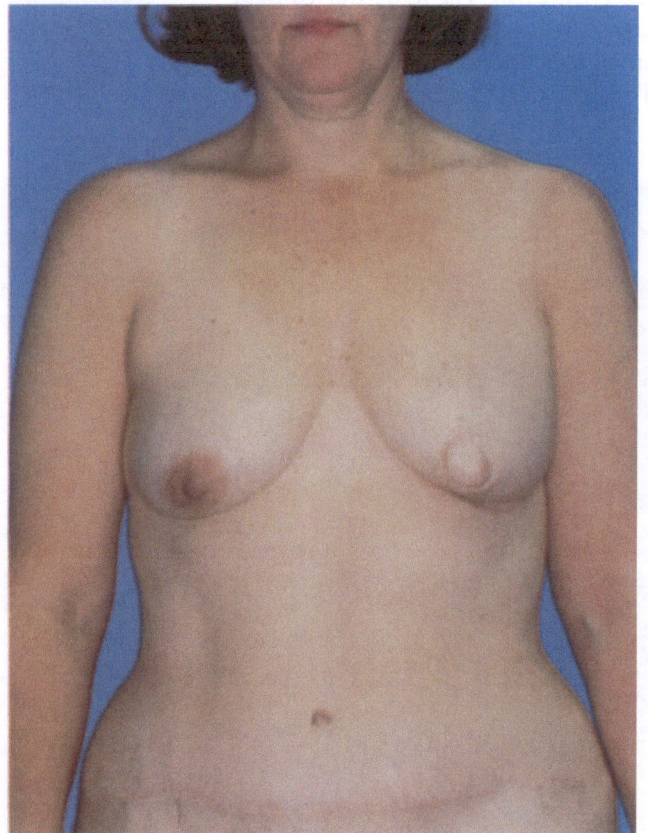

FIG. 20-4 (C) After revision, but before definitive nipple reconstruction.

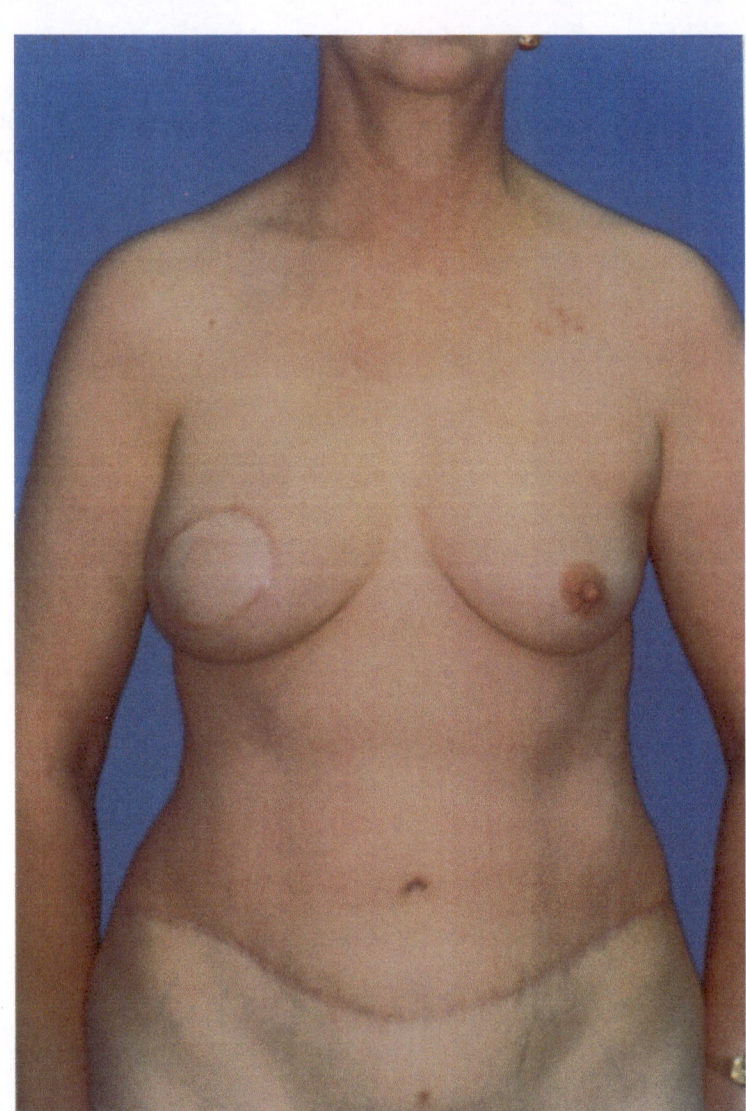

Fig. 20-6 (A) Patient after breast mound reconstruction with a free TRAM flap. The reconstructed right breast is too large. (B) Pattern for reduction of reconstructed breast, with use of the redundant skin as a "wrap-around" flap to create a nipple.

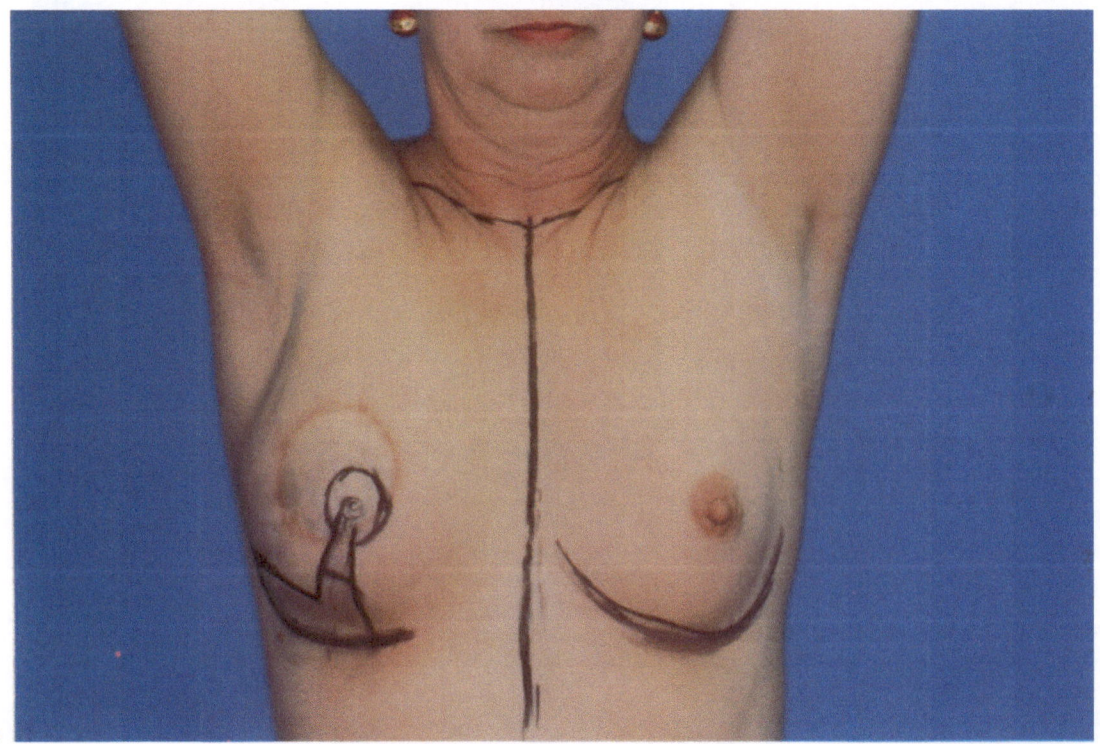

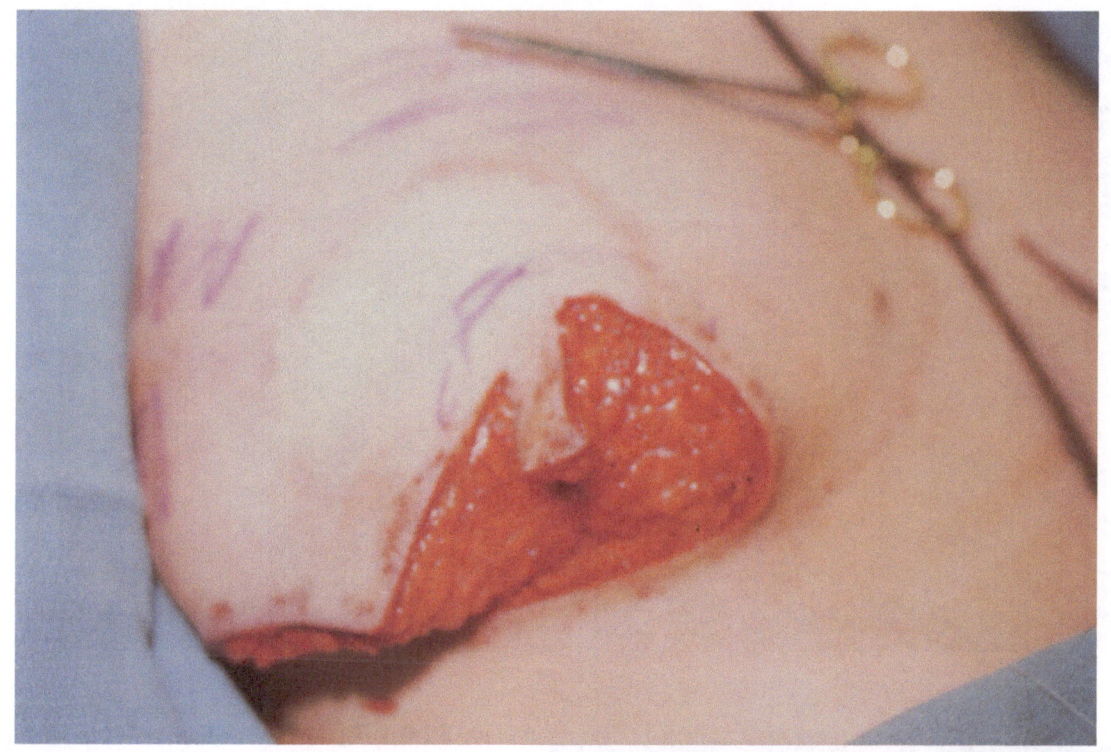

C

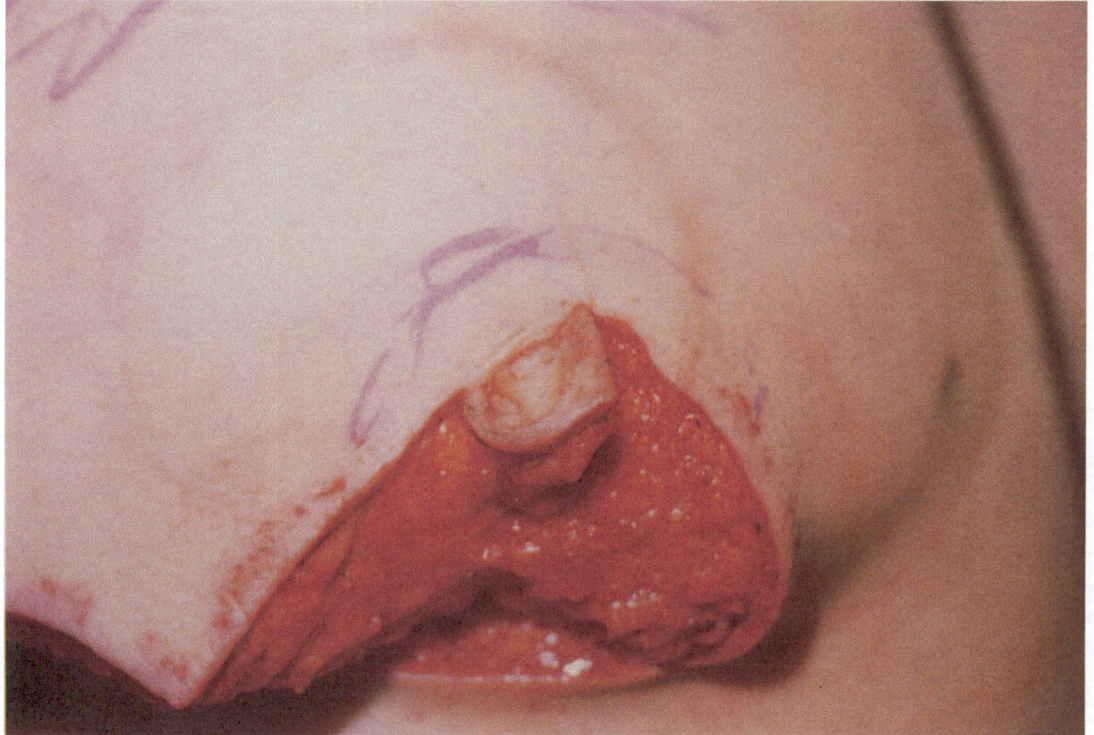

D

Fig. 20-6   (C) The wrap-around flap after elevation. (D) The flap is turned medially upon itself to create a projecting nipple.

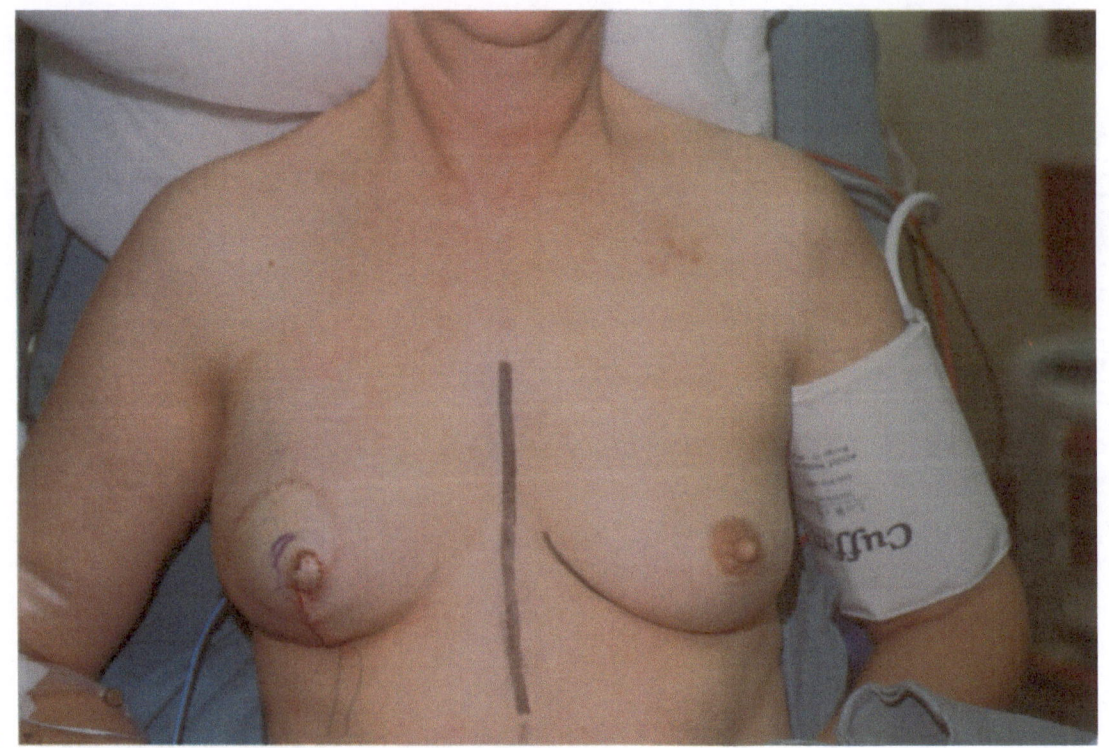

E

FIG. 20-6 (E) The immediate result in the operating room. (F) The same patient 3 weeks later.

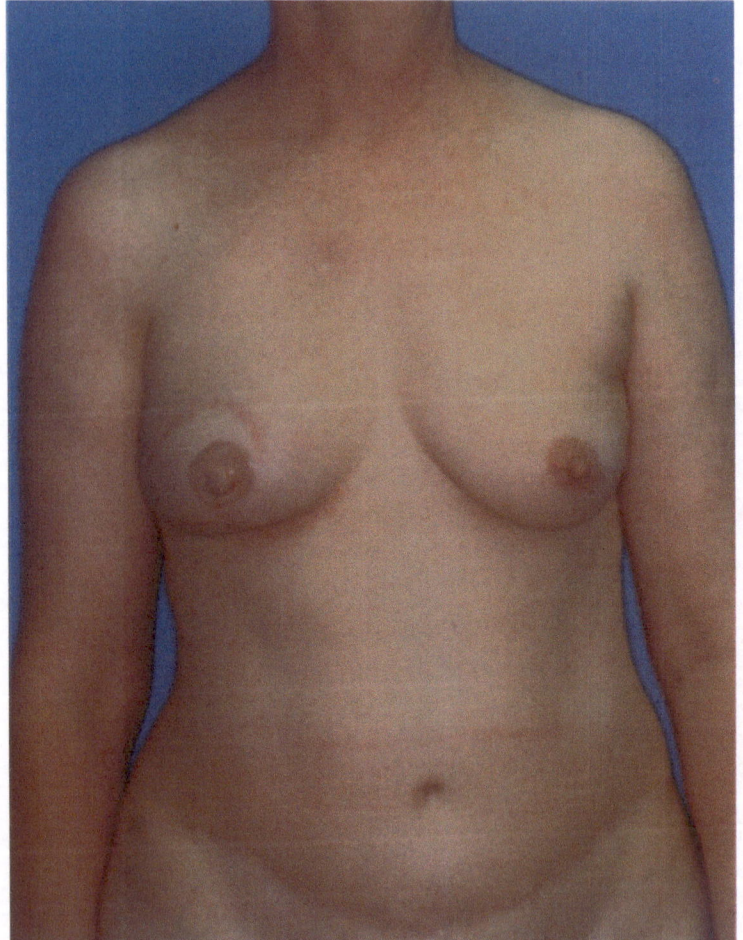

F

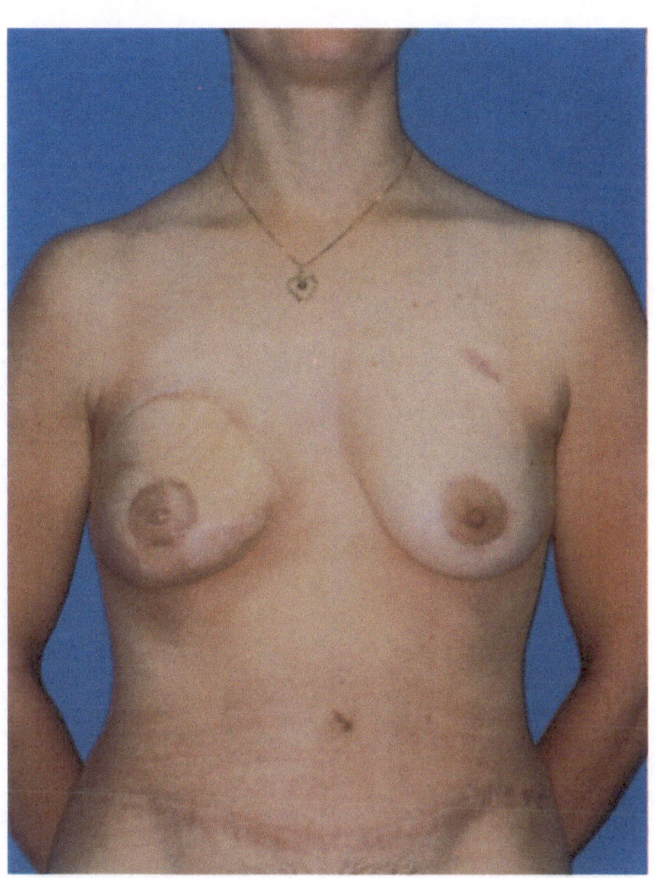

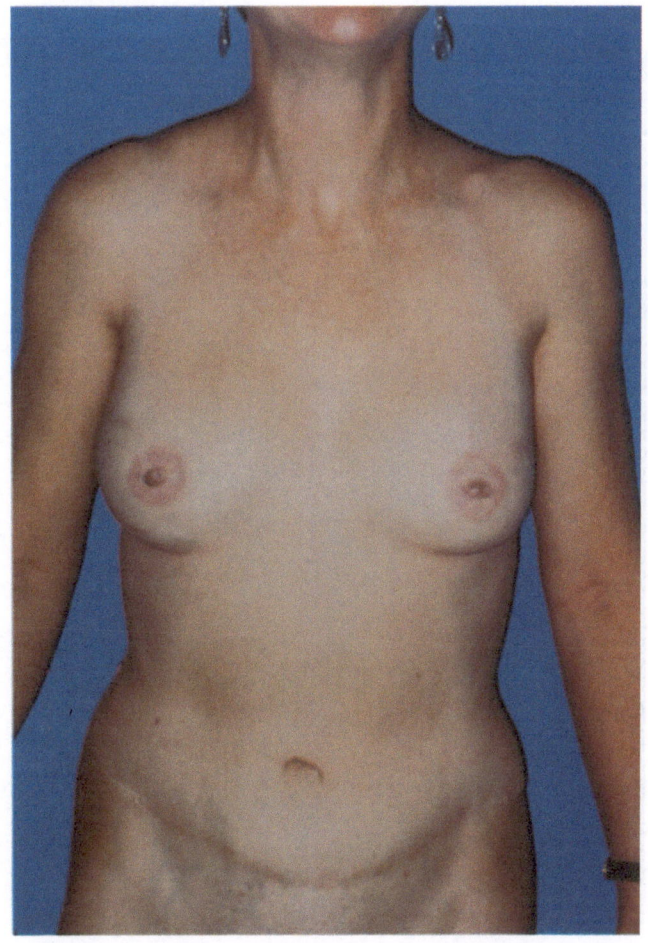

FIG. 21-11 Result of elective contralateral mastectomy and bilateral immediate reconstruction. The patient had cancer of the right breast.

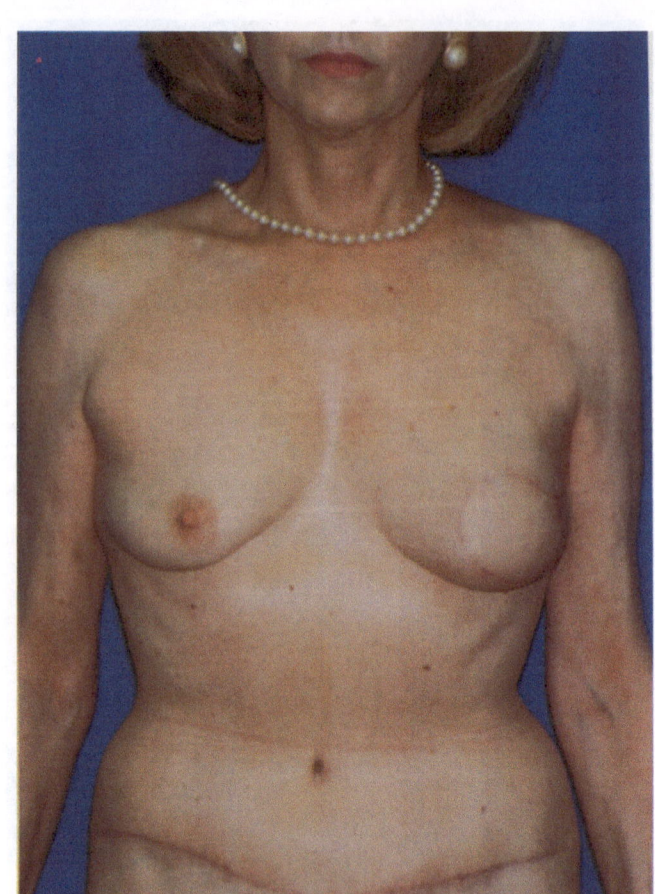

FIG. 21-9 (A) Patient with an immediate free TRAM flap breast reconstruction that is larger than her natural breast. She requested contralateral breast augmentation. (B) After augmentation with a small saline-filled implant, the symmetry is improved, and the patient was satisfied.

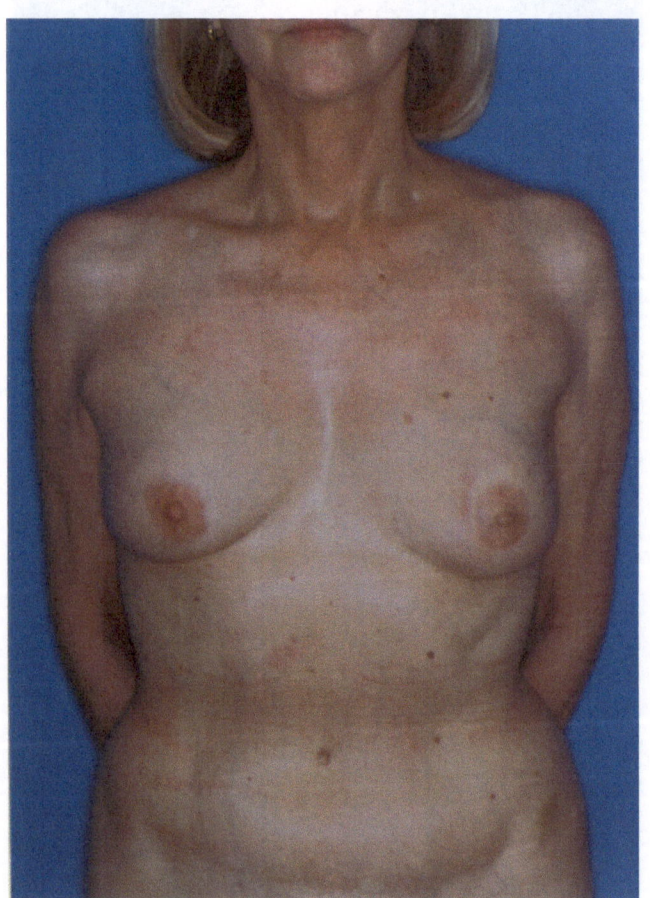

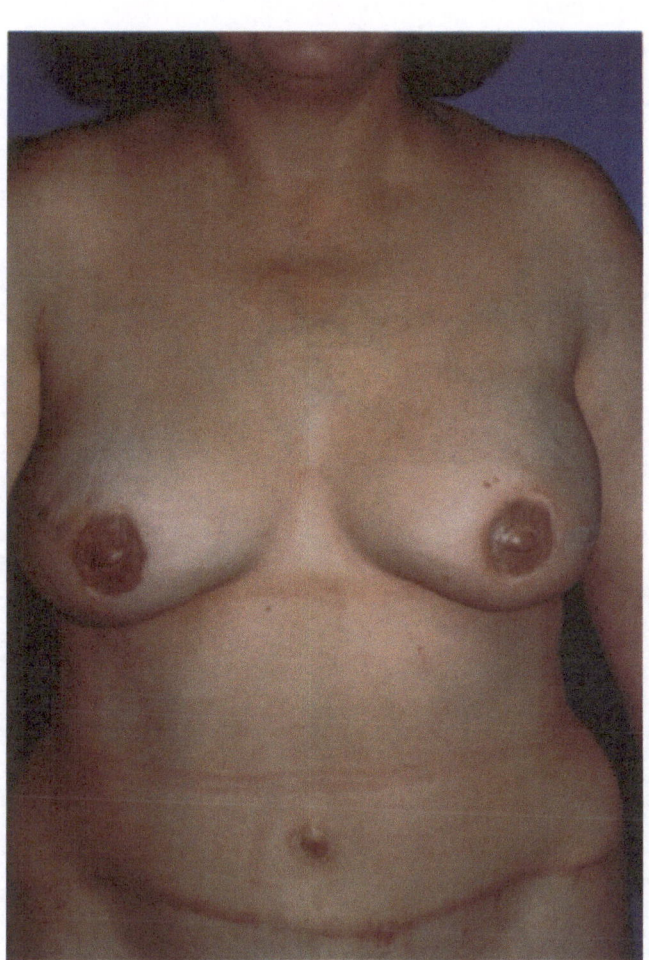

Fig. 21-12 Result of elective contralateral mastectomy and bilateral immediate reconstruction. The patient had cancer of the left breast.

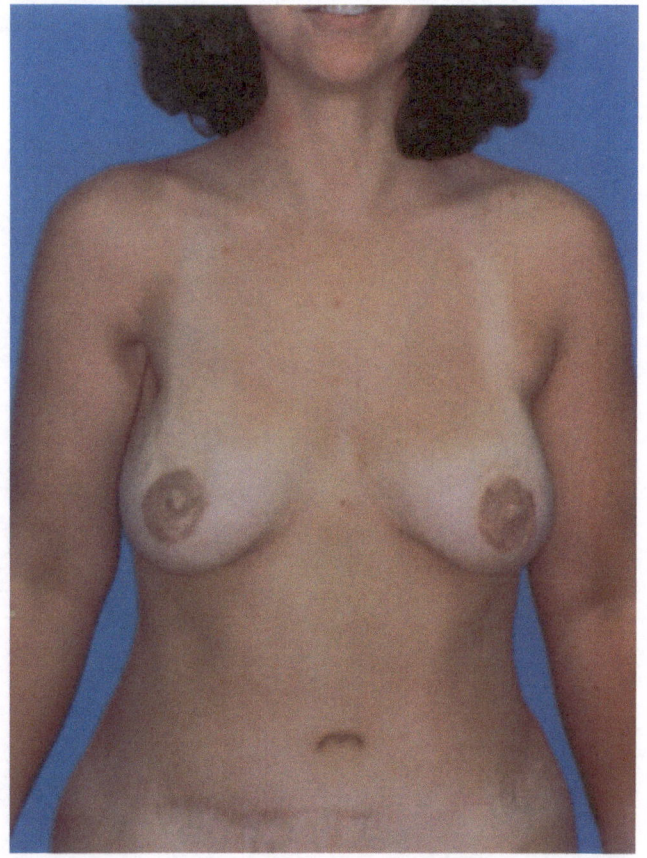

Fig. 21-13 Result of elective contralateral mastectomy and bilateral immediate reconstruction. The patient had cancer of the right breast.

A

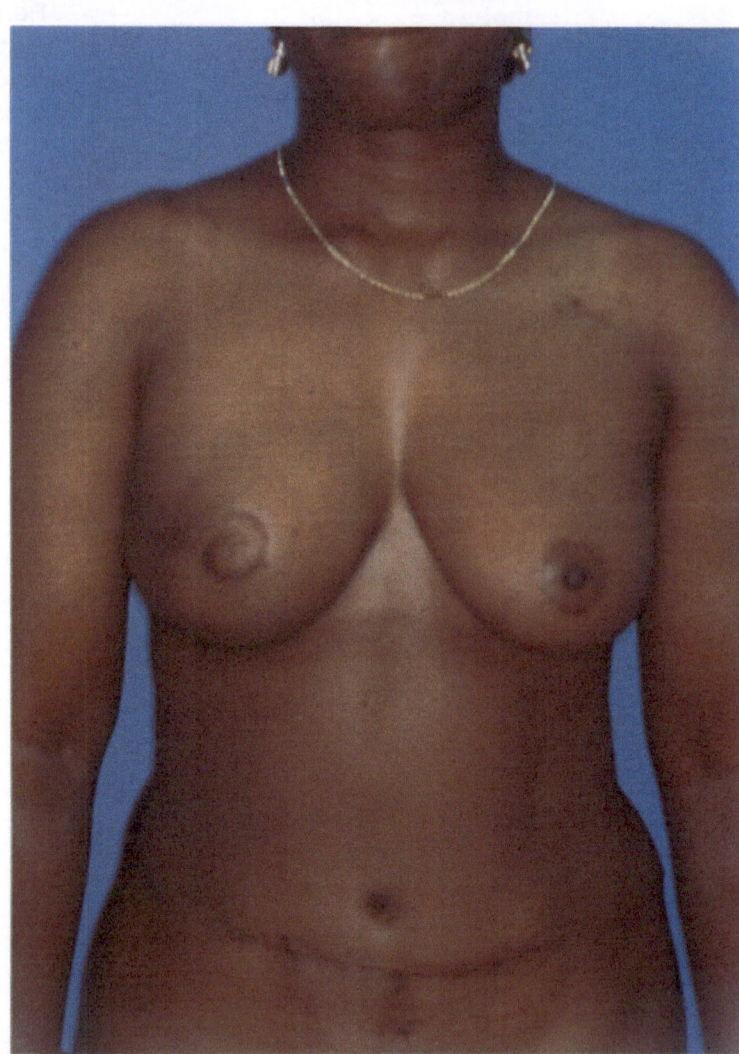

FIG. 22-22 (A) Patient after free TRAM flap right breast mound reconstruction and right nipple reconstruction with a wrap-around flap. The flap needs to be moved slightly lower and given more definition. (B) The design for a modified "star" flap with the base placed inferiorly.

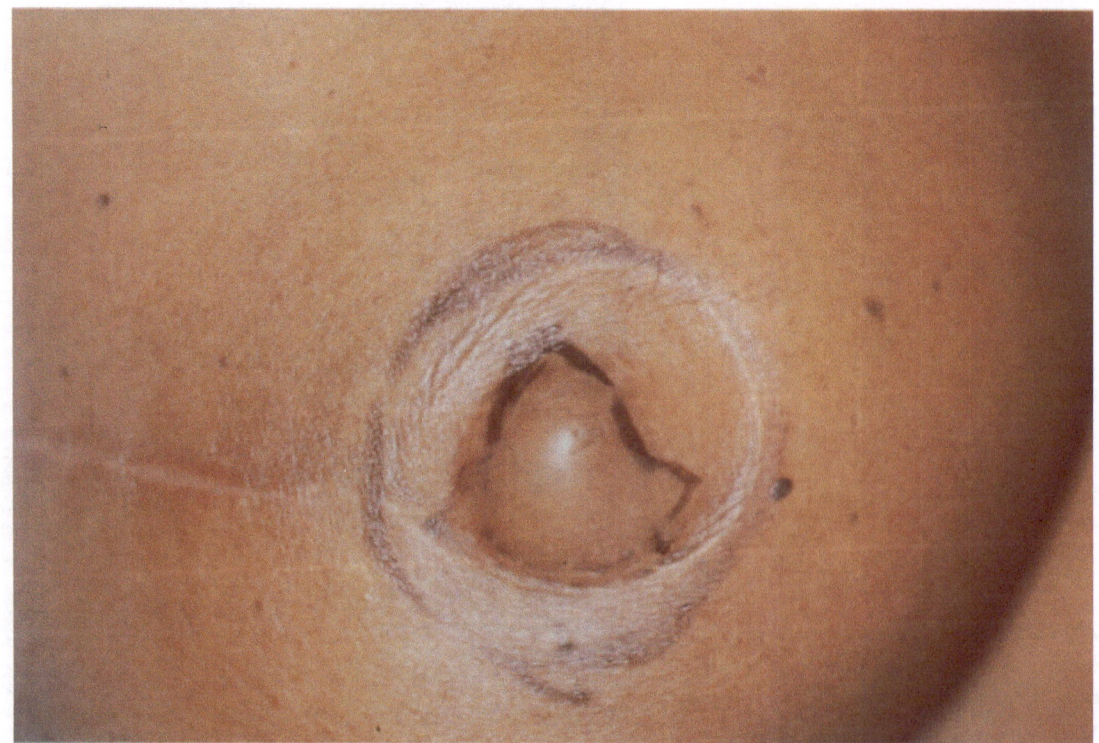

B

C

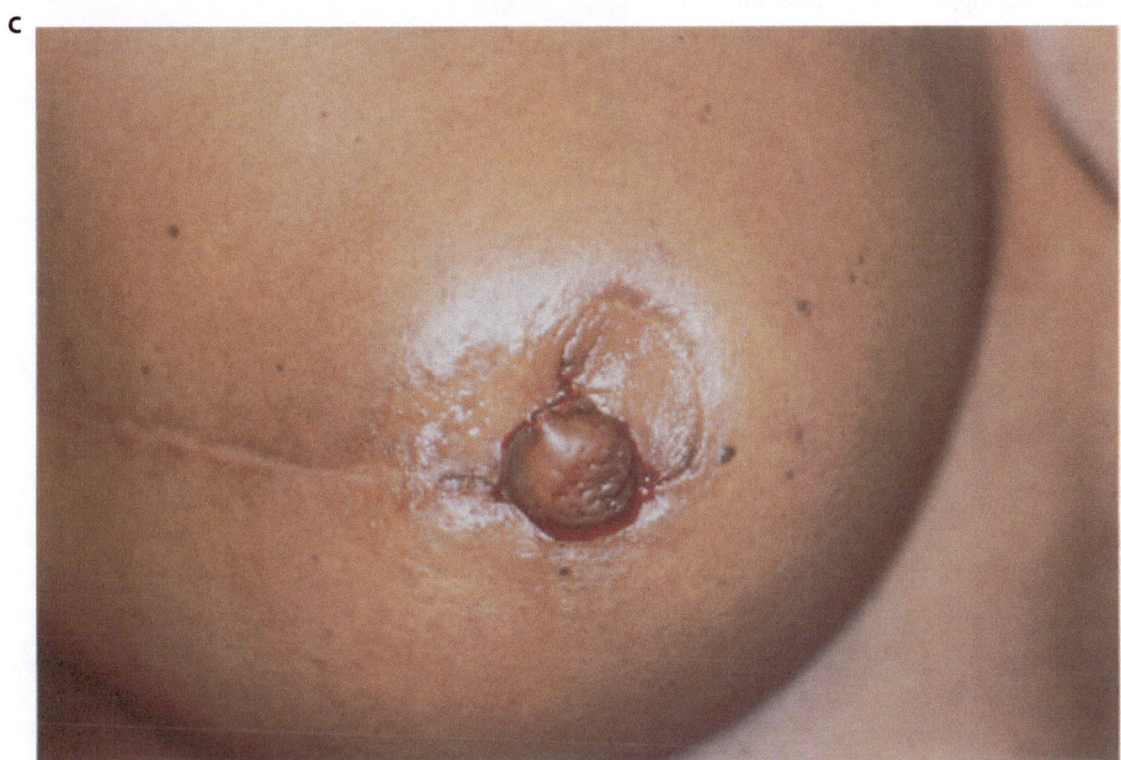

Fig. 22-22 (C) After completion of the star flap revision, the nipple has better definition. (D) The result of the nipple revision.

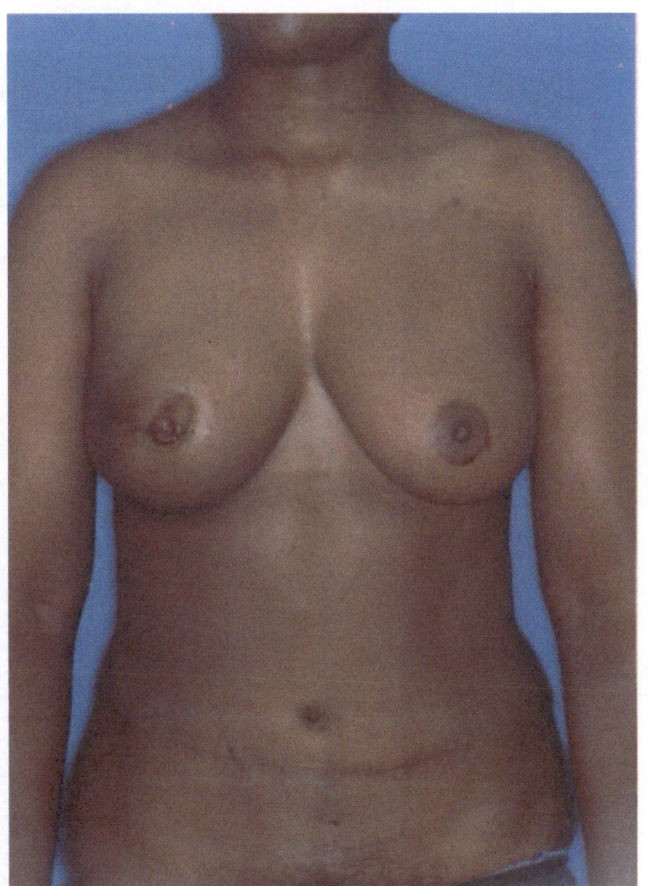

D

Fig. 22-4 A free TRAM flap breast reconstruction with symmetry of the breast mounds and nipples is very successful even though the breasts themselves do not have ideal shapes.

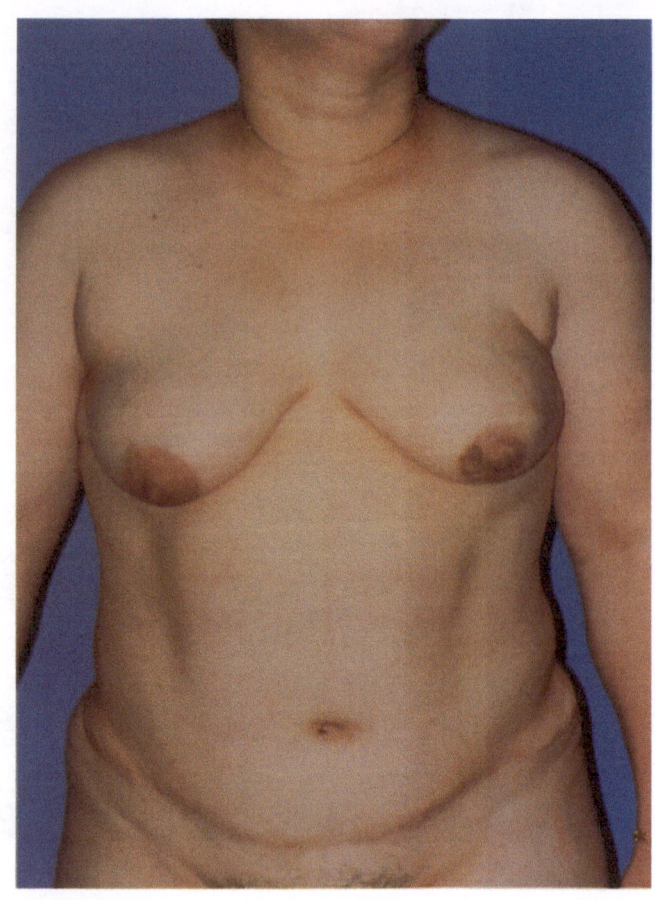

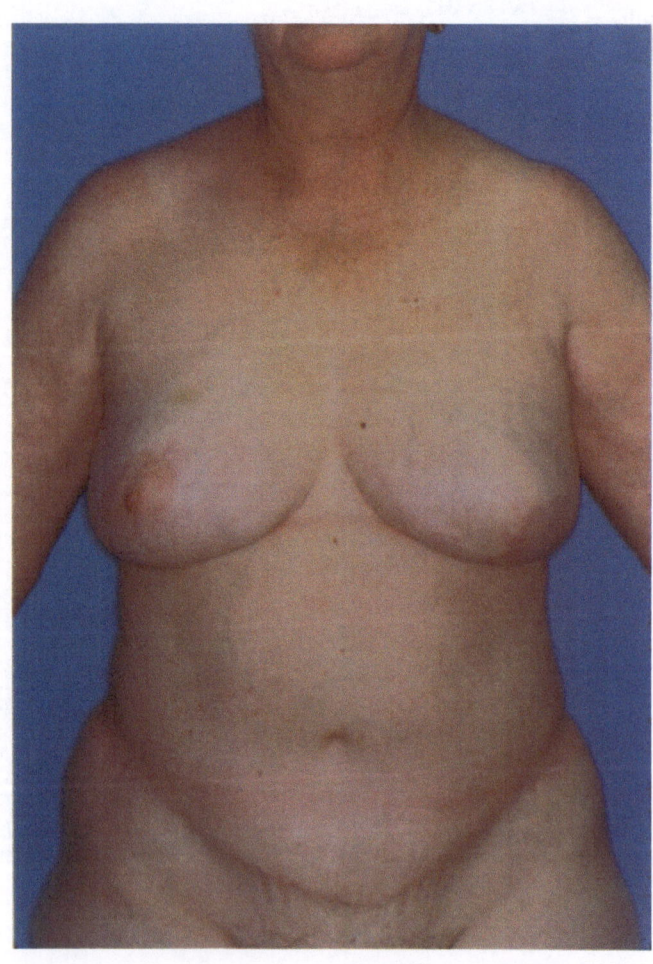

Fig. 23-4 (E) After another revision, the symmetry was restored.

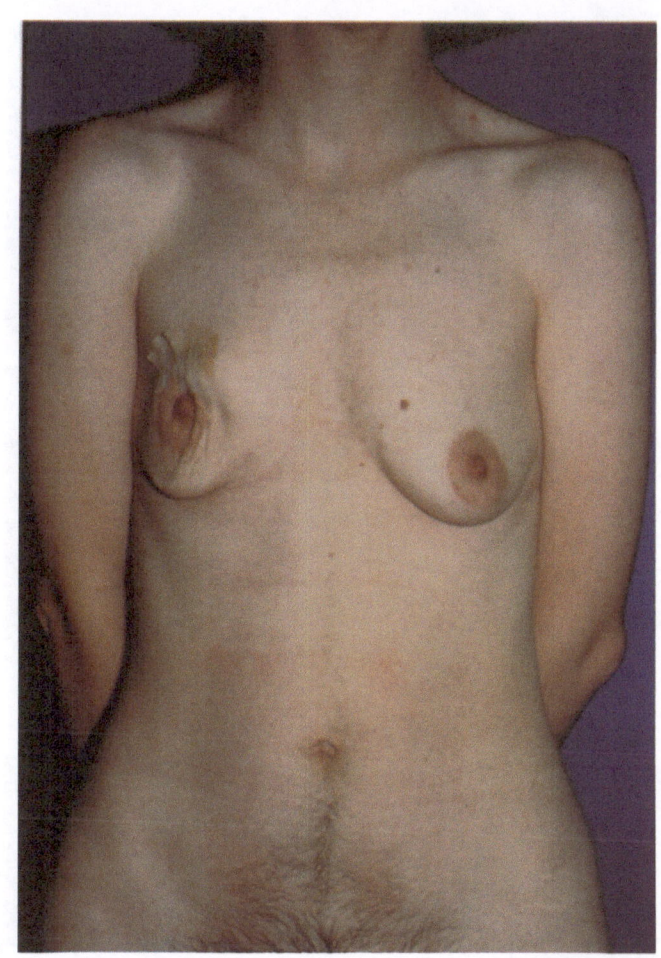

A

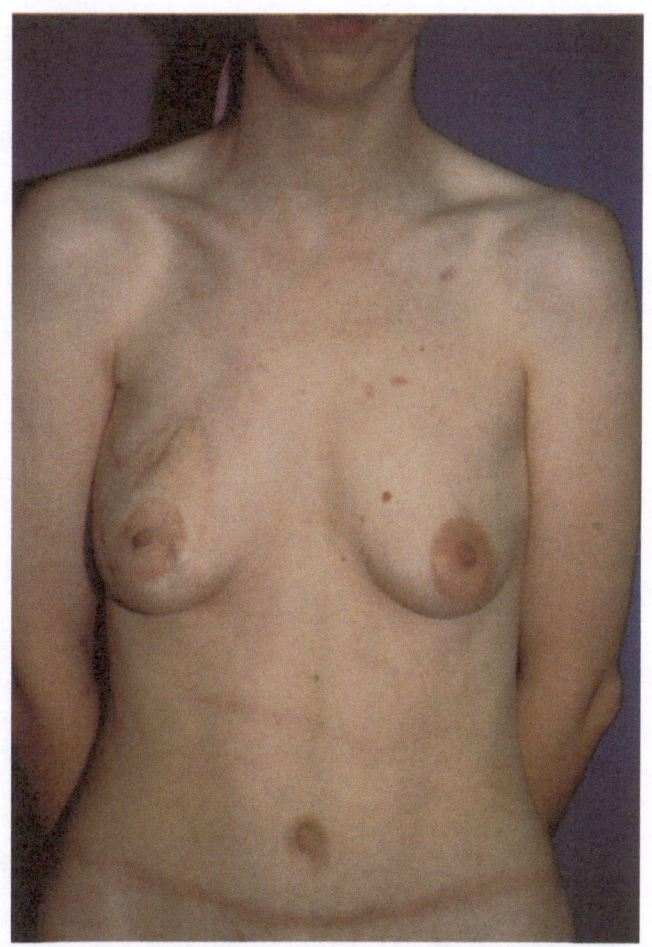

B

Fig. 23-3 (A) A 33-year-old woman after right breast biopsy, prior to mastectomy. (B) Same patient 1 year after immediate reconstruction of the right breast with a free TRAM flap.

FIG. 23-3 (C) Same woman 2 years later, following a successful term pregnancy. She did develop marked periumbilical striae, but otherwise there were no adverse effects.

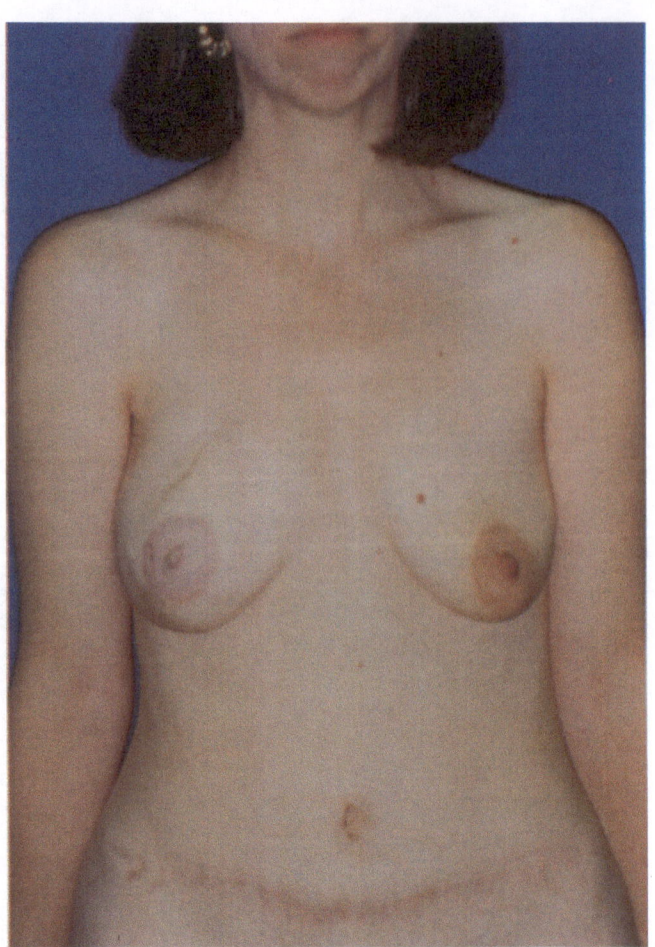

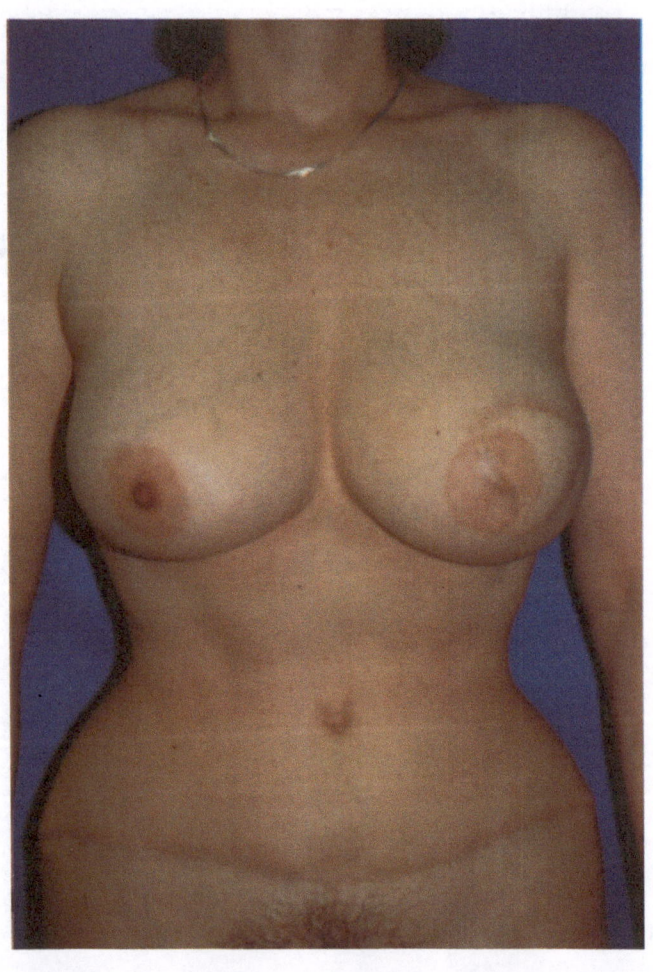

FIG. 23-6 Patient one year after immediate free TRAM flap reconstruction of the right breast. The scars are faded and very inconspicuous.

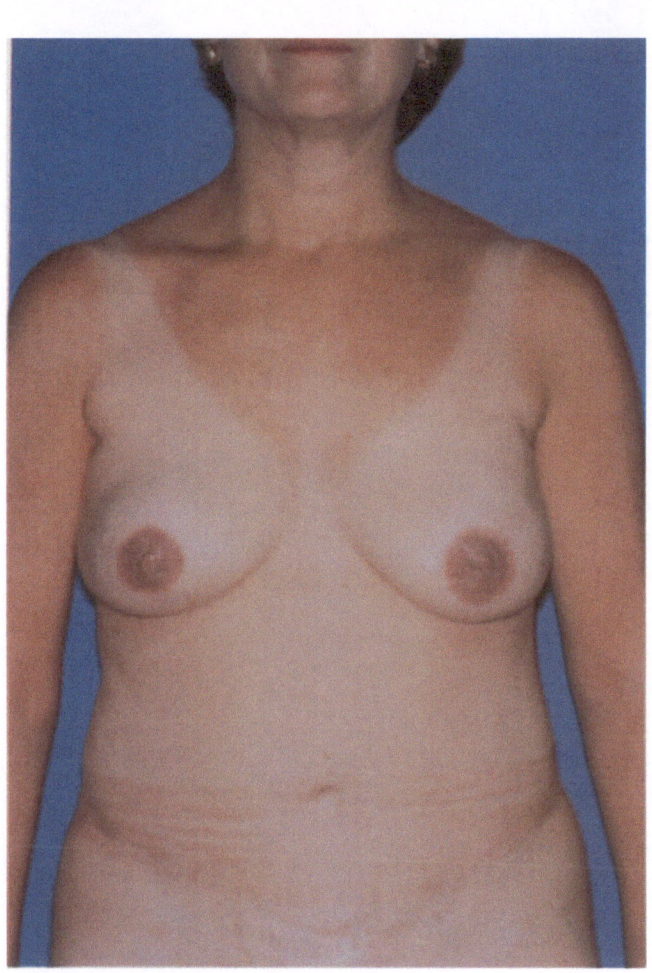

FIG. 23-8   Patient 5 years after bilateral immediate breast reconstruction with free TRAM flaps. The scars in the breast are barely visible.

FIG. 23-10   (A) Patient after reconstruction of the left breast, with tattooing to simulate natural pigmentation of the nipple and areola.

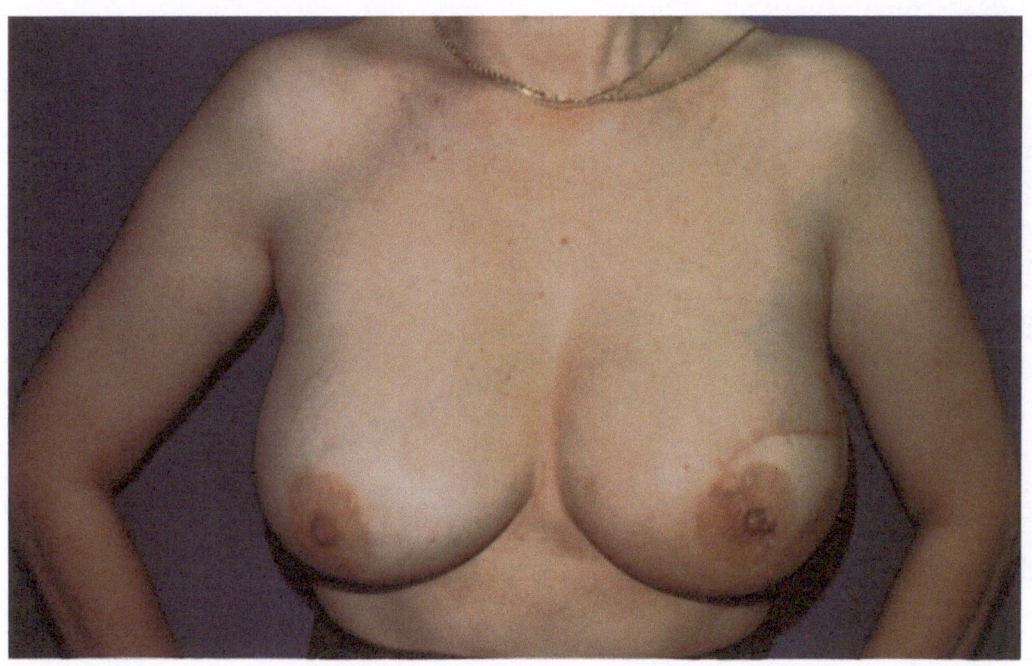

B

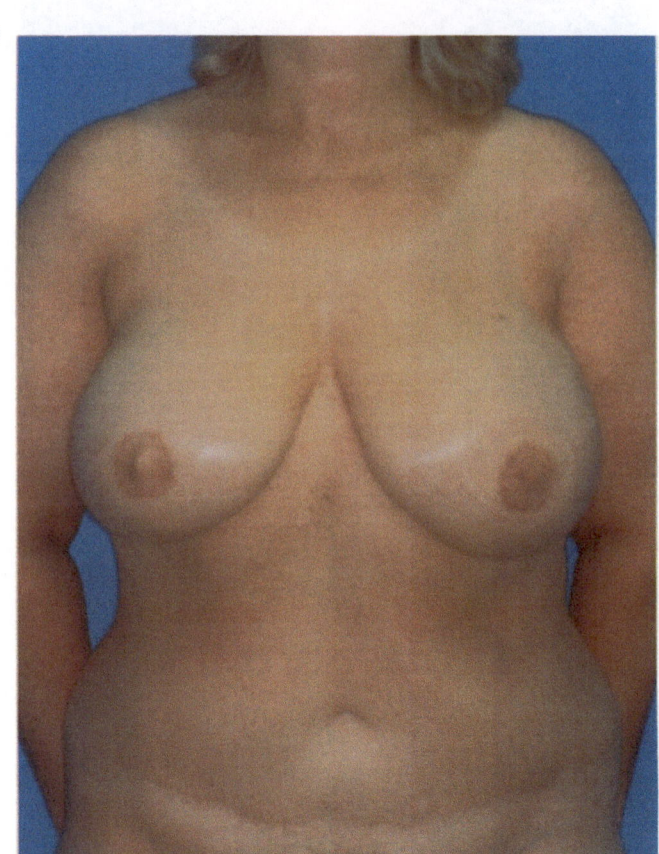

FIG. 23-10 (B) After 1 year, the tattooing has faded somewhat but the result is acceptable. (C) Five years after the tattooing, the pigmentation has almost completely faded away. Note that the patient has gained weight but in this case the breasts have remained symmetrical.

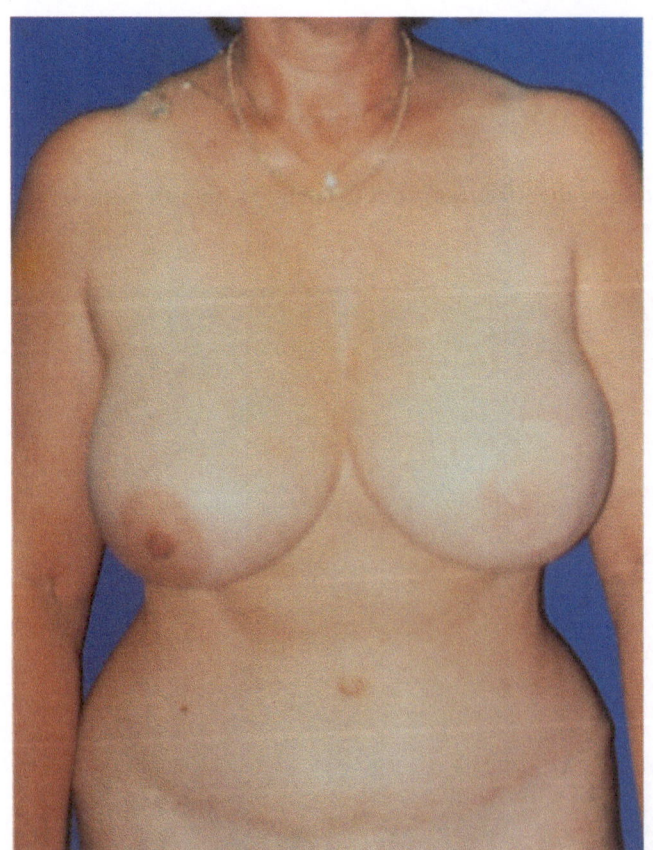

C

21 The Opposite Breast

The Importance of Symmetry

The goal of breast reconstruction is to make mastectomy patients look as normal as possible, especially in their clothing. Obtaining breast symmetry obviously contributes enormously to achieving that goal. It is rarely possible to reconstruct a breast mound that looks exactly like its opposite, natural counterpart on close inspection. Instead, the surgeon seeks to create an *illusion* of normalcy by creating a breast mound that is close enough in size and shape to the opposite breast that the observer is fooled, in part by his or her expectations, into believing that what is being seen is a real breast.

Sometimes the easiest way to achieve breast symmetry is to revise the opposite, natural breast.[1,2] This is especially indicated when the reconstructed breast mound looks better than the natural one, which commonly occurs when the opposite breast is excessively small or ptotic. In that case, surgery on the opposite breast may be indicated and will often provide an excellent result. Opposite breast alteration may also be indicated when changing the reconstructed mound to match the natural breast would be technically difficult, even when the natural breast has an attractive appearance. This is usually the case when the reconstructed breast mound has less ptosis than the natural breast, because lowering the reconstructed breast is so difficult. Whenever surgery is planned on an opposite breast, a mammogram should be obtained preoperatively so that if there is a suspicious lesion in the breast, biopsy can be incorporated into the planned surgery and will not require additional incisions.

Opposite Mastopexy

The most common cause of asymmetry after unilateral breast reconstruction is a lack of ptosis in the reconstructed breast. For this reason, mastopexy[3] is the procedure most frequently performed on the opposite breast. If opposite mastopexy will obviously be

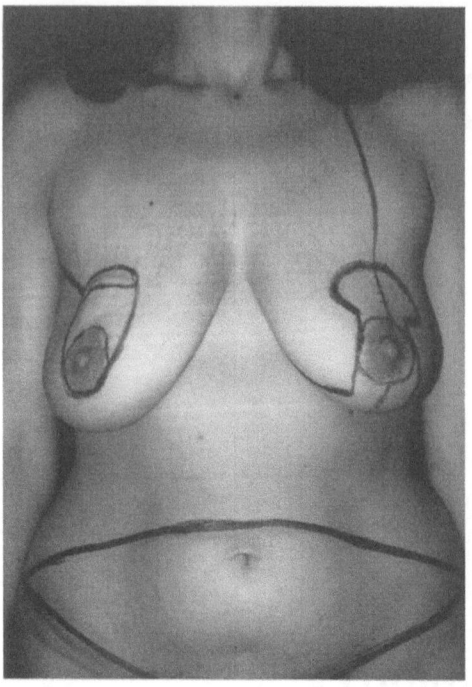
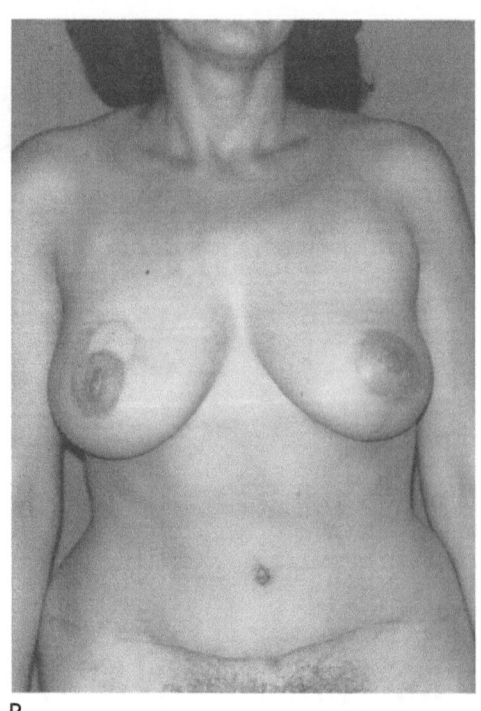

A   B

FIG. 21-1 (A) Patient with excessively ptotic breasts showing the operative plan. The nipple/areolar complex and biopsy scar were excised. (B) Result of immediate right free transverse rectus abdominus myocutaneous (TRAM) flap breast reconstruction and simultaneous left mastopexy.

required, it can be performed simultaneous with the breast mound reconstruction (Fig 21-1), eliminating the need for one subsequent surgical procedure. If the breast mound reconstruction is difficult or involves excessive time or blood loss, however, the mastopexy should be deferred.

To design a subsequent mastopexy, the surgeon marks ideal nipple position on the reconstructed breast mound. The breast meridian is marked on both sides, as are the clavicles, the sternal notch, and the inframammary fold. The mirror image of the ideal position of the reconstructed nipple on the reconstructed breast mound is marked on the natural breast, based on measurements from the clavicles and the sternal notch. The mastopexy is then designed around this newly determined nipple position (Fig 21-2). The desired distance between the nipple and the inframammary fold on the mastopexy side is calculated from the dimensions of the reconstructed breast mound (distance from inframammary fold to ideal nipple position).

In some cases, both the reconstructed breast and the natural one will need mastopexy or reduction. This situation arises when both breasts are ptotic and the patient requests that they be elevated and/or reduced. In that case (Fig 21-3), the nipple should not be reconstructed at the same time as the mastopexy or reduction. Instead, the surgeon should wait until the breast shaping process has been completed before selecting the location of the new nipple.

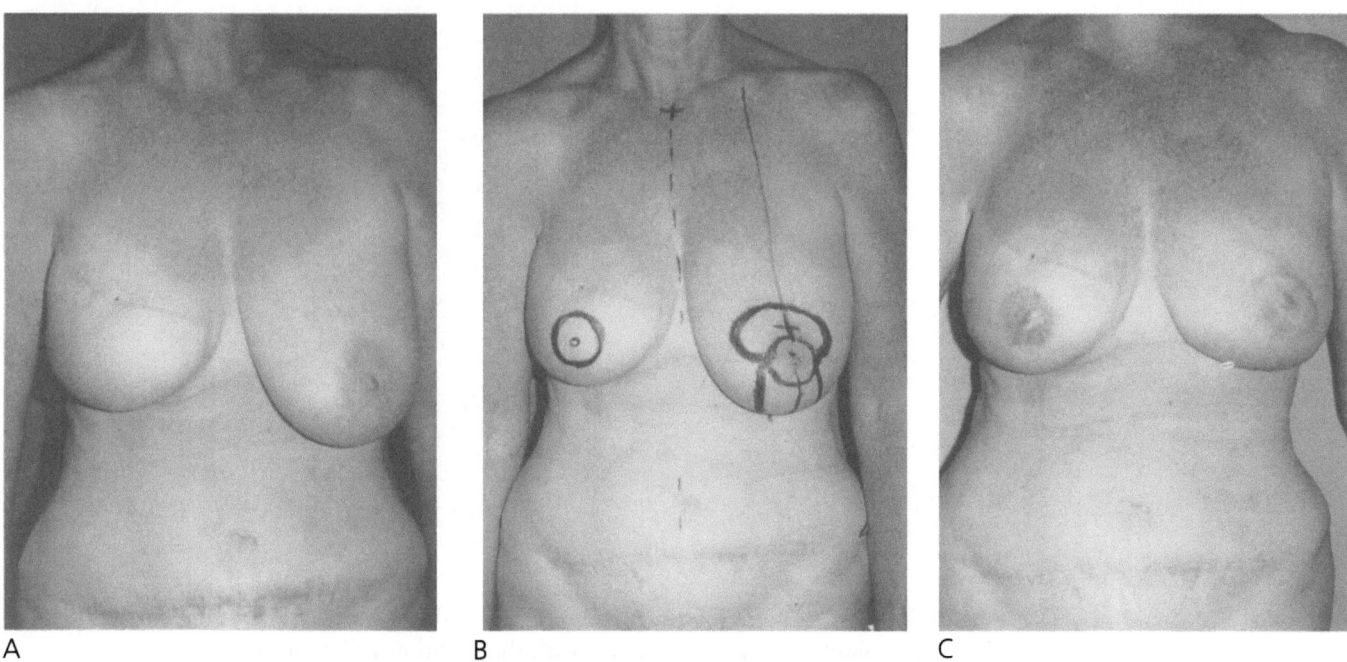

A   B   C

Fig. 21-2   (A) Patient with TRAM flap breast mound prior to revision. The natural breast is much more ptotic than the reconstructed one. (B) The ideal nipple position is marked on the reconstructed breast mound; then the mastopexy is designed around its mirror image. (C) Result of opposite mastopexy. (From Kroll SS: Options for the contralateral breast in breast reconstruction. In Spear SL, ed. *Surgery of the Breast: Principles and Art.* Philadelphia: Lippincott-Raven, 1998, pp. 653–658; Kroll SS, Miller MJ, Schusterman MA, Reece GP, Singletary SE, Ames F. *Ann Surg Oncol.* 1994;1:457–461. Used with permission.)

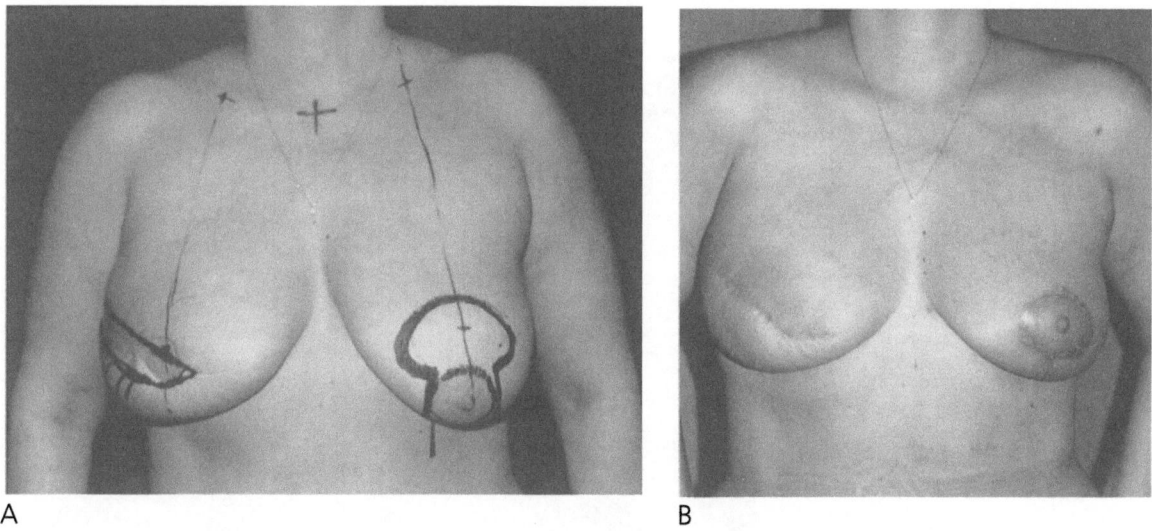

A   B

Fig. 21-3   (A) Patient with plan for simultaneous right breast revision and left mastopexy, without simultaneous nipple reconstruction. (B) Early result. The nipple site will be selected only after all breast shaping has been completed.

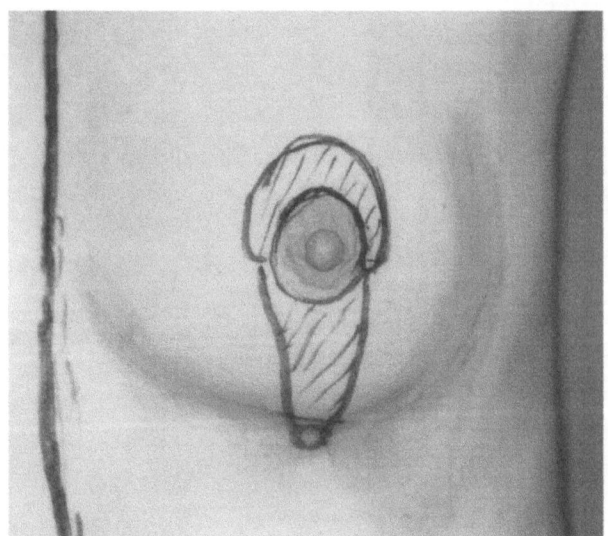

FIG. 21-4   Vertical pattern for mastopexy. This avoids the horizontal scar, but elevates the nipple/areolar complex less than is possible with the traditional Wise pattern.

If a considerable amount of elevation is required of the mastopexy, the choice of mastopexy pattern will be between a Wise pattern (Figs 21-1 and 21-2) and a vertical incision (Fig 21-4).[4,5] If only 1 or 2 cm of nipple elevation are required, however, a circumferential ("doughnut") or crescent mastopexy (Fig 21-5) is often a better choice.[6] The crescent mastopexy minimizes scarring in the lower part of the breast, but at the price of flattening the breast mound. In aesthetic surgery this flattening is ordinarily a

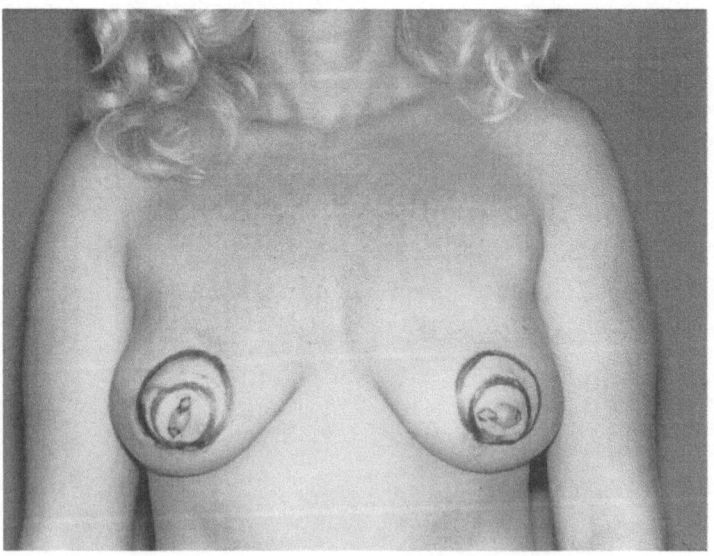

FIG. 21-5   Pattern for bilateral crescent mastopexy. This avoids all scars except the circumareolar ones but flattens the breasts.

disadvantage, but because lack of projection is a typical feature of a reconstructed breast mound, in this case the flattening can improve symmetry and therefore is usually desirable.

During the mastopexy, the patient should be placed in a sitting position on the operating table so that symmetry can be evaluated. Although a completely upright position cannot be achieved, a nearly upright position can be attained by combining back elevation with a reverse Trendelenburg position, allowing the surgeon to evaluate symmetry with reasonable accuracy. A temporary wound closure can be performed with surgical staples for this evaluation. If adjustments are necessary, they can then be made before final wound closure is performed with sutures.

One of the common but unfortunate sequelae of a circumferential mastopexy is widening of the scars. This can be improved by scar revision at a later time or prevented by using a permanent or long-lasting purse-string suture (Fig 21-6) similar, in principle, to the "round block" suture advocated by Benelli.[7,8] A purse-string suture will also reduce the tendency for the aerola to enlarge as a result of outward tension. Alternatively, eventual enlargement of the areola can be compensated for by making the areola somewhat smaller than desired and allowing it to expand when subjected to the tension of wound closure. This, however, does not avoid the problem of scar widening the way a permanent purse-string or blocking suture does.

Opposite Breast Reduction

If the opposite breast is larger than the reconstructed one, opposite breast reduction[9–12] is usually indicated. This is especially true if the opposite breast is too large and is causing neck or back pain, interfering with exercise, or causing rashes in the inframammary fold. Contralateral reduction also reduces the weight and ptosis required of the reconstructed breast, making reconstruction with a free flap safer and easier by reducing the necessary pedicle length. Often, when the breasts are excessively large, the patient will consider the reconstruction an opportunity to reduce breast size and obtain symptomatic relief, and may bring up the subject of opposite breast reduction herself. In such a case, it is generally preferable to perform the contralateral reduction at the same time as the initial breast mound reconstruction, provided that the breast mound reconstruction is not excessively lengthy or complicated by excessive blood loss. This allows fine-tuning of the reduction mammaplasty result at the time of the revision of the breast mound. In that way it is often possible to achieve good results after only one revision, minimizing expense and patient inconvenience (Fig 21-7).

If the reconstructed breast mound is smaller than the natural breast, reduction of the opposite breast can be indicated even when its size is not excessive. In such cases, symmetry could theoretically be achieved by enlarging the reconstructed breast, but this enlargement would require either an additional flap or the use of an implant. Reduction of the opposite breast is usually a much easier and more natural solution, and can achieve excellent results (Fig 21-8).

To accomplish opposite breast reduction, I generally use an inferior pedicle technique,[13,14] but any of the commonly accepted methods of breast reduction can be successfully used. The amount of skin excision is determined from measurements as de-

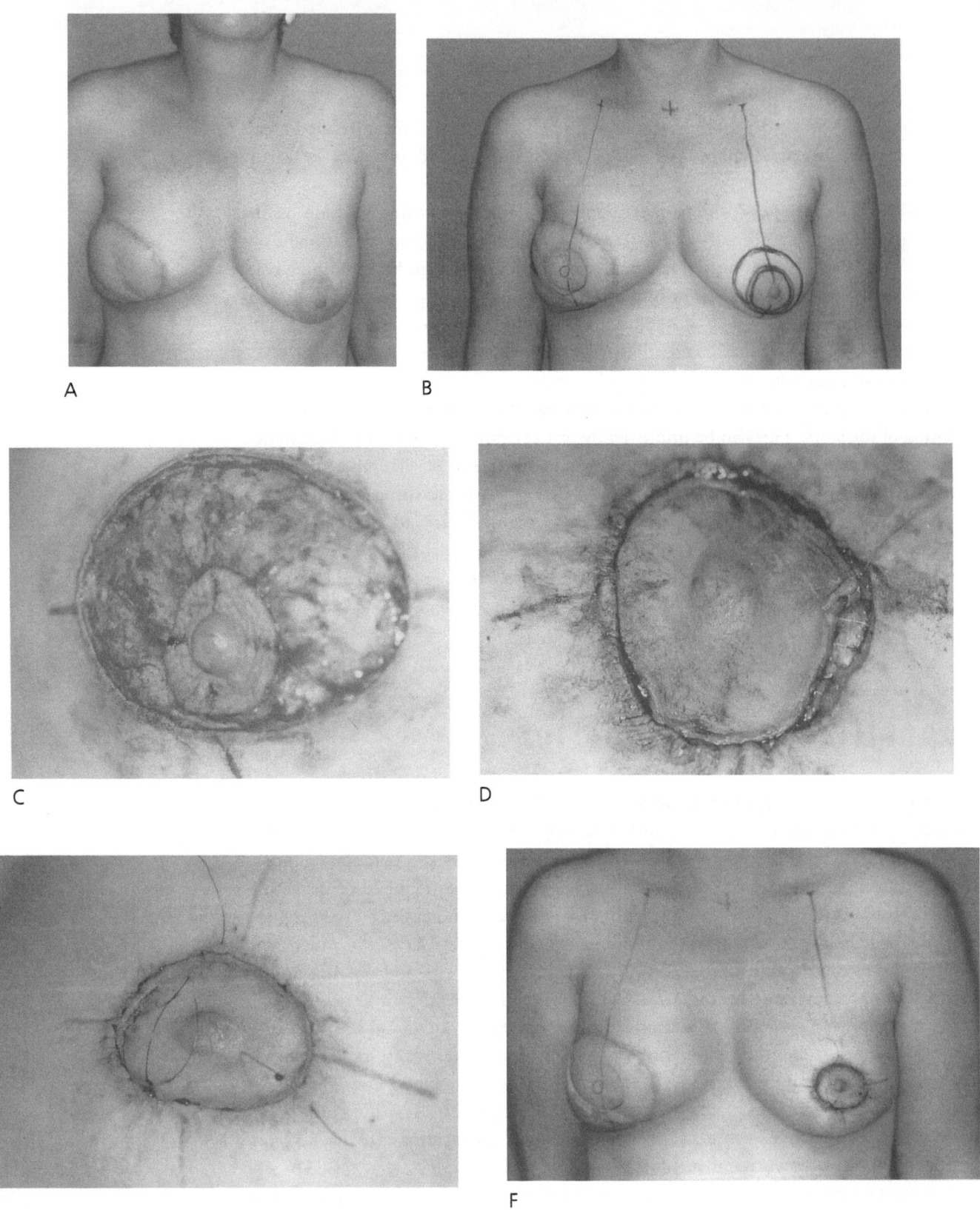

FIG. 21-6   (A) Patient with excess lateral fullness of the reconstructed right breast mound, which is also less ptotic than the opposite, natural breast. (B) Plan for revision of the right breast combined with crescent mastopexy on the left. (C) The excess skin has been removed, and markings have been placed in each quadrant to line up areola and surrounding skin. (D) A modified round block (or purse string) running suture is placed using a 2-0 monofilament absorbable PDS (polydioxanone) suture. The suture has not yet been completely tightened so it remains partly visible. (E) The purse string suture is tied so that the knot is buried well away from the incision. A layer of running subcuticular Prolene (polypropylene) suture is then placed to finish the repair. (F) The result is a moderate-sized areola that will not stretch or enlarge.

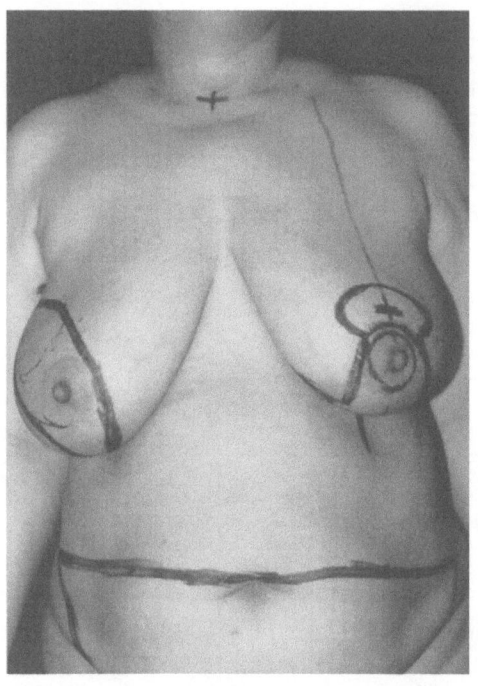
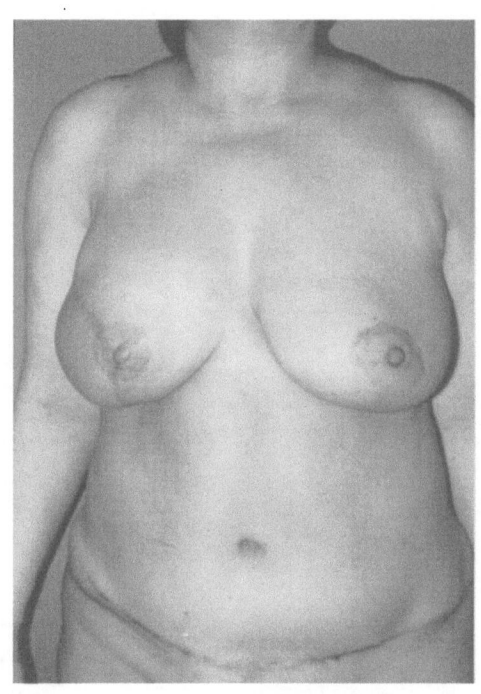

A   B

FIG. 21-7 (A) Patient prior to reconstruction. (B) After simultaneous breast mound reconstruction and opposite breast reduction. The symmetry is reasonably good. (From Kroll SS: Options for the contralateral breast in breast reconstruction. In Spear SL, ed. *Surgery of the Breast: Principles and Art.* Philadelphia: Lippincott-Raven, 1998; Used with permission.)

scribed above for mastopexy. The amount of glandular tissue that must be removed is determined by comparing the two breasts and excising tissue from the reduced side until symmetry is achieved. As in mastopexy, breast symmetry should be evaluated with the patient in a nearly upright sitting position. Whenever possible, a mammogram should be obtained preoperatively so that if there is suspicious breast tissue it can be removed during the reduction. Mammography should also be performed 6 months after the reduction so that a baseline film of the remaining natural breast will be available should mammographically suspicious lesions subsequently develop.

Opposite Breast Augmentation

Augmentation of the opposite breast can interfere with subsequent mammograms and subject the patient to risks associated with breast implants, such as capsular contracture, leakage, and periprosthetic infection. In theory, therefore, opposite breast augmentation is undesirable and is best discouraged if the opposite breast is not overly small. Nevertheless, many patients with small breasts will request such augmentation, especially if the reconstruction has created a pleasing breast mound that is larger than the natural breast. In such cases, especially if the natural breasts were very small, even a very small contralateral augmentation will often satisfy the patient (Fig 21-9). Because patient satisfac-

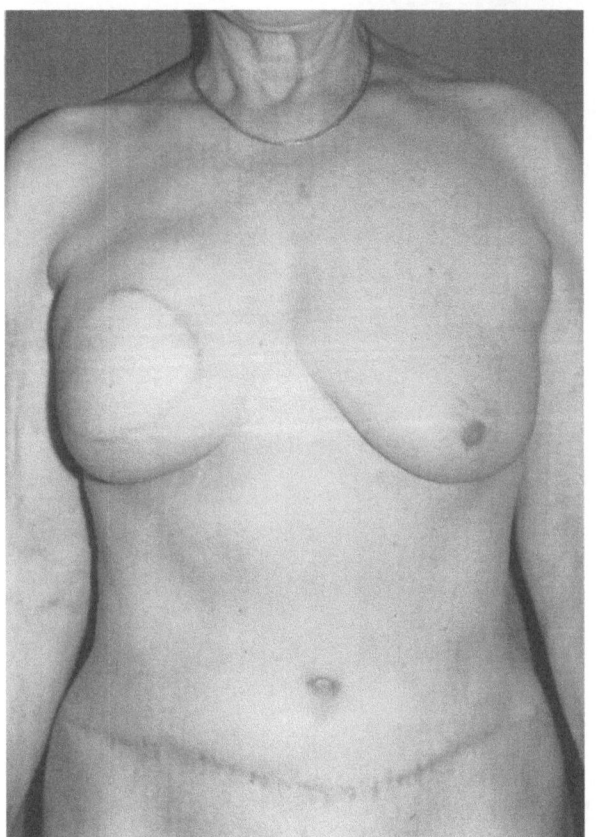

A

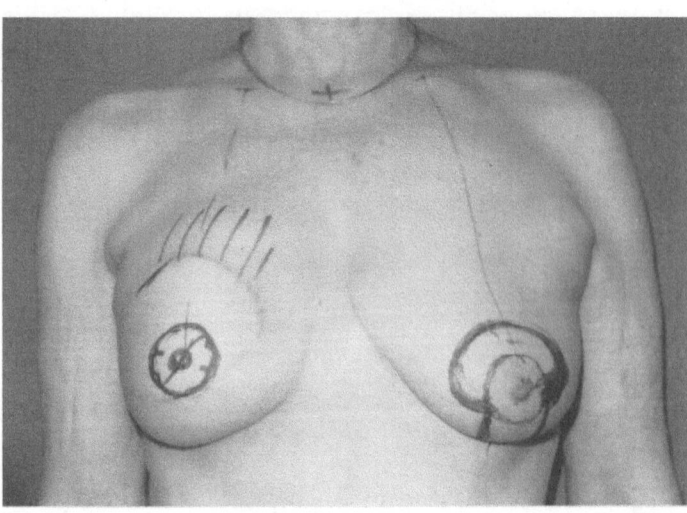

B

C

FIG. 21-8   (A) TRAM flap breast mound reconstruction prior to revision. The natural breast is larger than the reconstructed one. (B) The plan for left breast reduction using an inferior pedicle technique. The upper pole of the reconstructed mound also underwent suction lipectomy. (C) After the revisions, the symmetry is greatly improved.

tion is one of the goals of breast reconstruction, and because reduction of the reconstructed mound to a very small size may be technically difficult, opposite augmentation can be indicated in selected cases, especially when the patient is strongly in favor of it.

If a decision to perform contralateral augmentation is made, I prefer using saline-filled implants because the risk of capsular contracture is lower than when using silicone gel–filled implants. The implants are best placed submuscularly because that po-

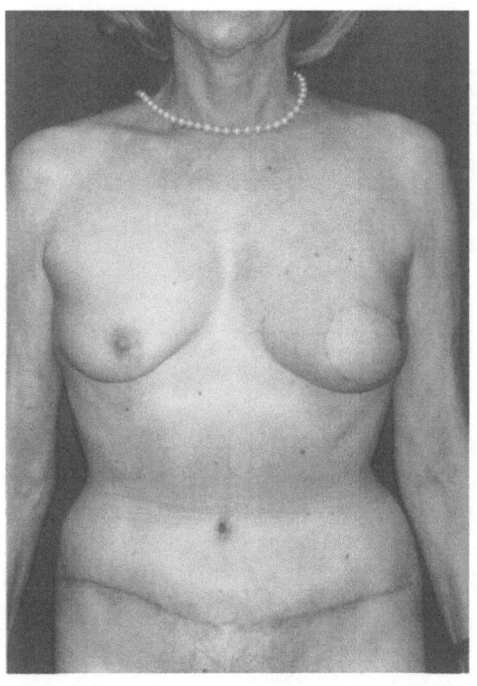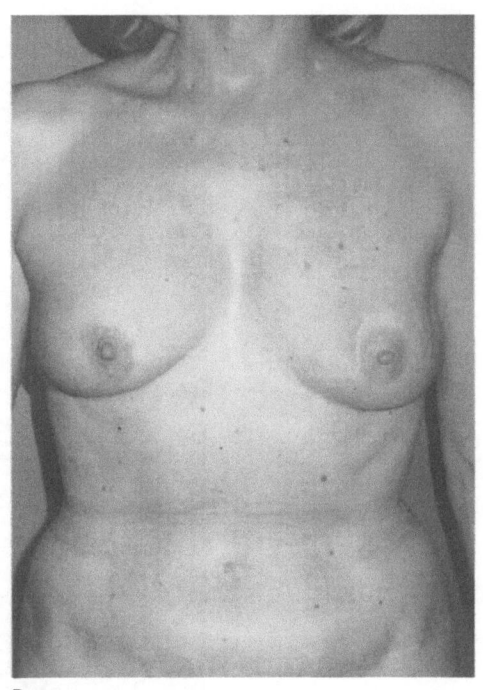

A   B

FIG. 21-9   (A) Patient with an immediate free TRAM flap breast reconstruction that is larger than her natural breast. She requested contralateral breast augmentation. See color insert, p. I-24. (B) After augmentation with a small saline-filled implant, the symmetry is improved, and the patient was satisfied. See color insert, p. I-24.

sition also reduces the incidence of capsular contracture, and interferes less with subsequent mammographic surveillance.

In most cases, the surgeon should select the smaller size implant that will achieve acceptable symmetry. This is because the ratio between the implant size and the amount of overlying breast tissue affects the risk of developing symptomatic capsular contracture. Because of the camouflaging effect of the overlying soft tissue, the smaller the implant and the more breast tissue covering the implant, the less likely it is that any capsular contracture that occurs will become symptomatic.

Elective Contralateral Mastectomy and Bilateral Reconstruction

Bilateral breast reconstruction is often more aesthetically successful than unilateral reconstruction[15] because it is not necessary to match a contralateral, natural breast to achieve symmetry. Especially if the two breasts are reconstructed with the same technique, symmetry is usually relatively easily achieved (Fig 21-10). Revision of the opposite breast is therefore not necessary. Because of the aesthetic advantages of bilateral reconstruction and because some patients with unilateral breast cancer are at high

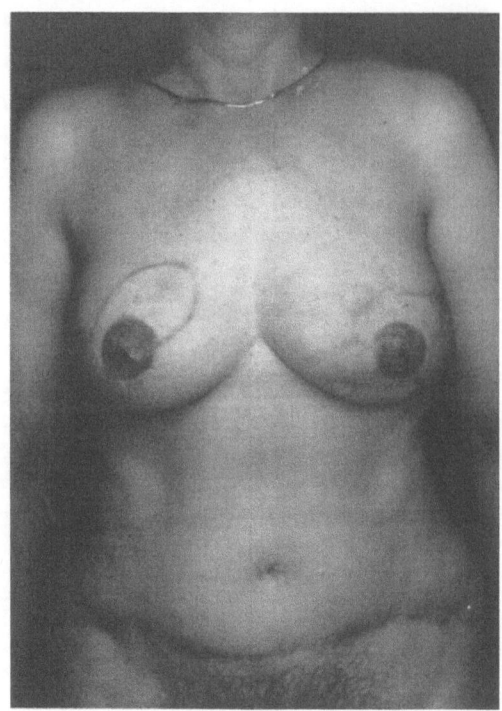

FIG. 21-10 Patient treated for bilateral breast cancer with bilateral mastectomies and immediate reconstruction. The symmetry is better than that usually seen after unilateral mastectomy and reconstruction. (From Kroll SS: *Clin Plast Surg.* 1998;25:251–259. Used with permission.)

risk of developing a second, contralateral primary tumor, some patients choose to undergo elective (prophylactic) mastectomy and reconstruction on the side opposite to cancer.[16]

Compared to the general population, all patients with unilateral breast cancer have an increased risk of developing a second primary malignancy of the opposite breast. For patients with ordinary ductal carcinoma, this risk is approximately 0.75% per year.[17,18] For certain patients, especially those with familial breast cancer, the *BRCA1* gene, or lobular carcinoma in situ, the risk can be much higher.[19] Other patients may not be at high risk of developing a tumor, but may have breasts that are difficult to examine and therefore may be unlikely to benefit from early discovery should a second tumor arise. Still other patients have numerous breast lumps and frequently have to undergo breast biopsy. For these and other reasons, some patients elect to undergo bilateral mastectomy and reconstruction, instead of unilateral treatment.

Because bilateral free transverse rectus abdominus myocutaneous (TRAM) flap breast reconstruction achieves such symmetric and aesthetically successful results, this approach can be very satisfying (Figs 21-11 through 21-14). It particularly appeals to younger patients, who have more years at risk than their older counterparts and who tend to be more concerned about their appearance. Among the advantages of this approach include relative freedom from worry about a second malignancy, avoidance of the possibility of having to go through an entire breast cancer treatment program a second time, avoidance of the need for subsequent mammograms, and (usually) excellent appearance and symmetry. Patients who have chosen to undergo elective con-

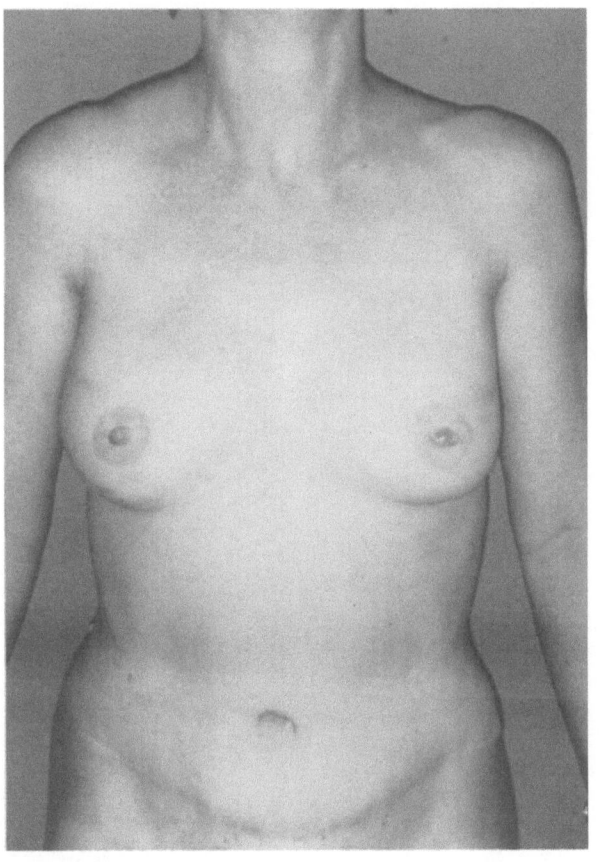

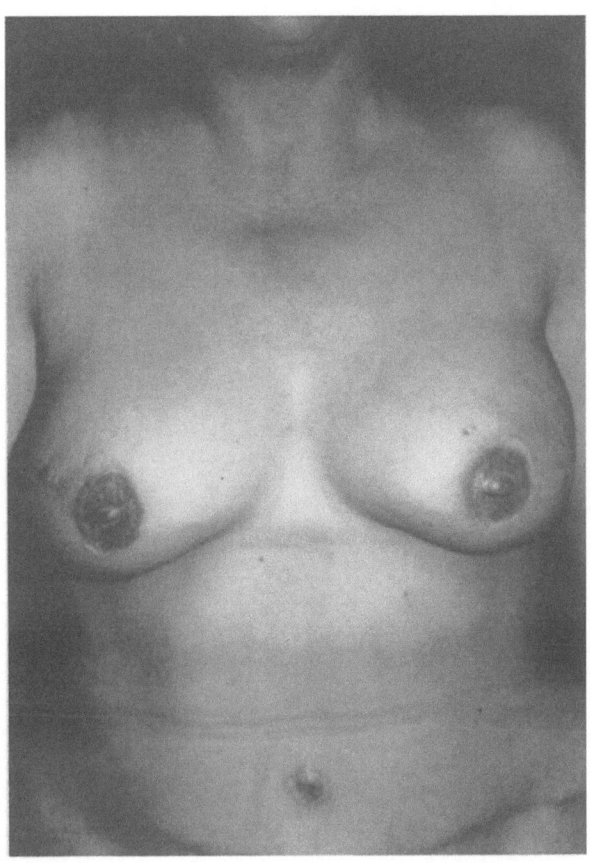

FIG. 21-11   Result of elective contralateral mastectomy and bilateral immediate reconstruction. The patient had cancer of the right breast. See color insert, p. I-23.

FIG. 21-12   Result of elective contralateral mastectomy and bilateral immediate reconstruction. The patient had cancer of the left breast. See color insert, p. I-25.

tralateral mastectomy and bilateral reconstruction have been among our most satisfied patients.

This approach is aggressive, however, and not without risk. Even in the most experienced hands, the possibility exists of a flap failure on the elective side or of a weakened abdominal wall because of bilateral TRAM flap harvest. In every case, nipple sensation will be lost in both breasts. Although development of a second primary malignancy after adequate mastectomy is unlikely, it is not impossible. Mammography may not be necessary, but routine self-examination is still required. Patients need to understand and accept all these risks and limitations preoperatively for elective contralateral mastectomy and bilateral reconstruction to be successful.

Another requirement for the successful use of this approach is a highly experienced reconstructive team. A flap loss rate of much more than 1% is not acceptable when the mastectomy itself is elective. Only reconstructive surgeons who are extremely confident of their ability to successfully reconstruct the breasts should offer this option. Even then, the operation should never be "sold" to patients. It should be provided primarily to those who are motivated to specifically request it. If the patient is at all reluctant, elective mastectomy should be avoided.

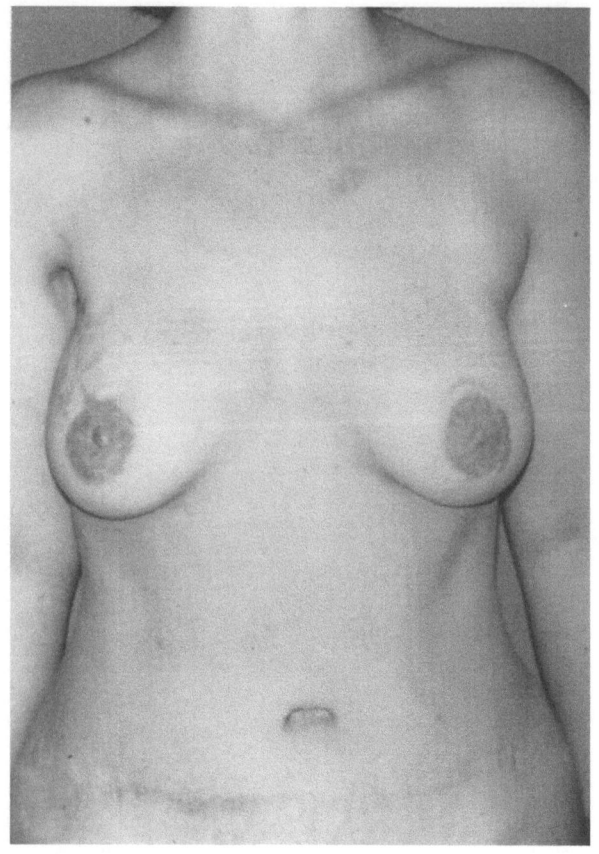

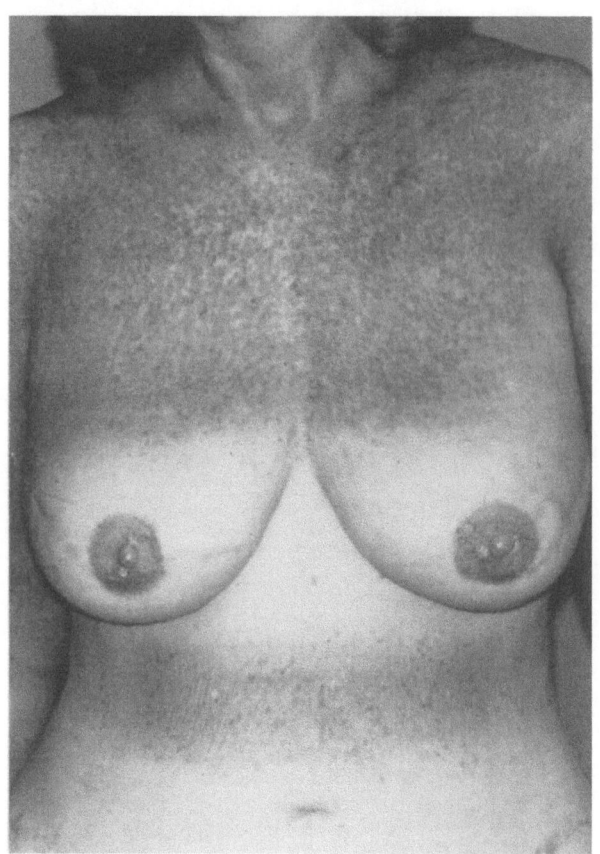

FIG. 21-13 Result of elective contralateral mastectomy and bilateral immediate reconstruction. The patient had cancer of the right breast. See color insert, p. I-25.

FIG. 21-14 Result of elective bilateral mastectomy and immediate reconstruction.

Summary

Whenever possible, if the normal breast is aesthetically attractive, the surgeon attempts to avoid disturbing it and tries to achieve symmetry by reconstructing a breast that imitates its opposite counterpart as closely as possible. If the opposite breast is too large, too small, or too ptotic, however, surgically altering it may be desirable. Even when the opposite breast is attractive, if it is larger or more ptotic than the reconstructed breast, contralateral reduction or mastopexy may be the most practical way of achieving breast symmetry.

In some patients who have a significantly elevated risk for developing a second, contralateral primary cancer or who have breasts that are especially difficult to examine, elective contralateral mastectomy with bilateral immediate reconstruction may be indicated. This approach is aggressive, entails risks, and should be undertaken only by experienced teams. It is capable of achieving outstanding results, however, and for selected patients is appropriate.

References

1. Stevenson TR, Goldstein JA. TRAM flap breast reconstruction and contralateral reduction or mastopexy. *Plast Reconstr Surg.* 1993;92:228–233.

2. Petit JY, Rietjens M, Contesso G, Bertin F, Gilles R. Contralateral mastoplasty for breast reconstruction: a good opportunity for glandular exploration and occult carcinoma diagnosis. *Ann Surg Oncol.* 1997;4:511–515.

3. Goulian D. Dermal mastopexy. *Plast Reconstr Surg.* 1971;47:105–110.

4. Lejour M. Vertical mammaplasty and liposuction of the breast. *Plast Reconstr Surg.* 1994;94:100–114.

5. Lassus C. A 30-year experience with vertical mammaplasty. *Plast Reconstr Surg.* 1996;97:373–380.

6. Spear SL, Kassan M, Little JW. Guidelines in concentric mastopexy. *Plast Reconstr Surg.* 1990;85:961–966.

7. Benelli L. A new periareolar mammaplasty: round block technique. *Aesthetic Plast Surg.* 1990;14:99.

8. Benelli L. Technique de plastie mammaire le "Round Block." *Rev Fr Chir Esthet.* 1988;13:7–11.

9. McKissock PK. Reduction mammaplasty with a vertical dermal flap. *Plast Reconstr Surg.* 1972;49:245.

10. Strombeck JO. Mammaplasty: report of a new technique based on the two-pedicle procedure. *Br J Plast Surg.* 1961;13:79–90.

11. Skoog T. A technique of breast reduction: transposition of the nipple on a cutaneous vascular pedicle. *Acta Chir Scand.* 1963;126:453.

12. Marchac D, Sagher U. Mammaplasty with a short horizontal scar. *Clin Plast Surg.* 1988;15:627–639.

13. Robbins TH. A reduction mammaplasty with the areola-nipple based on an inferior dermal pedicle. *Plast Reconstr Surg.* 1977;59:64.

14. Courtiss EH, Goldwyn RM. Reduction mammaplasty by the inferior pedicle technique. *Plast Reconstr Surg.* 1977;59:500.

15. Kroll SS, Coffey JA Jr, Winn RJ, Schusterman MA. A comparison of factors affecting aesthetic outcomes of TRAM flap breast reconstruction. *Plast Reconstr Surg.* 1995;96:860–864.

16. Kroll SS, Miller WJ, Schusterman MA, Reece GP, Singletary SE, Ames F. The rationale for elective contralateral mastectomy with immediate bilateral reconstruction. *Ann Surg Oncol.* 1994;1:457–461.

17. Rosen PP, Groshen S, Kinne DW, Hellman S. Contralateral breast cancer: an assessment of risk and prognosis in stage I (T1N0M0) and stage II (T1N1M0) patients with 20-year follow-up. *Surgery.* 1989;106:904–910.

18. Leis HP. Selective, elective, prophylactic contralateral mastectomy. *Cancer.* 1971;28:956–961.

19. Schrag D, Kuntz KM, Garber JE, Weeks JC. Decision analysis—effects of prophylactic mastectomy and oophorectomy on life expectancy among women with BRCA1 or BRCA2 mutations. *N Engl J Med.* 1997;336:1465–1471.

22 Nipple and Areolar Reconstruction

Goals of Nipple and Areolar Reconstruction

The purpose of nipple/areolar complex reconstruction is to make the reconstructed breast look as much as possible like a real breast. If there is an opposite natural breast, the goal is to fabricate a nipple/areolar complex that makes the reconstructed breast appear symmetrical with its counterpart. The surgeon tries to make a nipple that to casual inspection appears normal. With proper placement, this is not difficult to do and can significantly improve the result of any breast reconstruction (Fig 22-1).

It is vital to the success of nipple/areolar complex reconstruction that it be kept as painless, inexpensive, and convenient as possible. To this end, the surgeon should use methods that can be performed under local anesthesia in the clinic or office. If the reconstruction is painless, inexpensive, and convenient, patients are more likely to undertake it and ultimately will be more satisfied with their results. This outcome benefits both patients and the surgeon, and is worth pursuing vigorously.

Usually, it is a bad idea for plastic surgeons to talk their patients into having an operation. In my opinion, however, nipple/areolar complex reconstruction may be an exception to that rule. Many patients are satisfied with any breast mound that allows them to wear normal clothing, and they are willing to forego reconstruction of a nipple. Because nipple reconstruction is so simple and convenient, however, patients who would otherwise be reluctant to undertake nipple reconstruction are occasionally talked into it. I have found that these patients are often surprised at how much the nipple and areola add to the illusion of normalcy. They are usually grateful for the surgeon's encouragement and feel better about their body image. For this reason, I strongly encourage patients to undergo nipple reconstruction once their breast mound shaping has been completed, making it clear to them at the same time that my goal is to make them happy and that I will fully accept their decision if they choose not to have nipple reconstruction performed.

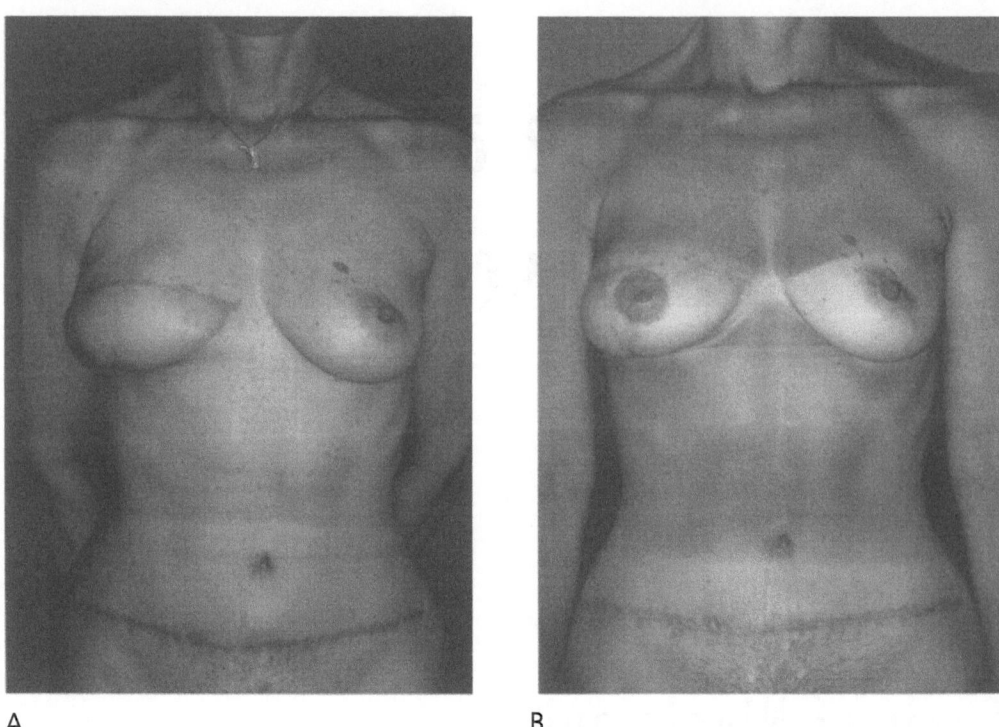

A   B

Fig. 22-1   (A) Patient after transverse rectus abdominus myocutaneous (TRAM) flap reconstruction of the right breast. (B) After revisions and nipple reconstruction, the symmetry is markedly improved. (From Kroll SS: Nipple and areolar reconstruction. In: Kroll SS, ed. *Reconstructive Plastic Surgery for Cancer*. St. Louis: Mosby, 1996:314–318. Used with permission.)

It is essential for the overall success of the breast reconstruction that the nipple and areola be located correctly. For this reason, nipple reconstruction is best deferred until breast mound shaping is complete. There are two reasons for this. First, determining the correct location for the nipple is much easier if the breast mounds have been made symmetric. Second, if nipple reconstruction is performed before all breast mound revisions have been completed, a subsequent change in breast shape might render the nipple position inappropriate. Although the surgeon may be tempted to reconstruct the nipple simultaneously with revision of the breast mound, because of the importance of correct nipple location that temptation should usually be resisted.

Planning the Nipple Location

The most important part of nipple reconstruction is determining the correct site for the nipple. Incorrect location has spoiled many otherwise excellent breast reconstructions (Figs 22-2 and 22-3), while other patients with relatively unattractive breasts have what they consider highly successful reconstructions because the symmetry, including that of the nipple, is so good (Fig 22-4). Sometimes the correct nipple location will be in the center of the flap skin that replaced the original nipple/areolar complex. At other times, however, that location would be incorrect and the nipple must be located elsewhere (Fig 22-5).

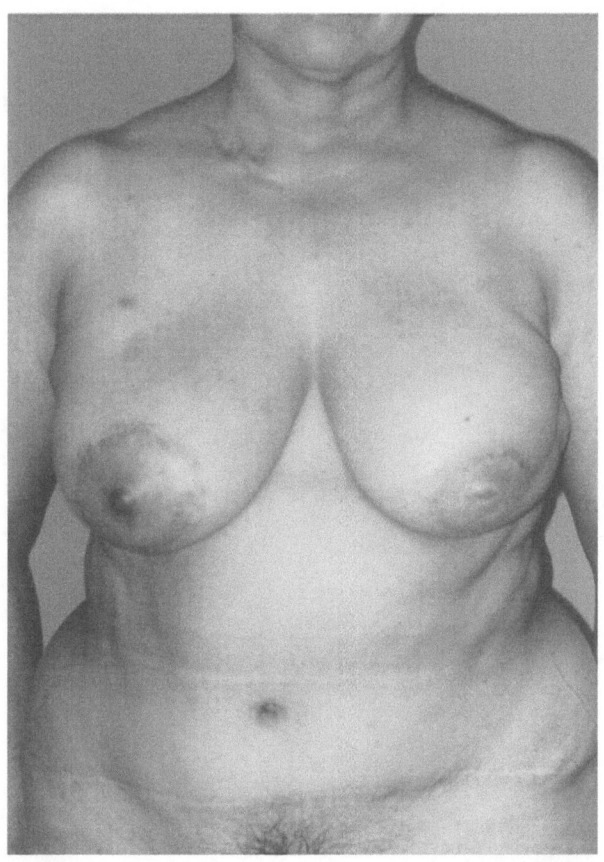

FIG. 22-2 Completed TRAM flap breast reconstruction with the nipple slightly out of position. The symmetry and aesthetic success of the reconstruction could have been improved by a more symmetrical areolar reconstruction.

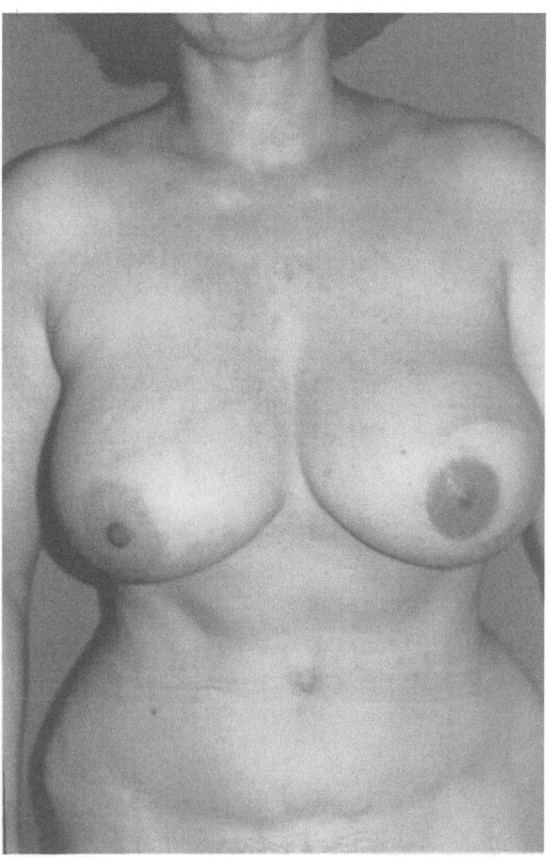

FIG. 22-3 Another completed TRAM flap reconstruction marred by incorrect nipple positioning. The nipple should have been lower and more lateral.

It is much easier to find the right placement for the nipple if the breast mounds are symmetric. In that case, the surgeon merely has to create a mirror image of the contralateral breast. In many cases, measurements from the midline and clavicle can help, but the final marking should be made by using artistic judgment, since the surgeon seeks the illusion of a normal breast rather than mathematical perfection.

In the case of bilateral reconstruction, nipple location is less critical as long as it is natural and symmetric. The nipple should be located slightly inferior and lateral to the actual center of the breast. It is better for the nipples to be too low and too lateral than too high and too medial, which would look unnatural.

Nipple location planning is more difficult when the breast mounds are asymmetric. Obviously, the surgeon would prefer to make the breasts symmetric, but for economic or technical reasons this may not be possible. In that situation, the surgeon must use artistic judgment to choose the nipple location that would be the least unnatural. This is accomplished by viewing the patient frontally and maintaining the same ratios between the nipple/areolar complex and the inferior, medial, and lateral breast borders as are present on the opposite, normal side (Fig 22-6). In this way, the surgeon may

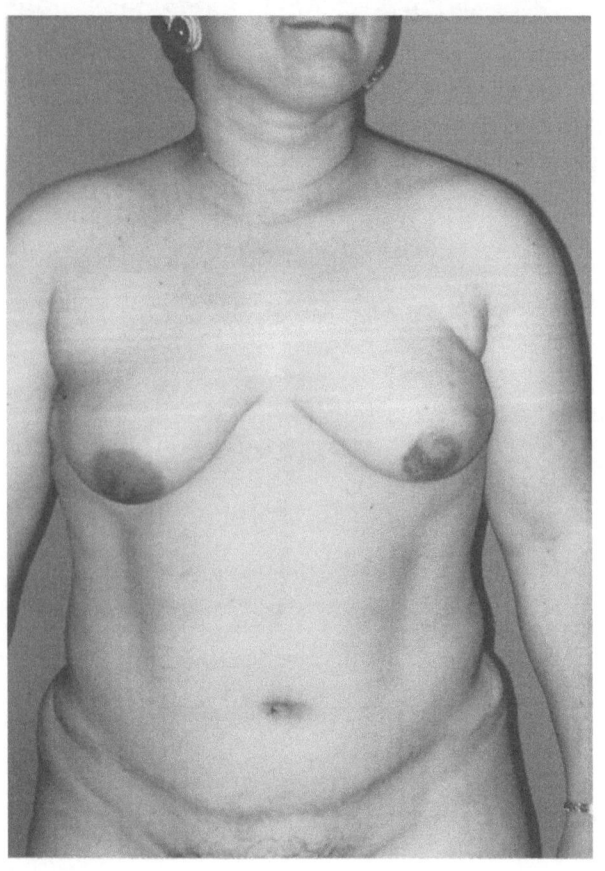

FIG. 22-4 A free TRAM flap breast reconstruction with symmetry of the breast mounds and nipples is very successful even though the breasts themselves do not have ideal shapes. See color insert, p. I-28.

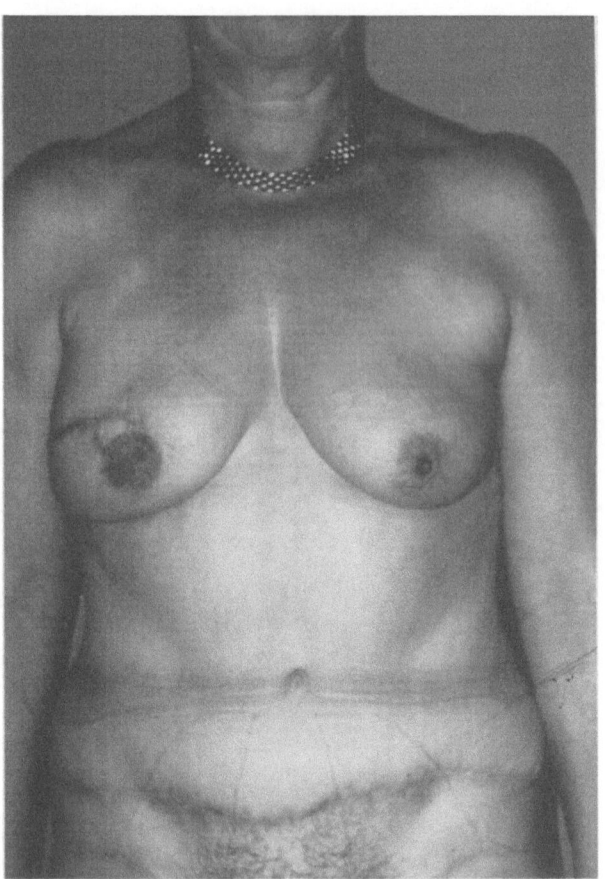

FIG. 22-5 In this patient, locating the nipple in the flap skin that replaced the original nipple/areolar complex would have led to a poor result.

create the illusion that the reconstructed breast is normal, only larger or smaller than its opposite counterpart.

Standard Nipple Reconstruction Methods

Most modern nipple reconstruction methods are similar in that they consist of small flaps of skin and subcutaneous fat that are elevated to project beyond the breast mound. The donor sites may be closed primarily or covered with a skin graft. The areola is created by tattooing[1,2] (usually at a later time) or by hyperpigmentation of a skin graft obtained from an area that is darker than the breast, such as the groin.

I find it useful to classify nipple reconstruction techniques into two groups: those that rely on one flap (such as the skate flap[3] or the star flap[4]), and those that rely on two flaps (the modified double-opposing tab [MDOT] flap,[5,6] the S-flap,[7] and others[8]).

The single-flap techniques have the advantage of simplicity. In the most basic form, a flap of skin and subcutaneous fat is elevated, and the donor site is closed to form a pro-

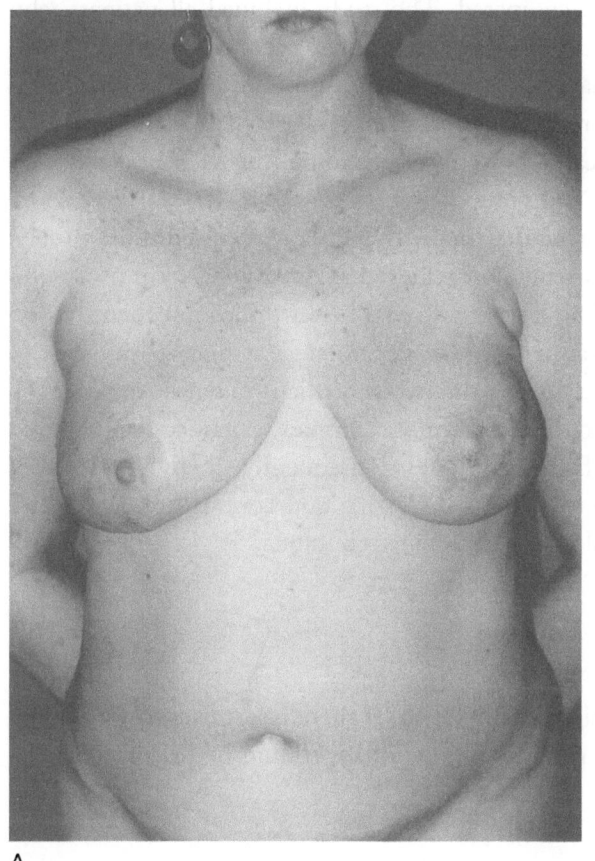
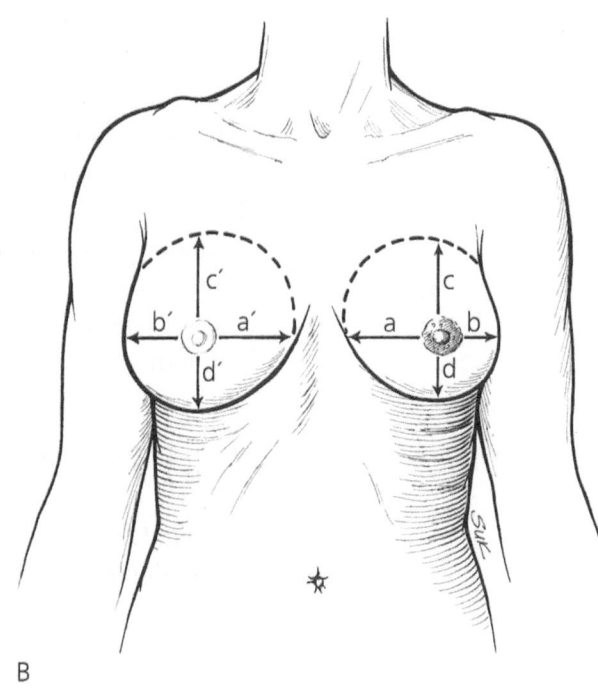

A

B

FIG. 22-6 When the breasts are not symmetric, the surgeon should try to maintain for each breast the same ratios of distances between the nipple and the medial, lateral, and inferior breast borders.

jecting nub, the raw parts of which can then be covered with a skin graft. Variations on this theme include extensions of full- or partial-thickness skin that are used to cover the raw areas of exposed fat. As these designs become more complex, however, they lose the advantage of simplicity. More important, they become at risk for insufficient flap blood supply and partial flap necrosis. The single-flap techniques also have the disadvantage of asymmetry. The donor site is located on only one side of the nipple, creating an asymmetric deformity when the nipple has been completed and the donor site closed.

The two-flap techniques have the advantage of increased blood supply; each flap is relatively short and therefore less likely to develop partial necrosis in its tip. They are also more symmetric than the single-flap techniques because the donor site is split into two parts, one on each side of the reconstructed nipple.

M. D. Anderson Cancer Center Nipple Projection Study

To determine which approach (a single-flap or a two-flap technique) was more effective in achieving lasting nipple projection, the two most popular methods of nipple reconstruction in use at The University of Texas M. D. Anderson Cancer Center, the star flap[2,4] and the MDOT flap,[5,6] were compared. The study included all patients who had undergone nipple reconstruction with these techniques between March 1, 1993, and December 31, 1995, and who had follow-ups of at least 6 months. The series consisted of 106 patients who had had reconstruction with MDOT flaps and 47 patients reconstructed with star flaps. The mean long-term projection of the MDOT flap group was 2.43 mm, while that of the star flap group was 1.97 mm ($p = 0.021$).

The conclusions of this study were that the MDOT flaps achieved more projection than the star flaps but that neither method achieved as much long-term projection as had been hoped for. Why the MDOT flaps achieved better projection than the star flap remains conjectural. It seems reasonable, however, to suggest that at least part of the reason is that the blood supply to each of the two short flaps raised in the MDOT technique is more reliable than that to the longer, more complex, extended flap required of the star flap (or any other single-flap) technique. Consequently, there is less loss of subcutaneous fat (from fat necrosis), less internal scarring and contracture, and better long-term projection from the double-flap (MDOT) technique.

MDOT Flap Technique

The MDOT flap technique is very simple (Fig 22-7). If there is a scar crossing the site of the nipple reconstruction, the long axis of the two flaps should be oriented parallel

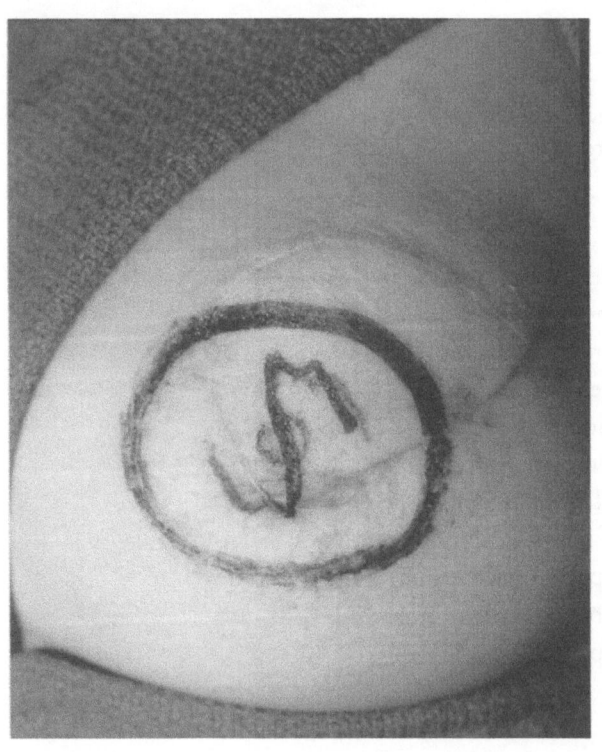

A

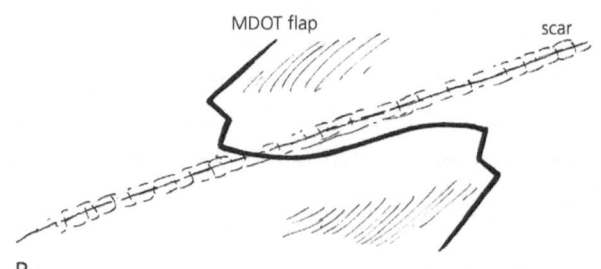

B

FIG. 22-7 Design of the MDOT flap. If a linear scar is present, the long axis of the flaps should be parallel to that scar. (From Kroll SS: Nipple and areolar reconstruction. In: Kroll SS, ed. *Reconstructive Plastic Surgery for Cancer.* St. Louis: Mosby, 1996:314–318. Used with permission.)

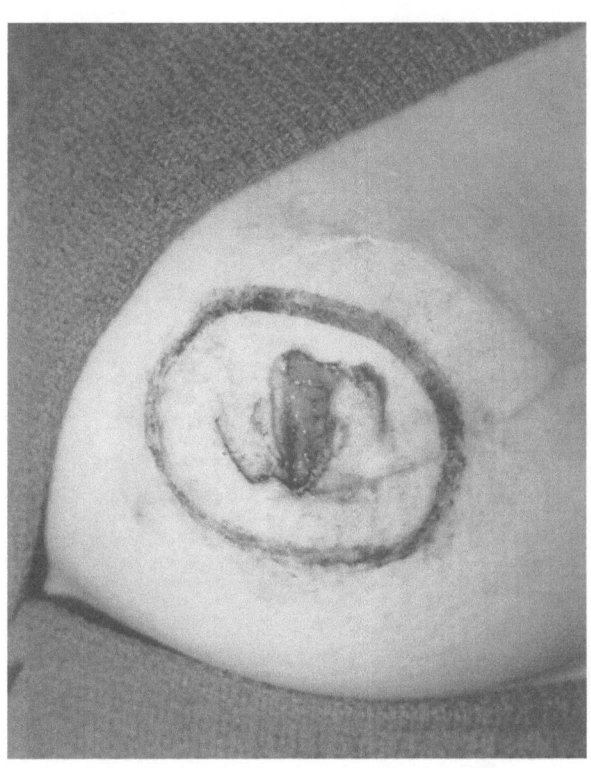

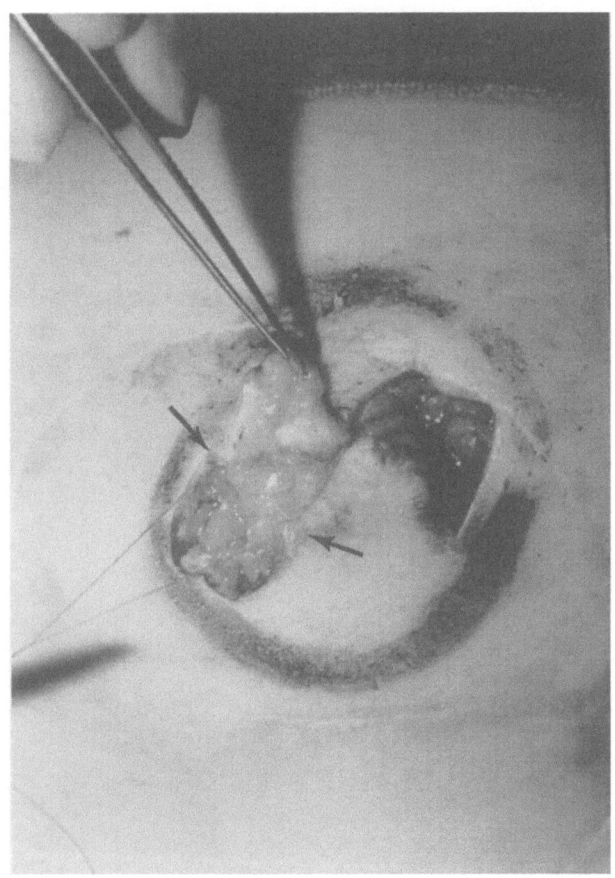

FIG. 22-8   The flaps are elevated with a thickness of approximately 4 mm.

FIG. 22-9   The key sutures are placed between the base of one flap (arrow) and a point halfway up the long side of the opposite flap (arrow).

to the scar to prevent the scar from interrupting the blood supply to the flaps. The width of each flap is approximately 18 mm (although sometimes this width is increased as described below). The skin is infiltrated with lidocaine 1% with epinephrine (1:500,000). The flaps should be approximately 6 or 7 mm thick, with only enough undermining to allow them to be moved into opposition (Fig 22-8).

The key sutures (buried dermal sutures of 4-0 Vicryl [polygalactin 910]) are placed from a point halfway along the long edge of each flap to the corner at the base of the short edge of the opposite flap (Fig 22-9). Once these two sutures are tied (Fig 22-10), they support each other's projection like two hands held in prayer and defne the nipple shape and position. The donor sites are then closed with buried sutures of 4-0 Vicryl.

The points created by the tip of each flap and its "tab" (which in the modified technique is not really a tab but an integral part of the flap) interdigitate with each other to create a rounded tip (Fig 22-11). The skin is closed with 5-0 chromic sutures. If the base is too tight when the skin is closed, one or two sutures can be released and the base on one side left partially open to heal secondarily. The results of the MDOT flap reconstructions are not perfect but usually they achieve reasonably good projection

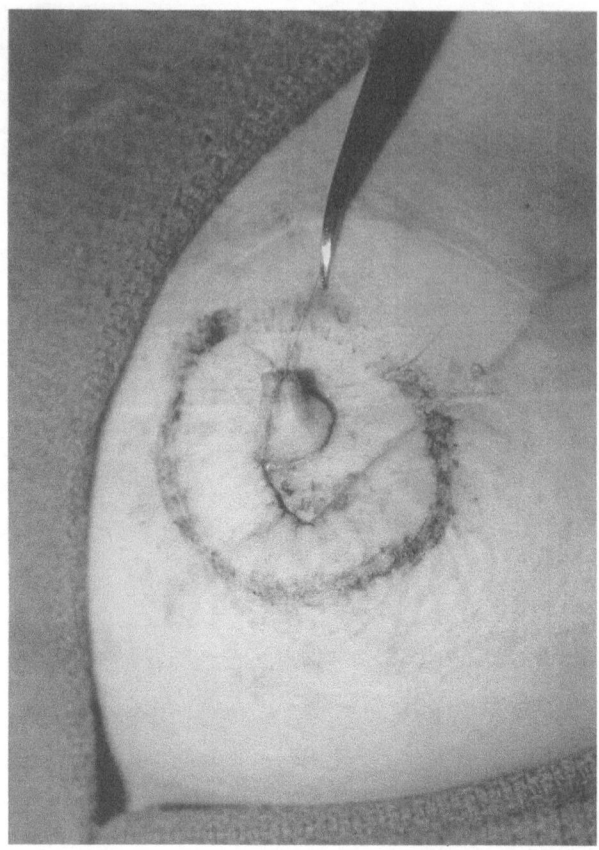

FIG. 22-10 When the key sutures are tied, the flaps are opposed and support each other's projection. The donor sites are then closed.

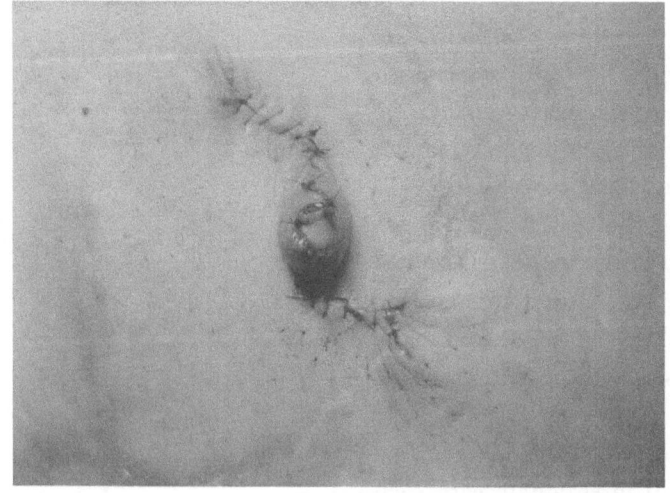

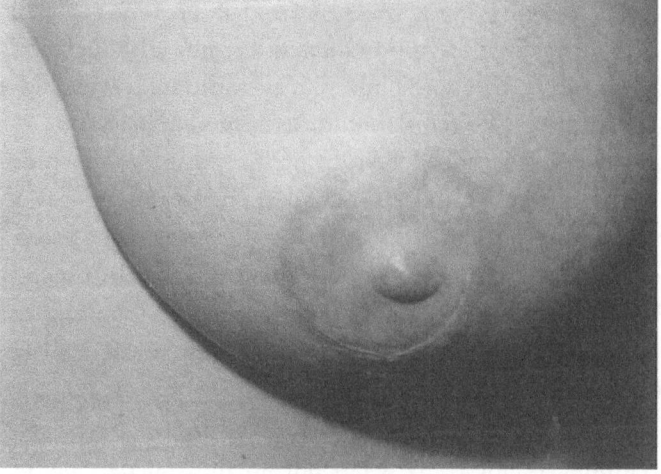

FIG. 22-11 The points of each flap and its tab interdigitate with those of the opposite flap to form a rounded tip.

FIG. 22-12 Result of nipple reconstruction with an MDOT flap.

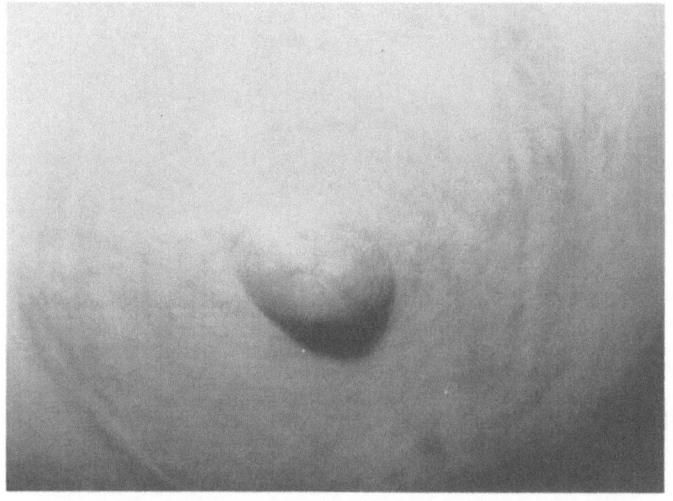

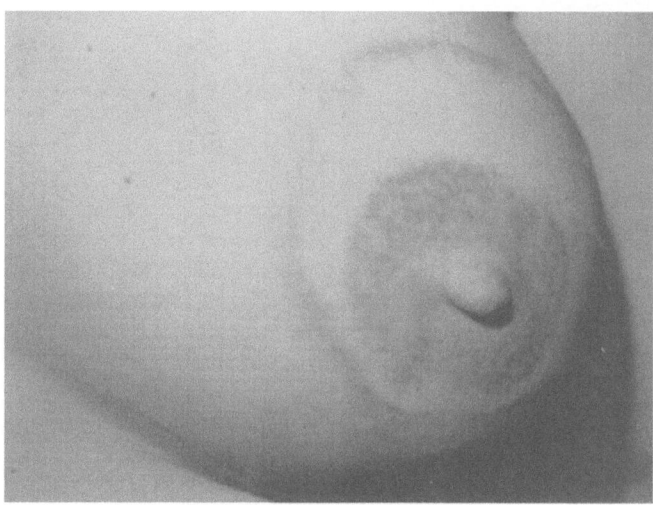

FIG. 22-13   Another result of nipple reconstruction with an MDOT flap.

FIG. 22-14   Excessive nipple projection after reconstruction with an MDOT flap. This much nipple projection is unusual.

(Figs 22-12 and 22-13). In a few unusual cases the projection has been excessive and the nipple has needed subsequent shortening (Fig 22-14).

Staging of the MDOT Nipple Reconstruction

In the nipple projection study described above, the long-term projection achieved by both nipple reconstruction methods was disappointing. Although unproven, it seems reasonable to believe that the loss of projection commonly seen after nipple reconstruction might be due to a loss of subcutaneous fat and other tissue caused by ischemia. If this hypothesis (that blood supply influences long-term nipple projection) is true, increasing the blood supply to the flaps further should improve nipple projection.

One way to improve blood supply to the nipple flaps is to make them wider. Over the past 2 years, I have been doing just that: designing the flaps as described above but making them 20 to 22 mm wide. This makes flap survival more certain and eliminates any risk of a tight closure at the flap base leading to flap strangulation. It does, however, create an oval nipple that must subsequently be revised (Fig 22-15) to make it more circular. This revision is performed approximately 4 weeks after the first stage of the nipple reconstruction, requires only local anesthesia, and usually takes only a few minutes (Fig 22-16).

It is too early to be certain that this approach has been effective, but the early results have been very encouraging. The nipples appear to have better projection that has been well maintained, at least during the first 6 months. The only disadvantages are the need for a second (although very minor) procedure and the fact that the wider flaps require more skin and therefore tighten the breast mound more than the 18-mm flaps. This is not important in patients with large or moderate-sized breasts, but can be significant when the breast mound is very small.

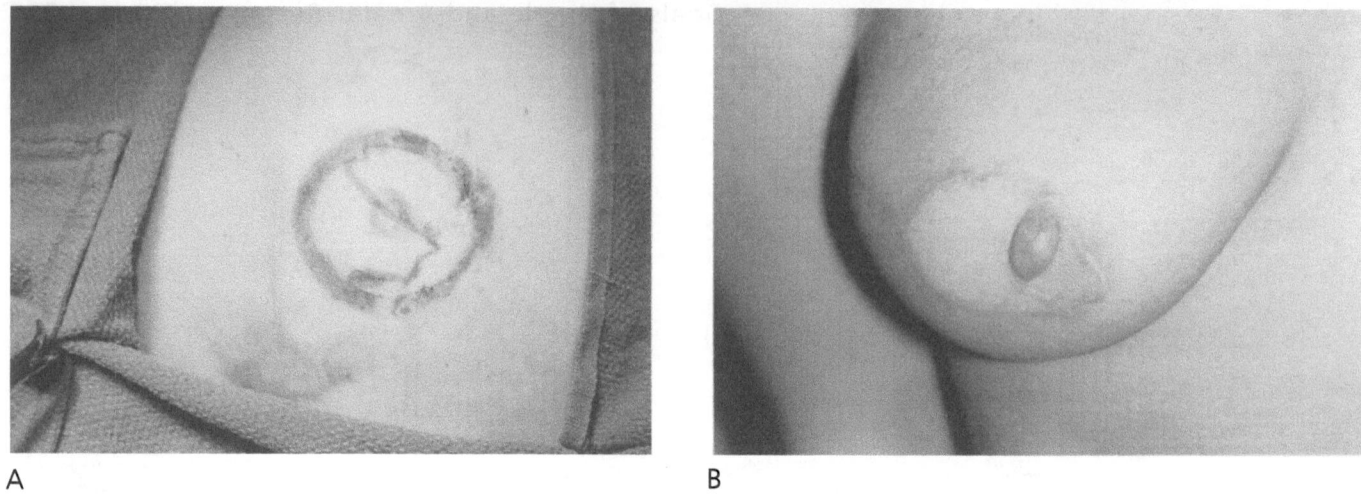

A   B

FIG. 22-15 (A) Bases of MDOT flaps are widened to improve the blood supply and thereby improve projection. (B) This creates an oval-shaped nipple that then needs revision.

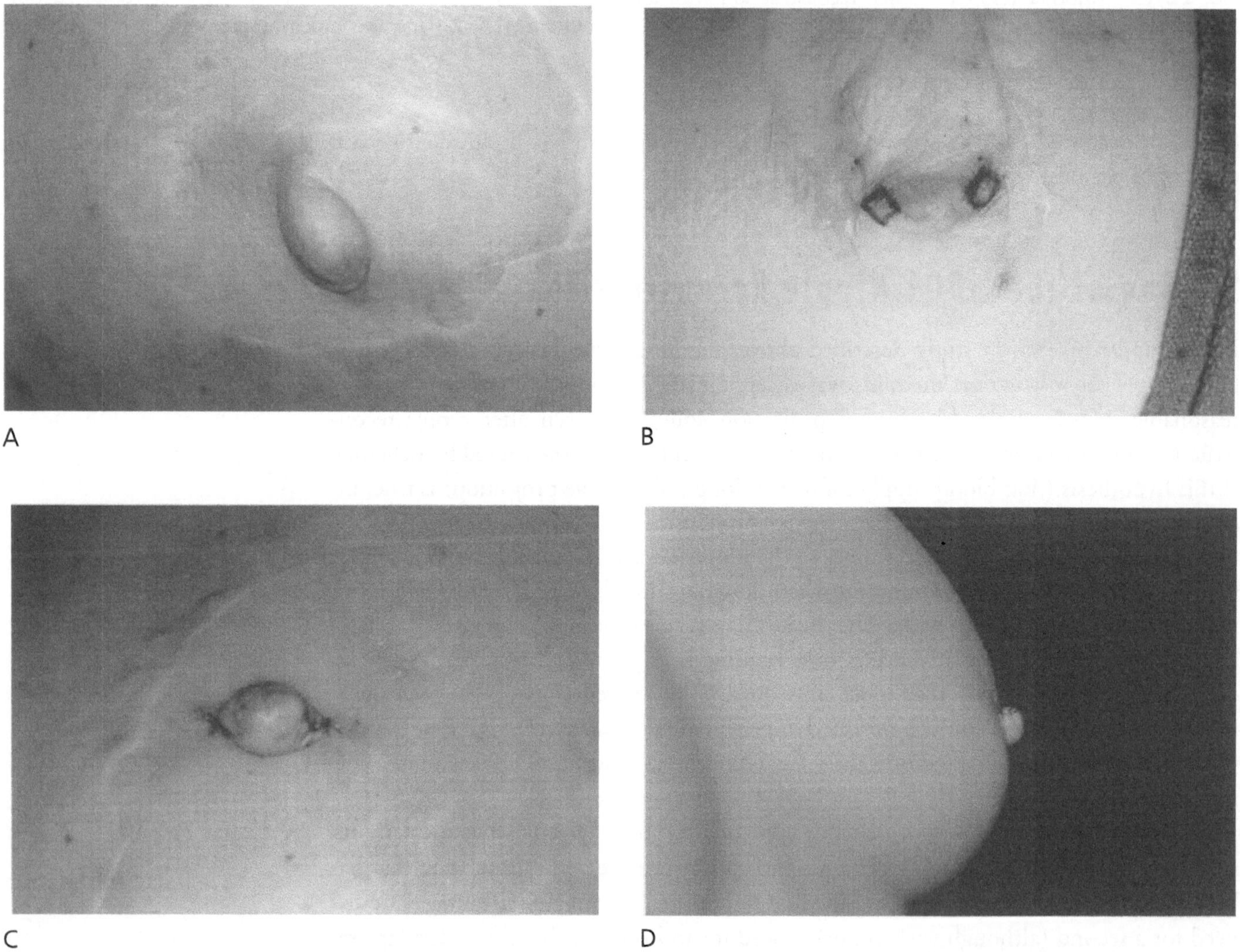

A   B

C   D

FIG. 22-16 (A) Oval-shaped nipple created by making the flaps of the MDOT flaps wider than 18 mm. (B) Plan for revision of the nipple, excising diamond-shaped pieces of skin and closing the diamonds parallel to the circumference of the nipple. (C) Result of such a nipple revision. (D) Side view showing that projection was well maintained.

Integrating Nipple Reconstruction with Breast Revision

Problems with Standard Nipple Reconstruction Techniques

Virtually all standard nipple reconstruction techniques borrow tissue from the breast mound to create a projecting nipple. In the past, the only alternative to this was to graft tissue from elsewhere, but although such methods do have advocates,[9,10] I have found that nipples created with such grafts usually look unnatural or have disappointing projection. In my opinion, grafts are not useful except for the patient who has an opposite nipple that is excessively projecting.[11] In that case, harvest of part of the abnormal nipple will make it less conspicuous and easier to match, even if the grafted reconstruction is itself unsuccessful.

All breast mounds reconstructed with transverse rectus abdominus myocutaneous (TRAM) flaps are relatively flat, and project less than a natural breast (Fig 22-17). This is because the TRAM flap itself is innately flat, and not cone-shaped, like a breast is. When tissue is taken from the breast mound to create a projecting nipple, the projection of the mound is reduced even further. Fortunately, this additional flattening is not problematic except in the very smallest of breasts. Nevertheless, it remains true that it is impossible to create nipple or breast projection out of nothing; so any projection that is achieved must always be taken from the existing breast

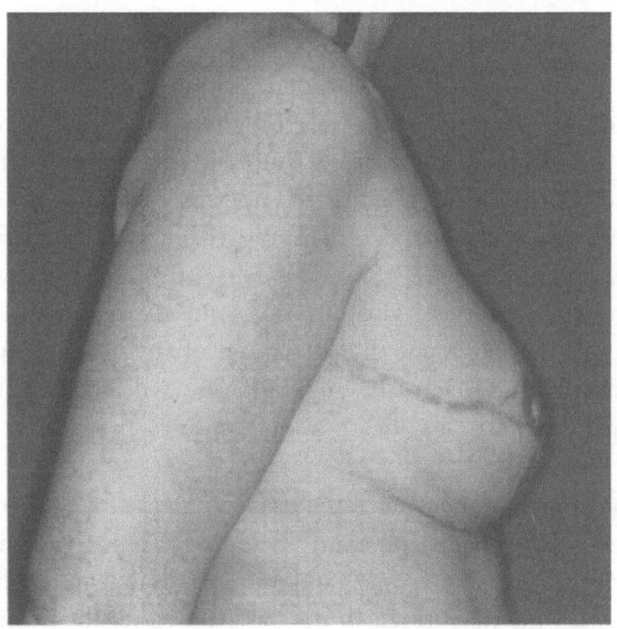

FIG. 22-17 Side view of another nipple reconstructed with an MDOT flap. The nipple projection is adequate. As is typical of a reconstructed breast mound, the projection of the nipple/areolar complex is less than that found in most natural breasts.

mound. Even the "keyhole" technique of Chang[12] and the similar "bell" flap of Eng,[13] which create the illusion of a projecting areola, do so at the expense of flattening the surrounding breast mound with a small circumferential (or "doughnut") mastopexy that is an integral part of the technique. The result, in my opinion, is no real net change in breast projection.

Creating Additional Projection

Breast projection can be created, in many cases, by reshaping the breast during secondary revision. This is only possible if the size of the reconstructed breast mound is excessive, and must be reduced as part of that revision. Fortunately, however, excessive breast mound size is common and in fact occurs most of the time. If the breast mound size must be reduced, some of the excess tissue that otherwise would be discarded can be used to increase breast projection and to reconstruct a projecting nipple.

This additional projection is achieved in two ways. First, tissue in the area near the areola is not always resected, but may be retained to increase the relative amount of tissue under the areola. Second, skin that would otherwise be discarded is retained as a flap, which is then wrapped around itself to create a truly projecting nipple. In part, the breast is reshaped as it might be in a conventional reduction mammaplasty.

The Wrap-Around Flap for Nipple Reconstruction

Inferior Triangle Resection

The best opportunity to create a projecting nipple with the wrap-around flap occurs when a triangle of tissue will be resected from the inferior pole. In this technique, the breast mound revision is designed like a superiorly based breast reduction. A triangular-shape segment of skin and underlying tissue is resected from the inferior pole of the breast mound (Fig 22-18), and medial and lateral breast flaps mobilized and sutured together. Preserving and burying some of the fatty tissue deep to the apex of that triangle will augment the projection of the breast mound in that area. In the inferior triangle resection, the augmentation will occur just below the nipple/areolar complex, a desirable location that mimics the projection of a natural breast.

The skin in the area of the apex of the triangle, instead of being discarded, is fashioned into a rectangularly shaped superiorly based flap. This flap is normally approximately 1 cm in width, 7 to 10 mm thick, and 3 to 3.5 cm in length. The flap is wrapped around on itself, with the tip sutured to the base (on either the medial or lateral side, depending on the surgeon's artistic judgment). The skin lying underneath the wrap-around nipple flap is then de-epithelialized. The layered skin closure of the breast mound reduction is then completed. The result is a nipple that projects beyond the limits of the previous breast mound.

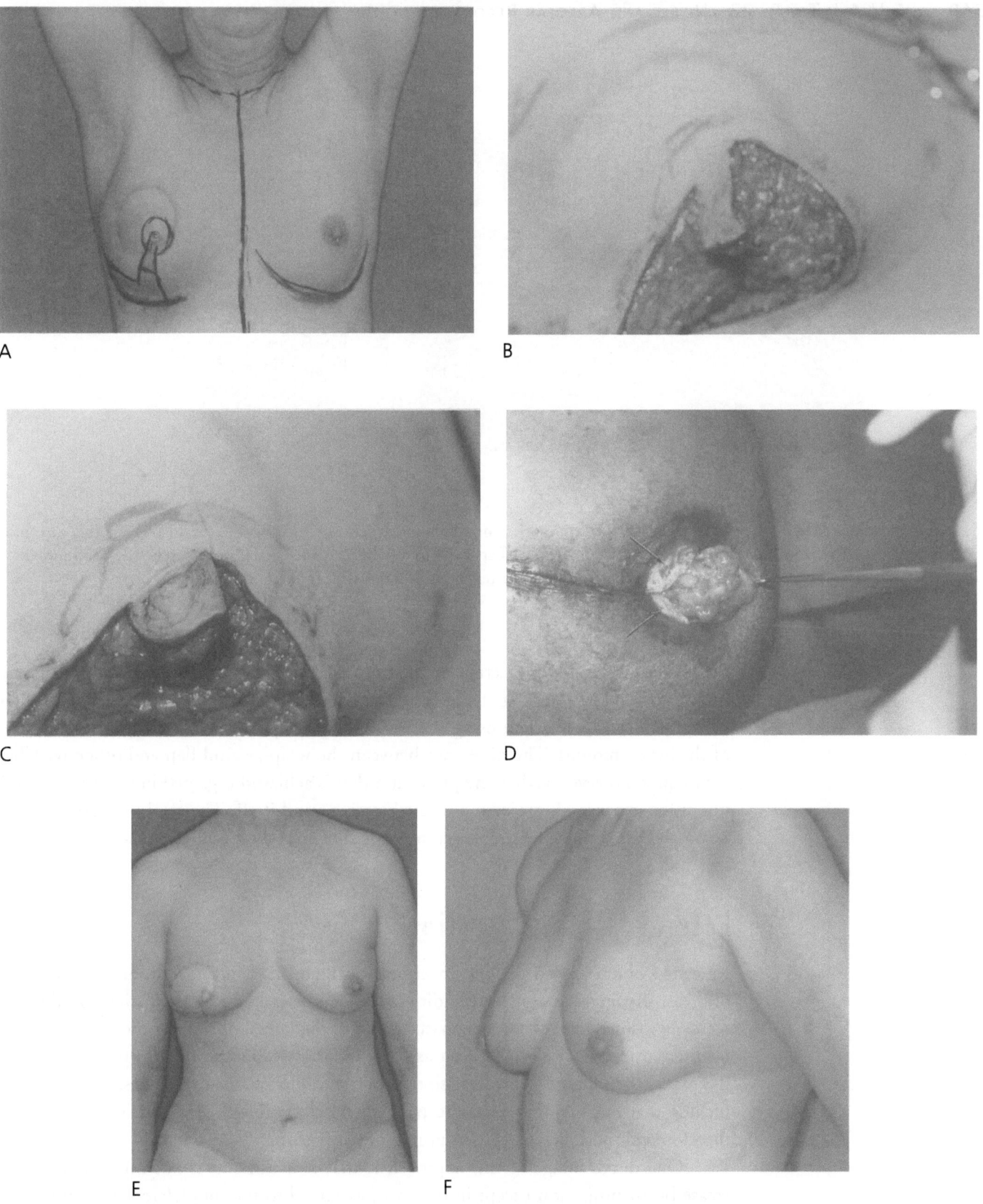

Fig. 22-18 (A) Plan for reduction of reconstructed breast mound by excision of a J-shaped section of skin and fat, along with creation of a rectangular superiorly based wrap-around flap for nipple reconstruction. (B) Subcutaneous fatty tissue is preserved in the apex of the triangle, just deep to the wrap-around flap, in order to increase breast volume just below the nipple/areolar complex. (C)The flap is wrapped around on itself to create a projecting nipple. (D) Breast mound skin underlying the nipple wrap-around flap (arrows) is de-epithelialized (in a different patient) so that the flap can adhere and heal to it. (E) Result of nipple reconstruction with the wrap-around flap. (F). Oblique view, showing that the projection of the breast mound and the nipple/areolar complex has been increased.

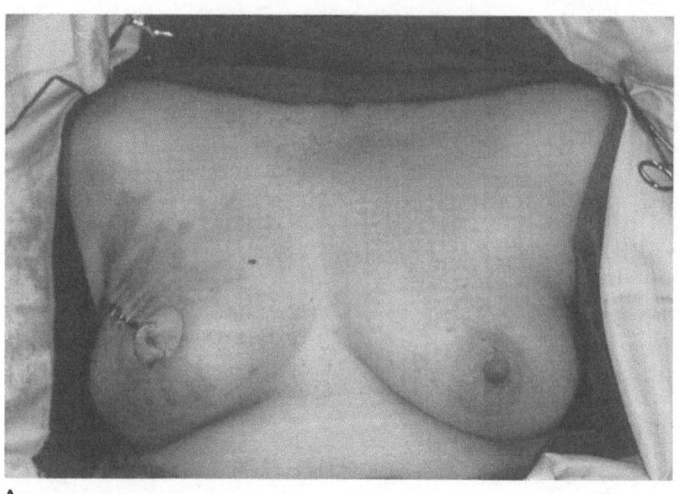
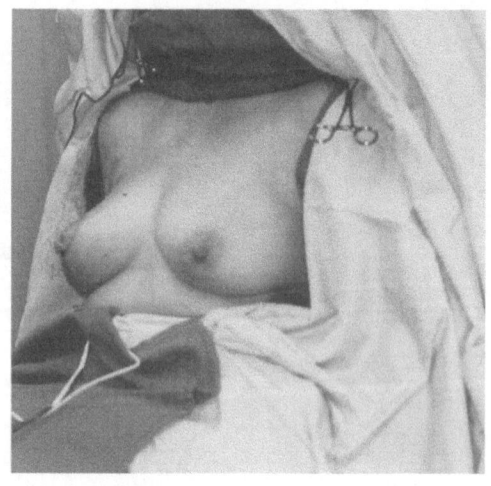

A   B

FIG. 22-19   (A) Intraoperative view of another nipple reconstruction with a wrap-around flap, in this case harvested from the lateral part of the breast. The flap has not yet been turned back upon itself. (B) Oblique view, showing that the breast mound has not been flattened at all by elevation of the nipple flap.

The measurable projection of the nipple created with the wrap-around flap may not be any greater than that achieved with other techniques. It may in fact be less than that which can be attained using the MDOT technique as measured from the surface of the breast mound. The difference between the wrap-around flap and other available techniques, however, is that any projection that is achieved is gained in addition to, and not at the expense of, projection of the breast mound itself. The total projection of the reconstructed nipple and areolar complex is therefore increased (Fig 22-19).

Lateral Ellipse Resection

Resection of a triangle from the lower pole of the breast is ideal from the point of view of breast shaping. It does create additional scars, however, and some patients find those scars objectionable. If there is an existing scar in the lateral portion of the breast mound (as there usually is, especially if an axillary nodal dissection was performed along with the mastectomy), an elliptical excision of breast mound tissue can be designed that will include that scar. In that case, the patient will trade the old scar for a new one and therefore will have no increase in visible breast scarring.

One disadvantage of this approach is that it is difficult if not impossible to increase breast projection except in the area just lateral to the nipple/areolar complex, an undesirable location. Consequently, little if any augmentation of breast mound projection can be achieved. Another disadvantage of the lateral ellipse excision is that the inframammary fold cannot be elevated, at least not by that technique alone. A wrap-around flap of skin and underlying fat, however, can still be created (Fig 22-20), so that the goal of achieving nipple projection without reducing breast mound projection remains attainable.

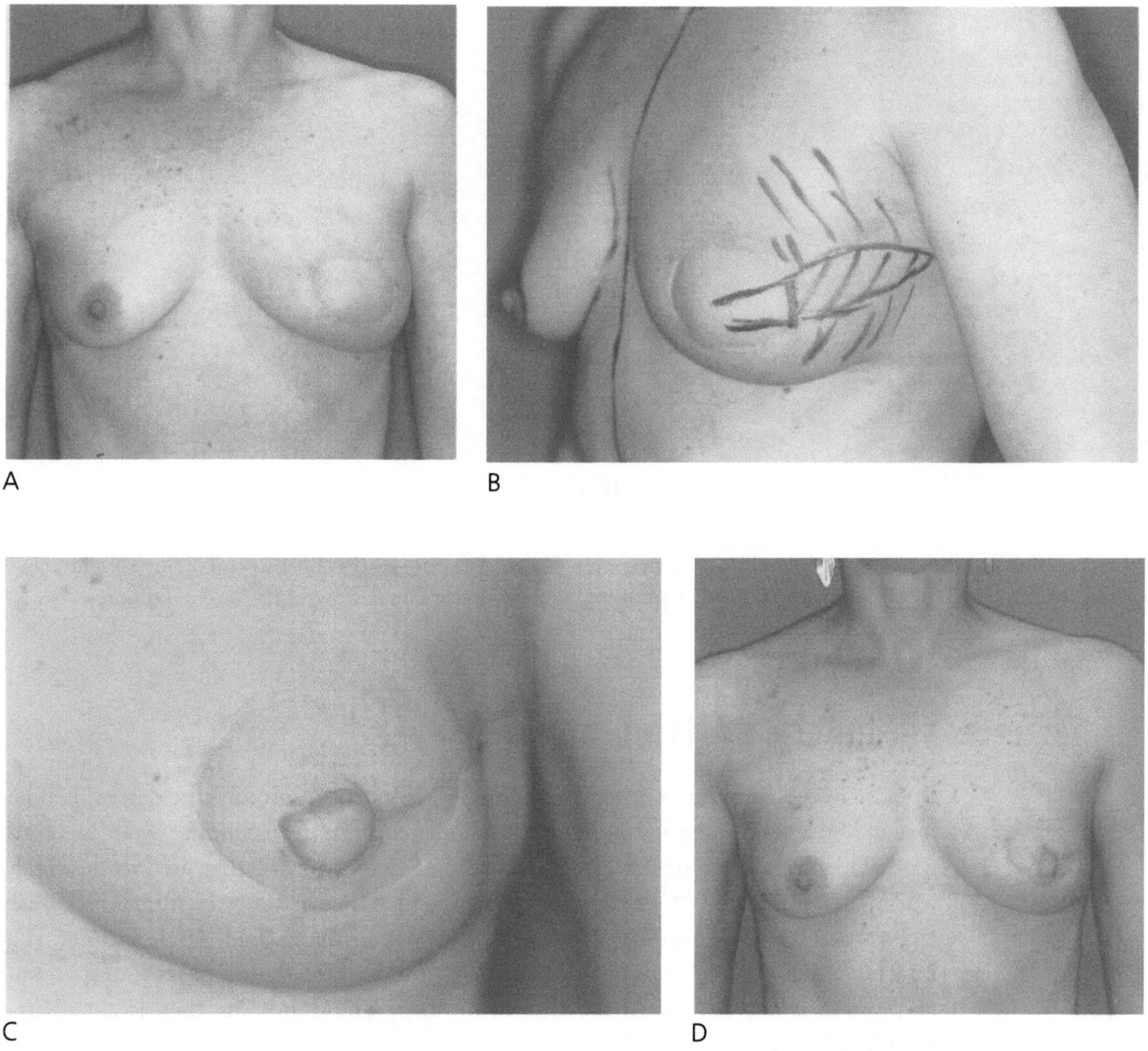

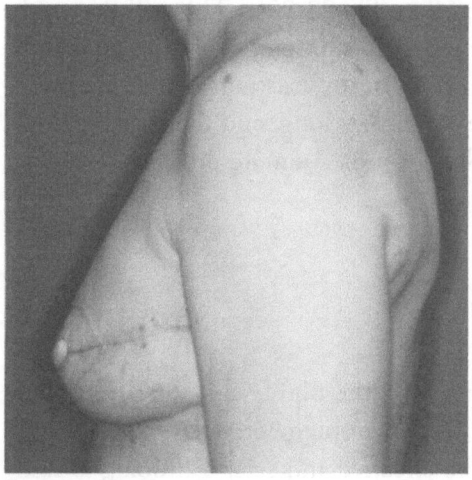

A

B

C

D

E

Fig. 22-20 (A) Patient after free TRAM flap breast mound reconstruction, with excess fullness laterally. (B) Plan for revision of the breast incorporating nipple reconstruction with a wrap-around flap and lateral ellipse resection. (C, D) Early result of wrap-around flap nipple reconstruction, before revision or tattooing. (E) Side view, showing the projection of the breast mound and the nipple that has been achieved.

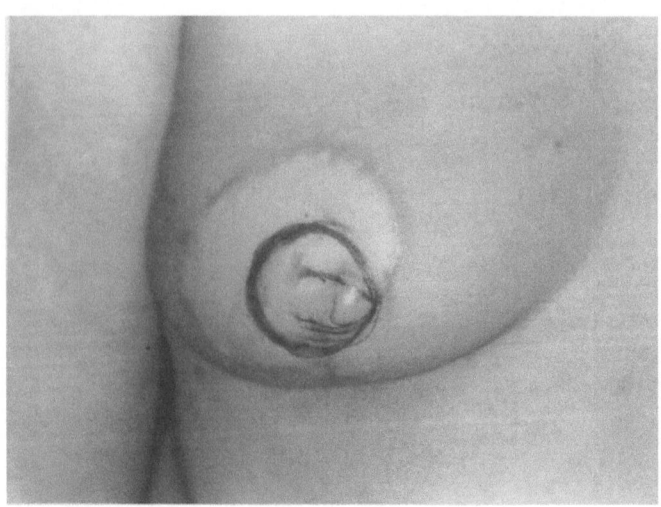
A

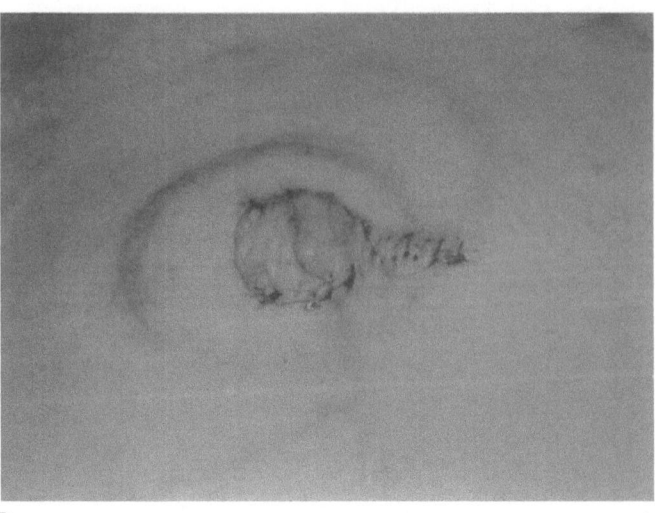
B

FIG. 22-21 (A) Plan for revision of nipple that will shift its location toward the base of the "inchworm" flap. (B) The flap is doubled upon itself to increase its projection and to shift its position, and the donor site is closed in a V-to-Y fashion.

Secondary Revision of the Nipple

Because in the wrap-around flap technique the nipple position must be determined before the breast mound revision has been completed, minor positioning errors are common. These errors can be corrected by creating a flap similar to that used in the "inchworm" flap of Puckett.[14] The base of the flap, which incorporates the nipple previously reconstructed with the wrap-around flap, is located at the desired nipple location (Fig 22-21). When the flap is doubled upon itself, the bulk of the nipple is increased and its position is moved toward the base of the flap. The donor site then is closed in a V-to-Y fashion.

Another approach to moving the nipple and at the same time increasing projection is to use a pattern like that of a small "star" flap (Fig 22-22).[2] This will flatten the breast mound very slightly but give better nipple definition and projection above the surface of the breast mound. Because of the scars already existing around the wrap-around nipple flap, the star flap should not be made very long, and the patient should be aware that partial nipple flap necrosis and loss of projection are possible.

Areolar Reconstruction

Areolar reconstruction is best performed by tattooing the nipple and the surrounding skin (Fig 22-23).[1,15] Medical grade tattooing, or "micropigmentation," equipment is now widely available and has been shown to be effective and safe. Tattooing is easily performed in the clinic or office under local anesthesia. If the color fades with time, the tattooing can be repeated as often as necessary.

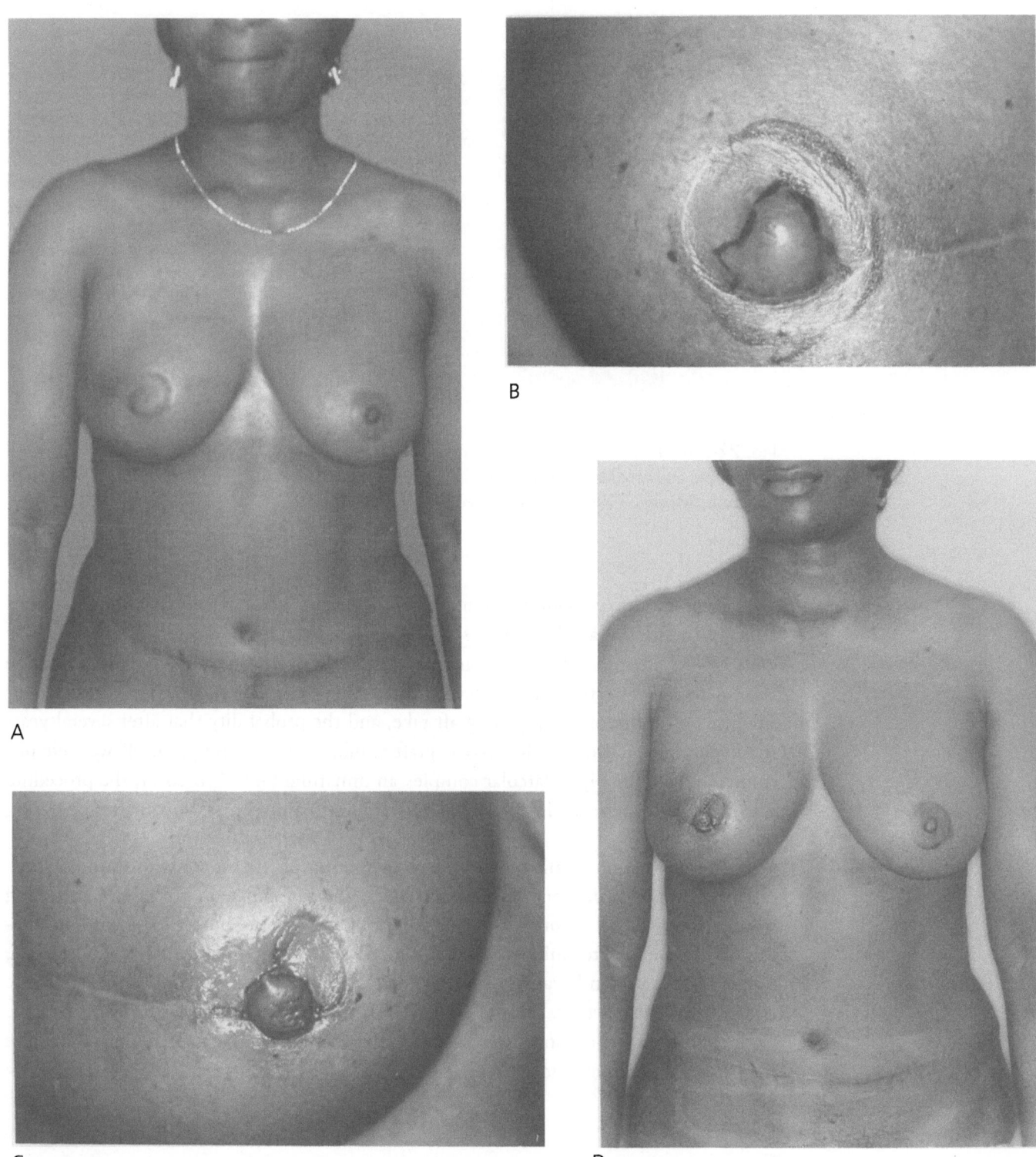

FIG. 22-22   (A) Patient after free TRAM flap right breast mound reconstruction and right nipple reconstruction with a wrap-around flap. The flap needs to be moved slightly lower and given more definition. See color insert, p. I-26. (B) The design for a modified "star" flap with the base placed inferiorly. See color insert, p. I-26. (C) After completion of the star flap revision, the nipple has better definition. See color insert, p. I-27. (D) The result of the nipple revision. See color insert, p. I-27.

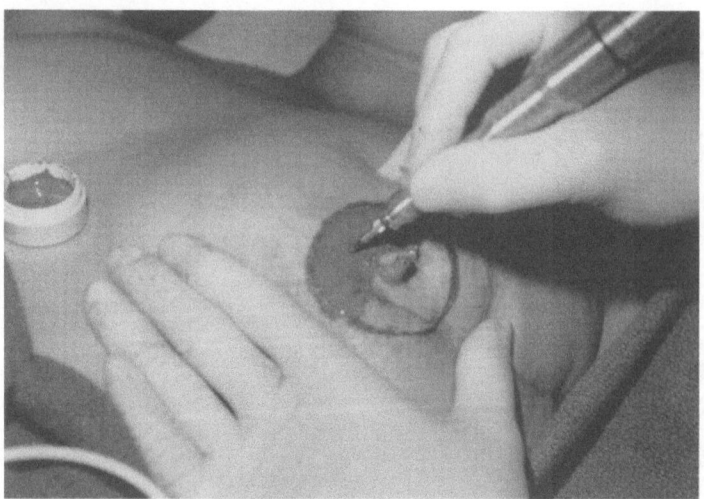

FIG. 22-23   Tattooing is used to pigment the nipple and to reconstruct an areola. (From Kroll SS: Nipple and areolar reconstruction. In: Kroll SS, ed. *Reconstructive Plastic Surgery for Cancer.* St. Louis: Mosby, 1996:314–318. Used with permission.)

Prior to the availability of micropigmentation, areolas were commonly reconstructed by placing a full-thickness skin graft from the groin around the nipple. The graft would subsequently darken and create the illusion of an areola. This technique was moderately effective but had several disadvantages. These included a painful donor site, the possibility of incomplete graft take, and the probability that after several years the hyperpigmentation of the areolar graft would fade. The nipple itself was left uncolored, giving the nipple/areolar complex an unnatural look. Moreover, the procedure was difficult to perform in the office and usually required a session in the operating room.

Reconstruction of the areola and pigmentation of the nipple with tattooing represents a major advance and has become the method of choice in our clinic. Tattooing is usually performed by our clinic nurses, who have become both expert with and enthusiastic about the technique. We generally delay the tattooing until 4 weeks after the nipple reconstruction because we believe that the tattooing is easier and more effective after the wounds have healed; the delay also prevents the tattooing from disrupting the wounds in the nipple donor site. Alternatively, the tattooing can be performed before the nipple flaps are elevated.[2,16]

Summary

The goal of nipple reconstruction is to make the reconstructed breast appear more normal and symmetric. Nipple and areolar reconstruction significantly improve the quality of the reconstructed breast and should be encouraged by the surgeon. To that end, it should be kept as simple, convenient, and inexpensive as possible. The most important step in nipple reconstruction is proper location. The location of the nipple should be determined only after breast mound shaping has been completed and is more likely to be correct if the mounds have been made symmetric.

There are many nipple reconstruction methods currently available. Of the standard techniques, we have found that the modified double-opposing tab flap gives the best long-term projection, possibly because the MDOT flaps have a better blood supply (for an equivalent amount of flap tissue) than nipple reconstruction techniques that rely on only a single flap. Nevertheless, many currently available techniques can be successful. If the breast mound needs reduction, however, both breast shape and projection of the nipple/areolar complex can often be improved by using the wrap-around flap technique. Areolar reconstruction and pigmentation of the nipple are best accomplished with tattooing, usually performed approximately 4 weeks after the nipple reconstruction has been completed.

References

1. Spear SL, Convit R, Little JW. Intradermal tattoo as an adjunct to nipple-areolar reconstruction. *Plast. Reconstr. Surg.* 1989;83:907–911.
2. Eskenazi L. A one-stage nipple reconstruction with the "modified star" flap and immediate tattoo: a review of 100 cases. *Plast Reconstr Surg.* 1993;92:671–680.
3. Little JW. Nipple-areolar reconstruction. *Advances in Plast Reconstr Surg.* 1987;3:43–78.
4. Anton MA, Hartrampf CR Jr. Nipple reconstruction with the star flap. *Plast Surgical Forum.* 1990;13:100–103. Abstract.
5. Kroll SS. Nipple and areolar reconstruction. In: Kroll SS, ed. *Reconstructive Plastic Surgery for Cancer.* Philadelphia: Mosby; 1996:314–318.
6. Kroll SS, Reece GP, Miller MJ, et al. Comparison of nipple projection with the modified double-opposing tab and star flaps. *Plast Reconstr Surg.* 1997;99:1602–1605.
7. Cronin ED, Humphreys DH, Ruiz Razura A. Nipple reconstruction: the S flap. *Plast Reconstr Surg.* 1988;81:783–787.
8. Hugo NE, Sultan MR, Hardy SP. Nipple-areola reconstruction with intradermal tattoo and double-opposing pennant flaps. *Ann Plast Surg.* 1993;30:510–513.
9. Amarante JT, Santa-Comba A, Reis J, Malheiro E. Halux pulp composite graft in nipple reconstruction. *Aesthetic Plast Surg.* 1994;18:299–300.
10. Tanabe HY, Tai Y, Kiyokawa K, Yamauchi T. Nipple-areola reconstruction with a dermal-fat flap and rolled auricular cartilage. *Plast Reconstr Surg.* 1997;100:431–438.
11. Bhatty MA, Berry RB. Nipple-areola reconstruction by tattooing and nipple sharing. *Br J Plast Surg.* 1997;50:331–334.
12. Chang BW. Reconstruction following mastectomy: timing, indications, and results. In: Cameron J, ed. *Current Surgical Therapy.* 5th ed. St. Louis: Mosby; 1995:570–579.
13. Eng JS. Bell flap nipple reconstruction—a new wrinkle. *Ann Plast Surg.* 1996;36:485–488.

14. Puckett CL, Concannon MJ, Croll GH, Welsh CF. Nipple reconstruction using the "inchworm" flap. *Aesthetic Plast Surg.* 1992;16:117–122.

15. Spear SL, Arias J. Long-term experience with nipple-areola tattooing. *Ann Plast Surg.* 1995;35:232–236.

16. Wong RK, Banducci DR, Feldman S, Kahler SH, Maders EK. Pre-reconstruction tattooing eliminates the need for skin grafting in nipple areolar reconstruction. *Plast Reconstr Surg.* 1993;92:547–549.

23 Follow-Up of TRAM Flap Breast Reconstruction Patients

I prefer to follow all of my breast reconstruction patients as long as possible. This is done both for my benefit and for that of my patients. I benefit by getting photographs of my long-term results and by learning how my reconstructions fare over time, as scars fade and sensation returns. My patients benefit because small problems that arise can sometimes be corrected early, before they become big problems. They also benefit because they can occasionally profit from new techniques for revision of their breasts that were not available at the time their reconstructions were initially performed.

Obviously, it is difficult for patients who live in other states or countries to come to my clinic for a follow-up visit. Nevertheless, I encourage them to return at least every few years, if possible, at their convenience. Often they have family or other medical care providers with whom they can coordinate visits to our clinic. Return visits should be kept as convenient and inexpensive for patients as possible, with a minimum of time spent in the waiting room. If the patient lives in or near Houston, I usually see her at 3 months, 6 months, and 12 months after the surgery. I then ask patients to return at yearly intervals for 2 or 3 years, then every 2 years indefinitely. If the patient comes from a long distance and this return visit schedule would be a hardship, however, I will accept any arrangement that is practical and that the patient will agree to. In some cases, I will have to be satisfied with receiving photographs by mail, taken by other plastic surgeons or photographers who work near the patient's home.

Abdominal Wall Integrity

Most abdominal wall bulges and hernias[1-3] will appear within the first 6 months after the transverse rectus abdominus myocutaneous (TRAM) flap surgery. For that reason, I allow my TRAM flap patients to begin attempting situps and other abdominal exercises after that time, if they wish. They should begin slowly, with abdominal crunches (partial situps), progressing to full situps and increasing the number of repetitions as tolerated. They should not have pain during the exercise; if the activity is painful it should be stopped and an alternative exercise that does not cause pain used instead.

Patients should not expect to feel completely normal until at least 2 years after the surgery. This does not mean that they will be in pain or disabled for all of that time, or even for a significant part of it. During exercise, however, they are likely to feel a tightness in their abdomen that will remind them that they have undergone a surgical procedure. This is normal, and patients should not be concerned about it. The amount of tightness will depend in large part on how much fascia has been removed during the TRAM flap harvest. The less fascia the surgeon removes, the less postoperative pain and tightness the patient will experience. For most patients, however, some tightness in the donor site is normal.

If there is a progressive sensation of weakness, however, even if the physical examination is normal a dehiscence of the internal oblique layer at the fascial donor site closure[4] should be suspected (Fig 23-1). If this has occurred, the patient will benefit from having this tissue separation repaired, because otherwise it can easily progress to become a "bulge" or "TRAM flap hernia" (Fig 23-2). It is best to repair this problem early, before the dehiscence has had a chance to grow wider. These problems usually arise within the first 12 months after performance of the TRAM flap, and should be looked for during that time. Late deterioration of abdominal wall integrity is uncommon.[2,3]

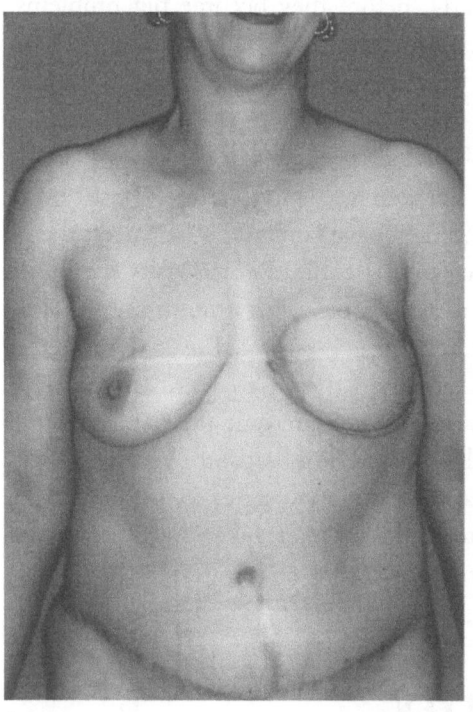
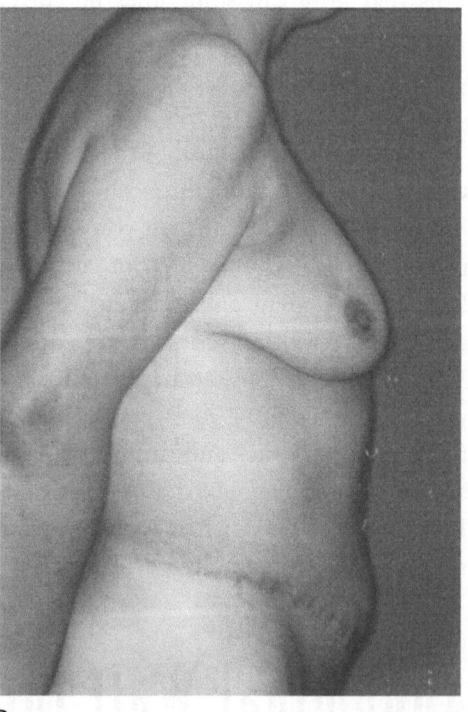

A   B

FIG. 23-1 (A, B) Patient who had minimal physical evidence of a bulge or hernia, but who complained of increasing localized discomfort and weakness at the site of the abdominal fascial repair. Surgical exploration of that site revealed a separation of the internal oblique fascia, which was then repaired.

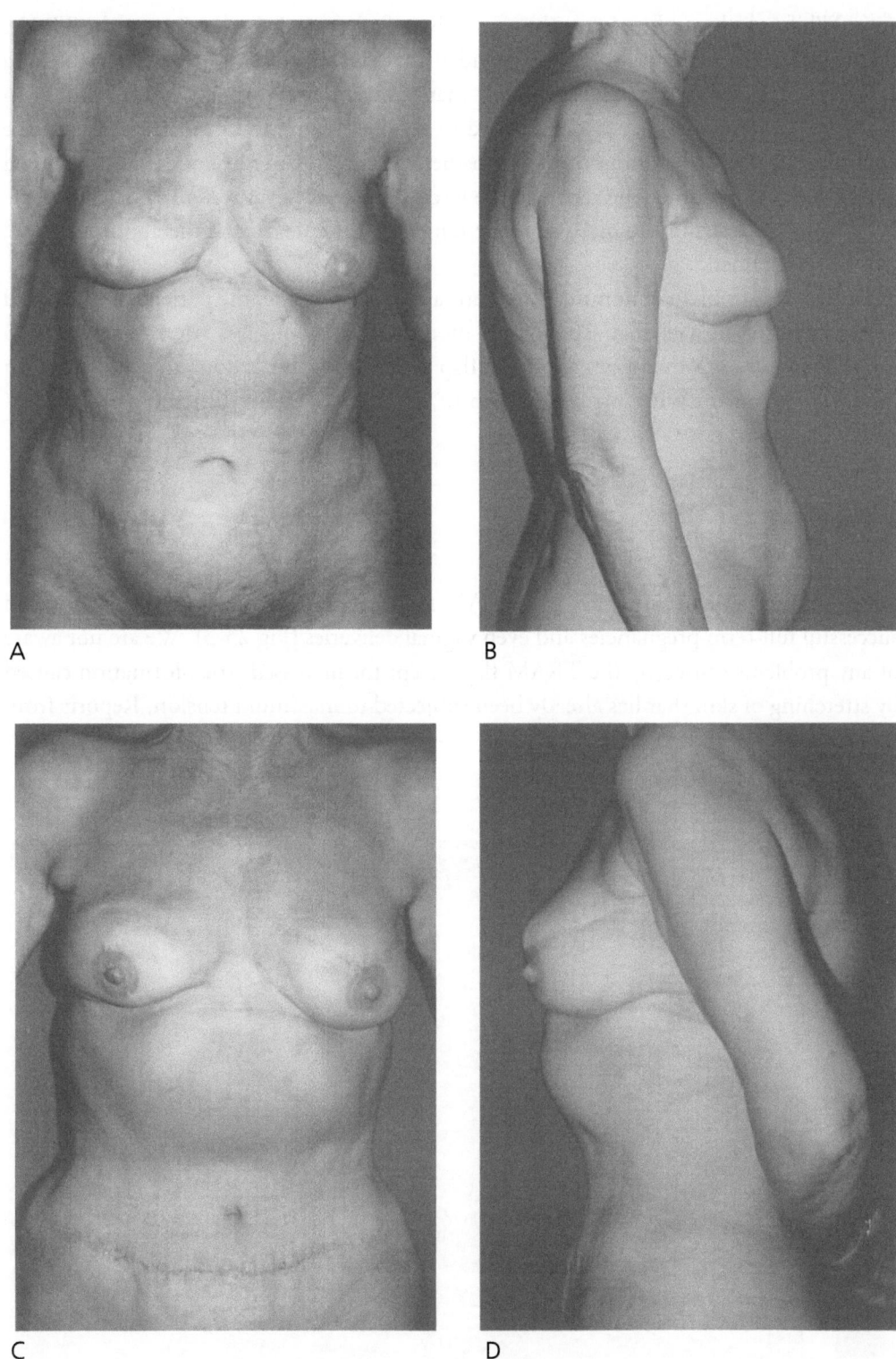

FIG. 23-2 (A, B) Patient with an abdominal "bulge," sometimes called a "TRAM flap hernia." This is caused by a dehiscence of the internal oblique fascia. The overlying external oblique fascia remains intact, but stretches so that the abdomen has a localized and symptomatic bulge despite the absence of a true hernia. (C, D) Same patient, after repair of the bulge.

While a bulge or hernia can be caused by a faulty repair at the time of the TRAM flap transfer,[5] in many more cases (provided that the surgeon was knowledgeable and experienced) it will be due to weak fascia that has been torn through by the sutures. In that case, repair of the defect as described in chapter 11 may be insufficient unless the abdominal wall is also reinforced with prosthetic mesh. The mesh should always be used as an overlay to reinforce the repair of the fascia, however, never to replace it. That way, if infection occurs and the mesh must be removed, the integrity of the abdominal wall will be maintained.

After repair of an abdominal wall hernia or partial hernia, the patient should avoid lifting anything heavier than 10 lb for 3 months, and should not attempt situps for 6 months, just as after the original TRAM flap procedure. This is done to avoid stress on the fascial repair until it is strong enough to tolerate it without difficulty.

Pregnancy

Several of our patients who have had TRAM flaps have become pregnant, and have had successful full-term pregnancies and even vaginal deliveries (Fig 23-3). We are not aware of any problems caused by the TRAM flap except for increased striae formation caused by stretching of skin that has already been subjected to maximum tension. Reports from

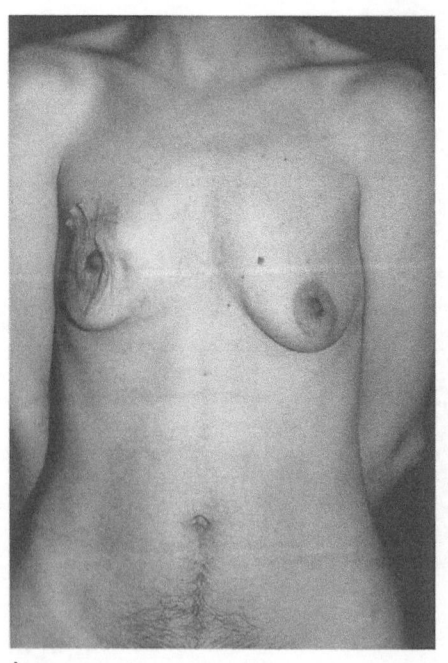 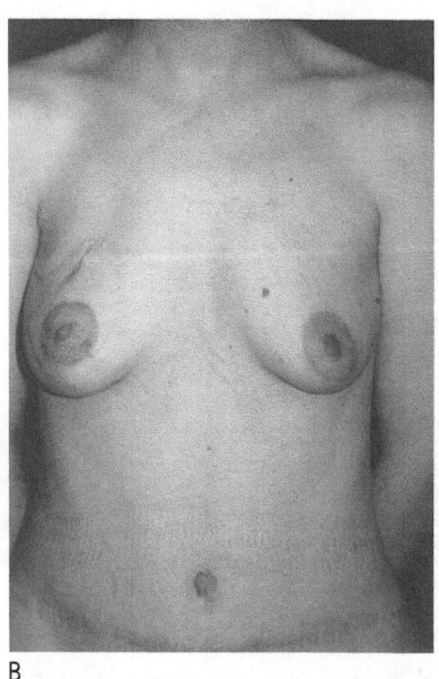 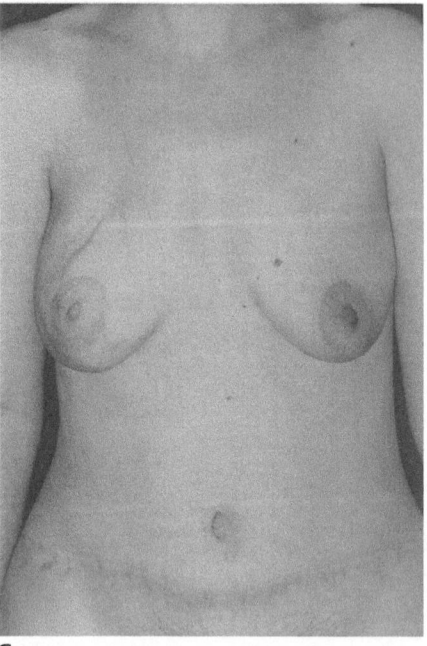

A   B   C

FIG. 23-3   (A) A 33-year-old woman after right breast biopsy, prior to mastectomy. See color insert, p. I-29. (B) Same patient 1 year after immediate reconstruction of the right breast with a free TRAM flap. See color insert, p. I-29. (C) Same woman 2 years later, following a successful term pregnancy. She did develop marked periumbilical striae, but otherwise there were no adverse effects. See color insert, p. I-30.

other institutions confirm this experience.[6] A TRAM flap is therefore clearly not a contraindication to pregnancy.

Despite this, I do not encourage my patients to become pregnant. Almost all breast reconstruction patients are also breast cancer patients, and some breast cancers will grow more rapidly and be more likely to recur if stimulated by estrogens. Although the prospect of having a new baby is appealing to many breast cancer patients, especially to younger ones, the possibility of having the baby and then developing recurrent malignancy as a consequence of the pregnancy has to raise strong concerns. If this occurs, the baby will be left without a healthy (or perhaps even a living) mother to raise and nurture it. It would seem to me that such an eventuality could cause not only a child-raising crisis but a strong sense of guilt not only in both parents but possibly, in later years, in the child as well.

Abdominal Pain

Patients who have had TRAM flaps are not immune to other medical problems, including intra-abdominal ones. Because of the rearrangement of abdominal tissues, pain from internal organs may not be felt in the usual places. In particular, the pain from acute or chronic cholecystitis may be referred to the right lower quadrant rather than to the right upper quadrant, its usual location. The surgeon should keep this in mind, and be sensitive to complaints of abdominal pain in patients who have had TRAM flaps. This is especially significant because women in the age group who are most likely to have had a TRAM flap are also highly susceptible to cholecystitis. It is also important because other physicians who are caring for the patient may be unaware of the change in symptom location that a TRAM flap procedure (or an abdominoplasty) can cause.

Abdominal Surgery

A previous TRAM flap is not a contraindication to abdominal surgery. If a hysterectomy is required, the abdominal donor site incision can be reopened and the abdominoplasty flap reelevated. A vertical incision can then be made through the fascia of the abdominal wall, either through the previous scar or in the midline. In this way, new visible abdominal scars are not required. If the vertical incision through the fascia is made at the site of the old TRAM flap harvest, care should be taken to include all the layers of the rectus sheath (especially the internal oblique layer) in the subsequent repair.

If Prolene or Marlex (polypropylene) mesh has been used to reinforce the abdominal wall, it will be intimately adherent to the fascia. The mesh can safely be ignored and an incision made through it as if it were fascia alone. When the intraabdominal procedure is finished, the layer containing mesh and fascia is closed just like any fascial repair would be. The wound should be drained, just as in the original TRAM flap surgery.

Weight Gain or Loss

Weight Gain

The reconstructed breast mound looks and feels like a breast, but it is actually subcutaneous abdominal fat and will behave as such if the patient gains or loses weight. In some women, the breasts will enlarge as much as their abdominal girth when they gain weight, and symmetry between a reconstructed and a natural breast will be maintained. In a few patients, the abdominal fat will enlarge less than the natural breast, and any added weight will show up in the buttocks and hips so that the natural breast will become larger than the reconstructed one. In most women, however, the abdominal fat will increase in size out of proportion to the breasts. In that case, the reconstructed breast will enlarge more than the natural one if the patient gains any significant amount of weight. Because weight gain is common in women of middle age, the surgeon will often be confronted by the problem of a unilateral TRAM flap reconstruction patient who was once symmetrical, but who has gained weight and no longer has breasts that match (Fig 23-4).

The best treatment for this problem of increasing obesity, by far, is weight loss. Obesity has many harmful effects aside from its effect on breast symmetry in reconstruction patients. Diet and exercise will reverse the asymmetry without requiring additional surgery, and will make the patient feel better as well.

If the patient cannot or will not lose weight, the reconstructed breast can be reduced. This reduction can be accomplished with liposuction, with standard breast reduction techniques, or with a combination of the two. The surgeon should insist, however, that the patient at least stabilize her weight before the surgery is undertaken. Otherwise, the frustrated surgeon will achieve symmetry in the operating room only to see it disappear as the patient gains additional pounds in the weeks and months following the surgery.

Weight Loss

If the patient loses weight, the size of the reconstructed breast mound will diminish (Fig 23-5). Sometimes this will be a good thing, and the symmetry will be improved. In some cases, both the reconstructed breast and the opposite, natural one will diminish in size at the same rate. In most cases, however, the reconstructed breast will become too small. The surgeon must always consider the possibility of disseminated systemic cancer, and be sure that the patient is being followed appropriately by an oncologist. If the weight loss is intentional, however, and not a manifestation of illness, the asymmetry can be addressed by augmentation of the reconstructed breast with a saline implant, or by reduction of the opposite side, if appropriate. As in the case of weight gain, the patient's weight should be stabilized before any surgical procedure is considered.

Scars

Scar formation varies tremendously from patient to patient. In some patients, the breast scars fade rapidly (Figs 23-6 through 23-8), while in others they remain prominent for

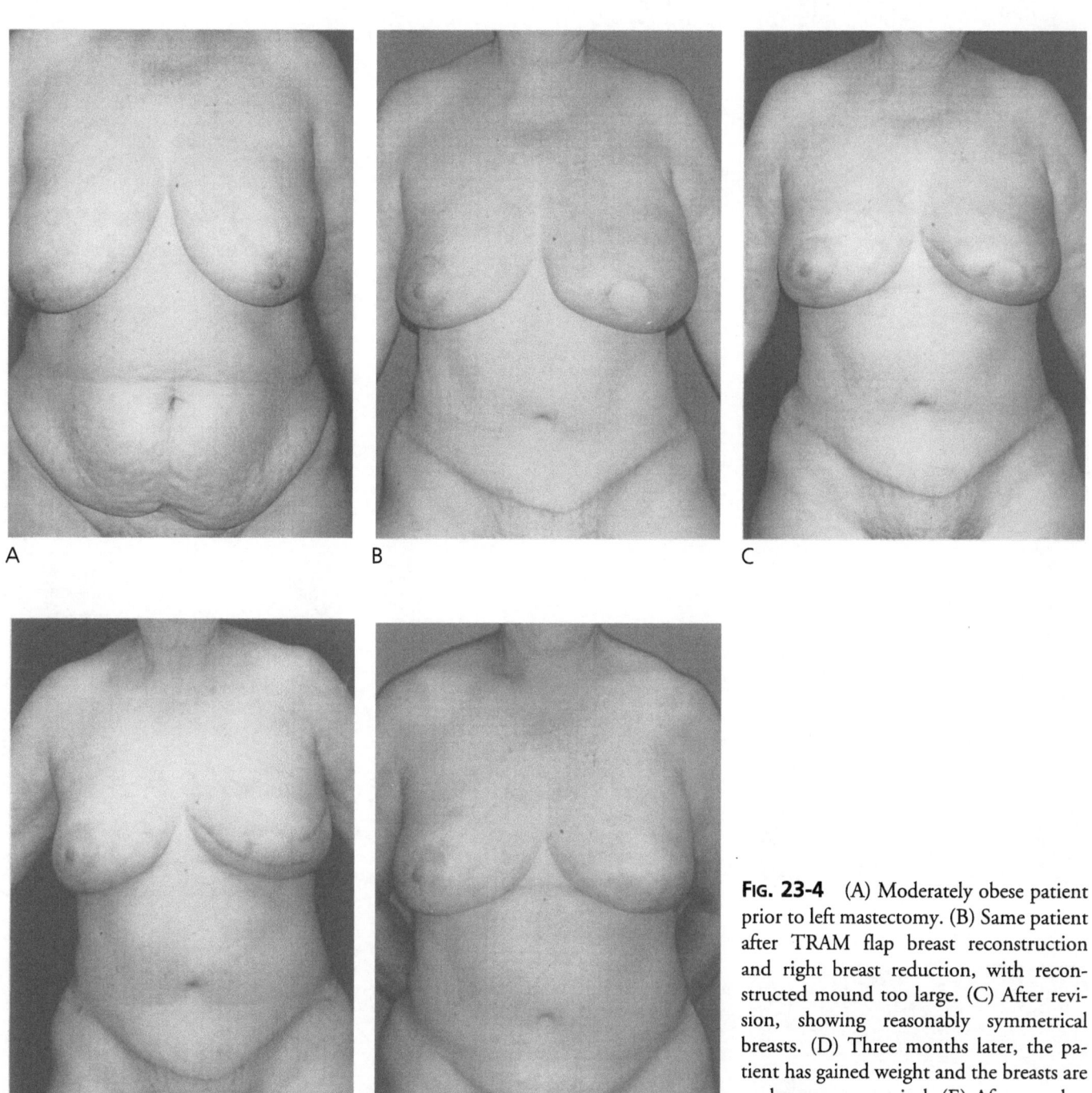

FIG. 23-4 (A) Moderately obese patient prior to left mastectomy. (B) Same patient after TRAM flap breast reconstruction and right breast reduction, with reconstructed mound too large. (C) After revision, showing reasonably symmetrical breasts. (D) Three months later, the patient has gained weight and the breasts are no longer symmetrical. (E) After another revision, the symmetry was restored. See color insert, p. I-28.

many years if not indefinitely (Fig 23-9). In most cases, all of the scars will improve with time. Abdominal TRAM flap donor site scars are usually more prominent than those in the breast, and also tend to widen because they have been closed under tension. This scar widening can be improved by secondary revision after the abdominal skin has stretched and the tension has disappeared. Most patients, however, are not bothered very much by the abdominal scars and only rarely do they request this revision.

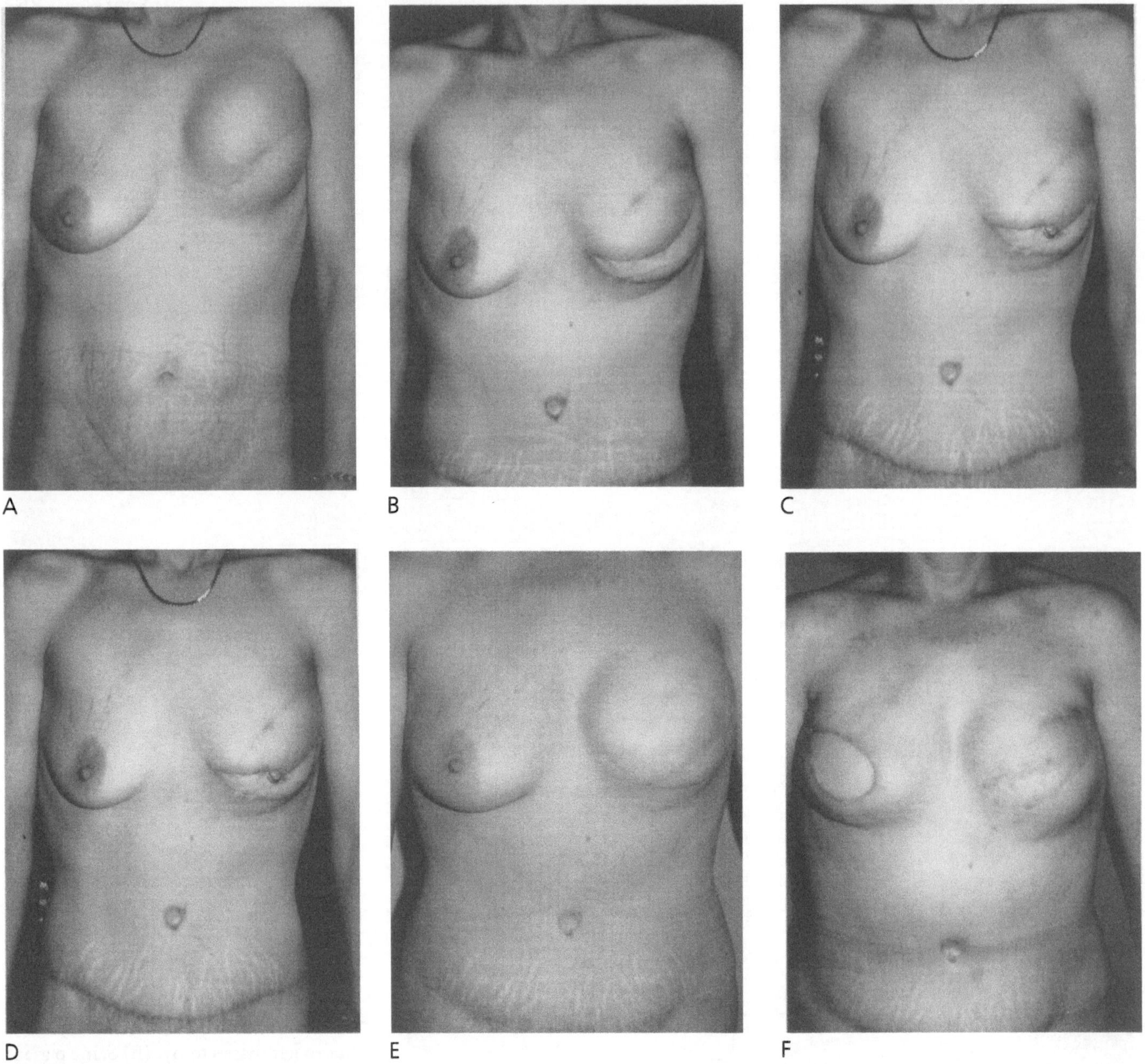

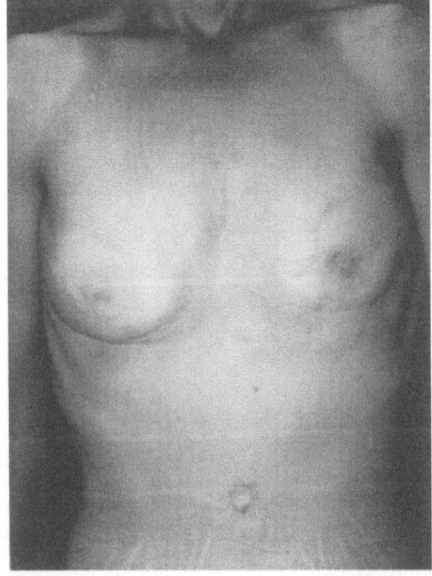

FIG. 23-5 (A) Patient after unsuccessful attempt at reconstruction with tissue expansion. (B) Three months after TRAM flap breast reconstruction, the reconstructed mound is larger than the opposite, natural one. (C) After revision and nipple reconstruction, the breast volumes are relatively equal. (D) Fourteen months later, after weight loss, the reconstructed breast is much smaller than the natural one. (E) After 2 more years, the patient has regained weight and the reconstructed breast is again larger than the opposite, natural one. (F) One year later, the patient developed a second primary carcinoma in the opposite breast. She was reconstructed with a superior gluteal free flap. (G) After 2 more years, the patient has again lost weight and the TRAM flap volume has almost completely disappeared. The volume of the gluteal flap, however, has been reasonably well maintained.

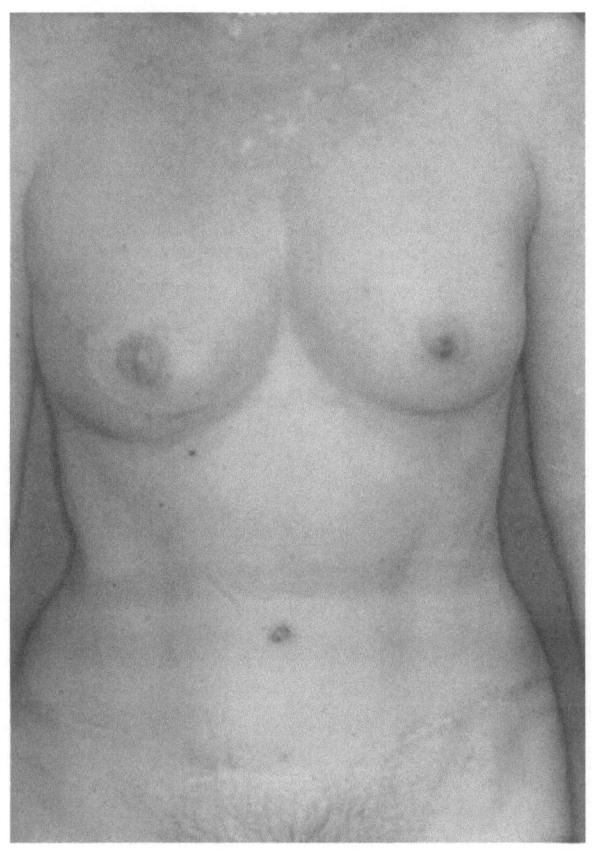

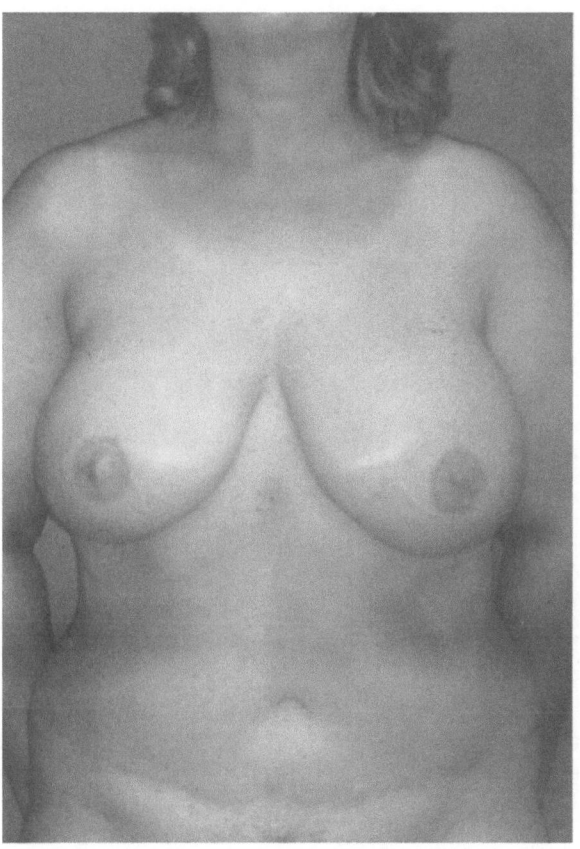

FIG. 23-6 Patient 1 year after immediate free TRAM flap reconstruction of the right breast. The scars are faded and very inconspicuous. See color insert, p. I-30.

FIG. 23-7 Patient 2 years after bilateral immediate breast reconstruction with free TRAM flaps. The scars in the breast are very inconspicuous. In: Spear SL, ed. *Surgery of the Breast: Principles and Art.* Philadelphia: Lippincott-Raven; 1998: pp. 547–553. Used with permission.

Nipple Projection and Pigmentation

Nipple projection typically decreases by at least 50% in the months following nipple reconstruction.[7] If it becomes inadequate, revision of the nipple can be performed. New local flaps can be raised to fashion another nipple "from scratch." If the breast is of adequate size, the nipple flaps should be made wider than in the first nipple reconstruction (as described in the previous chapter) to increase the blood flow to the flaps and reduce the probability that partial flap loss and loss of nipple projection will occur again. The patient should be warned, however, that her loss of nipple projection may well recur.

Reconstruction of the areola with tattooing[8–12] (micropigmentation) is convenient and effective, but tattoos often do fade with time (Fig 23-10). If the fading becomes objectionable, the tattooing can be repeated as often as necessary to restore the color of the nipple and areola. Obviously, this is less of a problem when the reconstruction has been bilateral and the fading is symmetrical.

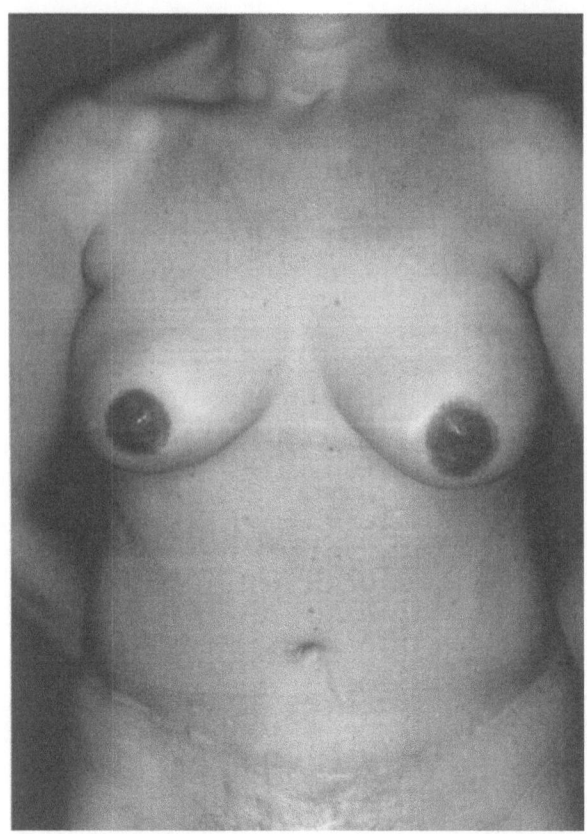

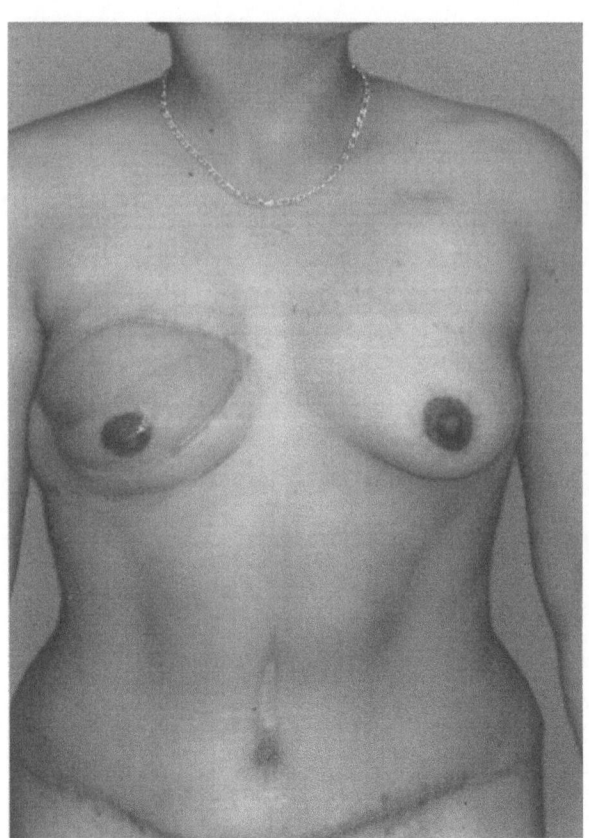

FIG. 23-8 Patient 5 years after bilateral immediate breast reconstruction with free TRAM flaps. The scars in the breast are barely visible. See color insert, p. I-31.

FIG. 23-9 Patient one year after delayed free TRAM flap breast reconstruction. The scars are moderately hypertrophic and the color match of the skin paddle to the surrounding breast skin is only fair. These scars will probably always be noticeable.

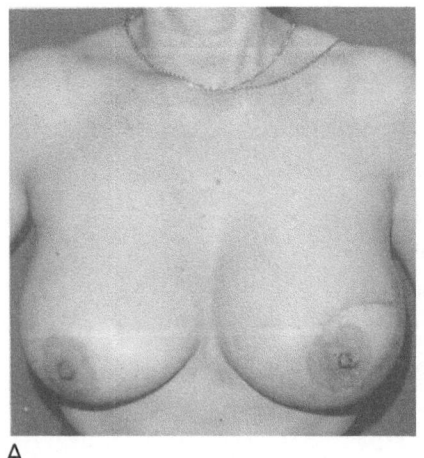

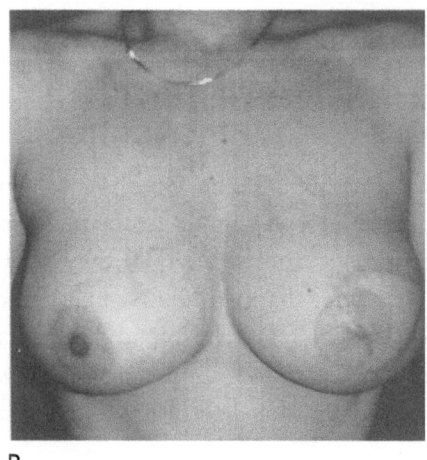

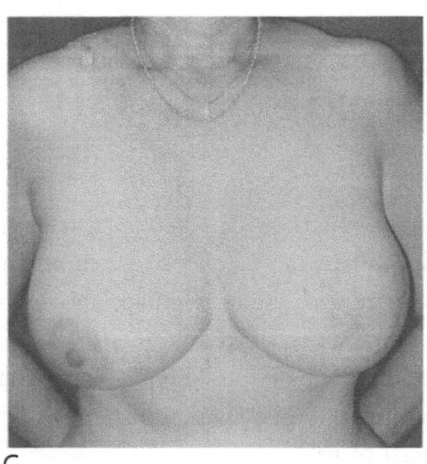

A

B

C

FIG. 23-10 (A) Patient after reconstruction of the left breast, with tattooing to simulate natural pigmentation of the nipple and areola. See color insert, p. I-31. (B) After 1 year, the tattooing has faded somewhat but the result is acceptable. See color insert, p. I-32. (C) Five years after the tattooing, the pigmentation has almost completely faded away. Note that the patient has gained weight but in this case the breasts have remained symmetrical. See color insert, p. I-32.

Cancer Surveillance

Almost all breast reconstruction patients will have had breast cancer and must be followed carefully to detect recurrent disease as early as possible. This is true even if the tumor was noninvasive (in situ). The surveillance is best managed by the patient's oncologist rather than a plastic surgeon. Regular mammograms should be obtained of the opposite breast since all breast cancer patients are at increased risk of developing a second primary tumor of the opposite breast. Whenever the opposite breast undergoes surgery for symmetry, a mammogram should be performed preoperatively so that if a suspicious lesion exists it can be biopsied as part of the procedure without making a separate incision. A second, baseline mammogram should also be obtained 3 to 6 months postoperatively so that any scarring caused by the procedure is identified and will not be confused with the development of malignancy at a later time.

Screening mammography of the reconstructed breast is of minimal value. This is not because local recurrences do not occur (in T1 and T2 patients our local recurrence rate at 6 years is 7%), but because when they do occur they are usually found just beneath the skin, where they can easily be detected by palpation. For this reason, it is important that breast reconstruction patients continue to practice regular self-examination. If the recurrence occurs deep to the breast mound, on the chest wall, it will probably not be detected by palpation until the tumor is quite advanced. Mammography will not detect it either, however, so that routine mammographic screening is usually not helpful.

I have seen one case of recurrent ductal carcinoma in situ that occurred in the subcutaneous tissue under preserved native breast skin that was not palpable but was detected by mammography. I consider this recurrence very unusual, but cannot state categorically that mammography of reconstructed breasts has no value. Mammography is intended as a screening tool for evaluating the interior parenchyma of a natural breast, however. As a screening tool for evaluating breasts reconstructed with abdominal fat, it probably is not cost-effective.

Management of Local Recurrence

When tumor does recur locally in the reconstructed breast, it must be widely excised. Provided that systemic disease is not present and the tumor is not aggressive, the prognosis may not necessarily be grave (Fig 23-11). The prognosis is obviously better if the tumor is slow-growing and if it has been many years since the mastectomy (implying a relatively low-grade tumor). Even when the interval between the mastectomy and recurrence has been short, however, long-term survival of the patient is not impossible or even unusual (Fig 23-12). In many cases, the recurrence simply represents persistent disease that was not adequately excised during the mastectomy; if it is subsequently removed in its entirety the patient may well be rendered free of disease.

After wide local excision of the recurrence, there will be a defect in the reconstructed breast. This defect can often be managed with local flaps (Figs 23-13 and 23-14) or by breast reshaping (Figs 23-15 and 23-16) using techniques similar to those described in chapter 19. Whether or not a successful restoration of breast shape will be

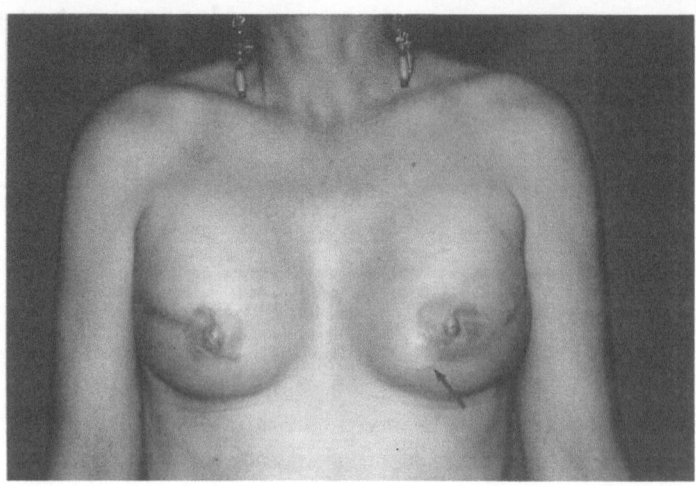

FIG. 23-11   Patient with bilateral breast reconstruction by tissue expansion who developed a local recurrence near her right breast incision 2 years after the mastectomy. After wide local excision of the recurrence, the patient remains free of disease 6 years later.

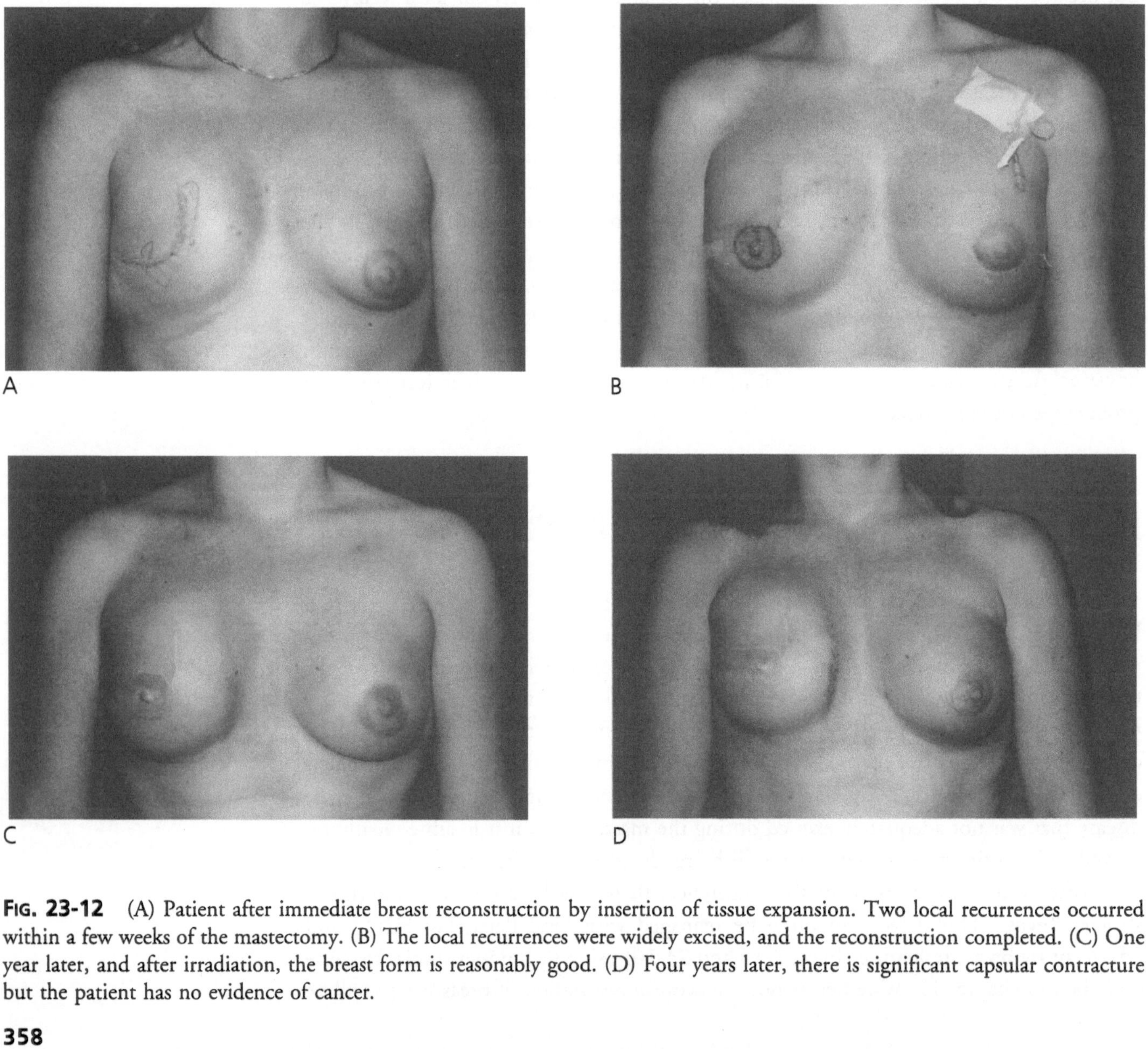

A

B

C

D

FIG. 23-12   (A) Patient after immediate breast reconstruction by insertion of tissue expansion. Two local recurrences occurred within a few weeks of the mastectomy. (B) The local recurrences were widely excised, and the reconstruction completed. (C) One year later, and after irradiation, the breast form is reasonably good. (D) Four years later, there is significant capsular contracture but the patient has no evidence of cancer.

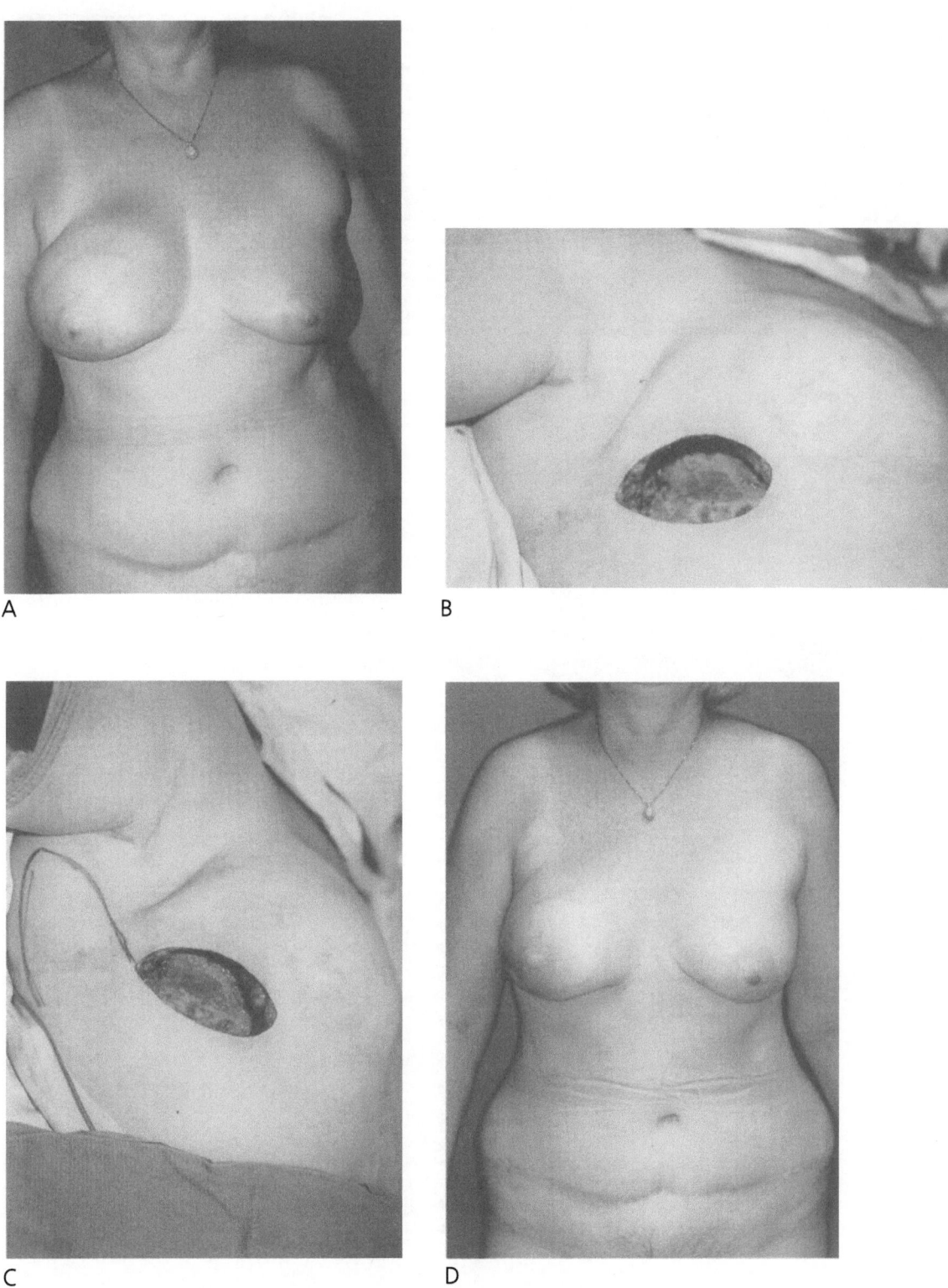

Fig. 23-13 (A) Patient after right breast reconstruction with a free TRAM flap. (B) A tumor recurrence was found and removed from the lateral part of the breast. (C) A local flap was used to shift tissue from the sub-axillary region into the breast. (D) The result was a breast reconstruction with a reasonably normal shape and symmetry. The patient remains clinically free of disease.

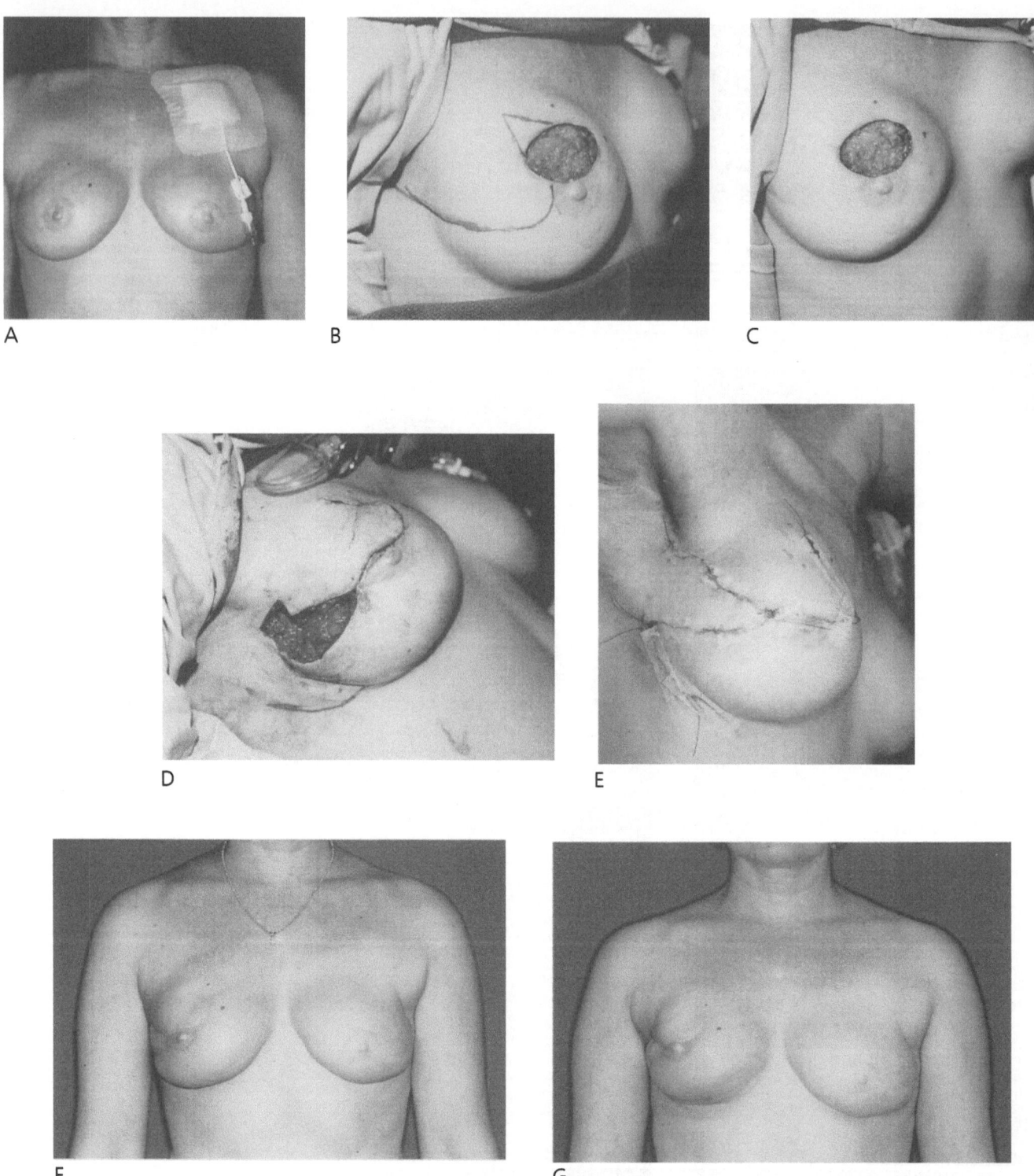

FIG. 23-14 (A) Patient who had an excellent bilateral free TRAM flap breast reconstruction at another institution, then developed a local recurrence in the right breast. (B) After wide local excision of the tumor. (C, D, E) The breast defect was repaired with 2 local flaps. (F) Six months later, the result was a reasonably good restoration of breast shape and symmetry. (G) After radiation therapy, and 1 year later, the right breast has developed radiation-induced fibrosis so that some symmetry was lost.

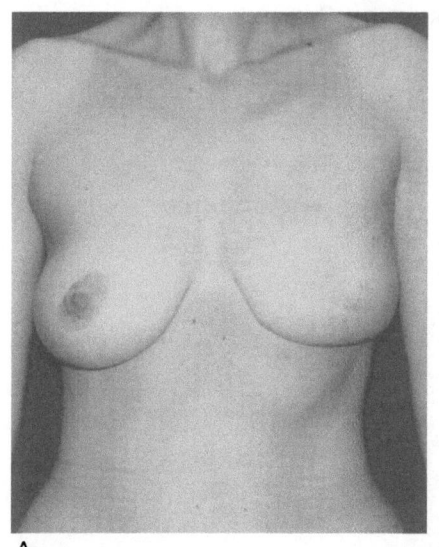

Fig. 23-15 (A) Patient 2 years after free TRAM flap reconstruction of the left breast. (B) Local recurrence was found by biopsy in the upper inner quadrant of the reconstructed breast. (C) Wide local excision was performed, leaving this defect. (D) A subcutaneously based island flap was designed in the lateral part of the breast. (E) The reconstructed nipple and areola were elevated as a superiorly based flap, and the island flap was mobilized. (F) The flap was advanced medially into the defect. The NAC was replaced over a de-epithelialized portion of the island flap. (G) The early result was a reconstructed breast with restoration of a relatively normal shape.

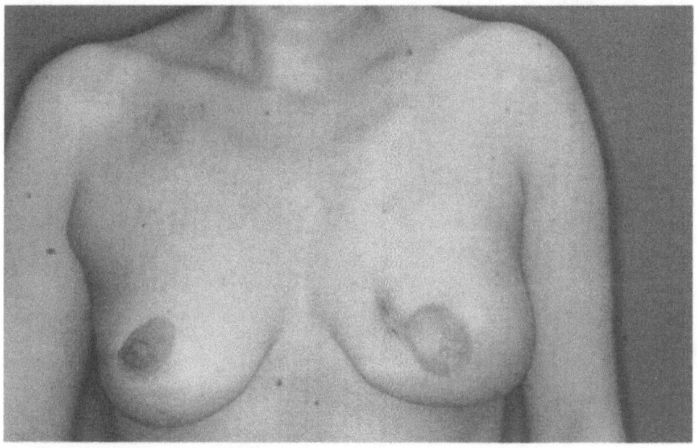

A

B

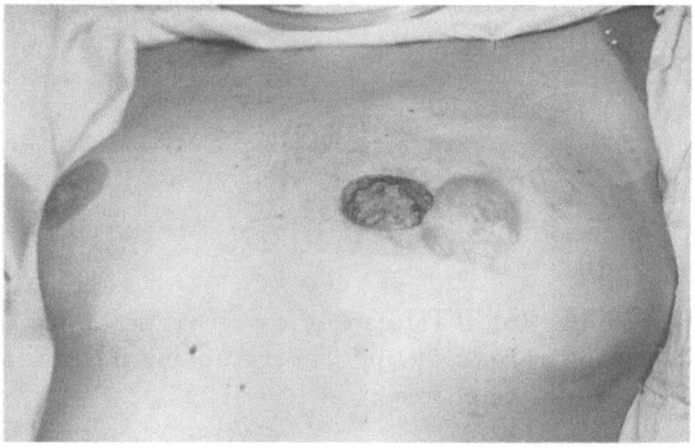

C

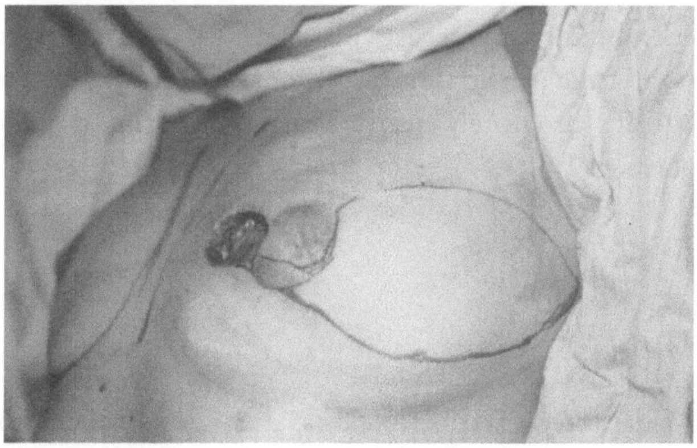

D

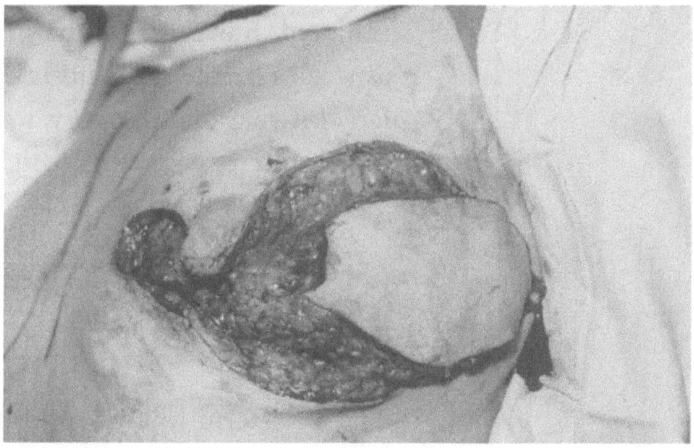

E

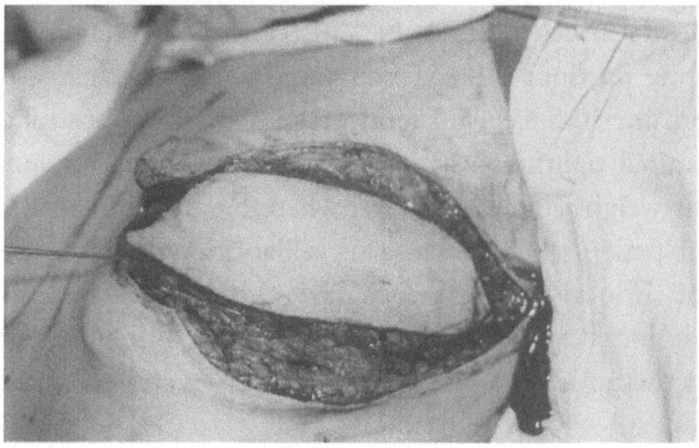

F

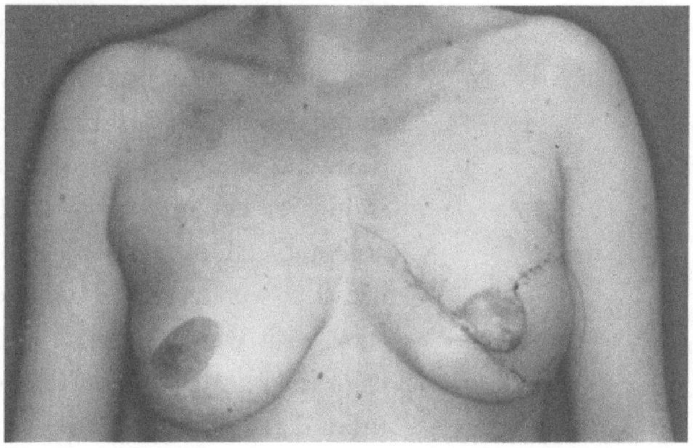

G

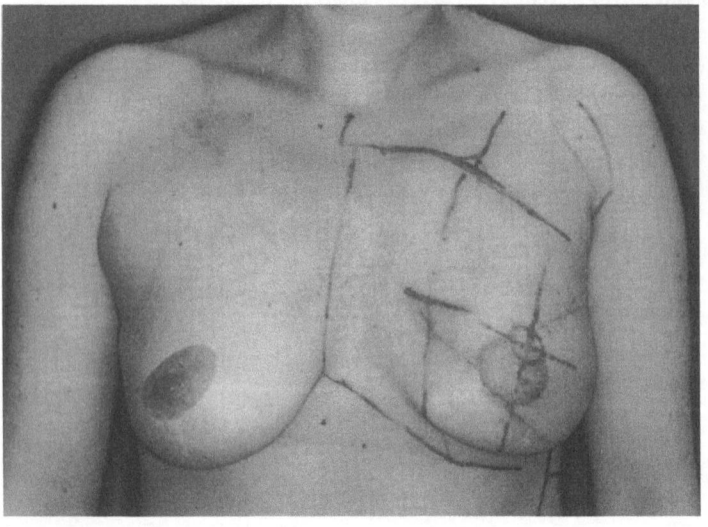

A

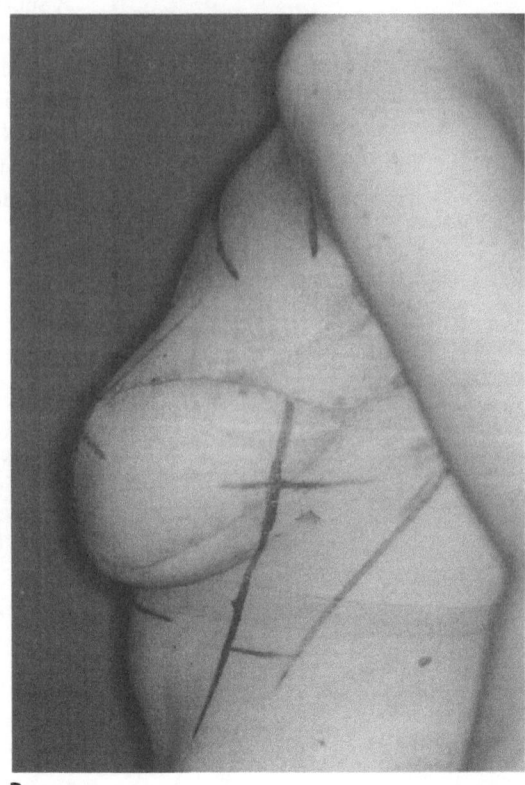

B

FIG. 23-16 (A, B) Three weeks later, the patient is marked for her impending radiation therapy. The effect of this therapy on her symmetry remains to be seen.

achieved, however, will be determined by the relative sizes of the defect and the breast as well as by the skill and imagination of the plastic surgeon. If the defect is sufficiently large, it may be necessary to reconstruct an entirely new breast mound using a technique different from the original one.

Summary

The long-term follow-up of TRAM flap breast reconstruction patients is beneficial to both patients and their surgeon. Problems of abdominal wall competence should be diagnosed and treated early and aggressively. Pain from cholecystitis can be felt in the right lower quadrant rather than in the usual location. Patients can undergo abdominal surgery without difficulty despite previous TRAM flap surgery, even if their abdominal wall has been repaired with mesh. Successful term pregnancy is also possible. Scars fade and symptoms of abdominal tightness usually improve with time. Patients should be encouraged to keep their weight stable, at a level where breast symmetry is acceptable. Unilateral breast cancer patients require close surveillance of the opposite breast as well as of the operated one. If local recurrence occurs, it should be excised locally with wide margins. This wide local excision will cause deformity, but in many cases the plastic surgeon can correct this, at least in part, using local tissues and/or breast mound reshaping.

References

1. Kroll SS, Schusterman MA, Reece GP, Miller MJ, Robb GL, Evans GRD. Abdominal wall strength, bulging, and hernia after TRAM flap breast reconstruction. *Plast Reconstr Surg.* 1995;96:616–619.

2. Mizgala CL, Hartrampf CR Jr, Bennett GK. Assessment of the abdominal wall after pedicled TRAM flap surgery: 5- to 7-year follow-up of 150 consecutive patients. *Plast Reconstr Surg.* 1994;93:988–1002.

3. Hartrampf CR Jr. Abdominal wall competence in transverse abdominal island flap operations. *Ann Plast Surg.* 1984;12:139.

4. Kroll SS, Schusterman MA, Mistry D. The internal oblique repair of abdominal bulges secondary to TRAM flap breast reconstruction. *Plast Reconstr Surg.* 1995;96:100–104.

5. Hartrampf CR Jr. In discussion: Drever JM, Hodson-Walker M. Closure of the donor defect for breast reconstruction with rectus abdominis myocutaneous flaps. *Plast Reconstr Surg.* 1985;76:563.

6. Chen L, Hartrampf CR Jr, Bennett GK. Successful pregnancies following TRAM flap surgery. *Plast Reconstr Surg.* 1993;91:69–71.

7. Kroll SS, Reece GP, Miller MJ, et al. Comparison of nipple projection with the modified double-opposing tab and star flaps. *Plast Reconstr Surg.* 1997;99: 1602–1605.

8. Spear SL, Arias J. Long-term experience with nipple-areola tattooing. *Ann Plast Surg.* 1995;35:232–236.

9. Spear SL, Convit R, Little JW. Intradermal tattoo as an adjunct to nipple-areolar reconstruction. *Plast Reconstr Surg.* 1989;83:907–911.

10. Eskenazi L. A one-stage nipple reconstruction with the "modified star" flap and immediate tattoo: a review of 100 cases. *Plast Reconstr Surg.* 1993;92:671–680.

11. Wong RK, Banducci DR, Feldman S, Kahler SH, Manders EK. Pre-reconstruction tattooing eliminates the need for skin grafting in nipple areolar reconstruction. *Plast Reconstr Surg.* 1993;92:547–549.

12. Hugo NE, Sultan MR, Hardy SP. Nipple-areola reconstruction with intradermal tattoo and double-opposing pennant flaps. *Ann Plast Surg.* 1993;30:510–513.

Index

Note. Page numbers followed by *f* and *t* indicate figures and tables, respectively.